Descriptive Psychopathology

Descriptive Psychopathology

The Signs and Symptoms of Behavioral Disorders

Michael Alan Taylor, MD
Nutan Atre Vaidya, MD

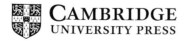
CAMBRIDGE
UNIVERSITY PRESS

CAMBRIDGE UNIVERSITY PRESS

Cambridge, New York, Melbourne, Madrid, Cape Town, Singapore, São Paulo, Delhi

Cambridge University Press
The Edinburgh Building, Cambridge CB2 8RU, UK

Published in the United States of America by Cambridge University Press, New York

www.cambridge.org
Information on this title: www.cambridge.org/9780521713917

First published 2009

Printed in the United Kingdom at the University Press, Cambridge

A catalog record for this publication is available from the British Library

Library of Congress Cataloging-in-Publication Data

Taylor, Michael Alan, 1940–
  Descriptive psychopathology : the signs and symptoms of behavioral disorders / Michael Alan Taylor,
Nutan Atre Vaidya.
      p.   ;   cm.
  Includes bibliographical references and index.
  ISBN 978-0-521-71391-7
1. Psychodiagnostics.   2. Neurobehavioral disorders–Diagnosis.   3. Psychology, Pathological.
I. Vaidya, Nutan Atre.   II. Title.
[DNLM: 1. Mental Disorders–diagnosis.   2. Neuropsychology–methods.   3. Psychopathology–methods.
WM 141 T244d 2009]
  RC469.T39 2009
  616.89'075–dc22
                                                                                    2008029842

ISBN 978-0-521-71391-7 paperback

For the next generation

Contents

Preface

"Of all Persons who are Objects of our Charity, none move my Compassion, like those whom it has pleas'd God to leave in a full state of Health and Strength, but depriv'd of Reason to act for themselves. And it is, in my opinion, one of the greatest Scandals upon the Understanding of others, to mock at those who want it." (Daniel Defoe, 1697)[1]

As in seventeeth century England, today's society continues to subtly mock those of us "deprived of reason". Mental health insurance in the USA is inadequate and less than that for other conditions. The psychiatrically ill are left in large numbers on the streets and alleys of our cities, a situation the medical establishment would find intolerable if the distress were due to heart disease. Sufferers are ridiculed in mass entertainment, equated to clowns, fools, and criminals. While the necessity of care by specialists is widely recognized for patients with stroke, epilepsy, dementia, and other "neurologic" disease, it is acceptable for almost any interested party to "hang up a shingle" and offer almost any kind of treatment to those of us "deprived of reason".

Yet the loss of reason and other psychopathology are expressions of brain disease and dysfunction, and this recognition has diagnostic implications increasingly important as more exact treatments are introduced. The need for diagnostic accuracy, however, is subverted by the poor validity of present-day psychiatric classification. Better delineation of clinical populations will reduce heterogeneity and thus facilitate the application of more specific treatments. The recent call to separate melancholia from other depressions[2] and catatonia from the psychotic disorders,[3] for example, provide the framework for the more specific treatments for these conditions. Obsessive–compulsive spectrum disorders identified within the impulse control category also warrant their own treatment approach to avoid mismanagement. Recognizing psychoses associated with seizure disorder avoids sufferers being considered schizophrenic or hysterical and receiving inappropriate treatments.

To accurately delineate psychiatric disease, however, requires in-depth knowledge of the signs and symptoms of behavioral disorders, i.e. descriptive psychopathology, and the examination skills to elicit clinically useful phenomena. Descriptive psychopathology, detailed here, considers the abnormal observable behavior and its subjective experience needed for this effort. Bedside assessment of cognitive functions complements the behavioral examination.

Hypothesized psychopathologic constructs (e.g. ego defense mechanisms, psychological reactions) represent a paradigm different from that of descriptive psychopathology. We do not discuss these ideas. For medical diagnosis, they are overly interpretive and lack objective definition. Their reliability is poor, and they are unhelpful in defining syndromes of the brain or in predicting treatment response and other clinical variables. In contrast, descriptive psychopathology can be reliably defined and its different patterns better predict pathophysiology and treatment response.[4]

Despite the detail we present, this book is not a dictionary of all psychiatric terminology. It is also not an encyclopedic compendium of the theories of the mind, or a wide-ranging dissertation on the psychology of behavior. We discuss theories and psychology only when helpful in clarifying the diagnostic or neurologic implications of psychopathology.

Thus, this book is not primarily written for the scientist or the theorist, although they should find it useful in defining their populations of interest. It is written to help clinicians in the care of their patients. Our approach is neuropsychiatric, derived from the understanding that all forms of descriptive psychopathology are observed in patients presently characterized as having neurologic disease (e.g. seizure disorder, stroke, and dementia), and that many classic neurologic signs and symptoms are in turn observed in patients recognized as having a psychiatric disorder. The separation of psychiatry and neurology is arbitrary. Both disciplines care for persons with brain dysfunction or brain disease. Their common ground is the clinical implications of the behavioral disturbances elicited by brain dysfunction. We delineate this common experience by detailing classic descriptive psychopathology and associated neurologic features. We show, often with clinical examples, how the presence of specific psychopathologic phenomena influences diagnosis. Within the limits of the present understanding of brain functioning, we also offer a neurologic understanding of classic clinical features as they affect diagnosis.

We divide the book into four sections.

In Section 1, we describe the problems and limitations of present classifications and through clinical examples show that they serve patients poorly. We illustrate that a command of the knowledge and skills of descriptive psychopathology provides more refined diagnosis and treatment.

As the study of descriptive psychopathology spans millennia, we review this history.[5] We detail the shifting tensions over the centuries between classification "lumpers" and "splitters" that led to present classifications. We next show that the "mental status examination" is better considered the "behavioral examination of the brain". The limited neuroscience of psychopathology is presented.

In Section 2, we describe the principles of diagnosis, and detail the examination style, structure, and techniques.

In Section 3, we define and describe psychopathology that goes beyond that found in present classification manuals, and show how the identification of these phenomena is of diagnostic importance. We present the behavioral domains of the examination in the order commonly addressed clinically. We start with chapters on general appearance, motor behavior, and emotion, areas of the assessment that rely heavily on inspection rather than extensive conversation.

In the chapter on motor disturbances we also delineate catatonia, and distinguish the motor disturbances of basal ganglia, cerebellar and frontal circuitry disease. We describe the differences in the speech and language problems encountered in patients with aphasia, mania, catatonia, and the "formal thought disorder" associated with psychosis. In the discussion of perceptual disturbances we detail the phenomena associated with temporal–limbic disease. We discuss delusions and aspects of abnormal thought content. The spectrum of obsessive–compulsive behaviors is presented as a more coherent picture than the present scattering of related conditions throughout classification. We detail the behaviors and cognitive impairment patterns of patients with delirium and different forms of dementia. We describe the dimensional structure of personality and personality disorder and how this approach is more productive than the present categorical system in predicting co-morbidities and in shaping behavioral treatments.

Lastly, in Section 4, we propose a re-structuring of present-day classification based on the psychopathology literature and its validating data. Our goal is to re-establish the best of the past within the framework of modern insights into brain function and psychopathology.

Nevertheless, present-day psychiatry retains much ambiguity. There are no laboratory tests that define psychiatric illness to the precision achieved in identifying specific strains of a virus or the number of trinucleotide repeats in a genetically based illness. Sustained pleasure for the psychiatric clinician must come from examining and making sense of diverse psychopathological expressions of illness and the satisfaction from using that understanding to shape treatments and resolve distress. "Figuring it out" and "getting all better" patients with complex patterns of psychopathology are experiences that sustain clinical practice. Telling the distraught mother and sister of an 18-year-old man who had been hospitalized for "encephalitis" and was considered "a hopeless case", but who in fact had a mood disorder and malignant catatonia that "We're going to get him all better, not just a little better" and then doing it, finally watching the previously mute and immobile patient walk out of the hospital with his family is an experience that cannot easily be achieved without a full understanding of descriptive psychopathology.

Defining psychopathology to delineate behavioral syndromes and to choose specific treatments is a practical effort for the trainee and the experienced clinician alike. All who accept the responsibility for the care of patients with behavioral syndromes should find useful information in this book. But our effort is aimed at those new to that responsibility – trainees in psychiatry, neurology, and neuropsychology. For them, our book offers a crossroad in their career journey, the path now less taken, but we think more rewarding than the cookbook psychiatry that has been created to complement present classification. Karl Jaspers expressed the same challenge more than 90 years ago in the prefaces to the 2nd and 3rd editions of his classic textbook *General Psychopathology*:

The opinion has been expressed in medical quarters that this book is too hard for students, because it attempts to tackle extremely difficult and ultimate problems. As far as that is concerned, I am convinced that either one grasps a science entirely, that means in its central problems, or not at all. I consider it fatal simply to adjust at a low level. One should be guided by the better students who are interested in the subject for its own sake, even though they may be in the minority. Those who teach should compel their students to rise to a scientific level. But this is made impossible if "compendia" are used, which give students fragmentary, superficial pseudo-knowledge "for practical purposes", and which sometimes is more subversive for practice than total ignorance.[6]

NOTES

1 Defoe (1697), cited by Hunter and Macalpine (1963), page 265.
2 Taylor and Fink (2006).
3 Fink and Taylor (2003).
4 Present classification does not predict treatment response. See the discussion in Chapter 4 and in Taylor and Fink (2006) chapter 1.
5 The Western interest in psychopathology dates from classical Greece, evolved in central Europe and France, captured the interest of physicians in Great Britain and then crossed the Atlantic to the USA and Canada. It is now worldwide. Chapter 2 provides a discussion of the history of Western classification of psychiatric illness. Medical traditions from Asia are not discussed because they have not influenced modern medical psychiatry.
6 Jaspers (1963), page x–xi.

Acknowledgments

Max Fink read many of the chapters offering substantive and language alternatives that clarified our intent. He suggested we discuss recent work that provides the framework for a more evidence-based classification.

Edward Simon also read parts of the manuscript and suggested changes to help less-experienced clinicians better understand the constructs of classic psychopathology.

Edward Shorter graciously read the chapters on history and classification, and offered many helpful suggestions and corrections.

Georgette Pfeiffer compiled the references and corrected and completed missing citation information.

The editors at Cambridge University Press were tireless in correcting the text and citations.

Any errors remaining are ours.

Section 1

Present, past, and future

Beyond the DSM and ICD:
a rationale for understanding
and using descriptive psychopathology

The straight jacket imposed on psychiatry by the introduction of [DSM-III] and its successors, reverberating in Europe with the [IDC-10] has had a profound effect on the practice of psychiatry. An earlier generation's more elegant constructions of a hierarchal basis for diagnostic classifications has disappeared, so that a patient now may end up with 3, 4, or even more DSM-IV diagnoses, and patients failing to fulfill one of the criteria for entry for a condition may be deemed not to be suffering from that condition, although logical clinical evaluation would suggest otherwise. Furthermore, many of the diagnostic inclusions are broad, ambiguous, and open to misuse in inappropriate settings . . . it seems the DSM-IV and its forerunners were created by committees which appear not to have been appreciative of the broad spectrum of conditions met with in psychiatric practice, and particularly in neuropsychiatry.[1]

Present-day psychiatry is dependent upon the *Diagnostic and Statistical Manual for Mental Disorders* (DSM) and *International Classification of Diseases* (ICD) classifications. The DSM has become the main reference source of recognized psychopathology and is the standard system for research subject selection worldwide. The ICD, rarely used in the USA, is favored in many parts of the world as a clinically useful document.[2] The ICD offers separate research and clinical versions in several languages.[3] Training programs in many parts of the world also rely on the DSM and ICD. Endorsed treatment algorithms are linked to classification labels. Manual category numbering is required for clinical documentation, and insurance reimbursement, and is referenced in legislative and legal proceedings. This dependence is accepted under the assumption that the manuals maximize reliability and contain validated conditions and groupings that encourage the best diagnostic decisions and treatment choices.

The dependence on the classification manuals has permitted a paradigm shift in psychiatry, particularly in the USA. The more leisurely psychological approach to patient care has been largely replaced by a primary care treatment model. Rapid diagnosis, followed by reflexive pharmacotherapy is encouraged

Developed from an article, Vaidya and Taylor (2006).

to accommodate high patient turnover. "I don't have enough time to see my patients . . . they only give me a half hour for intakes and follow-up visits" has become the mantra of psychiatry house officers.[4]

Applying the primary care model is facilitated by the ICD short descriptive prose or the DSM telegraphic lists. While the two systems differ in some categories (e.g. psychotic disorders, dementia, disorders in children and adolescents, and generalized anxiety disorder) and terminology (e.g. the ICD "organic" versus the DSM "secondary to" for syndromes with established etiology), both offer a skeletal view of psychopathology designed to be applied quickly.[5] The time-consuming detailed investigation of the unfolding of the patient's illness, the nuances of the sequence of symptom emergence, patterns of features, and the importance of some features over others is deemed superfluous and has been abandoned. Once diagnostic criteria are met, a treatment algorithm based on the DSM or ICD diagnosis is chosen. Treatment algorithms, often endorsed by an "expert" panel,[6] can be applied as if cooking recipes.[7]

Paralleling the format changes has been an expansion in diagnostic choices from a handful of syndromes in DSM-II (APA, 1968) and the ICD-6 mental disorders section to presently over 280 options. The expansion is meant to assure recognition of any psychiatric affliction,[8] implicitly promising that the classification contains all the known psychiatric conditions, that these conditions are sufficiently validated, and that the diagnostic criteria for each are reliable and sufficient to identify each condition. There should be no practical need to know more psychopathology than what is in the manuals. The promise, however, is unfulfilled, as validity is poor for many classification groupings (e.g. personality disorders, impulse control disorders) and the reliability of the systems is marginal.

The weakness in present classifications is illustrated in the startling and clearly implausible announcement that a study supported by the National Institutes of Mental Health in the USA determined that 55% of persons in the USA are at lifetime risk for psychiatric illness. In response, Paul McHugh, professor of psychiatry at Johns Hopkins and retired department chairman, blamed inexperienced interviewers relying on the DSM. He wrote:

In addition to relying solely on respondents' yes or no answers to a checklist, the investigators are committed to employing the official Diagnostic and Statistical Manual of Mental Disorders – Fourth Edition (abbreviated DSM-IV), which bases all psychiatric diagnoses on symptoms and their course, not on any fuller knowledge of the person. It is as if public health investigators studying the prevalence of pneumonia over time in the American population were satisfied to call every instance of a cough with a fever and a mucoid sputum a case of pneumonia.[9]

Training of descriptive psychopathology relies on classification manuals

The primary care model has elicited a metamorphosis in psychiatric instruction, notably in a reduction in the teaching of the *mental status examination* and descriptive psychopathology. Once the lynchpin of training, interest in psychopathology now focuses on how to recognize the clinical features needed to apply DSM or ICD labels. For example, in a 2002 mailed survey to all accredited psychiatry residency training programs in the USA ($N=149$),[10] of which 68 (45.6%) responded, while nearly 80% stated that they offered a course in descriptive psychopathology (often only one semester),[11] and another in the mental status examination (typically less than 5 h), less than 30% of respondents taught the classic features of psychopathology (e.g. catatonia, first rank symptoms), and less than 20% used any of the well-known psychopathology texts.[12] Twenty percent of programs offered no formal lecture series in descriptive psychopathology or mental status examination. Psychopathology was seen in many teaching programs as the signs and symptoms described in the present DSM, but nearly half did not provide classroom instruction or discussion of the features in the criteria, and those that did typically devoted less than 5 h to it. A 1991 survey of all psychiatric clinical tutors in the UK also found substantial reliance on the DSM for the teaching of basic psychopathology.[13] Surveys of the teaching of psychopathology in other parts of the world are lacking.

Problems in present classifications

Table 1.1 displays the problems in present classification. These are discussed in detail below.[14]

DSM and ICD reliability is weak

Reliability in diagnosis is its degree of precision, i.e. agreement among clinicians. If reliability is poor, validity of diagnoses (accuracy) is unclear.[15] Systematized "field trials" of the interrater reliability of the recent DSM and ICD iterations describe mixed results. Diagnostic agreement was also inflated by defining agreement as two clinicians placing the patient in the same diagnostic class rather than explicitly agreeing.[16] If the clinicians differed in the specific disorder within the class (e.g. if one diagnosed "schizophrenia", while the other said the patient had "delusional disorder"), agreement was accepted.[17] Such agreement is equivalent to clinicians agreeing that a patient has a respiratory problem, but not whether it is bronchitis or pneumonia, bacterial or viral or allergy-related.

Table 1.1. Problems in present classification

Problem	Effect
Reliability is weak	The "claim to fame" of recent DSM iterations is high reliability. Weak reliability insures idiosyncratic diagnosis
Encourages false positives and false negatives with over-inclusive diagnostic criteria	Some conditions are over-diagnosed (e.g. depression) resulting in false positives, research sample heterogeneity, and unneeded or dangerous treatment for patients. Some conditions are not recognized (e.g. catatonia), resulting in false negatives and inappropriate treatment
Offers false choices	False choices lead to the prescription of inappropriate treatments. Conditions such as schizophreniform have no validity. Dissociation, a symptom, is treated as a disease. Abnormal bereavement and puerperal depressions are given separate status
Omits or marginalizes established syndromes	Catatonia is incorrectly linked to psychotic disorders, melancholia is reduced to a modifying term, the different frontal lobe syndromes are not included
Diagnostic criteria are poorly defined	Terms such as "disorganized speech" encourage misdiagnosis (e.g. misidentifying a fluent aphasia as flight-of-ideas or formal thought disorder)
Checklist format limits meaningful examination	Items are incorrectly given equal weight. Type of illness onset, sequence of symptom emergence, and patterns of features are mostly ignored, resulting in misdiagnosis
Omits important discriminating psychopathology	Psychopathology associated with neurologic syndromes (e.g. psychosensory features and seizure disorder) are not mentioned, resulting in illnesses going unrecognized
Claiming theory neutrality, it avoids neuroscience and laboratory criteria	Patterns of features that indicate the involvement of a specific brain region or system are not included (e.g. features indicating right hemisphere disease). Laboratory assessments are not included as helpful criteria (e.g. hypothalamic pituitary functioning in depressive illness, CPK levels and response to lorazepam in catatonia)
Longitudinal criteria are not used	The pre-psychosis findings in schizophrenia are ignored, resulting in the over-diagnosis of the condition and research sample heterogeneity. The dimensional traits of personality are ignored, resulting in poor reliability and validity for the personality disorders

In the two DSM-III trials, the overall agreement for Axis I for adults was marginally acceptable (kappas of 0.68 and 0.72, with 0.70 the minimal agreement coefficient). For affective disorders they were 0.69 and 0.83. For schizophrenia, both trials obtained kappas of 0.81. The range among diagnostic classes, however, was broad and many had kappas near 0.50 (i.e. closer to chance agreement).[18] Kappas for children and adolescents were poor for most conditions, as were kappas for Axis II. Often, only a few patient vignettes per category were used, lessening the likelihood of meaningful agreement. DSM-III-R field trials have similar shortcomings (APA, 1987).

Assessments of DSM-IV also detail mixed results. The DSM-based clinical interview is reported to reliably identify patients with eating disorders,[19] symptoms and diagnoses in relatives of psychiatric patients,[20] and diagnoses from information obtained from personal interview or from an informant.[21] Other reports are less positive. For example, an assessment of 362 outpatients using the DSM-IV interview instrument for anxiety and mood disorder obtained good test–retest reliability for the two categories, but there was substantial overlap and "a common source of unreliability was disagreements on whether constituent symptoms were sufficient in number, severity, or duration to meet DSM-IV diagnostic criteria."[22] Participants also had difficulty categorizing clinical features presented randomly as representing an Axis I or II criterion, and in one study they misclassified 31% of Axis I criteria as representing an Axis II disorder and 25% of Axis II criteria as representing an Axis I condition.[23] They could not identify whether a feature was a symptom of disease or trait behavior. This is equivalent to not knowing whether the patient's cough represents a nervous tic or respiratory disease.

The DSM-IV field trials revealed diagnostic uncertainty. The mood disorder field trials of 524 patients from inpatient, outpatient, and community settings from 5 sites used structured interviews and reported good intra-site but only fair inter-site reliability with deteriorating reliability in a six-month retest.[24] Test–retest reliability is reported below for statistical reliability standards for psychosis, somatization, eating disorder, dysthymia, mania, generalized anxiety disorder, attention deficit hyperactivity disorder, and hypochondriasis.[25] Studies of the multiaxial systems of both classifications find poor agreement (i.e. which axis to place clinical features) and poor agreement on axes assessing environmental stressful events.[26]

The reliability of "bizarre" delusions, the hallmark of the criteria for the psychotic disorders, has also been found unsatisfactory.[27] An assessment for substance-induced psychiatric syndromes in 1951 acute psychiatric inpatients found a dimensional approach to have better reliability and predictive validity than the dichotomous DSM-IV strategy.[28]

ICD-10 field trials worldwide assessed over 15 000 patients at 112 clinical centers in 39 countries. Good reliability was achieved except for the personality disorders.[29] Independent examinations of 150 patients assessed with a European diagnostic instrument also found good reliability for schizophrenia,[30] mania, and major depression, but unsatisfactory reliability for schizoaffective disorder.[31] The validity of the psychotic disorders category, however, was questioned.[32] Systematic application of ICD descriptions to clinical samples also finds instability over time for the diagnosis of bipolar and recurrent depressive disorder.[33] The low interrater reliability for a depressive episode[34] and difficulties with the ICD depression subscales for endogenous and psychogenic depression[35] partially account for the diagnostic instability of the ICD mood disorder category. ICD reliability was found enhanced by the addition of clinical descriptions to the operational criteria, a strategy not used in the DSM.[36]

The mixed reliability results are particularly alarming because the field trial participants were intensively trained in the use of the system and examination instruments. Also, about 40% of the patient evaluations were done conjointly. These procedures are rarely used in clinical practice where diagnostic agreement among clinicians remains low.[37]

Further, while the assessment of patients by structured examination can obtain fair to good reliability,[38] this method has poor agreement with the more likely clinical circumstance of a clinician doing a semi-structured evaluation[39] or a standard clinical assessment.[40] Even when using semi-structured assessments, reliability is marginal for some diagnostic options.

Bertelsen (1999) cautions against the exclusive reliance on simplified list-based criteria. He points out that the best clinical approach is an initial comprehensive traditional clinical examination to first identify the syndrome followed by the matching of the findings to criteria for nosologic labeling, rather than reliance solely on the manuals.[41]

Classification validity is uncertain

Accuracy in diagnosis defines validity, i.e. the patient has the illness that is diagnosed. Poor validity leads to false positive and false negative classifications. A false negative occurs when the patient's illness is unrecognized. A false positive occurs when a patient is given a diagnosis he does not have. Present classification methods encourage both types of errors.

Diagnostic false positives

Diagnostic criteria in the manuals are mostly imprecise and overly broad, encouraging the identification of illness when none exists, or misidentifying one illness for another. The identification of over half the population in the USA as meeting such criteria for illness dramatically demonstrates the degree of false positive diagnosis inherent in using the DSM. Half of persons in normal bereavement also meet criteria for major depression, but neither the researchers nor the bereaved in the studies considered the state to be illness.[42] The major depression criteria of apathy and motor slowing are seen in frontal circuitry disease, while low energy, shyness, and anxiety are found in some persons with personality deviations. These patients may be misdiagnosed as depressed and needlessly prescribed antidepressant agents.[43]

The DSM diagnosis of major depression requires five or more items in any combination.[44] Depressed mood need *not* be present for the diagnosis of depression. A loss of interest or the inability to experience pleasure are acceptable alternatives. "Fatigue or loss of energy" and "diminished ability to think or concentrate" are choices. The criteria are not operationally defined (e.g. what degree of diminished concentration is needed to be a symptom and how concentration is to be measured, are not detailed). In the quest for diagnostic reliability, criteria are over-simplified, thereby lowering the bar for admission into the category of depression. Taken literally (which is a necessity to obtain expected reliability) the following patient meets DSM-IV criteria for major depression.

Patient 1.1

A 51-year-old man experienced substantial loss of interest and anhedonia for almost a year. He slept much of the day (hypersomnia is a criterion choice), and his movements and thinking were slowed (psychomotor retardation is a criterion choice). He had trouble concentrating his thoughts, and had no energy. He was pessimistic about the future. He did not want to kill himself, but he did not want to live in his present state. His symptoms caused "clinically significant distress and impairment in social functioning." His condition could not be explained as the "direct physiological effects of a substance . . . or a general medical condition." His general neurologic examination was normal, except for slowness of movement and thought. His symptoms began after his trailer home burned, destroying it and all his possessions. He was not burned and did not suffer significant smoke inhalation. Posttraumatic stress disorder was ruled out, because he did not have nightmares and was neither anxious nor ruminating about the event. Major depression was diagnosed by several clinicians and antidepressant medications were prescribed without improvement.[45]

On examination, the man's mood was reactive, and although subdued, he showed mildly diminished emotional expression rather than sadness or apprehension. A frontal lobe avolitional syndrome[46] was diagnosed and carbon monoxide poisoning hypothesized as the cause of his behavioral change.

CT scan showed bilateral basal ganglia calcifications, a finding consistent with the diagnosis of carbon monoxide exposure. Methylphenidate treatment improved his condition.

Patient 1.1 also meets criteria for "treatment-resistant depression", because he did not respond to two drug trials with different classes of antidepressants. However, about 10–15% of depressed patients labeled "treatment-resistant" are incorrectly considered depressed, and therefore do not benefit from antidepressant treatments.[47]

The DSM criterion A common to all the psychotic disorders is also problematic. Two of five features are needed, but sustained auditory hallucinations and "bizarre" delusions may stand alone. This provision is a vestige from the ideas of Kurt Schneider, who considered some psychotic features to be pathognomonic of schizophrenia if a neurological disease could not be recognized.[48] The identification in the 1970s of Schneider's "first rank symptoms" in patients with mood disorder and other conditions, however, demonstrated definitively that these features are not pathognomonic, but the error persists in DSM-IV. Consider Patient 1.2.

Patient 1.2
A 32-year-old woman was hospitalized because she barricaded her home and rearranged the furniture so that her two young children would not have to walk on the floor. She said she had overheard neighbors constantly plotting to electrify the floor and that she could feel static electricity. She was irritable and walked constantly throughout the inpatient unit on tiptoe and had several other catatonic features.

She responded to questions such as "What do you think is the reason for your neighbors doing those things to your house?" with:

"They're jealous, mean spirited, I'm the spirit of 1776, they see the spirit in me, I have an aura, an aura borealis, a whore (eyes filled with tears for a moment), a four by four."

Patient 1.2 meets the DSM criterion A for a psychotic disorder. She experienced sustained auditory hallucination (tactile also) and many would accept her delusional ideas as "bizarre". She also exhibited "disorganized speech", another criterion A choice. However, other psychopathology can be recognized. Her tiptoe gait is consistent with catatonia, and she exhibited other catatonic features, phenomena not detailed in the manuals.[49] Criterion A includes catatonia as a choice in the diagnosis of schizophrenia. Nevertheless, irritability and constant walking about the inpatient unit suggests hyperactivity or agitation and along with catatonia are consistent with a manic episode. She had grandiose delusions. Characterizing speech with such vague terms as "disorganized" is also poor practice.

Flight-of-ideas with clang associations describes her language better, and are features of mania. The patient was treated with lithium monotherapy and fully recovered.

False negative diagnosis and "not otherwise specified" (NOS)

The high proportion of patients receiving the DSM *Not Otherwise Specified* (NOS) choice further attests to the limits of the system.[50] To support treatment choices, the "catch-all" option permits clinicians to assign patients to a likely diagnostic category despite being unable to fit them to a specific illness descriptor (e.g. the diagnosis "psychosis, NOS" justifies prescribing an antipsychotic agent).

Use of the NOS choice occurs in several circumstances. Most commonly, the patient meets some but not all necessary criteria. When a patient has an established syndrome not recognized in the DSM, but has a clinical feature that suggests a diagnostic category, NOS is also applied. The frontal lobe avolitional and disinhibited syndromes, several seizure-related syndromes and the paraphrenias are not included in the DSM. Patients with these conditions go unrecognized and are typically labeled "psychotic disorder" or "mood disorder, NOS".[51]

Hirschfeld (2001) reviews the behaviors consistent with a *manic-depressive spectrum*, a construct not implicitly incorporated in the DSM. Such syndromes elicit the NOS suffix. The manic-depressive spectrum concept, however, leads to more effective treatment (e.g. mood stabilizers and antidepressants rather than psychotherapy alone) for many patients now considered as having personality disorders. *Cyclothymia* represents part of that spectrum.

The *Oneiroid Syndrome*, a dream-like state, known to European psychiatrists, but all but forgotten in the USA, is another example.[52] Recent reviews of the diagnostic usefulness of psychopathology associated with traumatic brain injury[53] and epilepsy[54] further highlight the omission of important syndromes.

The failure to define the catatonia syndrome illustrates another ICD and DSM shortcoming. Catatonia has strong linkage to mood disorder, more so than to schizophrenia. Yet, the DSM primarily places catatonia as a subtype of schizophrenia, while all patients with catatonia not clearly the result of a neurologic or general medical condition must be diagnosed as suffering from a psychotic disorder by the ICD. There are over 40 classic catatonic features and associated behaviors, but the DSM briefly mentions only 12 and the ICD fewer. Neither manual offers instructions on how to identify or elicit the features. A patient could easily have many catatonic features not elicited or recognized by the clinician trained to the DSM or ICD standard. It is not surprising that most DSM-trained clinicians think catatonia is rare despite the consistent finding that when systematically assessed, 10% of acutely hospitalized psychiatric patients, 40% of hospitalized manic patients, and many patients with developmental disorders meet criteria for catatonia.[55] Some catatonic and stuporous patients are mostly mute and cannot communicate the information needed to assess criteria. Patient 1.3 illustrates.

Patient 1.3
A 28-year-old woman became withdrawn and then mute over a period of several days. She sat staring for long periods, and when she did move, her efforts were slow. Without evidence of a general medical or structural neurologic cause for her condition, she was admitted to a psychiatric inpatient unit. Laboratory tests results revealed no explanation for her state other than dehydration. Her drug screen was negative. She was diagnosed "psychotic" "NOS". The brief psychotic disorder/schizophreniform/schizophrenia option was considered.

   A consultant elicited several catatonic features not identified in the DSM (Gegenhalten, automatic obedience, ambitendency) consistent with catalepsy, bradykinesia and mutism. IV midazolam in preparation for an MRI temporarily disinhibited the patient at which time she looked about the drab hallway to the MRI suite and said "Good, you're taking me to the basement incinerator. I deserve to die. I am a bad person." She described her depressed mood, hopelessness and desire to die. The MRI revealed no structural disease, and she was diagnosed as having melancholia with catatonic features. A course of lorazepam resolved her catatonia.

Some patients marginally match a large DSM or ICD category. Patient 1.4 initially diagnosed as having psychotic disorder NOS, with consideration of "late-onset schizophrenia", illustrates the need to recognize other forms of psychopathology.

Patient 1.4
A 63-year-old woman previously in good health stopped answering her phone. Concerned, her daughter went to the woman's house, but at first the mother would not open the door, saying that rays were being beamed into the house to gain control of her mind. She said her neighbors and their homes had been replaced by aliens from another planet and that the aliens were now probing into her mind and had started to gain control of her body. When she finally opened the door she screamed at her daughter, calling her an imposter and an alien. Once in the hospital she was unable to return to her room from the dining area, and angrily accused the nurses of hiding her room so that she could not find it.[56]

   The attending psychiatrist considered late-onset schizophrenia or psychosis, NOS as likely diagnoses. A consultant, however, recognized the woman to have Capgras syndrome, the delusion that familiar persons are imposters, often a sign of non-dominant cerebral hemisphere disease.[57] Delusions of replicated neighbors and homes (reduplicative paramnesia), experiences of alienation and control, and "losing" her hospital room (topographic disorientation) were also consistent with non-dominant cerebral hemisphere disease. The lack of other psychopathology (loss of emotional expression, avolition, auditory hallucinations, and speech and language disorders) further suggested the lesion was posterior. A right-sided parieto-temporal lobe stroke was demonstrated on brain imaging. Antipsychotic medication was withheld, and redirection and behavioral control became the focus of treatment. She was discharged a week later fully recovered.

False diagnostic choices

For a behavioral condition to warrant inclusion in the official classification of disease, it must meet long-established standards.[58] Its cross-sectional clinical features should delineate it from other conditions. The characteristic signs and symptoms should be validated by a characteristic course of illness or response to treatment, genetic predisposition, or laboratory markers. Present classification is replete, however, with examples that violate this standard, and many diagnostic classes are included without evidence warranting their recognition as disease entities. A patently false notion is the classifying of *brief, schizophreniform* and *schizophrenia* as three independent nonaffective psychotic disorders if they remain within their duration requirements, but as a continuum if their durations merge.[59] Follow-up studies of patients originally diagnosed schizophreniform find variable outcomes – some patients evolving to schizophrenia, while others develop a schizoaffective or mood disorder.[60] *Abnormal bereavement* and *puerperal depression* meet criteria for melancholia, and these depressions are no different in any meaningful way from melancholias occurring in other circumstances.[61] Nevertheless, they are classified by their circumstances as if they warrant independent status.

Conversion and *dissociative* disorders are also classified as distinct psychologically derived illnesses, despite evidence of great heterogeneity in samples of these patients and associations with a variety of neurologic diseases including seizure disorder and demyelinating conditions.[62] *Dissociative identity disorder* has also been associated with manic-depressive illness.[63]

Diagnostic criteria are categorical without dimensional considerations, and poorly defined

The DSM and ICD conceptually define many Axis I conditions as they do many general medical conditions (e.g. infection and bone fracture). The person is normal, then something occurs and the syndrome appears fully formed. While illness course is used to define unipolar and bipolar categories, longitudinal criteria such as age of onset and pre-episode features (e.g. schizoid traits) are not used in Axis I criteria. The magnitude of the omission is illustrated by evidence showing that many persons with schizophrenia have pre-psychosis childhood neuromotor, cognitive, and emotional difficulties that are identifiable and potentially useful in secondary prevention.[64] In one study of old "home movies" of young children at family gatherings, viewers experienced in childhood behavior who were unaware of the condition of the children in later years identified 90% of the children who became schizophrenic.[65]

The incorporation of a dimensional component into Axis I criteria has been proposed for future manuals.[66] The focus is on severity ratings of criteria to facilitate prognosis, monitor treatment response, and in the recognition of mild conditions. Patients would be given individual criterion and summed severity rating scores. This approach, however, will not solve the reliability and validity problems of classification, and does not address the necessary identification of the longitudinal emergence of disease.

Poorly drafted diagnostic criteria also limit the usefulness of the manuals. To bolster reliability, both systems over-simplify the descriptors of psychopathology such as delusions, hallucinations and language disorder. Although many forms of speech and language disorder in psychiatric patients are described in the classic literature, DSM-IV states: "Because of the difficulty inherent in developing an objective definition of 'thought disorder' and because in a clinical setting inferences about thought are based primarily on the individual's speech, the concept of disorganized speech has been employed . . ." (DSM-IV, p. 276). Not only does this approach lump most speech and language problems under one appellation, it assumes that the speech problems of patients derives from problems in thinking, when the classic literature and empirical studies show that this is not always the case.[67] Patient 1.5 is an example of how disregarding complexity endangers patients.

Patient 1.5
The behavior of a 60-year-old nursing home patient with a long history of manic-depressive illness changed over a week. Her mood fluctuated between high spirits and irritability. She became agitated and her speech was described as "disorganized and confused". At times she did not appear oriented to date and place. She was transferred to a psychiatric hospital with the diagnosis of recurrence of mania.

A consultant at the hospital noted that the patient's speech was spontaneous and fluent, without dysarthria, but she was paraphasic with agrammatisms and neologisms. She could repeat simple phrases, but at times she was non-sequitive

in her responses. She had naming problems and was circumlocutory. She did not have the circumstantial speech or flight-of-ideas characteristic of mania. Her change in speech and word usage was understood as a receptive aphasia syndrome following a stroke. Hypertension was considered contributory. At no time in the nursing home, hospital admitting area or initially on the inpatient unit was her behavior evaluated for anything other than mania, nor was her speech and language recognized as anything other than "confused". She initially received no evaluation for stroke. Once the diagnosis was made, psychotropic medication was avoided and her hypertension controlled. She was quickly able to return to the nursing home.[68]

The DSM and ICD formats limit meaningful examination

The checklist approach of the DSM and the brief paragraph offerings of the ICD are at best concluding summaries of the psychiatric examination. They are inadequate as guideposts to the examination. For example, illness onsets of hours, days, weeks and months have different diagnostic implications regardless of how the patient appears in the full expression of the disorder. Patient 1.6 has the cross-sectional features consistent with the diagnosis of schizophrenia, but the onset of his symptoms is distinctly not that of classic schizophrenia.

Patient 1.6
A 28-year-old man experienced auditory hallucinations (voices commenting and conversing) daily for years. The hallucinations were perceived as originating from a non-specific external source. The voices were loud, clear, and derogatory in content. They were most intense for several hours in the morning, but the patient would hear them occasionally in the early afternoon. He recognized that his experiences were a sign of illness, but when the voices were most intense, he believed them to be real and not self-generated. He did not work, had no future plans, and mostly kept to himself, worrying about the voices and fearful of their inevitable return. Emotional expression was intact, moods appropriate, and no speech or language disorder was noted. He was occasionally suspicious of strangers, assuming that they might be the source of the voices. He had never been depressed or manic. Meeting DSM criteria for schizophrenia, several antipsychotics had been prescribed, with minimal relief.

A consultant noted that the man's morning hallucinations typically began upon awakening. The patient would awake, become immediately frightened, and then hear the voices. After several hours, they diminished in intensity and ended. They recurred shortly after lunch. Because a nonaffective psychosis with preserved emotional expression is often associated with recognizable neurologic disease,[69] and hallucinations that are linked to a specific time of day, event, or stimulus are also most likely due to such disease, the hallucinations were considered post-ictal consequences of seizures that occurred upon wakening (when the afternoon voices occurred it was after a heavy lunch followed by a nap). Carbamazepine resolved the psychotic features.

The DSM and ICD do not incorporate the nuances described in Patient 1.6 despite many descriptions of the psychopathology associated with epilepsy,[70] and the high frequency with which depression, psychosis and personality change occur in epileptic patients. As a result, such patients come frequently to psychiatric clinics and hospitals for care. But their seizure disorder is unrecognized.

Patient 1.7 further illustrates how reliance on short lists of vaguely delineated symptoms and signs leads to misdiagnosis.

Patient 1.7
A 78-year-old woman lived independently until she was diagnosed as being depressed and prescribed buproprion. She progressively lost the ability to care for herself. "Confusion", followed by mutism and immobility, led her daughter to bring her to an emergency room. Thought to be experiencing a stroke, she was admitted to a neurology service. The MRI indicated mild old ischemic disease, but provided no explanation of her present state. The mutism and immobility resolved within an hour of admission. Over the next several hours the patient's state fluctuated from "confusion" to apparent alertness. It was "observed" that her episodes of confusion occurred when her daughter was present, but resolved when the daughter left the room.

The alternating periods of "confusion" and alertness were interpreted as evidence of hysteria or conversion disorder. The catatonic features noted in the emergency room and the previous diagnosis of depression were consistent with this conclusion and she was transferred to the psychiatry inpatient unit.

On the psychiatry unit, when lucid she showed reduced affective intensity, sadness, and psychomotor retardation. She was pessimistic about her future. Prior to hospitalization she had been eating and sleeping poorly. A psychiatry consultant noted the patient was subdued and appeared tired, but that she retained some humor, inconsistent with the degree of her depressive features. (The DSM does not consider patterns of features, but rather the number of features.) The consultant also noted that the patient's periods of "confusion" began abruptly and were characterized by not fully understanding the examiner's questions, although she could repeat some words and phrases. Some of her responses were non-sequitive. Others were laced with phrases that made no sense, odd sounding words and imprecise word usage (the DSM does not define speech and language disorders in specifics as do neurology texts. It considers episode duration, but not duration or fluctuations of individual features).

The patient's speech was recognized as episodes of transient sensory aphasia. Psychopathology from idiopathic disorders, however, does not typically begin in seconds, and aphasia from vascular disease does not come and go abruptly. Also, transient catatonia unrelated to a manic-depressive disorder is often due to recognizable neurologic disease. Non-convulsive status epilepticus was considered and confirmed by EEG. IV anticonvulsants resolved the patient's acute state.

The DSM and ICD offer a few clinical features as sufficient for each diagnostic class. The DSM requires a patient to exhibit a specific number of criteria for the diagnosis. The combinations of features, their characteristic onset, the relationships among different patterns, and the context in which symptoms unfold are rarely addressed. Although the duration of a syndrome in days, weeks or months is a common requirement to aid reliability, the more difficult assessment of the quality of symptom onsets (e.g. the rate of their emergence), the sequence of symptom appearances, and symptom pattern are not incorporated. Patient 1.8 meets DSM criteria for major depression, but the split-second change in psychopathology typically indicates a secondary syndrome.

Patient 1.8
A middle-aged man became profoundly gloomy, pessimistic and unable to work. He whined and tearlessly cried, pleading for help. He needed repeated reassurance. He made several serious suicide attempts (e.g. attempted hanging). The depressive episodes typically began suddenly in the late afternoon and slowly resolved by evening. They occurred daily. On several occasions a depressive episode lasted a week or more. A seizure disorder was recognized, verified by EEG. The illness resolved with anticonvulsant treatment.

Ignoring symptom patterns encourages misdiagnosis. For example, the DSM catatonia criteria[71] require two of five features to be met. If both excessive "purposeless" activity (item 2) and echolalia or echopraxia (item 5) are present, the patient is said to be catatonic. Manic patients, however, seem purposeless in their actions when in heightened excitement. They show echophenomena.[72] These criteria, as others, require the patient to receive a diagnosis of a psychotic disorder, and most likely that of schizophrenia. Such classification is followed by antipsychotic medication rather than treatments for mood disorder.

The inadequacy of relying on a few features for diagnosis and not obtaining the story of the patient's illness is further illustrated by the unique study of

Rosenham (1973). He recruited eight non-ill persons to seek admission to psychiatric facilities complaining of experiencing auditory hallucination of the words "empty . . . hollow . . . thud" over a period of several weeks. The remainder of their statements and answers to their examiner's questions were truthful and they acted in their usual manner. In 11 of the 12 presentations the "pseudo-patients" were hospitalized with the diagnosis of schizophrenia. The inpatient staff also considered them to be ill, although many other patients recognized the sham.

The DSM and ICD are non-theoretical systems in a neuroscience world

Classifying psychiatric patients by their shared signs and symptoms is traditional. Objectively observing and organizing this information is essential in the diagnostic process and the DSM and ICD take this position. Many clinical features can be understood within a neurologic framework, however, and many patients require assessment beyond the sketchy evaluation offered in the DSM and ICD manuals. Recognizing *psychosensory features*[73] in a patient with panic disorder, for example, directs the examiner toward a diagnosis of seizure disorder.[74] Identifying these features in a patient with manic-depressive illness influences treatment (the use of anticonvulsants as mood stabilizers rather than lithium) and prognostic concerns (the greater likelihood of chronicity and cognitive decline).[75] The presence of Capgras syndrome raises the possibility of a temporo-parietal stroke as seen in Patient 1.4.

Present classification does not incorporate the known brain and behavior relationships into diagnostic criteria because unlike some neurologic signs (e.g. hemiparesis, Broca's aphasia), most behavioral signs and symptoms are not localizing to brain sites. The behaviors do, however, reflect dysfunction in specific brain systems or are strongly associated with specific brain syndromes as well or better than are items included in present criteria. Subsequent chapters detail these relationships.

Summary

The framers of the latest DSM and the ICD classifications do not consider the manuals to be textbooks of psychopathology. They caution against their use by "untrained" persons. The DSM, nevertheless, has become the principal guide to psychopathology for an entire generation of psychiatrists in the USA and elsewhere, to the exclusion of works devoted to a fuller understanding of psychopathology. The DSM and ICD achieve adequate reliability only under structured circumstances and may elicit poor reliability for several categories in the typical clinical setting. The validity of many categories is weak. Sole reliance on DSM criteria and ICD brief descriptions leads to unacceptable false negative and false positive misdiagnoses and the overuse of the NOS category. Much discriminating psychopathology is not included in the classification, nor are recognized neurologic syndromes that are commonly seen in patients seeking help at psychiatric services. The result is that many patients are ill-served.

NOTES

1 Trimble (2002).

2 Mezzich (2002).

3 Sartorius *et al.* (1993, 1995).

4 Panzarino (2000); Doctor Taylor has been teaching psychiatry residents since 1969, Doctor Vaidya since 1989.

5 Hiller *et al.* (1994a,b); Slade and Andrews (2001); Peralta and Cuesta (2003a); Sorensen *et al.* (2005).

6 APA, (1996, 1997).

7 See the STAR-D (Rush *et al.*, 2006) "one size fits all" approach to the treatment of depressive illness and its report of results only marginally better than placebo (30% remitted in the first drug trial and an additional 18–25% in the second). Also see the treatment algorithms offered for manic-depressive illness (Nierenberg *et al.*, 2006) and psychosis (Schneider *et al.*, 2001).

8 Many of the DSM syndrome choices have sub-syndrome modifiers bringing the total to over 350 diagnostic options.

9 Paul McHugh: Overestimating mental illness in America, in A Nation of Crazy People? *The Weekly Standard*, Volume 10, Issue 39, 27 June 2005.

10 Taylor and Vaidya (2005).

11 In contrast, residency programs in the 1960s stressed the recognition of psychopathology. In the first year of residency (following a general internship) one of us (MAT) had a weekly 90-min seminar in descriptive psychopathology that ran for 10 months. This course was separate from other seminars in psychopathology.

12 Bleuler's *Dementia Praecox* (17.6%), Kraepelin's *Manic-Depressive Illness* (19.1%), Schneider's *Clinical Psychopathology* (17.6%); four programs (5.9%) used Jasper's *General Psychopathology*. One program each used Kahlbaum's *Catatonia* and Fish's *Schizophrenia*.

13 Macaskill *et al.* (1991).

14 Also see Wakefield (1997).

15 Reliability was expressed as a kappa statistic which corrects for chance agreement. Kappa is the proportion of agreement above or below chance. Zero is only agreement by chance. One is perfect agreement, while 0.50 is agreement half-way between chance and perfect agreement. A kappa of 0.7 is considered "good".

16 DSM-III Appendix F, pages 467–72.

17 One reason clinicians rely heavily on the NOS category.

18 See Kirk and Kutchins (1992) for a detailed presentation of the promotion of DSM-III and the field trial results.

19 Grilo *et al.* (2004).

20 Todd *et al.* (2003).

21 Schneider *et al.* (2004).

22 Brown *et al.* (2001).

23 Linde and Clark (1998).

24 Keller *et al.* (1995).

25 Keller *et al.* (1996); Bertelsen (2002); Blais *et al.* (1997); Woo and Rey (2005); Schneider *et al.* (2004); First *et al.* (2004); Sbrana *et al.* (2005).

26 Siebel *et al.* (1997); Willemse *et al.* (2003).

27 Flaum *et al.* (1991).

28 Ries *et al.* (2001).

29 Sartorius *et al.* (1993); Regier *et al.* (1994).

30 Jager *et al.* (2003).

31 Maj *et al.* (2000).

32 Bertelsen (2002).

33 Kessing (2005a,b).

34 Hiller *et al.* (1994a).

35 Vetter *et al.* (2001).

36 Sartorius *et al.* (1995).

37 Blashfield (1984).

38 Zanarini and Frankenburg (2001).

39 Benazzi (2003b). A structured interview is conducted using a pamphlet requiring the user to ask questions as written and in the order written, regardless of the clinical state of the patient. Follow-up questioning is limited. Semi-structured interviewing is closer to the traditional clinical examination. All items must be assessed, but the order and wording can be modified by the examiner. Follow-up questioning is permitted and essential.

40 Teeney *et al.* (2003); Becker *et al.* (2006).

41 Chapter 4 provides a discussion of the diagnostic process.

42 Clayton (1982); Taylor and Fink (2006), chapters 2 and 4.

43 Taylor and Fink (2006), chapters 3, 10, 11.

44 DSM-IV, p. 327.

45 Adapted from Taylor and Fink (2006); also seen in Atre Vaidya and Taylor (2006).

46 There are several frontal lobe syndromes, some of which have signs that overlap with mood disorder. See Chapter 3.

47 Starkstein and Manes (2000).

48 Taylor (1972); Abrams and Taylor (1973).

49 Chapter 7 provides a discussion of catatonic features.

50 Wilson (1989).

51 Holden (1987); Joseph (1999).

52 Kaptsan *et al.* (2000).

53 Pelegrin *et al.* (2001).

54 Onuma (2000).

55 Fink and Taylor (2003).

56 Adapted from Atre Vaidya and Taylor (2004), "The Cherry Pie Lady".

57 Bourget and Whitehurst (2004).

58 Robins and Guze (1970).

59 While their cross-sectional criteria are similar, they are defined by duration: brief psychotic disorder (<one month), schizophreniform disorder (>one but <six months), and schizophrenia (>six months).

60 Benazzi (2003a).

61 Taylor and Fink (2006).

62 Lalonde *et al.* (2001).

63 Savitz *et al.* (2004).

64 Erlenmeyer-Kimling and Cornblatt (1984).

65 Walker and Lewine (1990).

66 Helzer *et al.* (2006).

67 Landre *et al.* (1992); Landre and Taylor (1995).

68 Adapted from Atre Vaidya and Taylor (2004).

69 Davison and Bagley (1969).

70 Atre Vaidya and Taylor (1997).

71 DSM-IV, p. 289.

72 See Chapter 7.

73 Psychosensory features (e.g. dysmorphopsia, déjà vu) are signs of temporal–limbic disease and are described in the epilepsy literature and in studies of patients with manic-depressive illness. Atre Vaidya and Taylor (1997).

74 Vazquez and Devinsky (2003).

75 Atre Vaidya *et al.* (1998).

2

A history of psychiatric classification

The study of history is the best medicine for a sick mind; for in history you have a record of the infinite variety of human experience plainly set out for all to see; and in that record you can find yourself and your country both examples and warnings; fine things to take as models, base things rotten through and through, to avoid.[1]

Livy's awareness of the value of a historical perspective of human experience is echoed by modern medical historians.[2] In the preface to *The Origins of Modern Psychiatry*, Thompson writes:

A study of the history of ideas in any subject is important not only as an abstract field of enquiry, but as a method of retaining an appropriate perspective on the current status of the subject and proposed developments. In most cases "new" ideas have been thought of before . . . Psychiatry is a subject which is still developing and in order to understand present controversies and assess the adequacy of proposed changes an historical perspective is essential.[3]

The historical perspective reveals that changes in psychiatric classifications result from societal and theoretic processes more than from science. Demons, body humors, archetypes, and unconscious psychic forces dominated explanations for psychiatric illness for centuries. Social and political pressures buttressed some conditions (e.g. promoting posttraumatic stress disorder after the Vietnam war) while eliminating others (e.g. psychiatrists in the USA emerging from the turmoil of the 1960s voted to eliminate homosexuality as a diagnosis, defining it as a lifestyle choice). The notion of a mind–body dichotomy continues to influence present thinking (e.g. conversion disorder, shared psychotic disorder).

Throughout much of the second millennia CE,[4] classification also reflected experience with patients confined to asylums, focusing attention on severe illnesses. Marked deviations in personality were thus considered reflections of chronic mental deterioration.

Lastly, the clinical predisposition of the classifiers impacted the evolving classification, as some envisioned substantial heterogeneity among patients and pressed for new categories and subcategories while others sought parsimony and searched for common denominators and fewer categories. The influence of these "splitters" and "lumpers" mingled with theoretical constraints and social demands continues in efforts crafting new DSM and ICD iterations. Science has played only a modest role in the formation of classifications.

Empirical research, however, is not "theory-free". Every major shift in classification requires consensus, i.e. a best-estimate interpretation of the information at hand. Agreement is needed on what is to be classified and what factors will be used in sorting out patients. In psychiatric classification it must first be decided what is normal and what is not, what is deviance due to pathology or maturational variability and what deviance is the result of odd upbringing or other experience. This first step has never been resolved, even in the modern era where biology and genetics are so highly valued.[5]

For the clinician who cares for patients with behavioral disorders, however, a flawed classification system is better than none to avoid practice anarchy. The flaws in present classification affecting practice are detailed in other chapters. Understanding how the flaws emerged suggests corrective options. Those options are presented in the last chapter.

Theory drives description and classification

For millennia, philosophy dominated Western medicine's ideas about psychiatric illness.[6] In classical Greek literature and in the writings of Herodotus, madness was attributed to punishment by a deity, avenging demons, excessive drinking, and physical illness.[7] The Christian "Old Testament" pronounces madness and what can be considered neurotic disorders as god-sent. The Christian "New Testament" attributes these states to evil spirits.[8]

Despite the mythological views of causality, physicians of these eras described many recognizable behavioral disorders. Hippocrates (fourth century BCE) detailed familiar images of epilepsy, mania, melancholia, paranoia, and hysteria. Aretaeus of Cappadocia (first century CE) considered psychiatric disease to originate in the head and described melancholia and mania, manic-depression, alcohol-related and toxic states, and dementia. He grouped behavioral conditions by course and outcome, foreshadowing Karl Kahlbaum and Emil Kraepelin.[9]

Galen (130–200 CE), marshalling the knowledge of Western medicine, considered behavioral conditions to reflect brain disorder. Classifications of behavioral syndromes followed his formulations until the mid-nineteenth century, with perturbations in pulse and fever the main guidelines for separating syndromes. Epilepsies were well delineated. Melancholia was an established disorder and was understood to include episodes of mania. Catatonic stupor was reported.[10]

The humoral theory

Among classical Greek ideas, the humoral theory of disease and mental illness was the longest lasting. Hippocrates formulated four basic body substances, or humors: *blood, phlegm,* and *black* and *yellow bile.* In balance, these humors elicited health.[11] Imbalance led to illness and behavioral deviation. Diseases were grouped and named by the humor considered fundamental to their expression. "Melancholia", for example, refers to the belief that it was an expression of excess black bile (*melan,* black and *choleric* from the gall bladder). Temperament deviations were recognized as *sanguine* (an optimistic cheerfulness), *melancholic* (a pessimistic sadness), *choleric* (a general irritability), and *phlegmatic* (a tendency toward apathy). Chaucer, Shakespeare, Ben Jonson, and George Eliot, among many writers, relied on the humor construct in rendering fictional characters, and humoral descriptors of personality remain part of modern usage.

The humoral theory held sway until the end of the nineteenth century, accounting for treatments such as purging, blistering, bleeding, and cupping. George Washington, the first president of the USA, was excessively bled for what was likely a Strep throat, accelerating his death.[12]

Religious dogma

Religious dogma dominated Western thought from the fall of Rome until the modern era. Its influence on the formulations of mental illness and behavioral deviation was varied. Zilboorg, a psychiatric historian of the mid-twentieth century, paints the uniform picture of mental illness in the European Middle Ages as widely attributed to evil possession or sinful choice. He describes sufferers chained in dungeon-like structures, tortured, and burned as witches.[13] This was not always the case.

In addition to religious dogma, interpretations of behavioral syndromes included the humoral theory and physiological and psychological notions of etiology. The blending of such differing ideas was not troubling to medieval society. Celtic Ireland, while attributing madness to supernatural forces, also recognized it as illness and developed a detailed legal system for the care of the mentally ill (*the Bloodlyings Code*).[14] The early Anglo-Saxon tradition also advanced "cures" for persons with "troubling of foul spirits".[15]

The English legal system for incompetence was most advanced. The psychiatrically afflicted were characterized as either "natural fools" or "idiots" (developmentally impaired from birth or shortly thereafter), or as non compos mentis (all other behavioral disturbances). Adjudicated under the aegis of the Court of

Chancery with jury trials, persons from all walks of life could petition the court to confine a sufferer. Examinations were held that included tests of orientation, object recognition, digit span forward and backward, calculations, and biographic and declarative memory. While supernatural explanations were offered to account for the derangement, the most common documented explanations were physical illness or injury.[16]

Mesmerism

Mesmerism was another bogus explanation of behavioral disturbance. Franz Anton Mesmer, a late-eighteenth-century charlatan, introduced the idea of "animal magnetism" and claimed that he could cure neurotic ills with magnetism by placing sufferers in a contraption he called a *baquet*. His notions captured European thought even after being debunked in 1784 by a scientific committee lead by Jean Bailly, the revolutionist mayor of Paris, and that included Benjamin Franklin, American ambassador to France, and Lavoisier, the discoverer of oxygen. Mesmer's influence continued through the next century in Europe, evolving into the study of hysteria and the use of hypnosis by Charcot. In the USA, Mesmerism was adopted by Mary Baker Eddy who reformulated it into the Christian Science Movement.[17]

The notion of the unconscious

Ruminative, anxious states of doubt, and obsessive–compulsive behaviors were ascribed by fifteenth-century Arab physicians to too much love for philosophy and law, an early version of Janet's *idée's fixes*.[18] But T.B. von Hohenheim, a sixteenth-century professor of medicine at Basel, is credited as the first to suggest in a medical work an unconscious motivation to a behavioral syndrome ("unconsciously they [neurotics] have fantasies").[19] The idea of unconscious processes accounting for behavioral disturbances, however, did not fully emerge until the latter half of the nineteenth century when the mind–body dichotomy view of human behavior was widely accepted.[20] Theorizing centered on explanations for neurosis and hysteria.

Jean-Martin Charcot's notions profoundly influenced Freud. Freud did a fellowship in 1885 with the French neurologist at the Salpetrière, and Charcot's manipulation of patients by hypnosis[21] shaped Freud's construction of the dynamic unconscious. Charcot maintained that only persons with neurosis could be fully hypnotized. He led a generation of psychiatrists to accept the idea that easily manipulated and suggestible persons had brain disease, and he conflated these with patients with serious behavioral and neurologic impairment, the common denominator being the ability to be hypnotized.[22]

Pierre Janet also studied hysteria, introducing the term *idées fixes* as the underlying "subconscious" mechanism of neuroses linked to past psychologically

traumatic events. The neurosis emerged from the inability to integrate unconscious and conscious processes.[23] He considered hypnosis and dream analysis as
methods for identifying the neurotic unconscious' fixed ideas, and that the
exposure of these ideas with associated catharsis as curative.[24] These notions
influenced Bleuler's formulations of schizophrenia (see below).

Janet described *dissociation* as a hysterical condition in which intolerable
thoughts and feelings become independent from other mental functions and
are then expressed as dissociative states. This notion prevails in present classifications. He also associated hysteria and other neuroses with a hereditary or *constitutional weakness* in personality. He detailed the characteristics of hysterical
personality as the predisposing factor to neurosis.[25]

Janet was not alone in understanding unconscious mechanisms as underlying
neurosis and its cures, although Freud received the major credit. Auguste Antoine
Liébeault and Hippolyte Bernheim in Nancy, J. Milne Bramwell in England, and
Josef Breuer in Vienna, each treated neurotics with hypnosis as a form of psychotherapy before Freud's work became well-known.[26] "Psychic" treatments were
widely prescribed throughout Europe's private psychiatric clinics before Freud
dominated the field.[27]

Theories merge in the notions of neurosis and hysteria

Understandings of neurosis and hysteria included all the early theories explaining
human behavior. The theories were eventually blended with the fledgling understanding of the nervous system, foreshadowing modern efforts to reconcile
psychoanalytic and biological views of behavior into the "biopsychosocial" model
of psychiatric illness.

Hippocrates began the theoretical journey by attributing hysteria to a
wandering uterus and thus a condition exclusively seen in women.[28] Galen
rejected that notion, but accepted an "engorged" uterus as the cause.[29] In the
European Early Modern period, hysteria was considered of supernatural origin,
but still exclusively seen in women.[30] Reports were common of large groups of
people (also exclusively female) suddenly succumbing to supernatural forces.
Dramatic cases of chorea, St Vitus' Dance, Tarantism (a dance-like movement
disorder that in its cultural form is the dance, the Tarantella), and convulsive-like
syndromes were described. The true nature of these events is obscure.

One clue, however, comes from a presentation of 135 patients with chronic
encephalitis from the 1918 influenza pandemic who were admitted for psychiatric
disturbances to Manhattan State Hospital in New York City between 1920 and
1930.[31] Reasons for psychiatric hospitalization included "impudence and dis-
obedience", various odd motor disturbances, "excessive love of excitement",
"constant complaining", "meddlesomeness", "maliciousness", emotional lability,

non-melancholic depression, impulsiveness, sexual disturbances (including inappropriately increased libido, exhibitionism, paraphilia), compulsions (including kleptomania and pyromania), and neurasthenia. Such behavioral symptoms occurred years after the encephalitis. Physicians in earlier centuries would not have made the connection between the infection and the behavioral abnormality.[32]

Hysteria as an expression of demonic possession or psychic turmoil was challenged once physicians began to appreciate the linkage of the central nervous system to the rest of the body via peripheral nerves. The linkage offered a tangible pathway from "psychic" processes to "somatic" disease. Hysteria was seen as a nerve disease, and sufferers were said to be "nervous" or "suffering from nerves". Charles Lepois, a sixteenth-century writer, appears to be the first to attribute hysteria to a dysfunction within the brain.[33] He and Edward Jorden, a sixteenth-century British physician, also rejected the view that hysteria was of supernatural origin, but in his treatise on "the disease called the suffocation of the mother" Jorden continued the notion that the disorder was seen exclusively in women.[34]

Thomas Willis, the famous seventeenth-century British neuroanatomist, finally demonstrated through autopsy that the uterus was not involved in hysteria. He clinically equated hysteria and hypochondriasis, determining that both genders were afflicted.[35] Thomas Sydenham, in the late seventeenth century, diagnosed hysteria in women and hypochondriasis in men when unable to explain unusual medical symptoms. He included most of the psychiatric conditions that would later be termed neurotic under that umbrella.[36]

Robert Whytt, Scotland's first neurologist, also considered hysteria and hypochondriasis to be nervous system diseases. He, however, rejected mind–body dualism[37] and considered hysteria and hypochondriasis to reflect a constitutional vulnerability in temperament expressed when the person was under duress.[38]

George Cheyne also considered nervous disorders to result from "a nervous distemper" or following an accident. He linked hysteria and hypochondriasis to personality problems or to acute stress.[39] William Cullen, one of the most influential teachers of medicine of the eighteenth century and professor at Edinburgh, also delineated a group of diseases of the nerves without clear neuropathology, and introduced the term "neuroses".[40]

Many nineteenth-century physicians continued the effort to understand the nature and sources of the neuroses.[41] By late century, the notion was established that neuroses were acute, fluctuating behavioral syndromes that emerge under stress in persons with deviant personality and were therefore *personality illnesses.* An unconscious mechanism was considered a contributing factor.

In addition to hysteria and hypochondriasis, French and German clinicians of the mid-nineteenth century delineated the *phobic disorders* and *obsessional symptoms.* Pierre Briquet, professor of clinical medicine in Paris, detailed what is now labeled "somatization disorder".[42] He recognized that the condition also affected men, opined that it involved sensory and emotion-related brain regions, saw a heritable component in its etiology, and concluded that the illness diathesis consisted of emotional trauma impacting on a person with a vulnerable constitution characterized by traits of emotional lability and suggestibility.[43]

The concept of neurosis expanded with the experience of physicians caring for casualties of war. From observations of American Civil War wounded and his experience as an "electrotherapist",[44] George Beard merged a variety of chronic complaints centered on anxiety and fatigue as *neurasthenia* and *war neuroses*. Neurasthenia became the medical model for neuroses. It was believed the result of a weakness in the nerves, not the psyche. It became the fad diagnosis of the late nineteenth century.[45]

War neuroses evolved into the World War I "shell shock", with thousands of soldiers affected. The early-twentieth-century idea that the condition was the result of pressure concussion from artillery was soon rejected, and was replaced by a range of considerations from the personality vulnerability–stress diathesis model of hysteria to simple malingering to escape combat. Patients were described with neurasthenia and other anxiety disorders, loss of hearing or sight, anesthesia, and many motor features including convulsions, chorea, tics and dystonia, stammering, paralysis and contractures. These features could become chronic, and chronicity was also associated with cognitive difficulties, pain syndromes, sleep disorders, and neurasthenia with non-melancholic depression. In World War II these conditions were termed "combat neuroses".[46] From the Vietnam War we have "posttraumatic stress disorder" (PTSD).

Similar conditions, however, were observed in civilians. In the UK, trauma to the nervous system from the rigors of train travel was considered to play an etiologic role in the neurotic disorders.[47] Psychiatrists experiencing both world wars concluded that the presentations and pathologic processes of war-related neuroses were no different from neuroses related to acute stress in civilian life, and that the neuroses that emerged during war were no different than neuroses emerging during other experience.[48] The Veterans Administration in the USA forgot this understanding and subjected thousands of Vietnam combatants to specialized programs of dubious merit that encouraged chronicity and discouraged more appropriate treatment. Taylor and Fink (2006, p. 130) describe a melancholic veteran misdiagnosed as having PTSD who was denied treatment for depression and subsequently killed himself.

By the early twentieth century the neuroses were conceptualized as a few conditions that included hysteria and related states (conversion, somatoform and hypochondriasis), neurasthenia, phobic and obsessional syndromes, and the war neuroses. The grouping was shaped by the belief that they were expressions of unconscious conflict and ultimately included any condition considered the purview of the psychoanalyst.

The application of antidepressant agents, and anxiolytics for the treatment of anxiety disorders in the 1960s rekindled the idea that the neuroses were subtle brain disorders.[49] Pitts and McClure's seminal report[50] that under double-blind conditions lactate infusions induced typical panic attacks in patients with anxiety disorders but not in normal controls gave validity to a biologic understanding of neurotic disorders. Most of the psychoanalytically derived diagnostic designations were seen as invalid (conversion) or as symptoms rather than syndromes (hypochondriasis). This conclusion led to the expulsion of the neurosis category from later classifications. To appease the dominant psychoanalytic establishment, however, the designations were retained in several different categories. Their transfer did not improve their poor validity.[51]

Pre-nineteenth-century description and classification

Despite the dominance of theory over science, efforts continued to organize behavioral syndromes into a meaningful framework. Sixteenth- and seventeenth-century physicians were unable to do so, although they recognized epilepsy, mania (frenzy as well as what was likely catatonia), melancholia (which included the modern concept of mania), idiocy (combining developmental disorders and dementia), lunacy (a category of periodic mixed pictures), obsession and hysteria (the neuroses), and possession (a grab-bag of conditions with theological interpretations). "Mania" and "melancholia" became general synonyms for "madness", rather than well-defined terms, but at their core, the descriptions of that era capture the essences of mood disorder. That understanding was codified in Robert Burton's 1621 landmark *The Anatomy of Melancholy*,[52] the first psychiatric encyclopedia.

But the present-day convention of separating neuroses, personality disorder, and psychosis as if they derive from fundamentally different sources did not emerge until the late nineteenth century.[53] Neurosis denoted diseases of the nerves and muscles, personality deviation was considered degenerative nervous system disease, and psychosis, coined in 1845, denoted "mental disorder" which affected all spheres of personality leading to dementia.[54]

The evolving classification in the nineteenth century

The idea that mental illness was an expression of brain disease was not fully nor widely recognized in the seventeenth and eighteenth centuries as the older notions of humors and possession continued to influence medicine. In the early nineteenth century, however, neuroanatomy became a more established discipline building upon the work of Thomas Willis. Gall attempted to localize function with structure in his phrenology system of facial and skull configurations reflecting personality traits and cognitive functions. Bell and Magendie delineated the sensory and motor systems. The idea that mental illness (as opposed to neurosis) was brain disease gained currency.[55] Later in the century, a genetic influence underlying chronic degenerative brain disease gained favor. The model of general paresis and its dramatically different presentations sometimes seen in the same individual framed how psychiatric syndromes were considered and related to one another.

The original "splitters"

The efforts to formulate a classification led to the emergence in the nineteenth century of the struggle between the "splitters" and the "lumpers" that continues to the present. The splitters envisioned a classification comprised of many forms of distinct mental illness, just as is seen in disease of other organ systems. The lumpers, recognizing the lack of validating support for most of the separate categories, brought them together into one or a few groups. At present, the splitters are dominant.

John Haslam, the apothecary of the Bethlem Hospital in London[56] and a gifted objective observer was a splitter. He offered the first clear description of general paresis of the insane (GPI).[57] He recognized manic-depression and offered one of the first undisputed descriptions of schizophrenia.

William Hammond, professor of the diseases of the mind at the Bellevue Hospital Medical College in New York City and President of the American Neurological Association, also recognized hebephrenia a decade before Kraepelin expanded it into the dementia praecox notion.[58] Hammond's textbook is a marvel of accurate observation of syndromes and careful consideration of the demographic and epidemiological findings in psychiatric illness. His conclusions rival those of twentieth-century investigations bolstered by stringent methodology. Hammond's work, however, was influential only within the USA and only for a brief period.

In addition to hebephrenia, other syndromes also have long pedigrees. Jean-Etienne Esquirol, Phillippe Pinel's[59] pupil, introduced the term hallucinations, giving it the present-day definition and distinguished these phenomena from illusions. He detailed *monomanias*, and the delusional disorder and obsessive disorder syndromes of today.[60] His 1838 publication was the first modern textbook of psychopathology.[61]

Although manic-depression was well known for many years, Jean-Pierre Falret, Esquirol's pupil, and an expert on depressive illness and its associated suicide risk, introduced the concept of circular insanity (*la folie circulaire*) in 1854. Jules Baillarger, in a publication a few months later, used the term *folie à double forme*. These "rare" conditions were conflated by Kraepelin into his manic-depressive illness concept.[62] Baillarger also recognized the association between melancholia, stupor and what was to become known as catatonia.

Classification of mental disorders, however, remained uncertain and different systems were espoused across Europe. Johann Christian Heinroth, a German psychiatrist in the early nineteenth century, considered psychological and theological derangements to be fundamental to mental illness. Heinroth was more a fundamentalist theologian than an objective clinician.[63] But there was no general agreement on classification, with different versions (all elaborate) or schools centered about a prominent psychopathologist. The humoral theory, Galen's ideas about fever and pulse, and theological considerations continued to shape nosologies.

The early "lumpers" and the unitary notion of insanity

Wilhelm Griesinger was influenced by the neurophysiologist Hermann Helmholtz. He considered psychiatry a natural science, not a philosophical or theological discipline and rejected Heinroth's theological notions. He sought unity among psychiatric syndromes, viewing then as brain diseases. He wrote: "psychiatry and neurology are not merely two closely related fields; they are but one field in which one language is spoken and the same laws rule."[64] Griesinger's textbook of psychiatry inspired a generation of German neuro-psychiatrists.[65]

Griesinger took general paresis as a model of a single disease process expressed as several seemingly distinct syndromes. He applied this idea to the mental disorders. This *unitary psychosis* model (*Einheitspsychose*) came to dominate classification. Syndromes were considered stages of a single disease rather than different patterns reflecting different diseases. The sufferer passed through the stages of melancholia, mania, and amentia (delirium), ending in dementia. Griesinger and his followers were not perturbed by the awareness that while some patients experienced different episode types, others with the same presumed underlying illness experienced one or only a few types. An influencial contemporary wrote: "There is but one type of mental disturbance and we call it insanity."[66]

Because the major syndromes were thought to reflect the same underlying process, there was less need for classification and greater focus on etiology.

The return of the splitters

Henry Maudsley, a nineteenth-century British alienist, separated psychiatric syndromes according to presumed faculties of the mind (emotion and intellect) that were considered deranged in mental illness. Although his scheme was illogical as he included the same syndrome in several etiologic categories, his linking of insanity to specific mental domains foreshadowed Kraepelin's reliance on will, thought, and emotion in distinguishing dementia praecox and manic-depressive insanity.[67]

The nineteenth-century French psychiatrist Benedict Augustin Morel introduced the term *dementia praecox*. His characterization of the condition was incorporated by Kraepelin into the disease model that would become schizophrenia. Morel also classified psychiatric disturbances by the presence or absence of perceived hereditary factors.[68]

Daniel Hack Tuke, from a distinguished family committed to the care of the mentally ill, offered a classification that influenced late-nineteenth-century British thinking. Tuke's collaboration with Charles Bucknill resulted in the 1858 publication of the *Manual of Psychological Medicine* that became a standard textbook of psychiatry for the rest of the century. Tuke introduced the term "psycho-therapeutics" in 1872. He followed with the *Dictionary of Psychological Medicine* in 1892, a work of 128 contributors. In 1880 he became the editor of the *Journal of Mental Science*, the fore-runner of the *British Journal of Psychiatry*.[69]

Neurology and psychiatry had not yet fully separated, and in the latter half of the nineteenth century efforts were made to find the specific brain areas involved in the different behavioral disorders. This effort was an extension of Griesinger's labors to make the field more scientific and the earlier work of Willis (who considered different functions for white and gray matter), Dax (who associated a loss of thinking abilities to left hemisphere cortical injury), Broca (who characterized motor aphasia) and Meynart (who observed that motor functions were largely subserved by frontal brain regions).[70]

Carl Wernicke, professor of psychiatry and neurology at the University of Breslau, offered an extensive formulation of the relationship between brain structure and behavioral disturbance (*Grundrib der Psychiatrie* or Basic Psychiatry) that evolved from his study of aphasia. Wernicke forced his classification into his ideas of brain localization rather than basing it on more objective study.[71] Karl Jaspers called him a "brain mythologist" and compared Wernicke to Freud, writing that both made generalizations beyond the facts and produced only abstract constructions.[72]

The quest for localizing psychiatric disease to specific brain regions was continued by Bonhoeffer (acute reactive psychosis), Liepman (secondary psychosis) and Karl Kleist.[73] Kleist had the most success in seeing the association between psychomotor disturbances (e.g. catatonia, melancholia) and basal ganglia and other frontal brain region disease.[74] He also coined the term "cycloid psychosis" later elaborated by Karl Leonhard.

Much of nineteenth-century understanding of psychiatric illness was synthesized by Edward Spitzka, a New York City neurologist and President of the New York Neurological Society.[75] Spitzka considered psychiatric disorders as reflections of brain diseases and explicitly rejected the unitary psychosis model.

Spitzka offered a descriptive classification organized by what he understood to be either intrinsic brain disease or brain dysfunction resulting from disease in other organ systems. It took psychiatry in the USA another 90 years to recognize the value of this primary–secondary construct. Spitzka introduced the term *coarse brain disease* to characterize behavioral syndromes secondary to what we now defined as neurologic disease, differing from "mental disorders" only in the coarseness or identifiableness of the brain pathology. Among his rich descriptions and classification substantially ahead of his contemporaries, he recognized mania, melancholia, catatonia, benign stupor, delirium, a dementing process of late life suggestive of Alzheimer's disease, and "senile dementia", occurring shortly after the "involutional period", and likely frontal–temporal dementia. He described developmental disorders, hysterical insanity, a periodic insanity, and monomania (paranoia or present-day delusional disorder). His demographic and epidemiologic conclusions about the major psychiatric syndromes rival present-day understanding. Spitzka concluded, however, that while the ultimate understanding of the truth of psychiatric disease would derive from scientific inquiry, that goal was generations removed.

The emergence of present-day nosology (a compromise between splitting and lumping)

Karl Ludwig Kahlbaum's influence on psychiatric classification was underappreciated during his lifetime, and it remains so. He was never offered a professorship in a medical school.

Because the search for etiology of psychosis had been unproductive, Kahlbaum became a splitter. He rejected the unitary model and re-focused his attention to the delineation of syndromes. His 1863 textbook on classification was the first attempt to systematically organize mental disorders by their symptom patterns and course of illness rather than from some preconceived notion.[76]

Kahlbaum recognized an idiopathic, progressively deteriorating condition affecting all aspects of psychic life, an idea adopted by Kraepelin's for his concept of dementia praecox. Kahlbaum also defined idiopathic post-pubescent, circumscribed illnesses affecting *emotion*, today's mood disorders.[77] His disorders of *intellect* (e.g. paranoia, dementia paranoides) are today's delusional disorder. His disorders of *will* are exemplified by catatonia. Kraepelin adopted these formulations that became the foundation for early DSM and ICD iterations.[78] Neither Kahlbaum nor Kraepelin, however, was interested in the neuroses.

Kahlbaum's 1874 monograph on catatonia, or "tension insanity",[79] was a milestone in the evolution of psychiatric classification. With his pupil Ewald Hecker who delineated hebephrenia, Kahlbaum applied for the first time Sydenham's principles for establishing the diagnostic validity of disorders of unknown etiology to psychiatric syndromes. We strive to use these principles in present classification efforts.[80] Kahlbaum presented catatonia's distinctive clinical features and course along with autopsy findings of many of his patients as validation for catatonia being a distinct disease.[81] Hecker did the same for hebephrenia.[82]

Emil Kraepelin's early thinking was that of a splitter. He adopted Kahlbaum's classification system and most importantly the idea that insanity was not unitary but contained specific diseases. He wrote:

I got the starting point of the line of thought which in 1896 led to dementia praecox being regarded as a distinct disease, on the one hand from the overpowering impression of the states of dementia quite similar to each other which developed from the most varied initial clinical symptoms, on the other hand from the experience connected with the observations of Hecker that these peculiar dementias seemed to stand in near relation to the period of youth.[83]

He also wrote:

I kept Kahlbaum's and Hecker's ideas in mind and tried to collect those cases, which inclined towards dementia as "mental degeneration processes". Apart from Kahlbaum's catatonia, I differentiated between dementia praecox, which essentially corresponded with hebephrenia, and dementia paranoides with hallucinations, which quickly developed into mental deficiency.[84]

Kraepelin was trained in experimental psychology in Wilhelm Wundt's laboratory in Leipzig and was influenced by the prevailing idea of that era that the mind consisted of three domains: will, thinking, and emotion.[85] His initial formulation of dementia praecox was that of a disease that affected all three mental spheres. In later writing, he defined manic depression as a disease that primarily affected emotion. In his search for common themes in classification, the cross-sectional domains of the mind and the longitudinal illness course, Kraepelin became a lumper.

The effort began at Heidelberg University where he "first aimed at classifying the clinical pictures, which seemed to form connecting links between the acute affective mental disorders and the chronic course of insanity and put them into independent groups."[86]

Kraepelin's lectures,[87] which were organized around live patient presentations, show that his identification of dementia praecox relied heavily on the presence of catatonia. Some of his diagnosed dementia praecox patients would likely be considered manic-depressive by many modern clinicians.

In presenting a 25-year-old merchant who has been diagnosed with dementia praecox, Kraepelin instructs his students:

[He] ... had made himself conspicuous by putting leaves and ferns into his buttonhole. He takes a seat with a certain amount of ceremony, and gives positive, concise, and generally relevant answers ... he admits ... that he did not speak for some time ... he remembers most of the details of what he has been through ... he gradually becomes rather excited, grows rude, irritable, and threatening, and breaks out into an incoherent flood of words, in which there is a quite senseless play on syllables ... the patient intimates that he is the German Emperor and that the Grand Duke is his father-in-law ... He declines to obey orders ... he breaks off in his talk, and he intersperses it with curious snorting noises. His mood is changeable, but on the whole very much exalted. Often, more especially when he makes his jesting play on words, the patient bursts into a tittering laugh. His behavior shows no marked excitement. His deportment is pompous and affected. The diagnosis will have to rest principally on the peculiar aberrations in the patient's actions – the mannerisms, the play on words, the signs of negativism, and also on his emotional indifference. (Kraepelin (1904/1968), pp. 151–2)

And yet another patient was presented as suffering from dementia praecox or what was to become schizophrenia:

The patient was originally supposed to be suffering from maniacal-depressive insanity. His previous history and the alteration of excited and depressed moods seemed greatly to favor this view. But in further course of the case Katatonic symptoms came out prominently during both the stuporose and the excited periods. (Kraepelin (1904/1968), p. 153)

Without catatonia, Kraepelin's delineation of dementia praecox was tenuous. He later wrote:

I was forced to realize that in a frighteningly large number of patients, who at first seemed to have the syndrome of mania, melancholia, insanity, amentia or madness, the syndrome changed fairly quickly into a typical progressive dementia and in spite of some differences, the syndromes became increasingly similar. I soon realized that the abnormalities at the beginning of the disease had no decisive importance compared to the course of the illness. (Kraepelin (1987), pp. 60–1)

Catatonia became the face of dementia praecox. Kraepelin considered any patient with sufficient catatonic features to likely have dementia praecox. If the patient also had reduced emotional expression (emotional blunting) or characteristic aberrations in spoken language (formal thought disorder) he considered the diagnosis assured.

Special importance in the establishing of dementia praecox has, not without justification, been attributed to the demonstration of the so-called "catatonic" morbid symptoms.[88]

Hebephrenia, with its early onset and dementing picture, became the model for the longitudinal pattern of dementia praecox. But validity of dementia praecox rested on the validity of catatonia and hebephrenia and the value in linking them as a single disease with a deteriorating course. Present-day classifications follow Kraepelin's error.

Kraepelin added Kahlbaum's dementia paranoides with its onset later in life to the dementia praecox grouping, further complicating the construct of an early onset disease affecting emotion, intellect, and will that progressively worsened to dementia. He also recognized that some patients with dementia praecox recovered.[89]

While separating manic-depression from dementia praecox, Kraepelin expanded the construct by adding Kahlbaum's dysthymia group (melancholia and mania) and the Falret/Baillarger circular insanity with their later illness onsets, recurring episodes, and more optimistic outcomes.[90]

By the end of his career, Kraepelin had lumped most of the dementias occurring before age 50 and all of the various forms of mania, melancholia and circular mood disorders into two "functional" psychoses, dementia praecox and manic-depressive insanity, respectively. This formulation has become the bedrock of the ICD and DSM. Its weak logic (all conditions with the same longitudinal course have similar etiology), and faulty construct (the effect of the illness on the tripartite mind determining grouping) still adversely affects present-day efforts to delineate psychiatric illness.

The splitters and lumpers in confusion

Eugen Bleuler combined observation with theory, roiling Kraepelin's more clearly stated but poorly formulated classification. Bleuler accepted Kraepelin's idea that dementia praecox affected the three areas of the mind, but theorized that these fundamental or primary deficits resulted in psychological processes that elicited the accessory or secondary features of illusions, hallucinations, and delusions. Influenced by Jungian theory, Bleuler envisioned the fundamental symptoms to be found in all patients with schizophrenia while accessory symptoms were less universal and more fluctuating. But while Kraepelin envisioned one disease, Bleuler recognized sufficient clinical variability to warrant the idea of several disorders, one of which represented the majority of such patients.[91]

Bleuler's (1976, pp. 372–87) primary symptoms for schizophrenia were:

1 *Disturbances in associations* (with examples that correspond to rambling speech or word salad, answers that do not explain, portmanteau words, derailment, dereistic ["loss of contact with reality"] thinking, "obstruction" or deprivation of thought).

2 *Loss of normal affectivity* (from indifference to one's surroundings, family and friends to temporary reduction of emotionality *or* "contraindication in the

interplay of the finer feelings", poor modulation of mood, rigidity of affect, parathymias and loss of emotional rapport).

3 *Ambivalence* (synchronous laughing and crying, expressions of love and hate for the same person, catatonic indecision and ambitendency).

Psychiatrists in the USA during the 1950s and 1960s separated dereistic thinking as a primary symptom, changed it to "autistic thinking" and offered the mnemonic for schizophrenia of "Bleuler's Four As": associational loosening, autism, affective flattening, and ambivalence. By the late 1960s, these easily over-interpreted notions resulted in almost all psychotic patients in the USA being seen as schizophrenic.

Bleuler's broad and easily misapplied primary features of dementia praecox guaranteed clinical heterogeneity. His patients developed illness throughout adult life and not just in late adolescence. Many did not progress to dementia. He offered the term schizophrenia to replace dementia praecox, highlighting what he considered the more specific splitting of psychological functions that he found in his patients.

Thus, the present-day formulation that there are two "big" psychotic disorders, schizophrenia and manic-depressive illness was established over 100 years ago. However, while manic-depression was recognized for millennia, schizophrenia was relatively new to classification. Like a house of cards, Bleuler accepted Kraepelin's basic incorrect construct of the tripartite mind while Kraepelin built his ideas upon Kahlbaum's distinct but invalid disease notion of catatonia. Bleuler greatly influenced psychiatry in the USA, while Kraepelin's influence remained mostly European.

Early-twentieth-century skeptics

Early-twentieth-century psychiatrists were reluctant to accept Kraepelin's formulations.[92] The notion of a unitary psychosis still prevailed in German-speaking countries. Alfred Hoche compared the new formulations to an "attempt to clarify a turbid liquid by pouring it from one receptacle to another".[93] Many psychiatrists were alarmed by the lack of validating support for the dementia praecox construct and the broadening of the traditional vision of manic-depression. The phenomenologist, Karl Jaspers wrote:

No real disease entity has been discovered by this method of approach. We have no scientific knowledge of any disease which satisfies the claims made for a disease-entity ... the two disease-groupings of manic-depressive psychosis and dementia praecox are almost completely unknown so far as their causes and cerebral pathology are concerned. Their definition depends rather on the basic psychological form or on the course run (towards recovery or not) with varying emphasis placed on the one or the other. Whereas one set of investigators [Bleuler] pushes the initial outbreak into the foreground and thus makes the dementia praecox group impossibly wide, the other set refutes this and would rather emphasizes the course of illness (recovery with insight or not) and narrows down the dementia praecox group considerably ... the border between manic-depressive insanity and dementia praecox has vacillated considerably in a kind of pendulum movement without anything new emerging. Moreover both groups are so impossibly extended that we have to consider them victims of the same fate that in the last century overtook all disease-entities of psychological origin.[94]

Jaspers illustrated Kraepelin's flawed logic that the same outcome among syndromes is proof that the syndromes represent the same disease process. He criticized the lack of scientific support for Kraepelin's classification and the use of illness course as the fundamental criterion for forcing patients into the two putative diagnostic categories. Jaspers would have considered the present-day effort to find "the genes" and "the characteristic endophenotype" of schizophrenia to be misguided, akin to searching for "the gene and pathophysiology" of mental retardation.

Kraepelin's reliance on catatonia as the foundation of dementia praecox was another weak link in his formulation as the relationship of catatonia to mania and melancholia was well-known.[95] George Kirby, the director of clinical psychiatry at Manhattan State Hospital on Wards Island in New York City, wrote:

I wish to offer a brief discussion of the catatonic symptom-complex and especially of its occurrence in individuals who have also manic-depressive attacks ... Kahlbaum ... did not view the prognosis in these cases as particularly bad, in fact he rather believed that the tendency was toward recovery ... Kraepelin admitted that the catatonic forms ran a somewhat different course from other forms of dementia praecox ... It cannot be doubted that very marked catatonic symptoms occur in conditions other than dementia praecox, even in clearly organic psychoses ... Upon investigating recently the outcome of a large series of manic-depressive and dementia praecox cases, we found that a good many cases had been wrongly judged to be deteriorating types because of the presence of catatonic symptoms ... We have also shown that marked catatonic syndromes may appear in otherwise typical manic-depressive cases. In some cases a catatonic attack apparently replaces the depression in a circular psychosis. In cases showing both manic and depressive phases the manic-depressive features have the greater prognostic significance. There is little doubt that Kraepelin over-valued catatonic manifestations as evidence of a deteriorating psychosis, and that many of these cases have served to unduly swell the dementia praecox group.[96]

The empirical evidence gathered throughout the twentieth century overwhelmingly supports Kirby's comments linking catatonia to mood disorder rather than to schizophrenia.[97] Nevertheless, psychiatric interests in the USA were distracted by psychoanalytic notions and influential writers paid little attention to the catatonia–mood disorder association. Rather than presenting catatonia as a separate diagnostic category, they followed Kraepelin and Bleuler and linked it to schizophrenia in the DSM. The error profoundly affected subsequent thinking and research leading to the consideration of all so-called psychotic features to be evidence of schizophrenia, guaranteeing sample heterogeneity.[98]

The decline of psychiatric diagnostic standards in the USA

The influence of psychoanalysis

The uncertainties of psychiatric classification in the USA mirrored those of Europe, but by 1880 seven diagnostic categories were recognized: mania, melancholia, monomania, general paresis, dementia, dipsomania (alcoholism), and epilepsy. The neuroses were considered distinct from the other brain disorders.

The interest of the psychiatric establishment in the USA in psychopathology and classification, however, was more proprietary than substantive. Psychiatric syndromes remained theorized expressions of "mental" or "psychological" perturbation.[99] As psychodynamic theory came to dominated American psychiatry, attention to the biological aspects of psychiatric illness diminished. So too did concerns about classification and descriptive psychiatry. The focus became the dynamic understanding of the individual not the search for which illness group the patient best fit. Amid great pessimism about the lack of any successful treatment for the psychiatrically ill, many psychiatrists gravitated to the psychoanalytic movement exacerbating the split from neurology.[100] Freud's metaphorical language was also anathema to descriptive psychopathologists who sought more precise terms. Within a generation of Freud's 1909 North American lectures, the psychoanalyst became the face of psychiatry in the USA.[101]

Adolf Meyer, a leading psychiatrist in the USA in the early third of the twentieth century, contributed further to the decline in interest in classification by opining that psychiatric disorders were individualized "reactions", outgrowths of a person's unique biology and experience, and that efforts at classification were beside the point.

Efforts to provide a meaningful classification languished, and it was not until 1917 that the American Medico-Psychological Association and the superintendents of mental hospitals in the USA agreed on a unifying system that in time was to become the DSM.[102] In 1921, the association changed its name to the American Psychiatric Association, and through the organizing of the New York Academy of Medicine, the nomenclature of the "superintendent's document" was incorporated into the American Medical Association's classification of disease in 1933.

After World War II, the US Army offered its modification to classification. The World Health Organization quickly followed with the sixth edition of its international classification of disease (ICD-6) that for the first time included mental disorders. The categories were: psychoses (including mood disorders), psychoneuroses, character disorders, behavior disorder, and deficits in "intelligence". DSM-I, published in 1952, was based on ICD-6.[103] Many leading psychoanalysts oversaw the drafting of the DSM-I and the document reflected Freudian and Meyerian views of mental illness with syndromes labeled "reactions" and defined by ego defense mechanisms. The DSM-II, published in 1968 was similarly influenced.[104]

New treatments reveal a weak relationship between diagnosis and response

The concepts of Freud, Meyer and their followers would not have been so widely accepted had there been a contemporary competing biological model of psychiatric illness or effective treatments for psychiatric disorders. Early twentieth-century neuroscience technologies and laboratory procedures were primitive and no somatic treatment was established. In his 1907 Presidential Address to the American Medico-Psychological Association, the beginnings of the American Psychiatric Association, C. G. Hill noted that "our therapeutics is simply a pile of rubbish".[105]

The introduction of malarial fevers to treat central nervous system syphilis and its associated behavioral syndromes (1917), and the application of insulin coma (1933), convulsive therapy (1934), and leucotomy (1935) to treat patients with psychotic and mood disorders, challenged the psychodynamic model.[106] The initial success of these treatments in quickly relieving the most severe psychiatric conditions, and the sustained success of electroconvulsive therapy (ECT; introduced in 1938) changed clinical psychiatric practice and once again directed attention to the brain as central to psychiatric disorders.[107] New typologies were envisioned as the basis for more effective prescription of the available treatments.[108]

The therapeutic optimism, however, was of short duration, as the diagnostic categories of DSM-II were quickly recognized as poor guides for choosing the newly introduced medications.[109] Many psychopharmacologists described their frustration with DSM-II criteria for the selection of treatments.[110] One influential report examined 33 studies that had assessed medication treatments of depression, but could not find a diagnostic formulation that had predictive strength.[111] The DSM-II and ICD-8 classifications also had poor reliability, dramatically demonstrated in international studies.[112]

World War II alters psychiatry in the USA and UK

In the 1930s many European psychiatrists fled the growing influence of Nazi Germany. Some came to Great Britain and continued the continental interest in psychopathology and classification. Mayer-Gross educated a generation of British psychiatrists to the importance of clinical research. He, Elliot Slater, and Martin Roth incorporated rigorous scholarship in psychopathology in their classic textbook (1969). Slater became the influential editor of the *British Journal of Psychiatry*. Psychiatrists in the USA turned to it for scientific discussions of psychopathology. In contrast, several well-known psychoanalysts (e.g. Franz Alexander, Sandor Rado, Otto Fenichel) fled to North America, buttressing the psychoanalytic grip on psychiatric thinking in the USA.[113] European psychiatrists experienced in convulsive therapy also immigrated to the USA (e.g. William Karliner, Lothar Kalinowsky), but while electroconvulsive therapy has become the longest continuously used somatic psychiatric treatment, its early champions had little influence on classification.[114]

The psychiatric establishment in the USA, typically practicing from a leisurely psychoanalytic model, was ill-prepared for the numbers and severity of the war's psychiatric military casualties. The War Department responded by quickly training several hundred general physicians, so-called "ninety-day wonders", to provide the needed care. Following the war, many of these physicians became the leaders of academic psychiatry in the USA. Their "on-the-job" training led to a practical clinical approach to treatment and the acceptance of a stress-induced model of psychiatric illness. The understanding of the underlying pathology of psychiatric syndromes, however, remained psychodynamic.[115] Until the late 1960s all chairs of academic departments of psychiatry in the USA were trained analysts, and psychiatric housestaff were encouraged to obtain analytic training and undergo a training analysis.[116] Almost all psychiatric teaching programs, the field's most prestigious organizations, and agencies accrediting psychiatric training and treatment facilities were controlled by psychoanalytic leaders intolerant of dissent.[117]

After the war, interest in psychopathology in the USA was limited to large, under-funded state-run facilities. These were discredited by their poor treatment of patients and through films such as *The Snake Pit* that purported to show the "true" experiences of sufferers. The image of electroconvulsive therapy being administered in a dungeon-like setting to a tormented Olivia De Havilland became the poster for anti-psychiatry movements to the present.[118] The psychoanalyst and his couch was the image of legitimate psychiatric practice.[119]

The lack of interest and instruction in classification and psychopathology in the USA at that time is dramatically illustrated by Joseph Zinkin's experience in translating Bleuler's monograph, *Dementia Praecox or the Group of Schizophrenias*. In his preface, Zinkin writes:

It is one of the curiosities of psychiatric work in our time that one of the most valuable monographs in psychiatric literature [it was referred to in almost biblical terms as the definitive work on the clinical presentation of schizophrenia] has remained, for thirty years, untranslated from the original German. Although during this period practically every psychiatric bibliography made reference to Bleuler's monograph, often praising it as an outstanding work, very few psychiatrists, at least of my generation, had any personal knowledge of the Bleulerian text. Most, if not all, references to the Swiss work were second-hand; hence the frequent misunderstanding of what our author really had to say ... In asking many outstanding psychiatrists whether they would be interested in a translation of Bleuler's work, I almost invariably encountered the belief that it had long ago been translated. Everyone supposed that someone else had really read it.[120]

The interest in classification and diagnosis was weakened further by the social and community psychiatry movement. Emerging from the wedding of the psychoanalytic interpretation of behavior and the World War II experience, the guiding notion was that the psychological understanding of the individual could be applied to large populations explaining "the why" of societal problems that could then be addressed by community interventions. Psychiatric illness was deemed the result of societal forces acting adversely on the psyche, and not the result of individual brain diseases. Asylums were unlocked and voluntary admission was introduced in Great Britain. In the USA, patients in state hospital facilities were encouraged to return to "the community", but many ended up in city alleys and side streets. Community mental health centers, clinics and networks, and "therapeutic communities" sprang up in metropolitan areas across the USA with the implicit promise that public health concerns, poverty and other inequities would be resolved.[121] Recruitment of US medical students into psychiatry was never higher than during the peak of the community psychiatry movement in the 1960s, ebbing only with the ascendancy of biological psychiatry.[122]

Diagnostic confusion reigns

The Freudian and Meyerian rejection of grouping patients by their shared psychopathology, and the limited training in psychopathology of many academic leaders in psychiatry in the USA after World War II marginalized descriptive psychopathology.[123] Bleuler's reliance on his primary features to diagnose schizophrenia and the unavailability of his writing in English led to a decreased recognition of mood disorders and the over-diagnosis of schizophrenia.

It became obvious, however, that many patients diagnosed as schizophrenic recovered, belying the expected inevitable dementia or lack of full recovery. Efforts to separate "Good" from "Bad" prognosis schizophrenics followed. The former were characterized by preserved affect (good emotional expression and full volition), acute-onset episodes (less than 3 months from first inkling of illness to full severity), and episodes with intense emotion. "Bad" prognosis schizophrenics were characterized by emotional blunting.[124] Splitters and lumpers were once again struggling for a clear vision of psychiatric nosology.

The *schizo affective* construct combining schizophrenic and manic-depressive cross-sectional features, acute-onset episodes and a prognosis "intermediary" between dementia praecox and manic-depressive illness was offered by John Kasanin.[125] Research, however, indicated that much of the schizo affective category represented severe manic-depressive illness, not schizophrenia nor a third illness group.[126]

Gabriel Langfeldt proposed a *schizophreniform* disorder of "psychogenic origin" that was a "reaction" to stress and that presented with "schizophrenic" hallucinations and delusions and substantial affective features and had a good outcome.[127] The construct bears little resemblance to the DSM category other than having a better outcome than what is typically observed in schizophrenia. Langfeldt also proposed *reactive psychoses*, acute "psychogenic" psychoses emerging under stress with excellent prognosis. It was widely adopted in Scandinavia.[128] These syndromes were eventually conflated into the DSM category of *brief psychotic disorder*, but studies showed reactive psychosis to be early episodes of mood disorder.[129]

Karl Leonhard offered an even more elaborate formulation to account for the great variability in outcome among patients with psychosis. Leonhard's classification remains influential in German speaking countries. He is best known for his "cycloid psychoses" (anxiety–happiness, confusion, and motility types), characterized by periods of excitement and inhibition. They are reminiscent of Falret's *la folie circulaire*.[130]

Kurt Schneider introduced the term "first rank symptoms" and argued that these features were pathognomonic of poor prognosis, "true" schizophrenia when obvious neurologic disease was not present.[131] Schneider's influence was limited to German speaking countries until the early 1970s when he was re-introduced to psychiatry in the UK by Mellor and then in the USA by Taylor.[132] Subsequent studies, however, demonstrated their occurrence in mania and melancholia, as well as in schizophrenia, and that they were not decisive distinguishing features of the psychoses. Nevertheless, they form the basis of criterion A for schizophrenia in the present DSM and are treated as if pathognomonic.[133]

By the 1960s academic psychiatry in the USA had virtually abandoned the idea of manic-depressive illness. Almost every patient who experienced hallucinations, delusions, or catatonic features was considered schizophrenic. In one teaching hospital in New York City, no acutely admitted patient received the diagnosis of mania during the mid to late 1960s, and only a handful were recognized as having depressive illness. Influential professors opined that they had "not seen a manic in decades" and that it was likely that "mania never really existed, only agitated schizophrenia".[134] Several years later at the institution that rejected manic-depressive illness, a systematic series of studies using reliable research diagnostic criteria and external validating variables demonstrated that almost 30% of admissions (many the same patients from the era of "no mania") had acute mania and that many responded to lithium monotherapy.[135] Nearly 50% of patients diagnosed as schizophrenic were found to be misdiagnosed and to in fact have manic-depressive illness. However, it was not until after 1970 when lithium carbonate became widely available and marketed as a mood stabilizer did psychiatrists in the USA re-consider the existence of manic depression.[136]

The failure to recognize mania and severe depression became untenable following the publication of cross-national studies that compared diagnostic practice in the USA and Europe. Psychiatrists in the USA failed to recognize mania, psychotic depression, and personality disorder, commonly interpreting such conditions as schizophrenia.[137] One irony is the first reported psychiatric patient successfully treated with chlorpromazine in 1952. The 57-year-old man diagnosed as schizophrenic, was hospitalized for "making improvised political speeches in cafés, becoming involved in fights with strangers", and for several days "walking around the street with a pot of flowers on his head preaching his love of liberty".[138] Many clinicians today would recognize him as manic. Had the most famous anti-schizophrenia medication been first given to chronically ill psychotic patients rather than to a handful of treatment-responsive manics, the pharmacotherapy era might have been substantially delayed.[139]

Biometricians formulate classification: the triumph of the splitters

In response to the inadequate classifications, alternative operationally defined diagnostic criteria were proposed.[140] Their success encouraged the American Psychiatric Association (APA) to reformulate the DSM in the late 1970s.[141] The effort joined the departments of psychiatry at the Washington University in St Louis and at Columbia University's Psychiatric Institute. The former offered the Feighner criteria as a model of a few syndromes with reasonable validation. The latter, under the direction of the biometrics division of the institute offered a system that was centered on the computer-based diagnostic program, DIAGNO, and its related assessment instrument the SADS. The latter's overly simplified approach to psychopathology prevailed and defined the format of the DSM-III.[142]

The DSM-III proposal quickly became a political document fashioned to appeal to the widest audience to insure approval by the APA membership. Lacking a consensus theory of psychiatric illness, the formulation of the DSM categories was left to consensus among the members of each committee. Different committees relied on different sources, idiosyncratic personal clinical experiences, and different psychological and pharmacologic notions. For some disorders, a Kraepelinian template can be recognized (e.g. the schizophrenia criteria); for others a psychological formulation is apparent (e.g. dissociative disorders). The committees also represented diverse constituencies, and the final proposal was designed for accepted by advocacy groups (e.g. psychoanalytic and psychosomatic organizations), and the "typical" psychiatric clinician to assure passage by the APA membership's "up or down" vote on the proposed manual.[143] Dissatisfaction with the unscientific but democratically approved classification called for revisions in 1987 (DSM-III-R), 1994 (DSM-IV) and 2000 (DSM-IV-TR).[144] Another iteration is expected in 2010.

Major changes in DSM-III

DSM-III incorporated major changes in classification that are preserved in subsequent versions. It rejected short descriptive paragraphs (still the hallmark of ICD-10) for short lists of over-simplified diagnostic criteria to achieve better reliability. Neurosis and its historically sexist connection to hysteria and the uterus was eliminated, gaining support of APA feminist voters. Although many of the traditional neurotic disorders (e.g. anxiety disorders) were shown to be associated with abnormal brain functional imaging, electroencephalography, evoked potential and other laboratory measures, these findings were not incorporated into classification. Seeking not to offend psychoanalytically disposed members interested in "psychosomatic" disorders while not rejecting the biological evidence the DSM drafters presented the anxiety disorders without comment as to etiology, while other conditions were linked to psychological factors (e.g. posttraumatic stress disorder, conversion disorder, depersonalization, fugue). The old group of neuroses was separated into 9 classes and 78 diagnostic options, insuring a marketing niche for any influential membership group interested in neurotic conditions. The non-theoretical Briquet's syndrome, advocated by researchers at the Washington University School of Medicine in St Louis, was rejected for somatization disorder, a term used in the psychoanalytic literature.[145]

The *personality disorders* section was revised to follow the work of Mellon, dividing conditions into three categorical classes of different presumed severity. The extensive research indicating that personality traits are dimensional was ignored.[146]

The "organic disorder" category was replaced by a primary/secondary and then a "secondary to ..." scheme, giving recognition to modern neuroscience and the understanding that all behavioral syndromes derive from brain activities and all are therefore "organic".

The *psychotic disorder* category was changed. Delusional disorder was added as a separate condition, separating it once again after 100 years from the dementia praecox/schizophrenia syndrome. The duration-dependent brief/schizophreniform/schizophrenia notion was defined despite inadequate supporting evidence.

The well-documented *melancholia* concept was ignored,[147] but many depression choices were added despite little or no validation. By 1980, four major mood disorders were identified with 10 subtypes. For major depression, an additional three subtypes were listed with major and minor depressions given prominence despite poor validity. Manic-depressive illness was eliminated, replaced with unipolar and bipolar categories.[148] The bipolar/unipolar construct was immediately challenged, but without success.[149]

Other aspects of the new classification and its specific criteria were also challenged by clinicians who could not fit their patients within the defined categories. In response, new diagnostic classes were included in the 1987 revision (DSM-III-R) and again in the 1994 iteration (DSM-IV).[150] The number of recognized diagnostic entities dramatically increased (e.g. atypical, seasonal and postpartum depression).[151]

Conclusions

The history of psychiatric classification exemplifies the hackneyed comment "Two steps forward, one step back": a period of detailed and accurate observation followed by a period of distorted or forgotten ideas overwhelmed by theorizing and dogma. Hippocrates, Galen, Haslam, Kahlbaum, Hammond and Kirby on the one hand, the humoral theory, and religious and psychoanalytic dogma on the other. Throughout these cycles there have been tensions between the splitters and lumpers, shaping and reshaping classification.

The corrections in the nosology, regardless of which school of thought was dominant, evoke the aphorism: "The cure is worse than the disease." Most recently, the development of DSM-III was eagerly anticipated to replace an arbitrary and patently unvalidated system with an empirically derived classification providing "a common language" for the field. The resulting classification, however, has swollen into hundreds of categories and subcategories identified by simplistic lists of a few poorly defined signs and symptoms that encourage false positive and negative diagnostic conclusions. The splitters are now clearly dominant. The DSM-V iteration planned for the years 2007–10 is not expected to differ substantially, although there is some effort to organize the nosology to be more consistent with our present understanding of neuroscience.[152] Whether the neurosciences will offer sufficient data to define a more useful classification is unpredictable.

NOTES

1 Livy or Titus Livius lived in the first century BCE and wrote a history of Rome *Ab Urbe Condita* (*From the Founding of the City*) still used in studies of that period.

2 Hunter and Macalpine (1963), page ix.

3 Thompson (1987), pages 1–2.

4 Historians with a world view prefer the term "common era" or CE and "before the common era" or BCE to the Christian focused AD and BC.

5 Berrios (1999); Craddock *et al.* (2006).

6 There are other medical traditions. Ancient and recent Hindu medical tradition is voluminous, developing independently from the Greek, although reaching many similar conclusions. Older writings understood psychiatric disorders from a metaphysical perspective (Zilboorg, 1967, pp. 30–1). Arabian medicine offered familiar descriptions of several psychiatric syndromes. Avicenna (980–1037 CE) described melancholia in great detail (Zilboorg, 1967, pp. 121–7). However, because Western thoughts about medical illness and its treatments have come to dominate present thinking, the evolution of the classification of psychiatric disease is presented from that perspective.

7 Moss (1967).

8 Deuteronomy 28:28 and John 10:20, respectively.

9 Zilboorg (1967), pages 36–92.

10 Barrough (1583).

11 Moss (1967); Clarke (1975); medicine in India in the first millennium CE was also based on a theory of body humors in imbalance (Clarke 1975, p. 22).

12 Flexner (1969), pages 456–63.

13 Zilboorg (1967), pages 36–174.

14 Clarke (1975), pages 31–8.

15 Ibid., pages 41–5.

16 Neugebauer (1979).

17 Zilboorg (1967), pages 342–7; Eddy had some form of paraplegia that resolved following treatment by hypnosis (Pichot 1983, p. 61).

18 Zilboorg (1967), page 123.

19 Zilboorg (1967), page 200.

20 Scull (1981), pages 274–7.

21 James Baird, a British writer, is credited with re-introducing the term hysteria (Pichot, 1983, p. 61).

22 Shorter (1997), pages 84–6.

23 Zilboorg (1967), pages 363–78; Pichot (1983), pages 66–8.

24 Janet (1901).

25 Janet (1907).

26 Zilboorg (1967), pages 356–8; Freud also worked with Breuer.

27 Shorter (1997), pages 138–40; also see discussion in Chapter 14 on normal personality.

28 Zilboorg (1967), page 47; the uterus was considered to be untethered and when it moved upward toward the chest abdominal and respiratory symptoms emerged.

29 Zilboorg (1967), page 92.

30 Zilboorg (1967), pages 110, 130–3.

31 Bromberg (1930).

32 Cheyette and Cummings (1995).

33 Zilboorg (1967), page 260.

34 Hunter and Macalpine (1963), pages 68–75; Jorden (1603).

35 Hunter and Macalpine (1963), pages 187–90. Willis attributed mental illness to heredity, parents who were too young or too old, drunkenness, traumatic brain injury, epilepsy, stroke, and sudden fearfulness (Cranefield, 1961).

36 Hunter and Macalpine 1963, pages 221–4.

37 Hunter and Macalpine (1963), pages 389–92.

38 Whytt (1751), cited by Trimble (2004), page 3.

39 Cheyne (1733).

40 Hunter and Macalpine (1963), pages 473–9.

41 Griesinger (1862).

42 Pichot (1983), page 61.

43 Briquet (1859).

44 The delivery of low-voltage current to the head to relieve "nervous tension" was an established nineteenth-century medical practice.

45 Shorter (1997), pages 129–30. Until the recent inventions of the DSM, Beard's neurasthenia was the only contribution to psychiatric classification from the USA. Phrenology dominated medical school thinking in nineteenth-century USA. Benjamin Rush endorsed the humoral theory of illness and in 1812 wrote *Medical Inquires and Observations upon the Diseases of the Mind*. Although given the title "father of American psychiatry", Dorothea Dix and her efforts to improve the conditions of the psychiatrically ill had greater impact than Rush, and better deserves the title "Mother of American psychiatry" (Mora, 1992).

46 Ross (1941).

47 Erichsen (1882).

48 Kardiner and Spiegel (1941); Ross (1941).

49 Robinson *et al.* (1973).

50 Pitts and McClure (1967).

51 Several chapters present discussions of the problems with these designations (e.g. Chapter 6 on dissociations, Chapter 7 on conversion).

52 Burton (1621).

53 Beer (1996).

54 Feuchtersleben (1845) cited in Shorter (2005), page 65.

55 Zilboorg (1967), pages 245–341.

56 The "nickname" for the Bethlem Hospital for the "pauper lunatics" was "*bedlam*". The word remains in the English language to mean a great, uncontrolled uproar.

57 Haslam (1798).

58 Hammond (1883/1973), page 557.

59 Although an important reformer of the treatment of the mentally ill, Pinel was not unique in that effort and did not contribute to our understanding of psychiatric classification. In the UK, John Connolly and Robert Gardiner Hill temporarily reformed asylums in the mid-nineteenth century (Thompson, 1987, pp. 7–14). Vincenzio Chiarugi, an eighteenth-century Florentine physician, wrote the first treatise on the treatment of patients in asylums (Shorter, 1997, p. 10).

60 Zilboorg (1967), pages 390–1.

61 Esquirol (1838).

62 Falret (1854); Baillarger (1853); also see the translated paper by Sedler and Dessain (1983).

63 Shorter (1997), pages 31–2.

64 Cited by Zilboorg (1967), page 436.

65 Shorter (1997), pages 73–6.

66 Neumann (1859), page 167.

67 Maudsley (1867).

68 Pichot (1983), pages 17–20.

69 Thompson (1987) essay by E.H. Hare, pages 53–8.

70 Lanczik and Keil (1991).

71 Ibid.

72 Ibid.

73 Ibid.

74 Kleist (1914).

75 Spitzka (1887/1973).

76 Kahlbaum (1863).

77 Melancholia was placed in this category, but Kahlbaum used the term dysthymia for it. He also introduced the concept of cyclothymia as a low-grade form of manic-depressive illness.

78 Kraepelin (1913, 1971).

79 Kahlbaum used the term *Spannungsirresein*.

80 Robins and Guze (1970).

81 Kahlbaum (1874/1973); Kahlbaum's autopsy material indicates a variety of pathophysiologic processes consistent with the modern understanding that catatonia is a syndrome elicited by many conditions.

82 Hecker (1871); also see Sedler and Schoelly (1985).

83 Kraepelin (1971), pages 3–4.

84 Kraepelin (1987), page 59; also see Berrios and Hauser (1988) for a discussion of Kraepelin's early ideas on classification and disease. Kraepelin's progression in thinking is also seen in successive iterations of his textbook. The fifth edition (1896) presented the formulation of the two major disease entities defined by course as well as acute presentation. The fully defined manic-depressive insanity appeared in the sixth edition (1899). The ninth edition (1927) was over six times the length of the first.

85 Kraepelin (1987); DSM-IV diagnostic criteria for schizophrenia[85] retain the Kraepelinian imprint. *Criterion A* for schizophrenia requires the presence of 2 or more of 5 features. Delusions (item 1) and disorganized speech (item 3) represent Kraepelin's understanding of a defect in thinking. Negative symptoms (item 5) represent the defect in emotion. Catatonic behavior (item 4) represents the defect in will. Grossly disorganized behavior (part of item 4) reflects the socially inappropriate behaviors and inadequate self-care and self-control observed in many chronically ill psychiatric patients and are also consistent with Kraepelin's understanding of a defect in will. The examples of hallucinations in *criterion A* (item 2), however, do not readily fit Kraepelin's algorithm, as neither he nor Bleuler considered these phenomena fundamental to the illness, i.e. pathognomonic.

Consistent with Kraepelin's original formulation, the course of DSM schizophrenia is said to be prolonged (>6months), eliciting some permanent loss of function. Also see Shorter (1997), pages 100–9.

86 Kraepelin (1987), page 59.

87 Kraepelin (1968).

88 Kraepelin (1971), page 257.

89 Kraepelin (1971), page 4.

90 Kraepelin (1896).

91 Bleuler (1976), page 54.

92 Shorter (1997), pages 108–9.

93 Cited in Pichot (1983), page 74.

94 Jaspers (1963), page 567; Jaspers wrote the first edition of this seminal work bringing the principles of phenomenology to the field of psychopathology in 1913, when he was 30 years old. Like many German psychiatrists, he fled the Nazis in 1937 and settled in Switzerland.

95 Burrows (1976, pp. 184–6) described in 1828 a 22-year-old woman on her honeymoon who develops mania with catatonic features; it would be another 46 years until Kahlbaum delineated catatonia.

96 Kirby (1913).

97 Fink and Taylor (2003).

98 Taylor (1999), pages 271–5.

99 Freud (1984); Abraham (1927).

100 Scull (1981), pages 5–32.

101 Shorter (1997), pages 162–3; also see note 61. *The New Yorker* magazine's famous cartoons illustrate the dominance of the psychoanalyst. Throughout its existence every *New Yorker* cartoon about psychiatry depicts a psychoanalyst. The image of a man (always) in a comfortable chair, legs crossed, pad and pencil in hand and a woman patient (almost always) on the Freudian couch brings immediate recognition to the viewer (Mankoff, 2004).

102 American Medico-Psychological Association and the National Committee for Mental Hygiene, *Statistical Manual for Use of Institutions for the Insane*, New York (1918).

103 APA (1952).

104 American Psychiatric Association (1952). The formulation was modified in 1968 as the DSM-II.

105 Hill (1907).

106 As a counter to the success of ECT in relieving depressive illness, psychoanalysts theorized that the therapeutic effect was the result of the patient perceiving the treatment as punishment and thus an atonement for their delusional guilt (MAT, personal training experience).

107 Braslow (1997); Lothar Kalinowsky, an émigré from Germany via Italy, introduced ECT into the USA in 1940 (Shorter, 1997, p. 221).

108 See Taylor and Fink (2006) for a discussion of the forms of depressive illness proposed to respond to different treatments.

109 Klein (1989).

110 Healy (2002); Ban *et al.* (2002).

111 Nelson and Charney (1981).

112 Sandifer *et al.* (1969); Spitzer and Fleiss (1974).

113 Shorter (1997), pages 166–9.

114 See Shorter and Healy (2007) for a detailed narrative of the history of convulsive therapies.

115 Grob (1991); training in neuropsychiatry lasted 4 months.

116 Paula Clayton was the first appointed woman chair of a USA department of psychiatry (Minnesota in 1972). The number of women chairs has not substantially increased over the ensuing three decades despite the fact that more than 50% of the entering medical school classes in recent years in the USA have been women. Presently there are 10 (Atre Vaidya, 2006, personal knowledge as one of the 10).

117 Shorter (1997), pages 172–82; the influence remains in subtle form. All psychiatric residency training programs must still teach intensive, psychodynamic psychotherapy to remain accredited. Board certification examinations in psychiatry still require a working knowledge of psychodynamic theory and practice. In contrast, the prescription and use of ECT is almost never examined and no residency program has ever been challenged for not training its residents in the use of ECT.

118 Released in 1949 by 20th Century Fox.

119 These images remain to the present despite the fact that only about 5% or so of psychiatrists in the USA engage in a traditional psychoanalytic practice. Television's Tony Soprano sees an analyst for his panic disorder despite the fact that few present-day psychiatrists consider the condition psychological. Troubled young film heroes turn to Robin Williams or Judd Hirsch for relief, not to a character more typical of the modern medical practitioner.

  The French tradition illustrated by the writings of Henry Ey and Georges Lanteri-Laura blended philosophy into their ideas about psychiatric illness and have had minimal influence on the development of classification (Garrabe, 2005).

120 Zinkin's preface written in 1949 to the 1950 translation, Bleuler (1950).

121 Shorter (1997), pages 229–38.

122 Sierles and Taylor (1995).

123 Andreasen (2007).

124 Taylor and Abrams (1975b).

125 Kasanin (1933).

126 Taylor (1984, 1986).

127 Langfeldt (1939).

128 Stromgren (1974).

129 McCabe (1975).

130 Leonhard (1979).

131 Schneider (1959).

132 Taylor (1972).

133 The DSM permits the presence of hearing voices or one "bizarre" delusion defined in Schneider's terms as sufficient to warrant the diagnosis of schizophrenia. For studies demonstrating the prognostic implications of first rank symptoms see Taylor (1972); Taylor and Abrams (1973); Abrams and Taylor (1973, 1981).

134 This idea was taught to MAT as part of the residency program that produced the first edition of what was to become the standard "comprehensive" psychiatric textbook of Kaplan and Sadock.

135 Abrams and Taylor (1976a, 1981); Taylor and Abrams (1973); Abrams *et al.* (1974).

136 Baldessarini (1970).

137 Sandifer *et al.* (1969); Spitzer and Fleiss (1974); Gurland *et al.* (1969).

138 Delay *et al.* (1952).

139 Most patients of that era with the diagnosis of "acute" or "paranoid" schizophrenia were found to be manic-depressive and responsive to lithium or ECT as well as to some antipsychotic medications (Taylor *et al.*, 1974, 1975; Abrams *et al.*, 1974).

140 Feighner *et al.* (1972); Taylor and Abrams (1975a, 1978); Overall and Hollister (1979); Spitzer *et al.* (1980).

141 American Psychiatric Association (1980); DSM-III lists 265 disorders. The number is increased in DSM-IIIR (1987) to 292 and in DSM-IV (1994) as 295.

142 Spitzer and Endicott (1968); Feighner *et al.* (1972); Endicott and Spitzer (1978).

143 The vote was taken by its membership prior to the May 1979 annual meeting. As with many bills enacted in the US congress, few of the voters had read the proposal in detail.

Some writers continue to call for even greater diversity in the process of formulating the next DSM by including patients and their families on the drafting committees (Sadler and Fulford, 2004).

144 A planned revision of DSM-V is in progress.

145 Lipowski (1987).

146 Chapters 14 and 15 provide discussions of Axis II and the alternative dimensional approach to the understanding of personality.

147 See Taylor and Fink (2006) for a detailed discussion of melancholia, its history and pathophysiology, and its significance for the classification and treatment of patients with mood disorders.

148 Taylor and Fink (2006), chapter 1; proposed varieties of bipolar disorder are I, II, III, and IV (Akiskal and Pinto, 1999).

149 Chapter 16 provides a discussion of the mood disorder dichotomy.

150 APA (1994).

151 *Double depression* is the overlapping of two depression categories in the RDC, a major depressive disorder superimposed on an underlying chronic depression, or dysthymic disorder.

Seasonal affective disorder (SAD; Benazzi and Rihmer, 2000) was postulated as a depressive mood disorder that routinely worsened in the winter months. Treatment with bright light was proposed. The concept was incorporated in DSM-III-R in 1987 as a "specifier" for major depression and for bipolar disorder defined as "a regular cyclic relationship between onset of the mood episodes and a particular 60-day period of the year", especially the time from early October to late November. It is retained in DSM-IV.

Recurrent, brief depression refers to recurrent bouts of depression too brief to qualify as "major depression" or "dysthymia" in DSM terminology (Angst, 1997).

152 Kupfer *et al.* (2002); Helzer and Hudziak (2002).

3

The brain and psychopathology

The reader will find no other definition of "Psychiatry" in this book but the one given on the title-page: "Clinical Treatise on Diseases of the Fore-Brain". The historical term psychiatry, i.e. "treatment of the soul", implies more than we can accomplish, and transcends the bounds of accurate scientific investigation.[1]

The understanding that behavioral disturbances reflect biological events has growing acceptance. Theorists who place intervening constructs between the biology and behavior also recognize that at some level the brain generates behavior. Trained as a neuropathologist, Freud assumed his framework for the psyche had neurologic roots.[2] In discussing hysteria, he wrote: "A dynamic lesion is indeed a lesion [in the brain] but one of which no trace is found after death such as an edema, an anemia or an active hyperemia."[3]

The relationship between the brain and psychiatric illness, however, has been clinically marginalized, as the summing of a few clinical features now substitutes for diagnostic reasoning. This chapter provides an alternative framework to that approach, illustrating that the understanding of brain–behavior relationships is relevant to patient care.

The boundaries between normalcy and disease

Brain–behavior relationships define behavioral wellness as well as disease, and the boundary between behavioral wellness and disease is not always clear. Present classification deals with the ambiguities by arbitrarily separating behavioral disease (e.g. the DSM Axis I) from behavioral deviation (e.g. Axis II). The separation is not successful. Schizotypal, schizoid, and paranoid personality disorders, for example, reflect low-grade illness, not personality deviations.[4] Obsessive–compulsive personality disorder is also not trait behavior, but part of the obsessive–compulsive disorder spectrum.

Some have also argued that the exclusive focus on brain–behavior relationships as the basis for understanding psychiatric syndromes is unwarranted. The analogy is the computer and the fact that all software must run on hardware, and that glitches in software occur without hardware malfunction.[5] The analogy fails, however, because brain "programs" are as much neurological as are brain structures. Procedural memory (i.e. memory for motor, often skilled behaviors) is brain-based and understanding this is clinically relevant. There are many more sequences of movement than there are motor neuron pyramidal cells. Patient 1.1, who suffered carbon monoxide poisoning and lost his ability to knit, experienced a biological event to his brain that affected his skilled motor programming. Anesthetic agents produce temporary malfunction of brain programming without affecting the "hardware".

But while all behavior reflects the brain at work, behavioral disorders are more difficult to define. The DSM conceptualizes a "disorder" as a condition that is clinically significant and that causes distress or disability.[6] This definition fails because it is over-inclusive, incorporating as disorders non-illness such as demoralization, jealousy and revenge, and criminality. By the definition, normal pregnancy might be considered a disorder. Others have argued that a more precise definition of illness is: a condition that causes harm and that derives from dysfunction. Harmful dysfunction involves "something going wrong with the functioning of some internal mechanism, so that the mechanism is not performing one of the functions for which it was 'designed' by natural selection."[7] This conceptualization works for most presently recognized psychiatric disorders, but may fall short for some of the personality disorders.[8]

Confusion also arises from the fact that persons who appropriately receive classification labels are by definition deviant, but deviance has several fathers. Brain structural and physiological lesions (genetic and acquired), maturational variation, and indoctrination at odds with the cultural context cause deviation. Further roiling the conceptual waters is the fact that some deviation is advantageous (e.g. high intelligence, talent).

The social, political and health implications of these concerns have been discussed in depth elsewhere, and they impact patient care daily.[9] Descriptive psychopathology, however, focuses mostly on deviant behaviors assumed the result of brain dysfunction. It also addresses deviation of personality as a function of maturational variation.[10]

The brain behind the mental status

All behavior, no matter how complex, is an expression of the brain working. "The mind" cannot be separated from the body. Within a modern cognitive neuroscience framework, the mind becomes representative short-hand for brain processes within our awareness. Brain activity outside of subjective experience (e.g. maintaining blood pressure, posture) is recognized as neurologic. Memory, internal imagery, emotion, and thinking are subjectively experienced and are categorized as "mental", but they are no less neurologic than the homeostatic functions of the human nervous system.

For example, personal (biographic) memories, learned information, and skills are experienced as mental activity and in the early stages of dementias such as Alzheimer's disease sufferers characterize the loss of these memories as "losing their minds". What is experienced, however, is the effects of the degeneration of the neurologic structures subserving memory.[11]

Subjective experience is also engaged with visual imagery of things learned and experienced, and then recalled. The images are stored in long-term memory and are retrieved to create a short-term image that is useful in many cognitive activities (e.g. object and facial recognition, carpentry).[12] Retrieving the images is associated with left frontal region activation.[13]

Some images are generic (e.g. the image of a table, clock, and bicycle). These "Gestaltic" images are subserved by right hemisphere pathways. Cognitive assessment of right hemisphere functioning relies on testing the patient's ability to draw general images from memory (e.g. the face of a clock with the hands at 2:45). Other images are specific (e.g. the dining room table in your house, the clock on the living room mantle, your mountain bike). The generation of these images is associated with frontal activation, specifically in the anterior cingulate gyrus. This imagery is assessed when asking patients to describe their possessions and biographical-related environment.[14]

Subjective experience of emotional life is another hallmark of "the mind". Damasio (1999) suggests awareness of experiencing an emotion in response to external events, and the recognition that the emotion is internally generated, transient, and has been experienced before and will likely be experienced again forms the beginnings of conscious awareness of self. Nothing in human experience is more personalized than this recognition of being an independent living entity with a past and a future. Such experience, however, is fundamentally neurologic, and when the neurology subserving emotion is diseased, many psychiatric and neurologic conditions emerge. Even socially learned emotional responses reflect specific neurologic activity.[15] Although disgust is a universal human experience, what is disgusting varies widely within and across cultures. Almost stepping on a juicy beetle waddling across one's path might be disgusting to a Western professional rushing to work, but it is a lip-smacking, nourishing snack to a hunter-gatherer deep in a rain forest.

Laughter and humor also reflect emotional experience that seems characteristically human and "mental" in origin. But they are given high evolutionary importance by Darwin.[16] Laughter is a universal human behavior and one of the first social vocalizations of human infants, emerging between 2 and 6 months after birth. Congenitally deaf and blind infants laugh although never having perceived the laughter of others.[17] Despite substantial individual variability, laughter is a stereotypic, species-specific behavior. Its precursor is the "play-face" and pant-like vocalizations of apes in social play during their "safe times", and is considered an important evolutionary development in small hominid group cohesion. In humans, laughter and humor has been elaborated to support novel social functions, but it remains a brain-derived expression with reproductive (e.g. being emotionally attractive) and resource-gathering advantage (e.g. getting along with co-workers and superiors and in leadership strategies). The loss of the ability to laugh is always pathological.[18] Among patients with melancholia, regaining the ability to laugh (e.g. at the examiner's humor) is an important sign of the resolution of the depressive illness.

Cortical activities such as internal speech and verbal-based thinking are experienced as a significant part of mental life, but these thoughts are expressions of neurologic functioning. Internal speech is experienced throughout wakefulness as a running commentary on what has recently happened, what is happening, and what may happen. But the elements of internal speech are subserved by the same neurology as conversational speech. Functional imaging of normal persons to simple language-based tasks show different left cerebral hemisphere metabolic response patterns to each task. Hearing and speaking words as in conversational speech, generating words (ideas) as in "mental speech", and seeing words as in reading are all experienced as mental activity. But these functions and the brain areas subserving them are the same behavior–brain relationships associated with stroke and aphasia.[19]

The "mental status examination" is thus anachronistic. The behavioral and cognitive assessments incorporated in it do not characterize "the mind", but rather the brain, and the effort is best described as "the behavioral examination of the brain".

Brain disease and dysfunction as psychopathology

Although brain–behavior relationships are complex, broad relationships are understood and these are diagnostically helpful. A movement disorder will involve the motor system at some level, and more specific localization is likely with careful examination (e.g. basal ganglia versus cerebellar disease). A person with no speech or language disturbances but with misidentification delusions is more likely to have non-dominant than dominant cerebral hemisphere disease. Intense emotional expression, as in mood disorders, will be associated with amygdala activation.

Understanding established brain–behavior relationships strengthens the recognition of psychiatric illness when the pattern of psychopathology is ambiguous (e.g. avolitional frontal syndrome versus depressive illness; disinhibited frontal syndrome versus mania). The understanding helps identify neurologic disease when the disease's expression is mostly as psychopathology (e.g. psychosis due to strokes outside the motor system, many persons with partial complex seizures). For example, MacDonald Critchley's monograph (1953) on the parietal lobes describes patients hospitalized with recognized strokes in their right (non-dominant) parietal lobe. Many of these patients also exhibited classic psychopathology.

A woman said:

"I had a terrible shock this morning when I touched my left hand; I thought it was the head of a reptile." Asked where her left arm was, she said, "I don't know. Where is it? I don't feel it." When confronted with her left hand, she said, "That is someone else's hand." Whose is it? "It is not mine."

This patient exhibited a passivity delusion, *experience of alienation*, which was once thought pathognomonic of schizophrenia.[20] Her non-recognition of her hand and her illness is *anosagnosia*, or denial of illness.[21] From Critchley's description of her lesion it can be surmised that a slightly smaller lesion could have produced similar psychopathology without other stroke features. Such a patient coming to a busy emergency room today would likely be diagnosed as having psychosis (NOS) and an antipsychotic needlessly prescribed.

Another patient is described with the *Cotard syndrome* or delusion of nihilism.[22]

In an effort to recapture the feeling of her body which she believed she had lost, [the] patient ran naked into the grounds and flung herself into the snow. A similar "disappearance" or "rotting away" of the body has been encountered after focal cerebrovascular lesions.

Classic "psychological" symptoms also reflect disturbed brain function. *La belle indifference*, a patient's apparent lack of concern for severe symptoms, is observed in some persons diagnosed as having conversion disorder. But conversion disorders are also understood as subtle forms of neglect from right hemisphere dysfunction. Functional imaging techniques reveal brain abnormalities in such patients.[23] In studies of unilateral motor "conversion" contralateral frontal and thalamic hypometabolism is consistently reported.[24] This is the opposite of what occurs in voluntary movement and in subjects feigning paralysis.[25]

Functional brain systems and psychopathology

Brain functional organization guides understanding of brain–behavior relationships. The brain consists of several functional systems differentially affected by disease (e.g. herpes encephalitis often involves the temporal lobes). The systems

Table 3.1. Brain functional systems and their signature psychopathology

Functional brain system	Signature features
Frontal lobe circuits	Catatonia, perseverative and stereotypic behaviors; avolitional and disinhibition "frontal lobe" syndromes; basal ganglia signs, obsessive–compulsive behaviors; personality change
Cerebellar-pons	"Frontal lobe" syndromes; cerebellar motor signs
Dominant cerebral cortex	
Frontal	Broca's and transcortical motor aphasia; frontal lobe syndromes
Temporal	Wernicke's aphasia; psychosensory features; verbal memory problems
Parietal	Transcortical receptive aphasia; Gerstmann's syndrome;[26] astereognosia and graphesthesia
Non-dominant cerebral cortex	
Frontal	Loss of emotional expression (motor aprosodia)
Temporal–parietal	Capgras and Fregoli syndromes; reduplicative delusions Receptive aprosodia Visual–spatial and visual memory problems Psychosensory features and passivity delusions
Stress–response system[27]	Melancholia; anxiety disorders; circadian and ultradian rhythm perturbations
Hedonistic reward system[28]	Alcoholism and substance abuse
Arousal system	Stupor; delirium; sleep disorders

have signature signs and symptoms (e.g. localization of stroke by language impairment) eliciting different diagnostic considerations (e.g. partial complex seizure foci are more common in the temporal than parietal lobe).

Table 3.1 displays functional brain systems associated with psychopathology and their signature features. The neuroanatomy of the systems overlaps, facilitating disease localization. For example, severe psychomotor slowing is seen in both depressive illness and basal ganglia disease; the depressed patient, however, will not have a fine resting tremor, and unless also catatonic, muscle rigidity will not be present.

The recognition of the brain system involved in a patient's behavioral syndrome alters differential diagnosis and thus treatment options. Recognizing the frontal lobe avolitional syndrome encourages the prescription of stimulants while avoiding antidepressant agents.[29] Recognizing disturbance in the stress–response system in a depressed patient indicates melancholia and its treatment requirements. Identifying

Capgras and other misidentification delusions suggests structural non-dominant cerebral hemisphere disease that may resolve best without antipsychotic drugs.[30]

The frontal lobes and psychopathology[31]

Many characteristically human behaviors (e.g. personality, emotional expression, thinking and reasoning, expressive language, and the generation of ideas and voluntary movement) represent frontal lobe functioning. The frontal lobes subserve executive functioning, and guide the utilization of perceptions and memory. Executive functions include the recognition and solving of problems, the initiation of solutions, monitoring and self-correction of unfolding solutions, and the ending of solving actions when successfully completed.

Executive functioning deficits are common in patients with neuropsychiatric disease. Many symptoms of mania and melancholia represent poor executive and other frontal lobe dysfunction (e.g. the characteristic abnormal movements of mania and depressive illness, inappropriate social behaviors, and loss of efficiency in daily activities). The intrusive thoughts and repetitive behaviors of patients with obsessive–compulsive disorder reflect executive failure to regulate thought and action. Catatonia is the classic syndrome of motor dysregulation. The failure to recognize the unreality of hallucinations and the falseness of delusions is an executive function error.

However, the frontal lobes are not homogeneous structures. In addition to Broca's area and the supplementary motor areas, the frontal lobes are divided into prefrontal lateral and medial regions. Five parallel and anatomically separate circuits in each frontal region align roughly parasagitally and consist of a cortical area projecting to circuit-specific nuclei in the basal ganglia (striatum, globus pallidus, substantia nigra), which in turn project to circuit-specific nuclei in the thalamus, which send feedback projections back to the originating cortical area (Figure 3.1).

The five circuits are *motor, oculomotor,*[32] *dorsolateral, orbitofrontal* (*ventrolateral and medial*), and *anterior* cingulate, and each circuit has its signature features when dysfunctional. A lesion anywhere along a circuit compromises its function. Circumscribed syndromes are associated with discrete lesions within a circuit, as seen in small strokes. Complex syndromes are seen when the disease process involves more than one circuit as seen in traumatic brain injury and frontal lobe dementias.[33]

The dorsolateral circuit

Dysfunction in this circuit is associated with impaired executive function, reasoning and problem solving, new learning, recall, cognitive flexibility, idea generation, and using motor skills. When severe, diminished self-care is seen. Dysfunction in the circuit is associated with melancholic depressive states, schizophrenia, frontal lobe dementias, and an apathetic/avolitional syndrome (Table 3.2).

Table 3.2. Apathetic/avolitional syndrome

Apathy and avolition (emotional blunting)

Diminished spontaneity, verbal output (including mutism), and actions (akinesis)

Bradykinesia (slow movement), and bradyphrenia (slow thinking)

Loss of fluency and flexibility in thinking

Perseverative thinking and movement

Deficits in executive function (poor planning and loss of efficiency)

Deficits in new learning

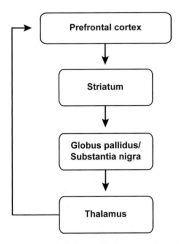

Figure 3.1 A frontal lobe parallel circuit

In patients with schizophrenia, executive function problems are also associated with the presence of negative symptoms (e.g. emotional blunting and avolition) and chronicity. The negative symptoms and the neurocognitive deficits, however, are distinct processes.[34] Both lead to behavioral and cognitive perseveration and an inability to adapt to novelty and changes in personal circumstances. Persons with autistic spectrum disorders prefer routine. The everyday lives of schizophrenics are often repetitive and devoid of new content. Similar deficits are found in children at risk for the psychosis before these signs of the illness occur. The deficits are relatively stable across the illness course.[35] In melancholia, dysfunction in the dorsolateral circuit is secondary to the intense activity in other frontal circuits and in limbic structures, and normalizes with proper treatment.[36] Re-engagement in daily activities and interests highlights the resolution of the depressive illness.

The orbitofrontal (ventral) circuit

This circuit has a lateral and medial subdivision. Dysfunction in the *lateral orbital subdivision* is associated with a disinhibited syndrome (Table 3.3) and is seen

Table 3.3. Disinhibited syndrome

Irritability
Emotional lability
Impulsiveness and distractibility
Witzelsucht (silly and shallow emotional expression)
Coarsening of personality
Loss of social graces
Tactlessness
Echophenomena and other stimulus-bound behavior
Utilization behavior

with traumatic brain injury and degenerative frontal lobes disease, particularly right-sided.[37]

Personality change and manic-like behaviors characterize persons with the disinhibited syndrome.[38] When severely ill, sufferers can be sexually inappropriate, aggressive and violent, and difficult to care for. As inpatients they disrupt meetings, frighten others, and their propensity to see an object and use it (utilization behavior) leads to discord (e.g. taking the property of others, going into other patients' rooms and lying on their beds, pulling fire alarms).

A "pseudopsychopathic personality" is also described and is characterized by distractibility and attentional problems, coarseness of manner, tactlessness, a disregard for social rules, excessive pleasure-seeking and high risk behavior.

Dysfunction in the *medial orbital subdivision* is associated with abnormal emotional expression including aggression, fearfulness and depressive illness. The subdivision has direct connections to the amygdala. Increased metabolic activity in the subdivision is associated with intense emotional expression and reactions to pleasant and unpleasant stimuli, and the mediation of autonomic changes accompanying emotional states.

Dysfunction in the orbitofrontal circuits is also associated with obsessive–compulsive (OCD) behaviors. The dysfunction is thought to disrupt frontal inhibitory processes resulting in the release of unwanted thoughts (obsessions) and associated procedural memory and its motor actions (compulsions). Structural[39] and metabolic (hypermetabolism)[40] abnormalities in the circuit are reported in such patients, as are deficits in visual–spatial recall, recognition, and motor sequencing.[41]

Serotonergic dysfunction is proposed in the pathophysiology of OCD.[42] Serotonin neuronal projections from the dorsal raphe nucleus modulate the forebrain and dopaminergic functioning, inhibiting repetitive behavior, impulsivity, and aggressiveness. This behavioral inhibition system also mediates responses to conditioned punishment and frustrative non-reward. The more active this serotonin modulation, the more behavior is inhibited. Disruption in the behavioral inhibition system is proposed as an explanation for the unwanted repetitive behaviors that are no longer responsive to conditioning stimuli.[43]

Anxiety is also proposed to play a role in the pathophysiology of OCD. The median raphe nucleus, another major source of serotonin neurons, projects to the limbic system and hypothalamus modulating noradrenergic functioning and flight/fight mechanisms. Dysfunction in this serotonin system is associated with high levels of anxiety that can elicit thoughts of danger and flight/fight behavior that disrupts cognition. OCD behaviors can result from disturbed serotonergic modulation of forebrain and limbic systems or from dysfunction intrinsic to these systems. Increasing serotonin modulation with selective serotonin reuptake inhibitor (SSRI) agents is reported helpful in alleviating OCD features.[44]

Species-specific repetitive automatic and dysfunctional complex feeding, grooming, social, sexual, and predatory behaviors are seen as animal models for OCD. Compulsive self-grooming and licking leading to fur loss and skin lesions in dogs (canine acral lick) has been successfully treated with SSRI agents. Other OCD-like behaviors in dogs successfully treated with SSRI agents are running in circles to grasp the tail, nail and foot biting, snapping at imaginary flies, repetitive chewing, and sucking on objects or bodyparts, polydipsia and polyphagia with pica, repetitive digging or scratching, pacing, and rhythmic barking.[45]

Some captive birds pick their feathers to the degree of self-injury and self-mutilation (i.e. "avian trichotillomania"). Some horses compulsively chew corral fences and "crib" (grasp the fence rail with their teeth and then lean back, tensing neck muscles while air swallowing, endangering their health). Pigs, cows, primates, bears, and elephants in captivity spend hours repetitively biting, chewing, licking, fur pulling, masturbating, and pacing. Great apes in captivity develop behaviors akin to eating disorders and engage in self-injury and self-mutilation and fur pulling.[46] Childhood onset OCD (about 30% of patients) is similar in presentation to these non-human behaviors.[47]

The anterior cingulate circuit

The ventral aspect of the anterior cingulate gyrus is associated with emotional expression and autonomic function. It has extensive connection with the amygdala, thalamus, nucleus acumbens (involved in hedonistic reward and the abuse of pharmaceuticals), and the ventral striatum (involved in craving and the anticipation of reward). In laboratory animals, lesions in this region are associated with an impaired autonomic response to conditioned stimuli and reduced aggression, increased shyness, emotional blunting, reduced motivation, and perturbed maternal–infant interactions.[48] Dysfunction of the anterior cingulate circuit is associated with marked apathy and stupor, akinetic mutism and other catatonic features, transcortical motor aphasia, and an inability to start and once started to stop actions (pathological inertia). Indifference to pain is also reported and is characteristic of catatonia. Diseases affecting this circuit include Parkinson's and Huntington's disease, progressive supranuclear palsy, and thalamic lesions. Increased metabolic activity in the region is associated with experiencing mood states.[49] Seizure foci in this area have been associated with childhood-onset OCD.[50]

Cerebral hemispheres[51]

Cortical organization

Multiple cortical areas are involved in the processing of the different aspects of sensory experience and the organization of the *multimodal* experience into the full perception of the immediate external environment. A functional hierarchy moves from primary cortex (receiving the various aspects of modality-specific stimuli), to secondary or *unimodal* association cortex (organizing the various aspects of the modality-specific stimuli into a more complex, fuller pattern), and tertiary or *heteromodal* association cortex (involved in multimodal sensory processing, linking modalities so that they "make sense"). A *supramodal* association area in the frontal lobe connects with subcortical networks and monitors, inhibits, facilitates and manages the heteromodal percepts that are being formed. This area also influences the executive control systems.[52]

Primary, secondary, and tertiary cerebral cortices configure the temporal, parietal, and occipital lobes of the cerebral hemispheres.[53] With their related subcortical structures they organize and make sense of the external immediate environment. This perceptual integration permits recognition of the distinction between self and the external world and an individual's location in three-dimensional space. The integrated perceptions and associated information are stored as memory.

Frontal circuits and the cerebellum utilize the information in memory to respond to external environmental needs. The hedonistic reward system helps maintain responses that were rewarding. The limbic system gives emotional salience (meaning) to perceptions and subserves flight/fight mechanisms. The arousal system provides the tone for these processes to occur, and through ultradian rhythms establishes wakefulness and restorative sleep.

Hemisphere functional asymmetry

The two cerebral hemispheres in humans are understood to process information differently.

The left hemisphere (by convention referred to as "dominant") in about 98% of the population is on macro- and micro-architectural levels structurally organized to most efficiently process high-frequency (dense) information, particularly language-related information. Discrete areas such as *Broca's* and *Wernicke's areas*, the *Planum Temporale*, and the *arcuate fasciculus* are identified in the dominant hemisphere.[54] Subcortical structures also subserve language, and patients with formal thought disorder are reported to have abnormal metabolic activity in left basal ganglia and thalamic nuclei.[55] Verbal memory and other dominant hemisphere functions are discussed below.

The right hemisphere (referred to as "non-dominant") is structurally organized to most efficiently process low-frequency information, particularly information that is visual–spatial. Lexical information in the images of words is high frequency. The low-frequency aspects of stimuli (e.g. their shape), the spatial relationships of objects within the environment, and the emotions of others are most efficiently processed by the right hemisphere. The right hemisphere functions holographically (it has more white matter and dendritic arborization than the left), and small lesions in the right hemisphere can go unnoticed. Correspondingly, environmental sounds are mostly low frequency, while speech sounds are mostly high frequency.[56] In normal persons, these different specializations are integrated through the corpus callosum.[57]

The right hemisphere is also more involved in arousal and the processing of emotion-related information. Right posterior regions subserve perception of emotion-related stimuli (receptive prosody) while anterior regions subserve the expression of emotion (motor prosody).[58]

The right hemisphere is also seen as processing "negative" avoidance-related emotion, while the left hemisphere processes "positive" approach-related emotions.[59] This laterality is also said to be more robust in women.[60] Some reports, however, find that while negative emotion stimuli are processed best by the right hemisphere, the processing of positive emotion occurs bilaterally.[61] The uncertain support for valence asymmetry reflects lack of attention to factors other than the emotional valence of the stimuli (e.g. physical aspects) and the laboratory setting in which stimuli are presented.[62]

Patients with right hemisphere lesions and the functional imaging studies of normal persons processing various aspects of language and conversation identify the right hemisphere as also having a specific function in understanding humor, sarcasm, metaphor, the non-literal meaning of statements, and the primary theme of a conversation. Subcortical and right hemisphere language-related structures are particularly relevant to the speech and language problems of psychiatric patients.[63]

An overlapping understanding of hemisphere lateralization is "novelty" versus "routine". The right hemisphere subserves exploratory processing of novel information that has no previously incorporated motor codes or action strategies. The left hemisphere subserves the processing of pre-existing representations and routine cognitive strategies. This view (modestly supported by clinicopathological and neuroimaging studies of non-ill persons) accounts for the fact that the right hemisphere has some linguistic functions (e.g. the processing of concrete rather than abstract words, understanding the "moral" of a story), while the left processes some non-linguistic information (e.g. recognizing the category to which an object belongs).[64] It also supports the idea of asymmetrical hemisphere activation in emotional states and why manias and depressions occur in the same individuals.[65]

Cerebral cortical regions

The temporal and parietal lobes of the left and right cerebral hemispheres have different functions consistent with overall hemisphere functional distinctions.[66]

Temporal lobe functions include: (1) understanding speech and environmental sounds; (2) reading and facial recognition; (3) providing emotional tone to sensory input; (4) new learning and long-term storage of sensory information (memory); and (5) triggering flight/fight and its physiologic support. Temporal lobe dysfunction is associated with mood and anxiety disorders, and memory problems. Many perceptual disturbances are associated with temporal lobe dysfunction. Left temporal lobe disease is associated with receptive aphasia.

Parietal lobe functions include: (1) awareness and abstract recognition (e.g. mathematics) of three-dimensional space and the relationship of the self to that space; (2) integrating semantic and visual sensory stimuli (e.g. vision and language); (3) linking somatosensory perceptions to motor performance and the guidance of motor actions in three-dimensional space; and (4) focused attention. Parietal lobe dysfunction is associated with many cognitive problems, syndromes of neglect and abnormal recognition (including several delusional phenomena), and problems with reading, writing, and naming.

Thalamic function is central to sensory integration. Sensory input and processing is physical. Only so much information can enter at one time. Receptors differ in their ability to handle amounts of information and in the speed in which the information is transduced. Information must travel along neural pathways of varying lengths and transfer speeds to reach cortical areas in different locations. Different cortical areas must exchange information. This kaleidoscope of sensory input must be integrated into a synchronized experience. The thalamus has several roles in this process.[67]

The thalamus is considered functionally to be a complex that includes the geniculate bodies and the pulvinar. All sensory information is processed through this complex. Thalamic function includes: (1) relaying somatosensory information to the appropriate area of the parietal cortex, maintaining body image; (2) synchronizing visual and auditory information with other perceptual modalities; (3) organizing all sensory information from a kaleidoscopic into a synchronized set of perceptions; (4) integrating sensory information in conjunction with a special multimodal sensory cortical area in the temporal lobes near the insula; and (5) providing tone to frontal circuitry and modulating attentiveness, wakefulness, and sleep.

The thalamus also links the cerebellum to the frontal circuitry and is involved in motor behavior as well as perception. Thalamic disease is associated with frontal lobe syndromes (disinhibited or avolitional depending on the lesion site in the thalamus), depression-like syndromes, dementia (when the lesion is extensive), amnestic syndromes, speech and language problems (subcortical aphasia and "formal thought disorder" seen in some psychotic patients), pain syndromes, body image disturbances, parietal lobe syndromes, abnormal emotional regulation, balance and coordination difficulties, and perceptual disturbances of disintegration (including hallucinations).[68] Thalamic neglect (the patient failing to respond to stimuli from one side) is also reported.[69]

To be useful, the complex perceptions generated by the sensory integrating system require identification. Thus, the system is linked to stored information (i.e. memory) that permits the recognition of objects, their function and names, the meaning of the perception, and the enrichment of the perception from linkage to autobiographic and other memory. The storage of information (encoding) and its retrieval is subserved by the hippocampus and its extensions, the mammillary bodies, and the entorhinal and the parahippocampal cortices. Alzheimer's disease initially disrupts the linkage between memory and perception leaving sufferers unable to identify familiar objects, places, and persons, and unable to understand the full meaning of what is happening around them.

Hemisphere differences and psychopathology

Understanding hemisphere functional specialization helps identify the neurology of psychopathological phenomena and psychiatric syndromes secondary to definable neurologic disease. For example, depressive-like syndromes are common following left-sided strokes in frontal circuitry and early in the course of neurodegenerative disease involving the basal ganglia (e.g. Parkinson's and Huntington's diseases).[70] These depressions are less likely to respond to antidepressant treatments, but may respond to stimulants.[71] Strokes in the right hemisphere are less likely to be associated with depressive syndromes, and when these occur the

Table 3.4. Psychopathology and lateralized cerebral hemisphere disease

Left (dominant) cerebral hemisphere disease	Right (non-dominant) cerebral hemisphere disease
Avolition, apathy and depressive-like syndromes with anterior hemisphere disease	Loss of emotional expression (motor aprosodia)
Speech and language problems; formal thought disorder	Denial of illness (anosagnosia); minimizing the illness (anosodiaphoria); the delusion of a doppelgänger (a double)
Pathological crying (with ablating lesions)	Experiences of alienation and control
Right-sided catatonic features	Capgras and Fregoli misidentification delusional syndromes (prosopagnosia)
	Reduplicative delusions (reduplicative paramnesia)
	Left-sided catatonic features
	Fantastic confabulations
	Eating disorders[73]

patient is more likely to have risk factors for depressive illness and co-occurring mood disorder.[72] Table 3.4 displays some of the associations between left and right hemisphere disease and psychopathology.

Motor system functioning and psychopathology

The motor system is a dominant feature of the brain. Composed of several units, it elicits whole-body, limb, and skilled movements, particularly of the hand and fingers. Normal movement also requires adequate sensory input that permits the recognition and localization of one's body parts.[74]

The *spinal cord* and *brainstem* convey the elements of simple and complex movements, reflexes, and motor sequences. Although disease in these structures is typically the focus of neurologists and rehabilitation specialists, their assessment is part of a thorough behavioral examination, and many psychopathological motor features are understood only after determining that the patient has adequate brainstem–spinal cord–peripheral nerve functioning.

Diseases of the brainstem disrupt the essential human behaviors of posture and walking, feeding and drinking, sleeping and waking, and sexual behaviors. Spinal cord and peripheral nerve dysfunction are features in many nervous system diseases that are mistaken for psychiatric disorder (e.g. conversion disorder, chronic pain). Assessing gait, muscle strength, vibratory sense and touch characterizes nervous system function to this level.

Brainstem and midbrain structures innervate the muscles of the face, mouth and throat. These motor structures can act independently of cortical control and their release is seen in emotional incontinence and pathological crying, and ictal and post-ictal chewing movements.

The *cerebral cortical areas* involved in basic movement include the primary motor area (Broadman 4), the supplementary motor area (SMA, Broadman 6), the primary sensory cortex (Broadman 3, 1, and 2), and the posterior parietal cortex (Broadman 5 and 7). Sensory and motor cortical–cortical fibers facilitate normal movement in addition to integration through the thalamus.

The prefrontal cortex, primary motor cortex, and the supplementary motor cortex use sensory information in their generation of skilled movements. A disconnection between motor structures and adequate sensory information (e.g. from a thalamic lesion or parietal lobe disease) can elicit catatonia.[75] The prefrontal cortex provides executive control of movement, planning, initiating and monitoring, self-correcting movements, and stopping movements when tasks are completed. Psychopathology is commonly associated with disease affecting the prefrontal cortex and associated parallel circuits.

The above structures move the body at will. There are many more movements, however, than there are pyramidal cell motor neurons, so movement relies on procedural memory (in essence, movement programs) that recruit the different combinations of pyramidal neurons needed for each task.

Once the movement program is initiated, the muscles of the upper limbs and shoulders are controlled primarily by a contralateral descending pathway, while the muscles of the trunk and legs are controlled by a second, mostly uncrossed but bilaterally integrated pathway, explaining why in stroke leg function often recovers better than that of the hand. The control of the arm and hand are also independent, explaining why many stroke patients can adequately reach for but poorly grasp or manipulate objects.[76]

The basal ganglia and cerebellum modulate movement. The basal ganglia and cerebellum provide input to the frontal cortices through the thalamus. They are essential in the learning of new motor programs.

The *basal ganglia* are an integral part of frontal lobe circuitry. They also have afferent and efferent connections to the limbic system and release motor programs for flight/fight. The basal ganglia fine-tune movement and provide procedural memory programs of learned motor sequences (e.g. riding a bike). They are involved in self-monitoring of conversational speech and participate in facial expression during conversation and spontaneous emotion.[77] They subserve attention, working memory and new learning, and sensory-motor and visual-motor sequencing. Disease of the basal ganglia typically leads to problems with motor function, cognition, and mood.[78]

The *cerebellum* has several cognitive as well as motor functions.[79] Posterior and lateral regions (primarily cerebellar neocortex) are relevant for cognition. Vermus lesions are associated with changes in emotional expression.

The cerebellar neocortex has direct reciprocal interaction with the contralateral prefrontal cortex via cortico-pontine and cortico-olivary projections, and by connections through the lateral thalamic nuclei. Cerebellar neocortex volume correlates positively with performance on tests of non-verbal reasoning in normal persons.[80] Right cerebellar cortex lesions can elicit left frontal deactivation, producing a fluctuating aphasic syndrome characterized by expressive and receptive agrammatisms.[81] Focal cerebellar lesions are associated with deficits in executive functioning, attention, and working memory.[82] The cerebellum also plays a role in word search and its dysfunction is associated with the paucity of speech seen in many patients with schizophrenia.[83]

The cerebellum acts in preparatory processes via altering cerebral blood flow or by differential enhancing of neural responsiveness of targeted brain areas (particularly the contralateral frontal circuitry) in the performance of a wide range of cognitive tasks. In cerebellar disease the ability to perform these tasks is not lost, but efficiency and coordination among tasks is diminished. This is termed *dysmetria of thought*.

The cerebellum has substantial afferent and efferent connections to the midbrain and limbic system and is also involved in emotional regulation and in movements associated with emotional expression. Cerebellar function, through the thalamus, integrates with prefrontal circuits in a variety of processes including motivation and emotional expression.[84]

Cerebellar vermus connections to the thalamus are ipsilateral.[85] In addition to coordination, the cerebellum modulates temporal–limbic activity, motor planning (trial and error learning of skills), new learning of procedural sequences (e.g. sports, dance steps), and speech and language (organizing some language elements and speech sound motor sequences).

The *thalamus* and cerebellum receive input from the brainstem, and the thalamus is the terminus for the reticular activating system. The thalamus is the lynchpin of the motor system. It links the sensory and motor systems, transfers cerebellar input to the frontal cortices, provides tone to the frontal lobes from the reticular activating system, receives input from the basal ganglia forming the circuits of specific frontal cortices, and connects to the limbic system, accounting in part for the association between strong emotion and motor behavior. Thalamic lesions are also associated with stupor and apathy. Morphologic changes in the thalamus have also been reported in patients with schizophrenia.[86]

A three-way view of the motor system

Since the mid-nineteenth century, neurologists have relied on the crossing over the midline of brain motor pathways and the lateralization of cerebral hemisphere functions to localize brain lesions. Left hemi paresis follows a right anterior brain lesion; right upper motor neuron signs predict left-sided CNS disease. Aphasia follows dominant hemisphere disease; visual–spatial problems are associated with non-dominant hemisphere disease. The examination for motor dysfunction is assessed from this *left/right view* with asymmetry indicating contralateral disease. This anatomic rule also applies to psychopathology, and asymmetrical psychopathology indicates contralateral brain disease.

The back/front view of the motor system recognizes the frontal circuitry as the front unit and the cerebellum as the back unit. Disorders of activity and motor regulation, catatonia, and basal ganglia signs are signature features of frontal circuitry dysfunction. Behavioral syndromes associated with these features indicate either intrinsic frontal circuitry disease (e.g. traumatic brain injury, Parkinson's disease, frontal–temporal dementia) or disruption of frontal circuitry function secondary to disease in related brain systems (e.g. temporolimbic disease). Bradykinesia (slowing of movement), bradyphrenia (slowing of cognition), and deficits in executive cognitive functions are also hallmarks of frontal circuitry disease.

The presence of basal ganglia motor signs (front) or cerebellar motor signs (back) delineate dysfunctional brain systems associated with many behavior syndromes. Patient 1.1 with an apathetic syndrome and loss of skilled motor ability due to basal ganglia disease (front) is an example. His behavioral change was interpreted as signs of depression, but his motor symptoms revealed the true different nature of his condition.

The top/bottom view of the motor system recognizes the frontal and prefrontal cortex and the parietal lobe sensory and associational cortices as the top unit and the basal ganglia and cerebellum as the bottom unit. Patient 1.1 illustrates bottom (basal ganglia) and front (also basal ganglia) disease.

Motor dysregulation signs are associated with prefrontal cortex disease and praxis is associated with parietal cortex functioning. These cortical areas represent the top. The presence of problems with motor regulation or dyspraxia but no basal ganglia or cerebellar signs indicates cortical disease.

Brain structures that subserve movement are so widespread that most diseases of the brain will impinge on part of that structure. The three views of the motor system permit the identification of many circumscribed brain conditions. Patient 3.1 illustrates.

Patient 3.1 (front/bottom)

A 78-year-old man had a two-year "depression" unresponsive to antidepressant treatment. He had no prior history of psychiatric disorder. The characterization of the onset of his condition was unclear, but it was neither abrupt nor prolonged. He and his primary care physician assumed he was depressed because he had no energy, had lost interest in his usual activities, slept too much, expressed feelings of worthlessness, and had "sad" thoughts about his condition. He was not suicidal, but he said he had no interest in living in his present state.

Examination found him euthymic with the ability to joke and laugh appropriately. He was neither anxious, nor psychotic. His speech and language were normal, except for mild circumstantiality, perseverative thought content, and mild word-finding problems. Motor behaviors including gait and regulation were normal except for a resting and postural tremor in his right hand. A frontal lobe avolitional syndrome was diagnosed and a left-sided, frontal, subcortical lesion hypothesized. A left caudate nucleus infarct was demonstrated on brain imaging and a psychostimulant improved his energy level, permitting the pursuit of his interests.

The neurology of emotion and psychopathology

Emotional experience is expressed continually throughout wakefulness and is both subjective (e.g. the recognition of the *valence* or type of emotion that is occurring and its physiological features) and overt (e.g. facial expression, gestures, and other motor behaviors reflecting the specific emotion). Emotion is evoked by both external and internal stimuli: immediate external environment, thoughts, and recall of experiences. The greater importance given to the evoking stimulus (i.e. its *salience*), the more likely an emotion will occur. The emotional response is modulated and elicits associated behaviors appropriate to the emotional situation.

Dysfunction in any of the phases of emotional perception and expression can emerge as psychopathology. Phobic objects and situations are assigned inappropriate salience (poor appraisal). In mood disorders the emergence of emotion may be unrelated to any obvious stimulus and the emotion expressed inappropriately intense and prolonged. Modulation breaks down. For patients with more circumscribed disease, the accurate perception of the emotion expressed by others (receptive prosody) or the inability to express emotion (motor prosody) is lost.

Ventral and dorsal emotion systems

Laboratory animal, clinicopathological, and functional neuroimaging studies indicate that the processes of emotional perception and expression are subserved by two neural systems.[87]

A *ventral system*, including the amygdala, insula, ventral striatum, and ventral aspects of the anterior cingulate gyrus and prefrontal cortex, identifies the salience of emotion-related stimuli and produces an immediate emotional response and its associated autonomic support. Sensory input to this system is from the thalamus to the amygdala.[88] Motor programs are accessed and appropriate movement to the emotional situation released. When dysfunctional, this system is central to the emergence of mood and anxiety disorders. The abnormal mood states observed in patients with epilepsy are associated with seizure foci in this system.

A *dorsal system*, including the hippocampus, and dorsal aspects of the anterior cingulate gyrus and prefrontal cortex, regulates the emotional state. Cognitive processes are integrated with and can affect and be affected by the dorsal system. When dysfunctional, this system fails to modulate normal and abnormal emotional states. Its intrinsic dysfunction may elicit avolitional or disinhibited syndromes. Executive control of emotion is compromised.

The generation of emotion

The generation of emotions reflects a rapid cascade. Potentially emotionally salient stimuli evoke activation and arousal. Activation is followed by appraisal, i.e. is the situation threatening, is there prey or predator present? This appraisal is immediate and bypasses the cortex. Following appraisal, the appropriate emotional response is generated.

Arousal and activation, subserved by the midbrain reticular formation and part of the thalamus, when over-active elicits anxiety. Under-arousal is associated with apathy and stupor. Dysfunction in the arousal subsystem of "go–no go" elicits bradykinesia, rigidity, and catalepsy. Dysfunction in an "effort" subsystem elicits avolition and emotional blunting.

Appraisal of emotion occurs within awareness (cortical) and out of awareness (subcortical). This process assesses stimuli for their relevance, immediately directs action in response to salient stimuli, and sends information to the hypothalamus (the head ganglion of the autonomic nervous system) to regulate associated autonomic support for flight/fight. The amygdala and the insula (a sensory integrating area adjacent to the mesial aspect of the temporal lobe) subserve this step.[89]

The *amygdala* modulates vigilance and attention to emotionally salient information.[90] The *insula* is involved in fear conditioning, conveying the representation of the aversive sensory experience to the amygdala for further "action". The insula is involved in the generation of social (secondary) emotions such as disgust, pride, humiliation, and guilt.[91] Excitatory lesions in the insula elicit gustatory hallucinations of unpleasant tastes, while ablating lesions are associated with impaired recognition of facial and vocal emotion.[92]

The amygdala also provides emotional coloring to memory by evaluating and modulating environmental cues based on their perceived salience. Amygdalecto-mized laboratory animals lose affectionate behavior, aggressiveness and sensitivity to social signals (analogous to emotional blunting). They respond to repeated stimuli as if they were novel. They do not become sensitized or habituated to stimuli (as seen in untreated patients with phobias).[93]

Bilateral amygdala ablation has the most profound effect. In monkeys, it is associated with placidity to the point of torpor, increased stereotypic masturbatory behavior and repeatedly putting objects in the mouth. This *Klüver–Bucy syndrome* is also seen in persons with severe bilateral temporal lobe disease (e.g. traumatic brain injury or degenerative disease). It is also reported as an aspect of temporal lobe partial complex seizures, and in such patients the syndrome is transitory.[94]

Expression and modulation of emotion involves prefrontal cortical planning.[95] Interactive with the hippocampus, the medial–dorsal prefrontal cortex inhibits the stress response cascade before it is fully released by subcortical structures (e.g. "*it's a bush not a mugger*").[96] Recurrent prolonged stress, however, is associated with hippocampal neuronal damage,[97] and inappropriate release of the stress response cascade driven by amygdala–hypothalamic hyperactivity. The failure of hippocampal feedback to inhibit the cascade over-rides cortical modulation, and is part of the pathophysiologic chain underlying melancholia.[98] Dysfunction in the related septal–hippocampal system that affects its capacity to inhibit the release of the fear response is proposed as a mechanism for anxiety disorders.[99]

The dorsal anterior cingulate is involved in discriminative attention. Dysfunction here is associated with attentional deficits and other cognitive difficulties.[100] Dorsomedial and dorsal anterolateral prefrontal cortical areas are involved in cardiovascular responses to fear-inducing stimuli. Dorsolateral prefrontal cortex areas are involved in executive function and the generation of ideas. Lesions here are associated with apathy, the loss of experiencing pleasure (anhedonia), and the loss of executive functions.[101]

Primary and secondary emotions

Primary emotions are experienced by all social mammals (e.g. humans, monkeys, wolves, dogs, and dolphins) and are seen in all human societies, appearing within the first year of life. In most species their expression is not lateralized to one hemisphere. In humans there may be some lateralization of function with more involvement of right hemisphere processes. Fear and anger are primary emotions. Happiness and sadness are common to primates, but whether other social mammals experience these emotions is unclear.[102]

Primary emotions provide a selective advantage in the evolution of the species. Fear alerts the individual for fight or flight. Anger is required for combat. Both fear and anger help maintain primate social hierarchies. Happiness and sadness also aid in the maintenance of social structures, particularly in the bonding of individuals within the group. Interacting with playmates and grooming mates elicits happiness. The loss of these individuals is associated with sadness.[103] Primary emotions also function by coordinating physiological, cognitive, and behavioral processes for immediate response to environmental requirements.[104] Psychiatric and neurologic illnesses that affect emotion affect primary emotion. Secondary emotions may also be perturbed in persons with personality disorder.

Secondary, or "social", emotions are variations or combinations of primary emotions, and may be unique to humans. Secondary emotions are elicited after a second appraisal beyond the immediate appraisal that generates primary emotions. This second appraisal is cognitive,[105] and is subserved by the cerebral cortices.[106] The content and trappings of secondary emotional experiences are learned. What stimuli elicit the secondary emotion, the intensity of the emotion and its associated behavioral display are influenced by culture.[107]

Secondary emotions also have biological importance. Pride (a variation of happiness in response to a sense of accomplishment) internally reinforces behavior leading to the acquisition of resources and power. Gratitude (happiness derived from appreciating another person's assistance in relieving one's anxiety) strengthens pair bonding and stabilizes relationships. Jealousy can be understood as an evolved protective response activated by threats to a valuable relationship (e.g. a mate) or a resource (e.g. a food source). It has a motivational function to initiate actions to deter the threat.[108] Because of their cultural content, the expression of secondary emotions also involves left hemisphere processes.[109]

The distinction between primary and secondary emotions has clinical relevance. Both mania and melancholia are characterized by measurable perturbations of the generators of primary emotion and require interventions that normalize the system and its associated abnormal stress response state. Cognitive interventions are minimally effective for these conditions. Secondary emotions, in contrast, have a substantial cortical component and non-melancholic depressive conditions characterized by themes of disappointment, low self-esteem, and unrealistic expectations are more amenable to cognitive-based therapies.[110] Present classification combines deviant expressions of primary and secondary emotions in the diagnostic criteria for major depression, explaining, in part, the heterogeneity in the category.

Chronic emotion

Acute emotional expression serves an evolutionary function. Chronic emotion is associated with chronic stress that elicits disturbed diurnal rhythms and a failure to shut off mediators of stress. Over time, chronic stress leads to wear and tear on the body: impaired immunity, atherosclerosis, obesity, bone demineralization, and atrophy of nerve cells in brain. These are reported in persons with manic-depressive illness and in patients with chronic anxiety disorders.[111]

The serotonin–noradrenergic–glucocorticoid system supports the stress response.[112] Under normal physiological conditions this assemblage protects the brain's adaptive systems against extreme fluctuation in sensory input. Impairment in this system, however, triggers brain changes associated with chronic anhedonia (e.g. the "concentration camp syndrome") and other depressive-like syndromes.[113] Under conditions of sustained or intense stress, neurochemical utilization eventually exceeds synthesis and reduction in amine function occurs. This reduction is mediated by the nature of the stressor (e.g. uncontrollable or not), experiential factors (e.g. prior exposure to acute stressors), or variables specific to the individual (e.g. age). Because of the reduced amine concentrations the individual is less prepared to respond to the demands of future stress. The more persistent the reduction in amine function, the greater the likelihood of structural pathology.[114]

Repeated stress in animal models elicits structural remodeling in brain regions involved in memory and emotions (e.g. hippocampus, amygdala, and prefrontal cortex) that is associated with impairments in memory, and the inappropriate expression of anxiety and aggressiveness.[115] Studies of humans experiencing prolonged and intense stress and the emotional response to the stress report such pathology.[116]

The neurology of manic-depressive illness

Manic-depression is a disease with substantial heritability that affects the limbic system and frontal circuitry. The ventral emotion generation system is directly affected, eliciting characteristic problems in behavior (see Chapter 8) and cognition, neuroendocrine and ultradian and circadian rhythm perturbations, and brain metabolic and structural abnormalities.[117]

Cognitive deficits are seen in acute mania and melancholia. For many sufferers, the problems remain even when symptoms resolve. While such patients do not exhibit overall decline in intellectual functioning, they do experience a *dysexecutive syndrome.*

Manic and hypomanic patients have problems in sustained attention, exhibiting deficits in both acquisition and retention of verbal and non-verbal memory.[118] Compared to patients with schizophrenia, manic-depressive patients have far greater visuospatial problems.[119]

Being euthymic does not guarantee good functioning. Of asymptomatic manic-depressive patients who are not demented, 30–50% nevertheless function poorly and have substantial impairment in several cognitive domains, including verbal memory and learning, oral fluency, visual organization and reasoning, and spatial orientation.[120] Manic-depressive patients with an early onset illness, who are psychotic, who are chronically ill and are elderly tend to have more diffuse and greater cognitive impairment.[121]

Neuroimaging studies correlate well with the cognitive deficits. Hypometabolism in the dorsolateral prefrontal circuitry is reported. Prefrontal and subgenu cingulate volumes are reduced. Findings of hippocampal and amygdala volumes are inconsistent, some studies showing reduction[122] while others report enlargement of these structures.[123] Most neuroimaging studies report some alteration in temporal–limbic and frontal structures.

Cognitive deficits observed in patients with depressive illness are associated with the neurotoxic effects of the abnormal stress response state affecting hippocampal/amygdala and frontal–subcortical systems.[124] Acutely, poor working memory and an inability to sustain concentration are reported. Cognition can be preservative, and sufferers have difficulty making decisions. When compared to other depressed patients, melancholic patients have impaired response selection, set shifting, and spontaneous recall.[125] The deficits correlate with severity of illness. More severely ill depressed patients exhibit more frontal and executive deficits, and a reversible dementia (pseudodementia) is seen in severely ill older melancholic patients. Verbal and visual memory and episodic memory impairment is associated with hippocampal volume loss that may become permanent.

The cognitive difficulties of melancholic patients usually remit with successful antidepressant drug treatment or electroconvulsive therapy. Many, however, continue to show deficits after remission.[126] Elevated cortisol levels, seen in many melancholic patients and most patients who are psychotically depressed, are associated with poorer cognitive performance especially related to verbal memory for lists of words and working memory.[127] Cortisol levels correlate with executive dysfunction and with difficulty in processing stimuli into storable information, leading to memory problems.[128]

Neuroimaging findings correlate with the cognitive problems.[129] Depressed patients have perfusion defects in temporal lobe and frontal lobes.[130] They also show hippocampal and caudate nucleus volume loss.[131] Frontal atrophy is also reported in patients with psychotic depression and first depressions occurring in late life.[132]

The neurology of hallucinations and delusions

Perceptual disturbances

Hallucinations and perceptual distortions are associated with lesions or dysfunction anywhere along sensory modality-specific pathways. Perceptual disturbances associated with neuropsychiatric disease, however, are most commonly related to temporal–parietal–occipital cortices and their linked subcortical structures.[133] As a rule, a hallucination in a specific sensory modality indicates dysfunction somewhere in that sensory system. The clinical challenge is determining if the phenomenon reflects a primary or secondary behavioral disorder.

Efforts to elucidate more specific relationships between perceptual disturbances and a brain lesion or dysfunction are disappointing because of the reliance on small samples with poorly described psychopathology. A typical study has almost as many authors as subjects.[134] The results from neurologic and psychiatric patients and normal individuals have been combined for interpreting underlying mechanisms, leading to confusion. For example, on functional MRI healthy persons exhibit intermittent and substantial increased activity in the auditory cortex during silence because they often subvocalize.[135] This activity is similar to patterns reported for patients while they are experiencing hallucinating voices. But if non-hallucinating and hallucinating persons have similar brain metabolic patterns under similar circumstances, the pattern does not explain the hallucination.

Generalizing findings is also risky, as many of the proposed relationships between perceptual disturbances and brain areas come from the epilepsy literature, where stimulation of specific cortices elicits hallucinations in that modality. An endogenous excitatory focus is also proposed for the perceptual disturbances seen in psychiatric patients, but has not been identified. The irritating focus, experimental or endogenous, may also not be linked directly to the associated perceptual disturbance as the involved area might influence "downstream" regions that more directly produce the perceptual disturbance.[136]

Patients with schizophrenia are also most often recruited for study. But it is uncertain whether the biological perturbations associated with hallucinations in these patients is specific to schizophrenia or also provides an understanding of the neurology of hallucinations found in other syndromes. The findings are also inconsistent for schizophrenia. Auditory hallucinations have been associated with reduced left temporal lobe volume in some patients,[137] but not in others.[138] Reduced metabolic responses to speech in the left but not the right planum temporale on functional imaging[139] is reported in other schizophrenics compared to normal persons.[140] However, these and similar studies are inconsistent in sources of subjects (chronically hospitalized, first-episode, post- or anti-mortem), quality of diagnosis (including or not including schizoaffective patients), and conditions under which the patients are assessed (tasked or at rest). No pattern of abnormality is consistent among studies of schizophrenic patients. Further, since schizophrenics also typically have speech and language problems, abnormal brain areas subserving language are expected. Any abnormality could be a function of the disease or its other features as well as contributing directly to hallucinosis.

While no single neuropathological mechanism can be said to explain hallucinations of any kind in any sensory modality, several modest associations can be made between the observed psychopathology and a neurologic area. In the functional imaging studies, the pattern is hypermetabolism unless otherwise specified. Visual hallucinations have been the most extensively studied in the "neurology" literature, while auditory hallucinations are most studied in the "psychiatric" literature.[141]

Visual hallucinations

Visual hallucinations are reported in normal persons under stress or who are fatigued (e.g. hypnogogic). They are reported in persons with lesions of the eye, visual pathways, and primary visual and association cortices. Many conditions are associated with visual hallucinations and visual perceptual distortions. In most patients where the pathology is within the brain, increased metabolic activity has been demonstrated by PET, SPECT and functional MRI.[142]

Elementary hallucinations of lights and shadows and visual illusions are reported in patients with occipital, occipital–temporal and anterior–medial temporal seizure foci.[143] Simple visual hallucinations (i.e. amorphic visual perceptions rather than a multifaceted scene) are reported with lesions along the visual pathways. Complex visual hallucinations are reported after electrical stimulation of temporal lobe cortex and in rare reports of the prefrontal cortex.[144] Complex visual hallucinations, however, have not been reported with occipital lobe seizure foci.[145]

Among the visually impaired, the content of complex visual hallucinations is reported to mirror the hierarchical structure of the visual system with content clusters of extended landscapes (ventral temporal lobe), grotesque disembodied and distorted faces (superior temporal sulcus face region), and small odd figures (visual parietal cortex projection area).[146] Complex hallucinations are typically described as vivid, stereotyped (the patient repeatedly experiences the same content), and can be dramatic (e.g. seeing monsters). Complex visual hallucinations are thought to occur from irritating foci acting on cortical integrating centers, defective visual processing, or as a cortical release phenomenon. Complex visual hallucinations are reported in patients with narcolepsy, brain stem vascular disease, L-DOPA/CARBA-DOPA toxicity, Lewy body dementia, migraine, epilepsy, hallucinogenic-induced states, delirium (particularly delirium tremens), and schizophrenia.[147] The presence of prominent visual hallucinations always warrants the search for an excitatory lesion in the visual system.

Auditory hallucinations

Auditory hallucinations are associated with lesions anywhere along the auditory pathway. Recent neuroimaging studies find that auditory hallucinations derive from a complex neuronal network involving frontal and temporal cortex.[148] How they occur, however, remains unclear.

Excitatory or ictal hallucinations are usually brief (few seconds), stereotypic, poorly formed, and typically not lateralized. Associated alteration of consciousness occurs before or immediately after the hallucinations. Hallucinations that appear to be release phenomena are typically fully formed, lateralized to the side of the lesion, and occur without any alteration in consciousness.[149]

Electrical brain stimulation of the temporal cortex in either cerebral hemisphere typically elicits auditory hallucinations. Spontaneous auditory hallucinations are commonly reported in patients with temporal lobe epilepsy. Complex auditory hallucinations (e.g. phonemes, music) are associated with temporal cortex stimulation or irritation. Elementary or simple auditory hallucinations (e.g. buzzing, mechanical humming, and unidentifiable sounds) are reported with lesions or stimulation of subcortical structures within the auditory pathways.[150] Auditory hallucinations occur across a range of non-illness and disease states, particularly those with reduced arousal, drug intoxication, delirium, and psychosis.

Dysfunction of the brain areas responsible for speech is associated with auditory hallucinations. The dysfunction is not always structural. Psychiatric patients often describe auditory hallucinations as either inside or outside the head. These two phenomena may originate from different brain areas. When the left *planum temporale* (the extension of Wernicke's area on the roof of the temporal lobe) is involved, hallucinated voices are perceived as external to the individual.[151]

Verbal hallucinations are reported when there is activation in the primary auditory cortex, *Heschel's gyrus*, on the left. Functional imaging also finds decreased metabolism in the left temporal gyrus and disruption of frontal–temporal connectivity.[152] When musical hallucinations are experienced, no such activity is seen in either the left or the right Heschel's gyrus, indicating that for musical hallucinations to occur the primary sensory cortex need not be activated. Spontaneous activity in the auditory neuronal circuit (network) other than primary sensory cortex is responsible for perceiving and processing musical stimuli.[153] The different brain areas subserving language and music are an explanation for why some aphasic patients who cannot speak fluently can still sing fluently.

Olfactory and tactile hallucinations

The neurobiological literature about tactile and olfactory hallucinations is scant and clinically unhelpful. Stimulation of temporal–limbic areas[154] in epileptic patients elicits these hallucinations. The brain areas responsible for olfaction and touch may also be involved.[155] Olfactory hallucinations have been reported in patients with migraine, epilepsy, temporal lobe hemorrhage, and brain tumors. Olfactory hallucinations are also seen in patients with schizophrenia, depressive illness, and eating disorder.[156]

Delusions[157]

There are no systematic studies assessing brain structural and functional neuro-imaging in persons with delusions, and the meager findings are inconsistent. There is no synthesis across methods and technologies used, the diagnoses of the patients studied, and important clinical features such as chronicity. Many studies do not differentiate between delusions and hallucinations, and lump them together as "psychotic features".[158] The only consistent finding is that delusional patients have disturbances in frontal–temporal–limbic networks.[159] This is neuro-logically consistent with the delineated phases of delusions (see Chapter 11), but non-specific as many forms of psychopathology are associated with dysfunction in these brain regions.

Many studies focus on delusions in patients with seizure disorder, schizophre-nia or Alzheimer's disease, confounding interpretation of findings are the results, the reflection of the disease process or the processes leading to the delusion. For example, Kimhy et al. (2005) construct a psychological theory of delusions based on cerebral blood flow studies that report that patients with grandiose delusions associated with excitement have increased cerebral blood flow[160] while patients with persecutory delusions have decreased cerebral blood flow[161] during tasks of self-assessment and self-relevance. The likelihood, however, is that the findings reflect differences between mania and schizophrenia, not the different content of the delusions.

Cerebral blood flow studies in patients with schizophrenia also commonly find abnormalities in the left prefrontal and temporal lobe cortex and in the left striatum, and are interpreted to represent the underlying process of persecutory delusions.[162] However, schizophrenic patients are identified by their abnormal speech and language and avolition, clinical features associated with left-sided frontal–temporal brain dysfunction. Thus, the cerebral blood flow findings likely reflect schizophrenia, not a unique pathophysiology for delusions. Similarly, in a series of studies examining the regional cerebral blood flow of patients with psychotic depression, the investigators delineated abnormalities they associated with illness severity and delusions, but the findings are also typically seen in non-psychotic patients with melancholia.[163]

Among studies of patients with schizophrenia, some examine first-episode patients while others focus on the chronically ill, making synthesis difficult. Further, the delusions studied are almost never defined by their form, so any pathophysiologic differences between primary or secondary delusions, for example, are lost. Finally, although the clinicopathological neurologic literature offers the clearest picture of the neurobiology of delusions, sample sizes are small and the form of the delusions studied are also not commonly detailed.

One theme throughout the clinicopathological literature, however, is that primary delusions are associated with lesions or dysfunction in the non-dominant cerebral hemisphere. MacDonald Critchley's patients with parietal lobe disease and delusions cited above demonstrate the association. Many case studies using different strategies (EEG, functional imaging, and lesion localization) have confirmed the correlation,[164] particularly for misidentification delusions.[165] For example, in 35 reported cases with imaging findings, 20 had right-sided and 15 bilateral lesions. Twenty-one were in the frontal and 13 in the temporal lobe.[166] In a study of 55 patients with Alzheimer's disease, Lee *et al.* (2004) reported bilateral abnormalities associated with delusional misidentification.[167]

A right-sided brain lesion or dysfunction is a common factor for many delusions of misidentification to develop.[168] In Capgras and Fregoli syndromes (delusions of impostors and false identification, respectively), poor facial recognition (temporal–parietal), an inability in self-assessment (frontal) and symptom recognition (anosagnosia) characterize the process, the patient unable to properly match a facial misperception with facial memory.[169]

The process by which a lesion in the non-dominant prefrontal or posterior–inferior parietal cortex elicits a delusion is unknown. Several psychological theories are offered to explain persecutory delusions, but these do not consider the clinicopathological findings implicating the right hemisphere, focusing instead on fragmented views of putative psychological processes in schizophrenia.[170] The conclusions of these studies are not warranted. For example, the theory of attentional bias to threat and hypervigilance as the cause of persecutory delusions is unsatisfactory, as hypervigilance could just as readily be the result of a persecutory delusion rather than its cause.[171] The idea that attribution bias elicits persecutory delusions fails for the same reason. The hypothesis is based on studies that report schizophrenic patients with persecutory delusions and patients with delusional disorder excessively attribute hypothetical positive events to internal self-generated influences ("its due to me") and hypothetical negative events to external causes ("its due to them"). Patients with other kinds of delusional content are reported to not show such attribution bias.[172] But the persecutory delusional state could just as well account for the attribution rather than the other way around. Another theory states that deluded patients more readily jump to conclusions than do non-deluded patients.[173] This idea fits the long-accepted notion that arbitrary thinking is the basis for delusions of any content and does not advance the understanding of delusional pathophysiology. Finally, "the theory of the mind" concept invokes the idea that humans naturally assume that other humans have minds similar to theirs and therefore they can understand and predict each other's behavior. Persons with persecutory delusions are said to have a deficit in this construct because they do not perform well on tasks concerning the "mental state" of others.[174] These studies, however, are weak and do not account for the effect of other features of schizophrenia influencing performance (e.g. poor executive function and other cognitive impairment).

Conclusions

Despite advances in neuroscience and countless efforts to correlate brain function and psychopathology, the specificity of the findings is extremely limited. Perturbations in prefrontal circuitry are associated with catatonia. Basal ganglia dysfunction is found in patients with OCD. Manic-depression is associated with an abnormal stress response and temporal–limbic dysfunction. The pathophysiologic cascades of these relationships, however, are mostly unknown.

Brain–psychopathology relationships are modestly helpful in delineating behavioral syndromes due to specific neurologic causes. Motor psychopathology assists in localization of brain disease. Avolition and apathy signal prefrontal circuitry dysfunction. Visual hallucinations and distortions suggest a lesion in the visual system. Misidentification and passivity delusions are associated with non-dominant hemisphere disease. Sudden and transient abnormal emotional expression is associated with subcortical and limbic lesions. Subsequent chapters detail the associations of specific psychopathologic phenomena and differential diagnosis.

NOTES

1 The quote is the opening paragraph from the author's preface of Theodor Meynert's 1885 text book in which he defined psychiatry as the clinical study of "the diseases of the forebrain" (Meynert, 1968). Meynert was a world-renowned neuropathologist making lasting contributions to that discipline, and the first professor of nervous diseases at the University of Vienna, where he was also the chief of their psychiatric clinic. Meynert's work and understanding that psychological events were epiphenomena of neurophysiologic events that were in turn dependent on specific neuroanatomic structures influenced many well-known neurologists of his day, including Wernicke. Freud studied under him and credited Meynert with shaping some psychoanalytic concepts.

2 Shorter (2005), pages 109–110.

3 From *The Complete Works of Sigmond Freud* (James Strachey, ed., The Hogarth Press, London 1966) cited in Koehler (2003).

4 Chapter 15 provides a discussion of these syndromes.

5 Wakefield (1997).

6 DSM-IV, pages xxi–xxii.

7 Wakefield (1997).

8 Chapter 14 provides a discussion of the nature of personality and personality deviation.

    Thomas Szasz has led a movement challenging the concept of "mental illness". He and others argue that there is no such thing as "mental illness" and that persons so labeled either have brain disease and thus have neurological illness, or they are deviant without brain disease and thus are being labeled by a society that does not tolerate the deviance (Szasz, 1974).

9 Wakefield (1997); Kendell and Jablensky (2003).

10 Chapters 14 and 15 provide detailed discussion of trait behavior.

11 Carbeza and Nyberg (2000).

12 Farah (1995).

13 Gardini *et al.* (2005).

14 Ibid.

15 Calder *et al.* (2000, 2001).

16 Darwin (1872).

17 Provine (2000).

18 Gervais and Wilson (2005).

19 Damasio and Damasio (2000).

20 Chapter 11 provides a detailed discussion of delusions.

21 Starkstein *et al.* (1992).

22 The most common association of the Cotard syndrome is melancholia (Taylor and Fink, 2006).

23 Black *et al.* (2004).

24 Mailis-Gagnon *et al.* (2003).

25 Spence *et al.* (2000).

26 Gerstmann's syndrome is defined by finger agnosia, right–left disorientation, acalculia, and dysgraphia.

27 The neuroanatomy subserving the stress response is well delineated in laboratory animals (Taylor and Fink, 2006, chapter 14).

28 Studies of laboratory animals show that this system arises in dopaminergic neurons in the ventral tegmental area of the midbrain. These neurons innervate the amygdala and limbic regions of the neocortex and the nucleus accumbens in the forebrain. All physiologically addicting drugs increase dopamine transmission in the nucleus accumbens, which mediates the biochemical effects of these agents (Taylor and Fink, 2006, chapter 14).

29 See Patient 1.1.

30 See Patient 1.4.

31 Salloway *et al.* (2001).

32 Dysfunction in this circuit is associated with abnormal eye movements such as the loss of smooth eye pursuit seen in patients with schizophrenia (Keedy *et al.*, 2006).

33 Chow and Cummings (1999).

34 Bowie and Harvey (2005).

35 Lewis (2004).

36 Taylor and Fink (2006).

37 Starkstein *et al.* (1988a); Braun *et al.* (1999).

38 Starkstein *et al.* (1988a).

39 Zald and Kim (1996a,b); Saxena *et al.* (1998).

40 Zald and Kim (1996a,b).

41 Zielinski *et al.* (1991); Cavedini *et al.* (2001).

42 Baumgarten and Grozdanovic (1998).

43 Zald and Kim (1996b).

44 Delgado and Moreno (1998).

45 Rapoport *et al.* (1996).

46 Brune *et al.* (2006).

47 Riddle (1998).

48 Phillips *et al.* (2003).

49 Mayberg *et al.* (1999).

50 Levin and Duchowny (1991).

51 Proverbio *et al.* (1997); Gazzaniga (2000); Tamietto *et al.* (2006).

52 Benson and Ardilla (1996).

53 The occipital lobes have no multimodal cortex. The visual multimodal cortex is mostly in the parietal lobe. This is because the demarcation of cortical lobes was originally based on gross anatomic structures that only approximated microarchitectural-based function. The occipital lobes process visual stimuli of movement, color and shape and begin organizing this information for further multimodal processing.

54 Damasio and Damasio (2000).

55 McGuire *et al.* (1998).

56 Sergent (1982); Taylor (1999, chapter 1).

57 Tamietto *et al.* (2006).

58 Borod (1992); Smith and Bulman-Fleming (2005). Not all studies find clear differences applicable to the understanding of states of illness (Borod *et al.*, 1998). Also see Ross (2000) for a review of prosody.

59 Ibid., and Lee *et al.* (2004); Sato and Aoki (2006).

60 Rodway *et al.* (2003).

61 Adolphs *et al.* (2001).

62 Bryson *et al.* (1991); Borod *et al.* (1998); Smith and Bulman-Fleming (2005).

63 Mitchell and Crow (2005).

64 Podell *et al.* (2001).

65 Taylor and Fink (2006, chapter 14).

66 Scheibel and Wechler (1990).

67 Contreras *et al.* (1996).

68 Scheibel (1997); Johnson and Ojemann (2000); Carrera and Bogousslavsky (2006).

69 Watson and Heilman (1979).

70 Starkstein *et al.* (1988b,c).

71 Taylor and Fink (2006, chapter 12).

72 Starkstein *et al.* (1988c).

73 Functional neuroimaging studies of patients with anorexia nervosa report right hemi-spheric hypoperfusion during illness which can be reversed after weight restoration (Kojima *et al.*, 2005).

74 Floel and Cohen (2006).

75 Fink and Taylor (2003).

76 Kolb and Whishaw (1996, pp. 121–45).

77 Chapters 9 and 8 provide discussions of psychopathology of speech and emotion, respectively.

78 Alexander *et al.* (1990).

79 Schmahmann (2004); Gottwald *et al.* (2004).

80 MacLullich *et al.* (2004).

81 Marien *et al.* (1996).

82 Gottwald *et al.* (2004).

83 Marvel *et al.* (2004).

84 Allen *et al.* (2005).

85 Ibid.

86 Lang *et al.* (2006).

87 Phillips *et al.* (2003).

88 Das *et al.* (2005).

89 Augustine (1996); Calder *et al.* (2001).

90 Davis and Whalen (2001).

91 Phelps *et al.* (2001).

92 Penfield and Faulk (1955); Calder *et al.* (2001).

93 Frijda (1986).

94 Lilly *et al.* (1983); Varon *et al.* (2003).

95 Tucker *et al.* (1995).

96 Lopez *et al.* (1999).

97 Salpolsky *et al.* (1990).

98 Taylor and Fink (2006, chapter 14).

99 Gray and McNaughton (2000).

100 Ochsner *et al.* (2001).

101 Tekin and Cummings (2002).

102 Parr *et al.* (2005).

103 Cyrulnik (2005).

104 Montanes and de Lucas Taracena (2006).

105 Lazarus (1991).

106 Damasio (1999).

107 Lazarus (1991).

108 Buss and Haselton (2005).

109 Ross *et al.* (1988, 1994).

110 Taylor and Fink (2006).

111 McEwen (2006).

112 Kalia (2005).

113 Kalia (2005); McEwen (2006).

114 McEwen (2006).

115 Wellman *et al.* (2007).

116 McEwen (2006).

117 Taylor and Fink (2006).

118 Osuji and Cullum (2005).

119 Osuji and Cullum (2005).

120 Atre Vaidya *et al.* (1998).

121 Atre Vaidya *et al.* (1998); Osuji and Cullum (2005).

122 Blumberg *et al.* (2003a,b); Kasai *et al.* (2003a,b).

123 Altshuler *et al.* (1998, 2000).

124 Egeland *et al.* (2005).

125 Austin *et al.* (1999).

126 Taylor and Fink (2006, chapters 10–12).

127 Gomez *et al.* (2006).

128 Egeland *et al.* (2005).

129 Schweitzer *et al.* (2001); Almeida *et al.* (2003).

130 Ibid.

131 Sheline (2000); Hickie *et al.* (2005).

132 Schweitzer *et al.* (2001); Almeida *et al.* (2003).

133 David (1999).

134 Woodruff *et al.* (1997) is illustrative: 11 authors, 15 patients, 8 controls.

135 Hunter *et al.* (2006).

136 Gloor (1990); Sveinbjornsdottir and Duncan (1993).

137 Barta *et al.* (1997).

138 Falkai *et al.* (1995).

139 Foundas *et al.* (1994).

140 Woodruff *et al.* (1997).

141 Stephane *et al.* (2001); Braun *et al.* (2003).

142 David (1999); Braun *et al.* (2003).

143 Gloor (1990); Sveinbjornsdottir and Duncan (1993).

144 Blanke *et al.* (2000); LaVega-Talbot *et al.* (2006). Complex visual hallucinations of the blind occurring in isolation and that are recognized by the patient as unreal is termed the *Charles Bonnet syndrome* (Braun *et al.*, 2003).

145 Bien *et al.* (2000).

146 Santhouse *et al.* (2000).

147 Manford and Andermann (1998).

148 Griffith (2000).

149 Cummings and Mega (2003).

150 Penfield and Perot (1963); Braun *et al.* (2003).

151 Hunter *et al.* (2003).

152 Stephane *et al.* (2001).

153 Dierks *et al.* (1999); Griffith (2000).

154 Penfield and Perot (1963); Halgren *et al.* (1978); Gloor *et al.* (1982).

155 Henkin *et al.* (2000).

156 Kopala *et al.* (1994).

157 Gilleen and David (2005).

158 Blackwood (2001).

159 Sanfilipo *et al.* (2000); Prasad *et al.* (2004a,b).

160 Sabri *et al.* (1997).

161 Blackwood *et al.* (2004).

162 Blackwood *et al.* (2001).

163 Skaf *et al.* (2002); Perico *et al.* (2005). See Taylor and Fink (2006, chapter 14) for a discussion of the functional imaging studies in melancholia.

164 Papageorgiou *et al.* (2004); Maruff *et al.* (2005); Ishii *et al.* (2006).

165 Forstl *et al.* (1991).

166 Malloy and Richardson (1994).

167 Lee *et al.* (2004).

168 Bourget and Whitehurst (2004); Likitcharoen and Phanthumchinda (2004).

169 Silva *et al.* (1993); Feinberg and Roane (2005).

170 Bentall *et al.* (2001); Gilleen and David (2005).

171 Blackwood *et al.* (2000, 2001).

172 Sharp *et al.* (1997); Blackwood *et al.* (2001).

173 Dudley *et al.* (1997); Blackwood *et al.* (2001).

174 Lee *et al.* (2004).

Section 2

The neuropsychiatric evaluation

4

The neuropsychiatric evaluation: principles of descriptive psychopathology and the diagnostic process

As one takes up mental alienation as a separate object of investigation, it would be making a bad choice indeed to start a vague discussion on the seat of reason and on the nature of its diverse aberrations; nothing is more obscure and impenetrable. But if one wisely confines one's self to the study of the distinctive characteristics which manifest themselves by outward signs and if one adopts as a principle only a consideration of the results of enlightened experience, only then does one enter a path which is generally followed by natural history; moreover, if in doubtful cases one proceeds with reserve, one have no fear of going astray.[1]

The principles of descriptive psychopathology

Descriptive psychopathology has long been the foundation for psychiatric diagnosis. Despite advances in neuroscience and efforts to define psychiatric syndromes by genotype and endophenotype, the delineation of behavioral syndromes remains centered on accurate description of their characteristic signs and symptoms.

Descriptive psychopathology has been equated with *phenomenology*, originally a philosophical effort to gain understanding of the human condition through critical analysis of subjective experience.[2] Karl Jaspers is credited with adapting the principles of phenomenology to the study of psychopathology, but using the discipline's early concern with outward appearances rather than inner meanings.[3] To best characterize the outward appearance of behavioral syndromes, Jaspers applied *objective observation* and *precise definitions* in assessing psychopathology. The definitions also required the *separation of the content of psychopathology from its form*, the form capturing best the characterization of the psychopathology. This approach diverged from phenomenologic philosophy,[4] although Jaspers and his followers also relied on the philosophy's focus on "empathic understanding" of the experiences of others.

Empathy in a psychiatric context meant the equivalent of "putting oneself into the other person's emotional and cognitive shoes". The goal was to so well understand the patient's experience that the examiner could recount what the patient was experiencing, the patient recognizing its accuracy. Obtaining the story of the patient's illness is the tangible method of empathic understanding (see below). Jaspers also searched for "meaningful connections" in what the patient was thinking. He applied this to the understanding of delusional phenomena, observing that the meaningful connection was broken between the patient's experience and the false conclusion.

The focus on outward appearance rather than inner meaning has become the stated ideal of recent DSM and ICD iterations. But many have argued that present manuals have gone too far. Andreasen laments that present classification systems are so severe that they represent "the death of phenomenology in the United States."[5] Others have called for a return to the philosophical methods of inner understanding of patients and their illnesses.[6] To minimize confusion, we use the term descriptive psychopathology rather than phenomenology, and we use it to mean the focus on observable and precisely elicited features of behavioral disorders.

Objective observation

Physical examination is invalid when based on interpretion. It is better to say "The patient is a 60-year-old man" than to say "The patient is an old man". Interpretation may be added ("looking younger than his stated age"), but without initial objective information, interpretation is idiosyncratic and has poor reliability. Any validity of the interpretation cannot be understood by other clinicians as it cannot be generalized to other patients who are unlikely to mirror the subjective observations of the first clinician.

Objective psychiatric examination is an extension of the medical physical examination. The focus is on behavior as an expression of brain function, the interactions between brain function and the rest of the body, and the influences of the environment on those interactions. Patient 1.7, the 78-year-old woman admitted in status epilepticus from the neurology service to the psychiatry service, illustrates how interpretive observation lead to misdiagnosis: because of the recent diagnosis of depression, it was assumed that her present symptoms were also "psychiatric" resulting in her seizures being unrecognized. Patients 4.1 and 4.2 are also examples of the dangers of distorting observation with interpretation.

Patient 4.1

A 56-year-old unmarried nurse stopped working to care for her elderly mother who was experiencing cognitive difficulties. But after six months, the daughter became less attentive, said she had no energy and had lost her eagerness to help. She said her sleep and appetite were poor, although she had not lost

weight. She appeared subdued and at times was tearful. She felt guilty for her inattentiveness.

Diagnosed as depressed by a psychiatric resident, an antidepressant was prescribed, but it had minimal effect. After three months of treatment the resident noted that the patient had developed "odd" movements and referred her to a neurologist.

The neurologist's report included the following: the patient looked mildly depressed as "anticipated from partial treatment", she had "frontal lobe" cognitive problems attributed "to the depression", and her movements were "cerebellar-like but psychogenic" because her depression and over-dependency on her mother (never getting married and stopping work to care for her mother) indicated a "conversion disorder, not a neurologic disease".

The patient's movements became worse and she was no longer able to care for herself. She was assessed for her ability to be hypnotized for treatment of her conversion, but was found to be a "poor" candidate.

A consultant noted that she had several severe features of cerebellar disease including ataxia of her head, trunk and limbs, intention tremor, dysdiodochokinesia, nystagmus, dysarthria, past-pointing, and dysmetria. Her performance on tests of executive function was within the dementia range. She was aware that she had substantial motor and cognitive difficulties and became tearful when discussing them. Cerebellar–pontine degeneration with a frontal lobe avolitional syndrome became the working diagnosis. Functional brain imaging was consistent with this conclusion, and further history revealed that the patient's mother and maternal aunt had similar conditions.

Patient 4.2

A 63-year-old woman confronted a new neighbor and accused him of spying on her, insisting that he was her old work supervisor. This altercation, her never marrying and living alone, and her vague history of a past psychiatric illness leading to family estrangement elicited the diagnosis of schizophrenia and the prescription of antipsychotic medication.

Her complaints of strange people in her room and someone leaving their food on her bed led to an increase in dosing. Severe rigidity, "disorganized" speech, irritability and an inability to care for herself quickly followed and led to hospitalization on a neurologic service. She became bed-ridden, mute, immobile, and febrile. Tachycardia was noted. She was no longer eating or drinking and IV fluids and tube feeding were begun. She was incontinent of urine and feces. An evaluation for encephalitis was unhelpful. Her condition worsened and she appeared obtunded. Arrangements for a hospice were made.

A consultant recognized the patient's acute condition as malignant catatonia/ neuroleptic malignant syndrome (NMS). The patient had a grasp reflex, Gegenhalten (negativism), and could be postured. A lorazepam challenge confirmed the diagnosis, temporarily relieving some of the rigidity, and permitting the patient to speak a few words. A course of bilateral ECT resolved the catatonia, although mild increased muscle tone and a mild resting tremor remained. The patient was able to dress, feed and care for herself. She could converse in a normal manner most of the time, and revealed that the "strange people" in her room were "little blue men" and that the food she saw on her bed was "bowls of fruit". At times, however, she briefly failed to respond and walked about the inpatient unit touching ordinary objects as if she did not recognize what they were.

The consultant re-defined the clinical features: misidentification delusions (the neighbor), Lilliputian visual hallucinations (the little blue men), basal ganglia motor signs, and a hypersensitivity to antipsychotics. Further questioning revealed a history of several falls and a concern several years before that she might be developing Parkinson's disease. A diagnosis of Lewy Body dementia was made.

Patients 4.1 and 4.2 had degenerative brain diseases for which there are no curative treatments. Those processes would have progressed regardless of the diagnostic label. How did the more objective diagnosis help? For Patient 4.1, it led to a change in the attitudes of her treaters. When she was believed to have a psychogenic movement disorder, her physicians treated her as the perpetrator of her condition and with perfunctory respect. When she was seen as the victim of a terrible neurologic disease, their attitudes changed markedly and she was treated more kindly. Appropriate arrangements were made for her continued care.

Patient 4.2 was being transferred for hospice care where death would likely have occurred within the next several weeks. Once recovered from her malignant catatonia/NMS,[7] however, she was transferred to an assisted living program where she remained active and happy. Her condition stabilized for the next several years and no further hospitalizations were needed.

Precise terminology

Information from the clinical evaluation needs to be organized into the medical record and communicated to others. Vague or ambiguous statements are unhelpful. It is unacceptable to examine a patient's heart and lungs and report "The heart beat wasn't normal . . . breath sounds were odd." It is also unacceptable to describe patients with behavioral syndromes in vague or ambiguous terms. To describe the patient as "bizarre or confused, or as having incomprehensible speech" suggests that the patient is not normal, but these terms, like other imprecise descriptors, encompass different behaviors having diverse diagnostic and neurologic implications. The following vignettes present the precise details needed for diagnosis.

Patient 4.3 (bizarre)

A 44-year-old man dressed as Robin Hood roamed his neighborhood robbing convenience stores, threatening store clerks with his bow and arrow, and then giving away the money he stole to strangers he met in the street. The patient was diagnosed as manic-depressive and responded to lithium monotherapy.

Patient 4.4 (bizarre)

A 39-year-old man pushed metal screws into his legs to ward off "rays" that he could feel were trying to control his mind. He was avolitional and had no emotional expression, spending the day in bed with a blanket over his head for further protection. He had a paucity of speech with many aphasic elements and a long history of chronic psychosis and the diagnosis of schizophrenia.

Patient 4.5 (bizarre)

A 33-year-old man was brought to the hospital by the police because he was acting like a wild animal, walking on all four limbs, growling, and trying to bite people in the street. In the hospital, he was mute and immobile, but could be postured. Catatonia was diagnosed.

The above patients had behaviors that a lay person would recognize as "bizarre". However, the silly playfulness of the Robin Hood image of Patient 4.3 is consistent with mania. The passivity delusion of Patient 4.4 is a "first rank symptom". First rank symptoms are often indicative of a more chronic illness, but are not pathognomonic of a specific disease.[8]

If the label "bizarre" is applied rather than the precise description, most clinicians would respond by prescribing an antipsychotic drug for Patient 4.3. The patient, however, did not require such an agent and responded to lithium monotherapy, avoiding the side-effects of the antipsychotic and receiving more specific treatment. Patient 4.4 was schizophrenic and required an antipsychotic, but in low doses, a common experience when schizophrenia is narrowly defined.[9] Patient 4.5's animal-like behavior and the subsequent mutism, immobility, and posturing are classic signs of catatonia. Antipsychotic agents can precipitate life-threatening malignant catatonia/neuroleptic malignant syndrome in such patients, and these agents are avoided in favor of initial relief with high-dose lorazepam followed by electroconvulsive therapy, the most effective and safest treatment for catatonia.[10]

Patient 4.6 (confused)
A 79-year-old woman admitted for a depression was found to be "confused" as she was disoriented to the date and day of the week. This characterization initiated an evaluation for a metabolic disorder. A more precise detailing of her cognitive problems, however, revealed that she could not repeat 5 numbers backward, or draw the face of a clock with the hands at 2:45. She could not remember three objects after a 5 minute delay. She rarely spoke, and never spontaneously. She often stared into space and postured. This image is consistent with frontal circuitry dysfunction and a mood disorder and encouraged the search for other features of depressive illness. IV lorazepam led to a temporary improvement in her cognition and motor problems. Bilateral ECT resolved her melancholia with stupor and catatonia.

Patient 4.7[11] (confused)
A 33-year-old music teacher could not recognize his students or his young daughter. He could no longer read music. He was unnecessarily treated for depression, conversion disorder and then psychosis, but his "confusion" was eventually recognized as visual agnosia and a signature feature of a degenerative brain disease. As motor and other difficulties developed, he was diagnosed with a form of Creutzfeldt–Jacob disease.

Cognitive processes mistakenly can be "lumped" together and the patient characterized as "confused" or "cognitively intact". Using screening instruments such as *The Mini Mental State Exam*[12] encourages this over-simplification. Patients 4.6 and 4.7 were both cognitively impaired, but with different patterns of problems implying different disease processes. Failing to recognize the frontal pattern of Patient 4.6's difficulties could have led to the diagnosis of dementia rather than depression. Proper treatment led to her full recovery.

Patient 4.8 (incomprehensible)
When asked how she was feeling, a 50-year-old woman responded "Fly-high, flee-pee, wee-wee. You see me." Her associations by sound (clang associations[13]) were consistent with her other features of mania (press of speech, hyperactivity and labile mood), and she responded to lithium monotherapy.

Patient 4.9 (incomprehensible)
A patient was found sleeping in a cardboard box on the shelf of a storage closet on the inpatient unit (bizarre). When asked "How come?" he replied "I'm sieged by them. They're holovisons. The cube guards the viscera blood." This

speech is paraphasic and sometimes referred to as driveling.[14] It is consistent with schizophrenia. The patient had other features of the illness (emotional blunting, experiences of alienation and control).

Patients 4.8 and 4.9 conversed without making sense; they had "incomprehensible speech". But clanging speech is often seen in manic patients with flight-of-ideas, and paraphasic fluent speech is characteristic of schizophrenia, and some aphasia due to stroke. The precise distinction led to different treatments, and for Patient 4.8, the more specific mood stabilizer. Delineating schizophrenia from a mood disorder also affects long-term planning.

Separation of form from content

The experiences of illness that patients relate, detailed description of devils and gods, flights in spaceships and other wondrous events can capture the examiner's attention. The psychoanalytic perspective gives credence to these descriptions as symbolic clues to understanding the patient's illness. For a medical diagnosis, however, the content of psychopathology is less important than its form. The form of psychopathology represents the illness to be identified. The content relates to the patient's experiences and less so from the illness, unless reflecting an abnormal mood (e.g. grandiose delusions in mania). In a stroke affecting speech, for example, different patterns of speech pathology can reveal the location of the stroke. The content of the speech is not relevant for the purpose of anatomic localization. Similarly for psychopathology, what the hallucinated voices are saying is not as diagnostically important as the fact that the patient is having a clear perception of someone speaking without external stimulation. Patient 4.10 illustrates how the form, but not the content, of psychopathology leads to the diagnosis.

Patient 4.10

A 38-year-old man heard angry shouting outside his apartment door. He heard someone say "let's get him". Fearing he'd be trapped, he opened his front door to escape. He saw several men at the other end of the apartment hallway fighting with knives. When they saw him, they rushed at him, shouting "Get him. Kill him". Terrified, he ran down the stairs and out into the street. The men pursued him, shouting and waving their knives. In a sudden, loud "pop" the men changed into dogs that rushed the man and began biting his legs. He could feel their bites and the blood running down his legs. He knew the dogs would soon bring him to the ground and devour him. He ran screaming down the street and turned into an alley. The alley had no way out. He turned to face the dogs. In a sudden loud "pop" the dogs changed into two policemen, who brought the patient to an emergency room.

When presented with this patient, medical students and junior residents have no difficulty recalling the weapons and animals involved in the story. They recall that the story starts in an apartment, moves to the street, and then into a blind alley. They recall that the changes in the pursuers occur with a loud "pop" and that the dogs change into two policemen. When then asked what the diagnosis is, they are often mystified. They also have trouble systematically and rapidly identifying the patient's psychopathology. However, when Patient 4.10's psychopathology is characterized by its form as *multiple, frightening hallucinations in multiple sensory realms, and delusions of persecution associated with great anxiety and agitation,* students immediately consider delirium and a toxic state. The patient had delirium tremens and was safely detoxified.

The content of a patient's delusion is also less important than the fact that the patient has a fixed, false belief. If a delusional patient says there is plot against him and that "The CIA is spying on me", while another delusional patient says "My employer is plotting to kill me because I know about their illegal activities", both patients have a persecutory delusion and are psychotic. Their content varies, but changes nothing about their diagnoses, treatment and prognosis.[15]

The story of the illness

The classification manuals present syndrome features as if all are of equal importance with no single combination more predictive of a diagnosis. How symptoms emerge and the sequence of emergence is not considered. This limited approach to psychopathology is the equivalent to learning the plot of *Hamlet* solely from a list of the cast of characters. Patients 1.6, the 28-year old man whose auditory hallucinations occurred for several hours upon wakening, and 1.8, the man who became suddenly despondent in the late afternoon, illustrate the need to obtain "the story" not just the list of present symptoms. Their seizure disorders were missed for years.

Rate of symptom emergence

One of the more important clinical variables influencing diagnosis is the rate of emergence of signs and symptoms. The sudden fluctuations in symptoms in Patient 1.7, the 78-year old woman in status epilepticus, was recognized as seizure-related. Episodes of primary mood disorders typically develop over several weeks; the early features of the first psychotic episode of schizophrenia can linger for months; and the cognitive decline in degenerative brain diseases can begin years before the dementia is recognized. "Overnight" behavioral change is most likely associated with a sudden environmental stress, toxicity, trauma, or a vascular brain event.

Sequence of events

The sequence of symptom emergence has diagnostic implications. For example, close attention is paid to the patient's initial experiences in an episode of illness to identify any seizure-defining aura. The sequence of emergence also clarifies if the behavioral syndrome is an ictal event or occurs before, after or between seizures. Such information solidifies diagnosis and influences treatment choice.[16] Recognizing the phases of migraine assists in preventative treatment planning.[17]

Detailed assessment of motor function *before* the prescription of psychotropic agents identifies illness that impacts the motor system and provides a comparison baseline should motor symptoms be recognized during treatment. It helps determine if the change in motor function is medication-induced.

Depressive features are common during the beginning weeks of the first psychotic episode in schizophrenia before hallucinations and delusions are fully formed, but unlike the early features in mood disorder, these early symptoms of schizophrenia are also associated with perceptual disturbances.[18] Early detection and rapid treatment can minimize the severity of the psychosis.

Persons with primary anxiety or obsessive–compulsive disorders are rarely without signs of these illnesses years before the full-blown syndromes emerge. Anxious–fearful personality traits, particularly a tendency toward behavioral inhibition, is characteristic. Persons whose anxiety or obsessive–compulsive disorder is associated with general medical or neurologic disease typically have no previous features of these conditions.[19] Following a stroke or after a myocardial infarction many patients have features of depression that represent demoralization, but it is those patients with previous mood symptoms that continue to experience a clinical depressive illness.[20] Patient 4.11 illustrates the importance of identifying the earliest features of an episode of illness.

Patient 4.11

A 38-year-old man was hospitalized after his wife found him in their bedroom holding a loaded gun to his chest. He had been hospitalized many times, always diagnosed as schizophrenic, his episodes characterized by irritability and delusions that his co-workers were plotting to harm him, information he gleaned from overhearing their conversations about him. Always treated with antipsychotics, episodes gradually resolved over several months. His irritability, leading to altercations with co-workers and threats toward his family, were the focus of his management. It was assumed that faced with another emerging episode, his despondency led to the suicidal act. There was no record from his many hospitalizations that the earliest features of an episode had been detailed.

The episodes, however, always began with him suddenly experiencing a sense of impending doom with physiologic signs of anxiety, followed by seeing a frightening, shadowy figure off in the distance. After several of these experiences a psychotic episode emerged. Of late, the small distant figure began to approach him, becoming larger and more ominous. When finally standing next to the patient, the figure was literally felt to be trying to enter the patient's body to "control" him. The patient concluded the "demon" wanted to assume his identity and that his only recourse was to let the demon enter his body and then shoot it. He did not think he would also die.

Recognized as experiencing classical signs of epilepsy (the patient had sustained a serious head injury several years before his first psychotic episode and before that was a high-functioning, stable person), the patient was treated with an anticonvulsant (a seizure disorder was confirmed on EEG), made a full recovery and remained well.

Pattern of symptoms

Present classification uses lists of unweighted symptoms as diagnostic criteria. If a patient has a certain number of features the threshold for illness is met, regardless of which features are present. A hypothetical example follows:

A patient is observed to have a grandiose delusion. He also meets the DSM catatonia criteria (two features are required) because he has excessive motor activity that is "apparently purposeless and not influenced by external stimuli", and "echolalia and echopraxia". Because he has both a delusion and catatonia he technically meets criteria for schizophrenia. Few experienced clinicians, however, would consider this patient to be schizophrenic and many would diagnose mania because of the pattern of features.

The pattern of features influences differential diagnosis. The pattern of psychopathology of Patient 1.1, the man who suffered carbon monoxide poisoning, was consistent with a frontal lobe syndrome, not depressive illness. The pattern of features in Patient 1.4, the woman with Capgras syndrome, was consistent with a right cerebral hemisphere stroke. The pattern of psychomotor disturbance (agitation or slowing), non-reactive apprehensive and gloomy mood, and vegetative disturbances (poor sleep, poor appetite, no libido), and evidence of circadian rhythm disturbances (night sweats, tachycardia) defines melancholia.[21]

Primacy of features

For the most part, present classification does not assign special diagnostic significance to any single feature, recognizing that there are no pathognomonic signs in psychiatric classification. An exception is in the criteria for psychotic disorders in which one feature is sufficient to secure the diagnosis of schizophrenia if it is a "bizarre" delusion (e.g. of control), or a hallucination of a continuous voice or voices. But hallucinated voices and delusions identified as "bizarre" occur in other conditions, including mood disorder, and are not sufficient for a valid diagnosis of schizophrenia. For major depression, one of five features must be "depressed mood" or "anhedonia", but anhedonia without other features of an abnormal mood is insufficient for the diagnosis of depressive illness.

Attributing special weight to a feature would also undermine the simplicity of the list system, requiring complicating subgroups or giving the feature the status of an independent required criterion. Nevertheless, the presence of some features substantially changes the differential diagnosis. These are discussed throughout the text.

Principles of diagnosis

Diagnosis is difficult. If the checklist approach is applied and the patient fails to have enough features, or has features not listed in the criteria, the "NOS" suffix is applied. Understanding the principles of diagnosis can provide better diagnostic resolution. These principles begin with *The Duck Principle*, *Sutton's Law*, and *The Rule of Parsimony*. To be applied, the clinician must be able to recognize typical syndromes, know the prevalence rates and other epidemiologic data of diseases, and know variations in disease presentation.

The Duck Principle

"If it looks, walks, and quacks like a duck, it's a duck!" Appling the Duck Principle to diagnosis recognizes that many diseases are "typical" in their presentation most of the time. If the patient's pattern of features is quickly recognizable as representing disease A, the Duck Principle indicates that the patient will likely have disease A.

Patient 4.12

A 63-year-old woman greeted the psychiatry inpatient unit director at the front door with a barrage of loud, rapid-fire demands. Despite his protestations that he first had to check-in, she persisted, following him to the nurses' station. Even with the door shut, she continued her comments through the glass.

Later that morning, she stood for some time with her hands up against the wall opposite the nurses' station as if holding it up. While doing this she loudly, but in good humor, rapidly spoke to each passer-by.

Recognized as the "Duck" of acute mania with catatonic features, lithium monotherapy was prescribed, and the patient, who for years had been diagnosed as schizophrenic, remitted and for the first time did not require an antipsychotic agent.

Sutton's Law

"Go where the money is." Sutton's Law is applied when the Duck Principle cannot quickly lead to the diagnosis. It derives from an interview with the famous North American bank robber of the 1950s, Willie Sutton, who when asked why he robbed banks, responded incredulously, "Because that's where the money is." Sutton's Law applied to diagnosis instructs that under most circumstances, the patient will have a common rather than a rare disease. The Zebra Principle is a corollary of Sutton's Law. It states that outside of sub-Saharan Africa, if you hear hoof beats it will likely be horses, not zebras. Again, common diseases are more likely than rare ones. Among patients 60–70 years of age who develop cognitive impairment over several months, depression is four times more likely to be the cause than Alzheimer's disease.[22] Patient 4.13 illustrates a tragic violation of both The Duck Principle and Sutton's Law.

Patient 4.13[23]

A 42-year-old woman became depressed. She was unable to sleep, became withdrawn, and refused to eat. She initially improved with tricyclic antidepressant treatment, but two weeks into therapy she became "confused", wandered aimlessly around her house, and fully withdrew from family and friends. CT-scan revealed cortical atrophy. A neurologist diagnosed Alzheimer's disease and recommended long-term care as he concluded that her condition was "hopeless".

Rather than confining her to a nursing home, her family cared for her at home for the next seven years. During that period she was mostly mute, stared, rarely moved, postured, and was incontinent of urine and feces. After many years, the illness was finally recognized as a mood disorder with catatonia and stupor. ECT resolved both and she resumed her role as a homemaker. But seven years of her life were "lost".

Severe depression can be confused with dementia from degenerative brain disease and when a depressed patient's cognitive functioning is markedly impaired, the term "pseudodementia" is applied.[24] Patient 4.13's initial depressive features and later catatonia, however, is a classic "duck" signifying a mood disorder. Even if missed, however, applying Sutton's Law will lead to the same diagnostic conclusion. Depression is many times more common than Alzheimer's disease in persons under 60 years of age. The most common cause of catatonia is mood disorder.[25]

The Rule of Parsimony

"The simplest explanation is usually the best explanation." The Rule of Parsimony tries to bring order to clinical chaos. When the patient exhibits several syndromes simultaneously, the rule encourages the clinician to search for a common process that accounts for as many of the syndromes as possible. One illness is easier to treat than two.

Patient 4.14[26]

An 87-year-old woman, living with her daughter, was functioning well, but taking "Triavil" (amitriptyline 75 mg plus perphenazine 12 mg) daily.[27] Emergence of mild oral–buccal dyskinesia led to a change to sertraline and risperidone. She became subdued, lost energy and interest in her usual activities, was unable to concentrate and said she felt hopeless and good for "nothing". She said god and the devil spoke to her and that she saw demons.

Additional medication changes had no benefit. She wandered aimlessly about the house or in the woods. She changed clothes and took showers repeatedly, stopped eating and drinking at the command of the voices calling her "evil", and threw away her credit card and diamond ring. She lost eight pounds in two weeks and began punching herself and twisting her arms to punish herself. She said she wanted to die.

[The "duck" is psychotic depression.]

Hospitalized, she received overlapping multiple psychotropic prescriptions. She required tube feeding, gastrostomy and bladder catheterization. A urinary tract infection elicited antibiotic prescription. Hyponatremia and left lower lobe pneumonia led to her transfer to another hospital.

On admission, she was agitated and disoriented and was described as "incoherent". She mumbled and complained of voices calling her "evil" and of seeing demons. She screamed and looked frightened. She was stiff and held her arms out as if carrying something. A grasp reflex and Gegenhalten was elicited. She was not febrile. A consultant diagnosed psychotic depression with impending malignant catatonia [the "duck"].[28]

An extensive evaluation ensued to identify a metabolic delirium. Rising CPK and dropping serum iron levels and the urging of the consultant led to the discontinuation of medications. Continued "confusion", fluctuating vital signs, hyponatremia, hyperreflexia, and bilaterally decreased breath sounds and rhonchi encouraged the search for an infection source.

Sudden screaming about mid-sternal pain and her hitting her chest led to a transfer to critical care. No evidence of myocardial infarction or pulmonary embolus was found and she returned to the psychiatry unit. A second episode of screaming and chest beating led to another fruitless transfer.

Back on the psychiatry unit, testing continued for a metabolic delirium. Using the two-channel EEG from the unit's ECT machine, the consultant demonstrated that the patient did not have EEG findings consistent with

delirium, and that the parsimonious diagnosis was psychotic depression with catatonia. A course of bilateral ECT quickly resolved the patient's melancholia and she returned home.

Although Patient 4.14 had several infections and likely medication overdose, her depressive features, psychosis, malignant catatonia, agitation and self-injurious behavior are all consistent with severe melancholia. A corollary to all the rules of diagnosis is: "If there is no likely harm, make the diagnosis with the best prognosis and the one for which there are good treatments."

Eliminating the possibilities to find the probable diagnosis

The Duck Principle, Sutton's Law and The Rule of Parsimony each indicate that clinical diagnosis is basically "betting the odds" on the "favorite": "Of all the conditions that afflict humans, which one is most likely affecting my patient?" The process of elimination occurs rapidly, and much of it is automatic. If the patient is male, pregnancy, uterine and ovarian problems and all other female gender-specific conditions are immediately eliminated. If the patient is prepubescent, the differential diagnostic list is markedly different from that of a person over age 65, even if both patients have many common symptoms. Anxiety, tremor, and muscle stiffness are consistent with basal ganglia disease, but while Parkinson's disease immediately comes to mind if the patient is age 65, in a 14-year-old patient Wilson's disease and illicit drug use must be considered first.

An onset over a few hours evokes a different set of diagnostic choices (e.g. stroke, intoxication) than onsets developing over days, weeks, or months.

For some behavioral conditions, laboratory tests are helpful (e.g. waking and sleep EEG, structural and functional neuroimaging, assessments of the hypothalamic–pituitary axis functioning), and some tests are definitive (e.g. genetic testing for Huntington's disease, serologic testing for HIV and syphilis), but testing should not be random. Tests should be linked to the differential diagnostic list generated by the principles of clinical diagnosis. Patient 4.15 illustrates.

Patient 4.15[29]

A 14-year-old girl was admitted to a psychiatric inpatient unit complaining of hearing voices telling her to kill people she didn't like. She recently brought a knife to school to kill a boy, and a month before tried to stab a girl. The voices, keeping her awake at night, had been experienced intermittently over the previous 14 months. She reported feeling "sad, irritable, and angry", and said she worried constantly, but denied other features of melancholia or mania. A previous hospitalization two years before led to the diagnosis of conduct

disorder. Although the patient also said that she had been experiencing hearing music in her head for the past three years, no EEG or neuroimaging were done at that time.

On the index admission the girl was described as well-groomed, exhibiting a "sad flat affect", delusions that people were talking about her, hallucinations of voices telling her to kill others and then herself, and visual hallucinations of unfamiliar persons.

Although important information is not provided in this published vignette (e.g. motor behavior, the presence of psychosensory features), the big picture (the duck) is of a young person with hallucinations in several sensory fields, irritability, and persecutory delusions. The differential diagnosis must include drug intoxication, psychotic disorder, and seizure disorder. The evaluation for seizure disorder, although a clinical-based diagnosis, typically includes EEG studies, serum prolactin levels following defined seizure-suspected events, and functional imaging. The published report goes on to detail that during an EEG assessment:

... the patient reported hearing a voice associated with a shining light and was noted to have a yawning spell. The EEG showed epileptic discharges and serum prolactin obtained at that time was elevated. Valproic acid was prescribed and lead to remission.

Conclusion

Psychiatric diagnosis remains an art, although medical science can help in the identification and treatment of sufferers. The application of the rudimentary criteria in present classifications, however, has become the primary method in psychiatric illness identification despite its well-known shortcomings that ignores the traditional methods of medical diagnosis.

An alternative to the reliance upon the DSM and ICD is to first apply the principles of descriptive psychopathology in recognizing, eliciting, and thinking about the signs and symptoms of behavioral syndromes. Second, to consider the diagnostic and neurologic implications of the psychopathology to identify the illness, permitting the application of the most appropriate treatments. Lastly, the patient's symptoms can be matched to criteria in the manuals for official purposes.

NOTES

1 Pinel (1806/1962), original preface cited by Zilboorg (1967), page 329.
2 Taylor and Heiser (1971); Mullen (2007).

3   Friedrich Beneke, a philosopher-psychologist at the University of Berlin, wrote about the "phenomenology of psychopathology" in 1824. He championed phenomenologic empiricism as a method for studying "psychic life". He considered psychopathology as deviations from the norm and foreshadowed Jung (Harms, 1967). Beneke's influence remained within Germany.

4   Berrios (1993).

5   Andreasen (2007).

6   Mullen (2007).

7   See Fink and Taylor (2003) for the evidence for neuroleptic malignant syndrome as a form of catatonia that requires treatment for catatonia to obtain maximal recovery.

8   Tohen *et al.* (1992).

9   Klein and Davis (1969).

10   Fink and Taylor (2003) detail the risks of precipitating a malignant catatonia/neuroleptic malignant syndrome in catatonic patients by the administration of antipsychotic agents.

11   He suffered from the Heidenhain variant of Creutzfeldt–Jakob disease (Kropp *et al.*, 1999).

12   Folstein *et al.* (1975).

13   See Chapter 9.

14   Ibid.

15   The separation of form from content was not the concern of all psychopathologists. Bleuler distinguished delusions seen in melancholia from those of dementia praecox by content (Bleuler, 1976, p. 92).

16   Taylor (1999, chapter 10).

17   Ibid., Chapter 10.

18   Chapman (1966).

19   Carmin *et al.* (2002); Pinto *et al.* (2006).

20   Taylor and Fink (2006), chapters 6 and 12.

21   Taylor and Fink (2006).

22   Taylor and Fink (2006), chapter 6.

23   Adapted from Fink and Taylor (2003), Patient 4.4.

24   Emery and Oxman (1992).

25   Fink and Taylor (2003).

26   From Taylor and Fink (2006).

27   Combination preparations are expensive and offer no dosing flexibility. *Triavil* preparations only provide adequate antidepressant dosing when the antipsychotic is overdosed.

28   In the old-old, fever is not always present in NMS/malignant catatonia as well as in infection (Fink and Taylor, 2003).

29   Modified from Ramsey (1999).

5

The neuropsychiatric evaluation: examination style, structure, and technique

In writing the history of disease, every philosophical hypothesis whatsoever, that has previously occupied the mind of the author, should lie in abeyance. This being done, the clear and natural phenomena of the disease should be noted – these, and these only. They should be noted accurately, and in all their minuteness; in imitation of the exquisite industry of the painters who represent in their portraits the smallest moles and the faintest spots . . .[1]

The behavioral evaluation is neither amorphous nor mysterious. The evaluation follows a medical model and all the ground rules for competent history-taking and physical examination. Manner, style, and examination structure are similar to what should be expected of any caring clinician. Psychiatrists typically spend more time with patients than most other physicians, but at its highest level, the behavioral evaluation and examination are a specialized part of a thorough general medical and neurologic assessment. It relies on questions, comments, and interactions rather than palpation, percussion, and auscultation, but the motor and cognitive parts of the examination, also require "laying hands" on the patient.

The examination focuses on behavior and what it reveals about the patient's brain function, much like the cardiologist's examination focuses on the heart and the history and physical examination signs and symptoms that reflect cardiovascular function. The behavioral evaluation is therefore within the context of an assessment of all organ systems and the immediate environmental impacts on those systems. Clinicians other than psychiatrists who also evaluate patients with behavioral syndromes should follow the same guidelines described here.

Examination style

A conversational interaction

The evaluation is a semi-structured conversation between the patient and the examiner. The examiner has specific evaluation goals, topics to cover, and examination tasks for the patient. The examiner also responds to the patient's spontaneous questions and comments. The roles of patient and examiner are clear and incorporate role-specific, socially appropriate behaviors. The examiner "sets the ground rules" and controls the evaluation to achieve its goals. The patient commonly voluntarily submits to the evaluation. When the patient does not cooperate, special rules of interaction and techniques are needed (see below). The examiner is also allowed to touch the patient and ask highly personal questions. The patient is permitted to be rude.

Assessing the patient to complete a form or a checklist of features encourages perfunctory, often stilted examination (see below). Less formality and no medical jargon are best. A style that suggests a helpful, avuncular trusted neighbor eases the patient's anxiety and self-consciousness.

The examiner's manner

Patients expect physicians to look and act like "the doctor". In the 1960s, particularly in the USA, the nature of psychiatric illness and the role of the psychiatrist were debated. Some saw psychiatric conditions as pejorative labels thrust upon persons that society considered odd.[2] Many considered psychiatric illness the result of social deprivation and created the community mental heath system to counter the effects of poverty and social inequities. Psychoanalytic theory was applied to large groups as well as to individuals, and psychiatry was viewed as a tool for social reform. In this paradigm, psychiatric nurses, social workers, and psychiatrists were considered to have similar skills for implementing behavioral change, and the demarcation of their roles was blurred. They dressed in "civilian" clothes and interacted with "clients", not patients. Therapy was the lynchpin for change, while pharmacotherapy was considered adjunctive.

The biological nature of many psychiatric disorders, however, is undeniable, and the care of suffers requires a foundation in medicine. Psychiatrists in hospital and clinic settings who look like "the doctor" (e.g. wearing hospital coats) present an image instilling confidence, and subtly communicating to the patient that he has a medical condition. A general physical examination needs to be done. The co-occurrence of behavioral, general medical and neurologic disease is common, and psychiatrists need the diagnostic knowledge and skills to recognize these conditions in their patients.

A good "psychiatric manner" is the same as is needed to achieve any good doctor–patient relationship. "Open-ended" questions (e.g. "Tell me about your family") are used to elicit the patient's spontaneous perceptions of his difficulties and to gather "big picture" information. Closed-ended questions (e.g. "How many brothers and sisters do you have?") elicit the details and clarify the patient's information. Consideration, respectfulness, kindness, sympathy, knowledge and skills, confidence, and flexibility enhance the patient's positive feelings for the examiner, the medical opinions offered, and the treatments prescribed. The substantial "placebo effect" seen in clinical trials reflects the importance of the interpersonal qualities of the treaters.[3] In clinical practice it is an ally, eliciting early reassurance that the condition will resolve with continued treatment. A good doctor–patient relationship maximizes the placebo effect and compliance.

Examination setting

Patients with behavioral syndromes are encountered in all clinical settings and often under difficult circumstances. In emergency rooms, safety is the primary concern for both patient and staff.[4] While "panic" buttons in examination rooms are necessary, their use is "too little, too late". The situation is already violent. Quick assessment of the potential for violence, using techniques to minimize injury (see below), and a ready escape route, provide the best insurance against assault. The same pertains on inpatient units. When the threat of violence is palpable, the rules of safety supercede the need for privacy, and the patient is seen in an open area or with other staff and, if needed, security personnel present.

For non-violent patients, examination rooms are best configured so that the patient and examiner do not directly face each other as this positioning is threatening to some patients. Chairs set "kitty-corner"-style present a more informal, anxiety-reducing image. Patients who have suffered childhood abuse may feel claustrophobic in a small examination room. In hospital consultation settings, the patient is often bed-ridden and the psychiatrist stands. If appropriate, holding the patient's hand or placing a hand on the patient's shoulder during the examination is reassuring.

Examination ground rules

Most patients seeing a psychiatrist for the first time have the "movie" image in mind. Many reluctantly come to the assessment at the urging of their family or general medical physician. Helping the patient to understand the ground rules of the evaluation reduces tension. The identity of all persons present and the purpose and procedures of the examination are explained. Permission is requested for the examination phase requiring touching the patient. For very anxious patients or those with cognitive difficulties, the presence of a family member can be invaluable. If asked to wait outside the room, it is helpful to bring the family member back in to discuss the findings and recommendations. Before this discussion, the patient is asked if any information is "off-limits", and such wishes are honored, unless not informing the family member presents a danger to the patient or others. Before ending the evaluation, what needs to be done next is discussed.

Asking questions and eliciting information

The procedural skills of the physical examination take time to learn. In the general medical examination, how and when to test reflexes, cerebellar function, liver size and consistency, for example, are precise over-learned manipulations of the patient. Examining the brain is no different. Questions, comments and social interactions are the probes, palpations, and percussions of this part of the medical examination, but they are no less precise and also require practice. Specific language is presented below, in the chapter appendix, and in subsequent chapters.

The examination should be conversational. Medical jargon should be avoided, and colloquialisms and idioms used freely. Most patients will recognize their medications by their trade names, not generic names.

Mentioning current events and mundane matters such as the weather early in the introductory phase of the examination, and using humor appropriately eases patient anxiety. Inpatients expect the same questions that have previously annoyed them, and can be disarmed by the unexpected personal approach, such as with Patient 5.1.

Patient 5.1

A 50-year-old manic man agreed to participate in a teaching conference, but on the morning of the conference was irritable and mostly uncooperative. The resident warned the examiner that the patient was likely to bolt with the least provocation.

When the patient entered the room, the examiner stood and greeted the patient, introduced himself, asked if the patient would sit in the chair that was positioned for him, and when both he and the patient were seated, said "That's a great hat you have on. I like the colors. Where did you get it?" The patient smiled broadly and after a brief discussion about his hat, spontaneously began telling the examiner about his illness.

Stating the obvious is often better at putting the patient at ease than beginning with socially stereotypic greetings. Most patients in critical care settings, indwelling tubes everywhere, and under an array of monitors, have little patience for the automatic "How are you today?" Articulating the patient's present experience fosters confidence that the examiner knows what "is going on". Helpful openings are "I'm doctor XX, are you as uncomfortable as you look? . . . You look like you're in a lot of pain. How bad is it?"

Examination structure

Although a good examination appears conversational, it is systematic and thorough. It has a structure. It follows a reasoned sequence. Chapters 6 through

Table 5.1. Behavioral domains in the neuropsychiatric examination

Domain	Considerations
General appearance and socialization behavior	Gender, age, ethnicity, body habitus, level of arousal, manner, hygiene, grooming and dress; species-specific, gender-specific, culture-specific, and contextually specific social behaviors
Motor behavior	Activity, gait, motor regulation and catatonia, dystonia, dyskinesia, dyspraxia, compulsions and other perseverative actions and movements, basal ganglia and cerebellar symptoms
Emotional expression and volition	Volition, emotional expression, prosody, mood lability, intensity and appropriateness
Speech and language	Conversational speech, articulation, speech production and organization, cortical and subcortical aphasia, reading and writing, speech organization, formal thought disorder
Perceptual disturbances	Distortions and psychosensory features, illusions, hallucinations
Delusional phenomena and thought content	Suicidal and violent thoughts, culturally deviant ideas, over-valued ideas, obsessions, delusional mood, primary and secondary delusional ideas, delusional perceptions, delusional memories, confabulation and fantastic confabulation
Cognitive functioning	Level of arousal, concentration, executive functions, cognitive flexibility, ideational fluency, thinking and problem solving, visual–spatial function, verbal and visual memory, procedural memory
Personality	Dimensional trait behaviors (e.g. persistence, reward dependence, harm avoidance, novelty seeking)

15 follow the sequence of the examination from behavioral domains that focus on observation and inspection through those that require more intrusive interactions (Table 5.1).

   Although each domain of the examination is systematically covered, the examination begins with what is most appropriate under the clinical setting and the acuity of the situation. A calm, alert, and cooperative patient will respond to a matter-of-fact introduction followed by "What's been happening that has brought you here today?" A modestly anxious patient can feel some relief from the recognition of that anxiety from an opening comment such as "I know this is an upsetting situation and that you're nervous, but tell me what has been going on that has led to . . .". Specific techniques are needed for the severely anxious, agitated, or psychotic patient.

To avoid oversights and confusion, once a domain is introduced (e.g. past illness, hallucinations during the present episode), it is best to stay with the topic until all aspects of it are assessed. Determining "the big picture" first facilitates the gathering of details in an understandable fashion.

"So, over the past several weeks things have been getting worse?"

"Have I got it right, the panic attacks come in bunches when you are also feeling gloomy?"

"Over the years, have your difficulties been about the same or are they changing?"

If the patient endorses a symptom it can be used to assess for other features.

"Has your depression affected your general health . . . your sleep . . . your appetite?"

"Can you see the people talking about you? Do they do anything to you physically?"

"Do you do anything to relieve the tension from those repeated thoughts?"

Once the domain is covered, summarizing the results for the patient helps segue into the next topic.

"As I understand it, this depression is like the others, but a bit worse. But has there ever been a time when a depression just changed into an excited or high-energy period? . . . Have you ever had an unexpected or unusually high-energy period unconnected to a depression?"

Special examination techniques

Some clinical circumstances require specific techniques. The conversational style may no longer be effective. Observation and inspection are sometimes all that is possible, but these aspects of the evaluation are often the most important. For example, the stuporous, bed-ridden patient who is mostly mute still provides the following information: approximate age, gender, habitus, level of grooming (e.g. finger and toe nails, hair cut and coloring), signs of old and new trauma, the presence of tattoos and body piercing, signs of many general medical conditions (skin coloring, the presence of jaundice, heart and lung signs, liver and spleen features, thyroid size), signs of many neurologic disorders (e.g. paralysis, paresis, abnormal reflexes, some cranial nerve signs), and many catatonic features. Knowing this information substantially focuses the differential diagnosis. More active examination techniques are presented in Table 5.2.

Examining for risk of violence

The aggressive and assaultive patient is a special challenge. Behavior that results in injury to a person or damage to property is violent behavior. Self-injury is often

Table 5.2. Techniques for difficult examination situations

Situation	Technique
Agitated patient	Divide the examination into multiple brief encounters; walk with the pacing patient; initially avoid anxiety-provoking topics; use the voice's lower register[5]
Hyperverbal patient with press of speech or flight-of-ideas	Increase examination structure and use typical general medical physical examination procedures to redirect the patient; also redirect the patient's associations with comments such as "I'd like to know more about that later, but right now can you help me with . . ."; use mostly closed-ended questions; speed up the rhythm of questioning; repeatedly come back to the topic at hand so that the content does not "get away"; speak in a whisper to gain attention as it is impossible to out shout a manic. For patients with substantial frontal lobe distractibility, use a third party in the room as a foil (ask that person the questions as the patient may interrupt with the answers, i.e. "How old do you think Mr. Jones is?" . . . "I'm 42.")
Hypoverbal patient with psychomotor retardation	Slow the rhythm of questioning; reduce the number of questions; use closed-ended concrete questions that do not require decisions (e.g. "Are you losing weight?" rather than "Are you gaining or losing weight or is it about the same?"); divide the examination into several short periods; do most of the examination in the late afternoon for the patient with a diurnal mood swing and less afternoon bradykinesia and bradyphrenia
Hypoverbal, avolitional patient	Same as for hypoverbal patient above; use typical general medical physical examination procedures and "paper and pencil" cognitive tasks as probes for assessing behavioral domains
Suspicious patient with persecutory delusions	Immediately recognize any anger and offer assistance; obtain the patient's "story"; orient wording of questions to the patient's viewpoint; avoid judgmental-sounding phrases
Delirious patient	Direct history-taking is a "lost cause" (medication sheets and laboratory test results often reveal etiology), focus on observation, inspection, and the general medical and neurologic examinations; interact with the patient to stimulate responses that may reveal strengths and weaknesses; asking for over-learned personal information (e.g. telephone number, address, birthdate) may gain the patient's attention

Table 5.2. (cont.)

Situation	Technique
Demented patient	History-taking is limited by the degree of cognitive decline; brief concrete questions and comments in the voice's lower register help the patient to understand, minimizing anxiety; avoid sudden movements; bedside cognitive assessment requires additional techniques
Patient in a panic attack	The patient cannot be "talked out of it"; use similar techniques as above for demented patient; explain slowly what procedures will be done; a few milligrams of lorazepam is worth a thousand words[6]
Patient with antisocial personality disorder	Such patients are dangerous, avoid confrontation (see below); invoke "hospital policy" as explanations for why unreasonable demands cannot be met

Table 5.3. Violence risk factors

Recent history of violent behavior

Experiencing persecutory delusions (particularly of being poisoned or of jealousy), or angry command hallucinations

Alcohol or stimulant drug intoxication

Having an illness associated with increased violence risk (e.g. traumatic brain injury, antisocial personality disorder, chronic illicit drug use, manic-depressive illness, epilepsy, dementia)

included in the definition of violent behavior. Verbal abuse, shouting and irritability, while hostile and on occasion precursors to violence, are not defined as violent behaviors. Criminal violence requires the act to violate the law and the perpetrator to have had intent and the "mental" capacity to understand the nature, wrongfulness, and consequences of the act. Such behavior is a societal, not a medical, concern.[7]

Preventing violence is the best technique, yet every year many mental health professionals are injured by patients because they either do not recognize the signs of imminent risk, or they do not follow the behavioral and procedural rules needed to minimize risk. Table 5.3 summarizes factors associated with increased risk of violence in clinical settings. Men who abuse drugs are most likely to be violent in emergency room and outpatient settings. Men under age 40 who abuse drugs or who have a developmental disorder, and women over 70 with cognitive dysfunction are most likely to hurt staff members in hospital settings. In communities, young men from low socio-economic backgrounds are most likely to be violent.

Table 5.4. Behavioral signs of imminent risk of violence

Escalating irritability in a previously violent person

Pacing and shouting

Exhibiting threat behaviors (e.g. clenching fists, baring teeth, punching the air, palm of
the hand, wall)

Menacing or threatening staff or other patients

Extreme psychotic excitement

Table 5.5. Behavioral strategies to reduce and control violence risk

Good respectful care; structured inpatient and outpatient programming with low expressed
emotion[8]

Do not see patients with imminent risk factors alone; consider the same protection for
those with high risk factors; do not confront such persons, use security personnel to enforce
hospital policy; search all patients in the emergency or admitting areas for weapons; patients
with high risk factors for violence should be in hospital clothes before admission

Have uniformed security in emergency rooms and quick-response teams for inpatient
needs; have panic buttons in outpatient examination rooms, and rooms with easy
escape routes

When a patient is violent: clear the area of patients and staff; keep away from the patient (10–15
feet), keep the patient talking, get the patient to sit, get the patient to eat or drink

Table 5.4 summarizes the signs of imminent risk of violence, and Table 5.5 summarizes behavioral strategies to control or reduce the risk of violence.

The examiner's response to the aggressive patient can often determine the outcome. Consider Patients 5.2 and 5.3.

Patient 5.2

A 35-year-old manic male inpatient was demanding immediate and special attention from the nursing staff. His resident physician left the nursing station to "reason with him" and "calm him down". She approached him quickly and stood facing him. After a brief verbal exchange, he slapped her face. With the aid of security personnel, he was placed in seclusion.

Patient 5.3

A 43-year-old physically imposing, newly hospitalized psychotic man was approached by a team of physicians and students making morning rounds. His resident physician introduced him to the attending, and briefly explained who the other team members were and what they were doing. The patient

began complaining about his treatment on the unit and quickly became angry. Face flushed, jaw jutted, fists clenched, he took several steps toward the attending.

The attending immediately dropped his eyes, slumped against the wall while slightly turning away from the approaching patient, and held his hands together in front of his abdomen. The patient immediately stopped his approach, looked perplexed, and walked off.

Face-to-face direct eye contact is an aggressive posture recognized by most primates. Although Patient 5.2's resident was trying to placate her patient, her quick movement and face-to-face posture triggered an assault. In contrast, the attending physician's rapid assumption of a submissive posture immediately terminated aggression.

Delirious patients and patients with altered arousal because of a seizure process may be violent. The violence is not premeditated, and can be sudden and without warning. The patient is unaware of the act, and may have no memory of it. Such violence typically occurs when the patient comes into contact with an object and attacks it, or when someone trying to help touches the patient, and the patient fearfully strikes out at the restraining touch. The delirious patient frantically fighting his restraints is another example. Unless the patient is engaged in self-injurious behavior, or is attacking someone or property, it is best to stay clear of the patient until the process is over, or the patient can be safely restrained. Patient 5.4 illustrates.

Patient 5.4

A 33-year-old, physically imposing Marine with martial arts training was hospitalized after several months of being increasingly uncooperative and irritable at work, and then smashing much of the furniture in his house and trying to attack his wife. He denied all such actions. He was diagnosed schizophrenic and an antipsychotic was prescribed. As the dose was increased, however, he became increasingly threatening to staff and patients and was transferred to a locked inpatient unit.

The unit psychiatrist examined the patient in his small office. Initially both patient and physician were seated, but as the evaluation proceeded, the patient became agitated and began to pace, blocking the examiner's exit. The patient's voice suddenly became staccato, his facial expression blank, and he stopped responding. The examiner remained seated, quiet, and still until the pacing stopped and the patient's normal voice resumed. They then both exited the office. The patient was diagnosed as epileptic, the antipsychotic medication was stopped, and the patient then responded fully to an anticonvulsant.

Table 5.6. Factors important in suicide assessment

Melancholia with anxiety, agitation, or psychosis
Melancholia in manic-depressive illness
Psychosis with command hallucinations of self-harm
Male >50 years old
Co-occurring heavy alcohol use or abuse
Co-occurring chronic pain from general medical or neurologic illness
High afternoon cortisol levels or cortisol non-suppression to dexamethasone
Impulsive personality traits

Examining for suicide risk

Even if a patient does not express suicide intent the risk of suicide is still assessed. The mildest questions can elicit intent:

"Have you been feeling so badly that you'd just as soon go to sleep and not wake up? Would others be better off if you were dead? Have you been thinking a lot lately about death?"

Depressed patients may deny suicidal pre-occupation even to the most direct questions:

"Have you thought of harming yourself? Have you made a plan to kill yourself? If you had the chance would you kill yourself now?"

Table 5.6 displays the factors associated with increased suicide risk.

History-taking

The big picture

The present illness is the most recent chapter in the patient's life's story. History-taking is learning about the preceding chapters. Plot, important characters, and major themes provide the "big picture". Recognizing the big picture permits the full appreciation of the patient's present situation and what can be done about it. Details are important only within this context. Thus, there are treatment and risk of relapse implications if the patient with a mood disorder has had none or several previous episodes, or if episodes are occurring with increasing frequency. The exact number of episodes over several decades of illness, however, is not important. After five episodes, the big picture is "frequent episodes". Table 5.7 displays some "big picture" patterns to consider.

The patient's biographic story offers diagnostic clues (e.g. exposure to industrial toxins, parental psychopathology), and reveals the patient's strengths and

Table 5.7. Big picture illness patterns

Age of onset (childhood, adolescence, young adulthood, middle age, >60)

Episodic or continuous illness

Frequency of episodes (one, few, intermittent, or many)

Changes in course (frequency and length of episodes increasing, form of episodes changing)

Inter-episode function (full recoveries, modest decline, substantial decline after early episodes, progressive decline [rapid, slow, step-wise])

---

weaknesses used to shape treatment (e.g. level of education, skill levels, family and friend supports).

Neuropsychiatic illness

Linking questions about past episodes to the patient's present complaints makes the effort important for the patient, rather than appearing to be for the examiner's benefit.[9] Questioning about personality traits and illness associated with personality deviation is detailed in Chapter 14. Questioning about previous episodes begins with characterizing the big picture:

"Have you ever experienced anything like this before? . . . Is this time different in any way? . . . Is this time the worst? . . . Over the years, have the [characterization of the episode] been getting more frequent/longer/more severe? How are things when you are not ill?"

Questions determining specific forms of illness are asked next and are presented in Appendix 5.1. Some lead-in questions are:

"I knew a patient who had similar experiences to what you've been telling me and at that time [he/she] also experienced . . ."

"When patients have [the patient's prominent clinical concern], they also experience [the examiner's concern]. How about you?"

"With all the things that have been happening to you, do they ever affect [the examiner's concern]?"

Symptom rating scales

Symptom rating scales are used worldwide. Designed primarily to encourage systematic and thorough collection of clinical information for research, they are used to assess syndrome severity, symptom change over the course of treatment, and as a data source structure to help establish syndrome and subject group characteristics. Their psychometric properties, however, are often more sophisticated than their psychopathologic content, and most do not contain most of the phenomena covered in this text. Some specific scales are briefly discussed in the end notes.[10]

Structured examination instruments such as the Schedule for Affective Disorders and Schizophrenia (SADS) permit the collection of large amounts of information for research purposes by relatively unskilled interviewers. The instruments, however, are unwieldy for clinical use and cover limited psychopathology. Their structured approach is interpersonally robotic, and ignores most of the examination principles covered in this text.[11]

Because symptom rating scales are used clinically to assess severity and symptom change during treatment, all trainees should be experienced with the content and use of the commonly employed scales to help shape their skills in the systematic and objective assessment of their patients. Clinician-generated scales are also helpful, the clinician listing and rating the features identified in the initial examination, and then periodically re-assessing the patient using that list.

Whether applied to clinical assessment or in research, a rating scale's designed purpose should determine its use. For example, the Beck Depression Inventory is a psychotherapy assessment instrument that does not have adequate specificity when used in the care or study of hospitalized patients with depressive illness. The Hamilton Depression Rating Scale is a better scale for use in patients with severe depression, but it is a severity scale, not a diagnostic scale, and should not be used to distinguish subgroups of depressed patients. The Montgomery–Asberg Depression Rating Scale was specifically designed to assess behavioral change in treatment trials. But like most scales used to measure symptom change during treatment, it offers only a limited measure of outcome.[12]

Self-rating scales are intended to provide evaluations with the minimal use of professional time, and thereby expense. They do not replace skilled examination. They are of little use when the patient is severely ill, a child, or cognitively impaired.

Summary

The behavioral examination of the brain remains an art. But art is based on principles and crafted skills. It is neither haphazard, nor casual. An effective behavioral examination that elicits valid diagnosis has a structure and employs specific techniques. The interpersonal skills of the examiner can ameliorate the anxieties of the patient and family, and a semi-structured conversational manner is an effective model. However, the examination is not therapy. Although an effective examination instills confidence in the examiner and encourages compliance, its purpose is to establish the diagnosis and the gathering of other information needed for effective treatment.

NOTES

1 Thomas Sydenham, cited following the forward of Frank Fish's *Schizophrenia* (1962).

2 Szasz (1974).

3 Taylor and Fink (2006) chapter 10.

4 Cembrowicz and Shepherd (1992).

5 The voice tends to rise in pitch when a person is anxious as the vocal musculature tenses. Demented patients may still be able to perceive this, increasing their own fearfulness.

6 Some clinicians believe that benzodiazepines elicit a paradoxical excitement in some patients. The literature for this effect is almost non-existent. This has not been our experience. Any subsequent excitement is associated with low doses that disinhibit the patient (as happens in the early stage of alcohol intoxication). Adequate dosing elicits sedation, and benzodiazepines are widely used to treat the post-anesthesia emergence delirium.

7 For a detailed discussion of violence, see Volavka (2002).

8 Expressed emotion refers to the intensity level of critical emotion-laden interactions among persons within a group, including families and staff. High expressed emotion, criticism, importunate advice, and uproar among patients, staff, and members of the patient's household increases the likelihood of relapse (Bebbington and Kuipers, 1994).

9 Assessing personality traits is also done at the time information is collected about the patient's past. This assessment is detailed in Chapter 14.

10 The Hamilton Rating Scale for Depression (HAMD), the best known symptom rating scale, is the most widely used to assess depressive illness. Published versions include 17, 21, and 24 items. Scores of 13, 17 and 21 and higher are, respectively, consistent with a diagnosis of depressive mood disorder (Hamilton, 1960; Taylor and Fink, 2006, chapter 5). In many studies, remission is defined as a persistent score of 10 or less for the 24-item scale, and 5 and 7 or less for the shorter versions. A score of zero can be achieved in patients who are adequately treated.

The Montgomery–Asberg Depression Rating Scale (MADRS), like the HAMD, is an observer-rated instrument designed to assess response to antidepressant treatment (Montgomery and Asberg, 1979; Taylor and Fink 2006, chapter 5). A score >35 identifies severe depression, while a score <10 is consistent with remission. In persons over age 65, a score greater than 21 is evidence for a mood disorder (Zimmerman *et al.*, 2004).

The Beck Depression Inventory (BDI) is widely used as a self-rating scale of the severity of depressive illness (Demyttenaere and Fruyt, 2003; Beck *et al.*, 1961). It correlates weakly with the HAMD, and is overly influenced by personality traits (Enns *et al.*, 2000). A "psychological/cognitive" factor derived from the BDI reflects its origin as an instrument in psychotherapy evaluation. The BDI is not useful in assessing melancholia or the severity of depressive illness in hospitalized patients. It may, however, be sensitive as a screening instrument for outpatient samples (Vinamaki *et al.*, 2004).

The Zung Self-rating Depression Scale, the Carroll Rating Scale and the Bech–Rafaelsen Melancholia Scale are other self-rating depression instruments. The Newcastle Endogenous is similar to the HAMD and the MADRS. There are many depression scales (Taylor and Fink 2006, chapter 5), but fewer instruments that measure acute mania. These are similar in form and limitations to the depression scales (Young *et al.*, 1983; Berk *et al.*, 2007).

Rating scales have been developed for almost every diagnostic class, and most of them rely on the overly simplified clinical features listed in the classification manuals. The Brief Psychiatric Rating Scale (BPRS) has a 10- and an 18-item versions, both widely used in schizophrenia research. The BPRS is unsophisticated, offering basic categories only (e.g. hallucinations, agitation) to measure general symptom severity. The BPRS is sensitive to symptom change and so is also used to monitor treatments (Hafkenscheid 1993).

As the BPRS offers only one item specific to negative symptoms, several instruments have been developed to assess this aspect of psychopathology. They are helpful in teaching aspects of emotional blunting (see Chapter 8), and several reliable instruments are available (Abrams and Taylor 1978; Berenbaum *et al.*, 1987; Bell *et al.*, 1992). Some of these also measure positive symptoms (e.g. hallucinations, delusions), and replace the BPRS (Andreasen, 1982; Bell *et al.*, 1992; Santor *et al.*, 2007).

Catatonia rating instruments are now available (Bush *et al.*, 1996; Braunig *et al.*, 2000), and are helpful in teaching the many features of catatonia and in assessing the response of patients with suspected catatonia to a lorazepam challenge test (1–2 mg IV). A positive test confirms the diagnosis and indicates treatment (Fink and Taylor, 2003).

11 Endicott and Spitzer (1978).

12 Mortimer (2007).

Questions for past illness

Melancholic depression

"Was there ever a period in your life when you felt emotionally terrible . . . overwhelmed, worried all the about the littlest of things and gloomy or crying all the time?"

"Has there ever been a time in your life when for days or weeks you felt constantly apprehensive and down in the dumps? . . . Were you feeling that way every day, all of the time? . . . Was there any relief for you, anything that could make you forget your worries and cheer up?"

"Did this depression affect your general health . . . sleep . . . appetite . . . interest in sex (for women, menstrual cycle)?"

"What sleep problems did you have . . . falling asleep/staying asleep? When you awakened was your heart beating fast . . . were you sweating? . . . Did you ever get a restful sleep?"

"Did you lose your appetite and lose weight? Can you recall if you were constipated? Did you feel like you were slowed down? Were there times when you could hardly move? Were you able to concentrate? Were you able to get your work done OK?"

"When people feel the way you describe yourself, it changes the way everything looks and feels. Did this happen to you? Did you hear things that frightened you . . . household noise, or sounds in the street? Did you hear people whispering or talking about you in a frightening way? Did you have ideas that somehow people were talking about you behind your back or plotting to harm you in some way?"

"Did things get so bad that you just wanted it all to stop, even hoping you'd go to sleep and never wake up?" Did you think about harming, killing yourself? Did you have a plan? Did you try to kill yourself?" (If so, details are obtained.)

Questions about the "psychological" features of depression are less defining of severe illness,[1] but are still asked"

"When you were depressed, did you overly blame yourself for things that others thought were minor or not your fault at all?"

"Did you think many of your difficulties were due to other people not understanding you or them acting badly?"

"When you got depressed, did you lose interest in activities that are usually fun for you? . . . did you get overly pessimistic, like the glass is always 'half empty' . . . did you lose all your energy and desire to do things . . . did you feel you let people down?"

Mania and hypomania[2]

"Have you ever experienced periods where for days or weeks you had unusual energy, were full of ideas, were thinking faster than usual, talked a lot and could do a lot with little sleep? . . . If I had seen you then, would I have noticed a 'hyper' sort of a person?"

"During those periods of increased energy, were your thoughts racing? . . . Were you always 'on the go'? . . . Did you have lots of plans? . . . Looking back on it, were some of those plans unrealistic, or did they get you into financial or other difficulties? . . . In those periods did you find yourself feeling that you had special abilities or powers other people do not have?"

"Were there periods where for days or weeks when your emotions got the better of you and you were too emotional, too hyper, too high, but were not drunk or using drugs?

Manic-depressive patients may not recognize past manias, but they will remember the consequences of their behavior. Helpful questions are:

"When that [the episode] happened, were people upset, angry or frightened of you . . . were the police called . . . did they bring you to the hospital . . . did they put you in restraints?"

"Do you have periods where for days or weeks you become short-tempered and more aggressive than usual, even yelling and arguing with people or getting into fights? . . . Were friends and family members frightened by the way you were?"

Psychosis[3]

"In the past have you ever been troubled by suspicions that you were somehow in danger . . . that people were talking about you behind your back or plotting to hurt you?"

"In the past have you ever experienced seeing or hearing things that didn't make sense or were strange or unusual, like hearing voices when no one was nearby, seeing visions or frightening things that seemed real, but others said were from your imagination 'playing tricks on you'?"

Sleep disorder[4]

Sleep disorders are common, particularly in persons over 50 years of age. Sleep apnea, restless leg syndrome, and non-REM sleep stereotypy impact general health and are associated with mood disorders and neurologic disease, complicating management of many behavioral conditions. Questions include:

"Have your present difficulties affected your sleep? How is your sleep when you are otherwise feeling well?

"Do you snore loudly? How does your [bed partner] awaken you?[5] Do you fall asleep during the day at work, or when driving your car?"

"Are you a restless sleeper? Do you kick off the bed covers?"

"Do you ever have sudden sleep-like experiences during the day? Are you fully alert during these periods? What have people said that you do during these periods?"

The time of night difficulties occur has diagnostic implications. Non-REM disorders tend to occur in the first third of the night. Patients with non-melancholic depression often have initial insomnia, but then may sleep through their alarm. Patients with melancholia have delayed sleep onset (>20 mins) and reduced REM latency (their first REM period occurs shortly after sleep onset). They do not have restorative sleep and wake anxious, sweaty, and with tachycardia. Questioning assesses these details.

Migraine and cluster headache[6]

"Do you have frequent severe headaches? . . . How often do these occur? . . . How long do they last? . . . Do you have any warning that you are going to get a headache (e.g. odd skin sensation of the headache spot, stuffy nose on the side of the headache onset)?"

"Where on your head do the headaches begin? . . . Does your vision change with the headache (e.g. seeing a herringbone pattern, shimmering lights, arcs of light)? Do you experience the visual symptoms you've told me about at times when you don't have a headache? . . . Have you ever had sudden, but temporary loss of full vision (tunnel vision, loss of acuity, everything looking grey)?"

"Do the headaches come in bunches? . . . Is there anytime of the year when they are more likely to occur?" (the weeks around the summer solstice is a peak).

"Is there anything you've noticed that triggers a headache (e.g. late luteal phase of menstrual cycle, long exposure to strong florescent light, frequent or long air flight)?"

Seizure disorder[7]

"Have you ever had 'blackout spells', or episodes were you couldn't account for a short period of time? . . . Have you ever found yourself someplace where you didn't remember how you got there (in a different room in the house than remembered, in a building, but only recalling being in the street or parking lot outside the building)?"

"Have people told you that you have 'spells' you don't remember where you seem 'spaced out' or unresponsive or where you do something odd or some repeated action? . . . Have you ever had 'fits' where you pass out and fall, injuring yourself? . . . Have you ever had 'fits' were you were told your arms and legs were shaking, or where you lost control or your bladder, or bit your tongue?"[8]

Cognitive decline[9]

"Of late have you been worried about your memory? . . . Have your friends or family expressed concerns about your memory? . . . How has your concentration been? . . . Have you recently had more trouble than you expected learning something you wanted to know?"

Table 5A.1. Past experiences with present illness implications

Past experience	Implications
Difficult gestation or delivery	Anoxia or fetal brain damage resulting in ADHD, conduct disorder, school academic and behavioral problems
Maternal perinatal depression	Increased risk for early onset depressive illness in exposed children
Childhood febrile convulsions	Seizure disorder in adult years
Delayed motor, speech, and socialization landmarks	School and behavioral problems; increased risk for schizophrenia
Frequent or severe Strep infections	Increased risk for PANDAS (Pediatric Autoimmune Neuropsychiatric Disorder Associated with Streptococcal infection)
Chronic and substantial parental discord (including divorce)	Increased risk for depressive illness
Chronic child abuse	Increased risk of being an abusive parent and to have depressive illness
Parental psychopathology	Increased risk for depressive illness
Traumatic head injury	Increased risk for seizure disorder and manic-depressive-like syndromes
Severe injury leading to loss of a body part or permanent loss of function	PTSD
Illicit drug use	Increased risk for psychosis

"When having a conversation, have you been having any trouble finding the words you want to say, or have you found yourself losing your train of thought? . . . Have you found yourself forgetting to remember to do things, and have had to increasingly keep lists or notes to yourself to help remember?"

Past experiences with preset illness implications

Some experiences have substantial diagnostic implications, increasing risks for several conditions (Table 5A.1). The assessment of their presence is part of a thorough evaluation.

Many of the experiences in Table 5A.1 cannot be recalled. If the patient's mother, or an older sister, is not available to provide information, family lore may be helpful.[10] Questioning includes:

Pregnancy and postpartum problems

"Do you recall your mother telling you that she had a difficult pregnancy when carrying you? Did she mention her labor or delivery or how your health was at birth?"

"Has anyone in your family suffered from difficulties similar to yours? Do you recall your mother or anyone else saying that after your birth or during her pregnancy with you that she had a depression or other difficulties? Did she or anyone else see a psychiatrist, psychologist or social worker for emotional problems? Were they ever treated with medication . . . shock treatment?" (Details about any illness, treatments and outcomes are then obtained.)

Childhood health

"How was your health as an infant? Do you recall anyone saying that they were worried about your health? Did anyone say that when you were young you had high fevers and that sometimes these lead to fits or convulsions?"

"Do you recall anyone mentioning to you how old you were when you started walking and talking? Did they say that they were concerned about how you were progressing as a young kid?"

"Do you recall being sick a lot as a child? Were you ever in a hospital as a child? Do you recall having Strep throats? Did anyone mention if these were more severe than the usual ones? Did you have any after-effects from them as far as you recall?"

Family and abuse

After determining the members and their ages, and their relationship to the patient,[11] helpful questions are:

"Can you tell me about your family when you were growing up? . . . How did they get along?"

"Were you a happy child? Were you hit or hurt in any way?" (Details are then obtained.)

"How long did all that go on?"

Head injury

Many patients have had a head injury, but only substantial injuries are associated with later behavioral difficulties. A period of unconsciousness greater than 20 mins and the presence of abnormal neurologic features immediately after the injury presage future behavioral disturbances, as does the length of the period of amnesia following the head trauma. The longer the period of this anterograde amnesia, the more severe the brain injury, and the more likely later behavioral problems will occur. The amnesia occurs because the post-injury brain is not adequately processing and storing new information.[12] The image of this period can be elicited by such questions as:

"After your injury was there a period of time that you don't remember well . . . that seemed fuzzy? Did it feel like you were half-asleep? Do people tell you that back then you didn't seem to remember from one event or conversation to the next? How long did this experience last?"

"Have you ever had a head injury where you were knocked out? What happened?"

A blow to the head that is damaging (e.g. being hit with a blunt object) produces trauma beneath the impact. In head injury where the head is in motion and hits an object (e.g. in a fall, being thrown from a moving vehicle), the injury will be coup-counter-coup.

Sometimes head trauma elicits a post-concussion syndrome. Questions assessing this include:

"After your head injury, were you dizzy or unsteady on your feet for any period of time? Were you sick to your stomach? Did you have headaches? Were you feeling anxious for no specific reason? Did you tire easily? Did you find yourself feeing gloomy or being tearful?

Posttraumatic stress syndromes

Severe injury leading to loss of a body part or permanent loss of function almost always elicits an acute stress reaction and bereavement. Helpful questions include:

"Have you ever been seriously injured? What happened? Did you find yourself reliving [the injury] a lot? Could you put it out of your mind? Did it give you nightmares? How long did this last?"

"Have you ever been assaulted or had some other terrible experience?"

When the PTSD is prolonged beyond a year, the trauma likely precipitated an anxiety disorder in a vulnerable person.[13]

Drug and alcohol abuse

The use of prescribed and non-prescribed pharmaceuticals should always be assessed. Information about the former provides a quick image of the patient's general health, while the latter yields both differential diagnostic and treatment-shaping information.

Tobacco and caffeine: patients with depressive illness have a fourfold increase in tobacco use.[14] Manic-depressive patients may overuse caffeine. Caffeine in high doses slightly lowers seizure threshold, and epileptics should avoid it.[15] Sensitivity to caffeine, or caffeineism, is part of the differential diagnosis of anxiety disorder and can be identified with questions such as:

"Do you drink beverages containing caffeine?" If so, "Does the severity of your anxiety have highs and lows during the day? When you are becoming anxious, can you put your finger on a cause? Does the anxiety affect you physically? Does it make you jumpy . . . produce an empty feeling in your stomach . . . make your muscles twitch . . . is it associated with a change in the way you see colors (a bluish tinge), or does it produce a metallic or odd taste?"

Alcohol: the CAGE questions taught in most medical schools in the USA as an assessment for alcohol abuse have low sensitivity,[16] and thus elicit too many false negative conclusions about the patient's alcohol use.[17] Many alcoholics do not drink in the morning, or have a DUI. Many never have trouble stopping drinking, because they have never thought of stopping. The DSM approach also elicits too many false negative conclusions.[18] Alcoholism is defined when the patient continues to drink heavily despite health, employment, or interpersonal difficulties directly related to the consumption of alcohol. Assessment is directed to the amount (estimate ounces) consumed daily and the potential consequences. A person who continues to work, has never been arrested for public intoxication or for driving under the influence of alcohol, and who only drinks at night after work, but does so daily *to frequent intoxication* is an alcoholic, and will ultimately have alcohol-related health and other problems.

Illicit drugs: a patient's use of illicit drugs is a threefold problem. Illicit drug use is a crime that carries heavy legal penalties. Illicit drug use can cause brain damage (e.g. white matter small vascular-related bradyphrenia and executive function decline from prolonged cocaine use, recurrent chronic psychotic disorder from hallucinogen use, and basal ganglia dysfunction and movement disorder from ecstasy) and other health problems (e.g. fatal arrhythmia, stroke, seizure, and placenta previa from cocaine use, chronic obstructive pulmonary disease (COPD) from heavy cannabis use). Illicit drug use also interferes with all psychiatric treatments leading to non-compliance, and has adverse pharmacodynamic effects for drug therapies.[19] Questioning focuses on the age of onset of use, approximate frequency of use, and acute adverse reactions from use. The earlier the onset, the heavier the use, the more severe the adverse reaction, the more likely the patient's present illness is related to brain dysfunction from illicit drugs. Substances that are specifically addressed are: LSD, PCP, cocaine and crack, ecstasy, methamphetamine, volatile solvents, opiates and opioids, hallucinogenic mushrooms, mescaline and other organic hallucinogens, and cannabis.

NOTES

1 Taylor and Fink (2006), chapters 1–4.
2 Goodwin and Jamison (1990).
3 Taylor (1999), chapter 9.
4 Taylor (1999), chapter 16.
5 A quick assessment of the quality of a couple's relationship is the manner used to awaken the snorer. It ranges from a gentle pat or shake to kicking and punching.
6 Taylor (1999), chapter 16.
7 Taylor (1999), chapter 10.
8 Although tongue biting and urinary incontinence are consistent with a grand mal seizure, they do not always occur with generalized seizures. They almost never occur with ECT, although a generalized brain seizure is induced.
9 Taylor (1999), chapter 12.

10 One of us (MAT) was the principle investigator on a large project that gathered information from first-degree relatives of patients with either schizophrenia or a mood disorder. Whenever possible, relatives were personally interviewed, but they also provided information about the patient and other relatives. Mothers gave the most and the most reliable information. Older sisters were the next best source. The information from patients' fathers was highly variable in quality and quantity.

11 Obtaining the ages and names of close family members accomplishes two things. First, it provides some assessment of the patient's biographic memory and cognitive difficulties. Second, the ages of the family members can be compared to the age of risk for diseases in the differential diagnosis, and whether they are in the risk period. For example, if Huntington's disease is a consideration, but the health of the patient's parents is unknown and the patient's siblings appear healthy, healthy siblings over age 60 are unlikely to have the illness, but healthy siblings under age 30 are yet to enter the peak risk period.

12 Levin *et al.* (1985).

13 Peleg and Shalev (2006).

14 Covey *et al.* (1998).

15 Kaufman and Sachdeo (2003); Bonilha and Li (2004).

16 CAGE is a four-item screening acronym assessing for alcoholism and standing for *cutting down, annoyed by criticism, guilt feelings,* and *having eye-openers.*

17 Fink *et al.* (2002).

18 Chung and Martin (2005).

19 Enevoldson (2004); Winger *et al.* (2005).

Section 3

Examination domains

6

Psychopathology of everyday behavior and general appearance

With the growth of psychopharmacology and the development of biochemical and neuro-physiological research, the need for careful description of the clinical phenomena in psychiatry is greater than ever before. Without good clinical knowledge research in psychiatry will be fruitless.[1]

A person's general appearance is revealing. A graphically tattooed woman with spiked purple hair and metal nose, ear, and lip studs is likely to be deviant in other ways.[2] A clean-shaven, middle-aged man in a three-piece Brooks Brothers suit is more likely be a professional or in business than the drummer in a rock band. Self-decoration, choice of clothing, demeanor, and similar factors provide clues to temperament and social class, and sometimes to illness. Non-verbal cues during employment interviews (e.g. dress, posture) predict the outcome of the interview.[3] The voting public in the USA apparently places great store in such information, although subliminally, as inferences of competence based solely on the facial appearance of federal senate candidates predicted the election outcome in 68.8% of the races of 2004.[4]

The initial "big picture"

The general appearance "big picture" is always defined first, and may be charac-terized by a single striking feature (e.g. the patient is pregnant, devoid of all body hair, or is mute and immobile). Most often, however, it is an image blending many details. Observing the patient outside the examination room setting *before* formally starting the evaluation provides this information. Emergency room care-givers, for example, often rely on the big picture in assessing acuity. A supine patient with ankles crossed, hands crossed behind the neck, or folded over the abdomen is unlikely to have any acute, life-threatening condition.[5]

In the waiting area, is the patient sitting calmly reading a magazine, watching other patients, or pacing, fidgeting, or talking to himself? In the emergency room, is the patient cooperative, or causing a disturbance? Observations are made about dress, grooming, and alertness before meeting the patient.

Does the hospitalized patient interact with others in common areas, the dining room, and hallways? Is the patient disruptive and loud or passive and reclusive? The following images and their implications illustrate.

An elderly, disheveled, white-haired woman slouched slacked-jawed in her chair not interacting with other patients and staff is the image of depression, dementia, or over-sedation.

A middle-aged woman with a furrowed brow [a worried look] sitting outside the nursing station continuously rocking and wringing her hands, seemingly oblivious to her surroundings, is the image of melancholia. The furrowed brow produces a crease between the eyebrows termed "the omega sign" (like the Greek letter Ω). Along with Veraguth folds (prominent upper eyelid folds sloping down from the midline), it forms the image of a profoundly sad face.

A young adult man engaging one patient after another in animated conversation suggests mania or a histrionic substance abuser.

A teenage boy standing at attention for hours at the front door of the inpatient unit saluting persons entering the unit is catatonic, and the playfulness of the salute suggests associated manic-depressive illness.

A middle-aged man, irritable and sluggish, staying in bed all day with blankets over his head, is an image frequently associated with cocaine withdrawal.

A plethoric, middle-aged man with a shock of white hair, broken small facial blood vessels, and a "beer belly" characterizes chronic alcoholism.

Interactions with other patients, staff and family members also reveal the patient's temperament and strains in relationships. An example of the last situation follows.

The two grown daughters of a severely depressed, newly hospitalized patient were early for a meeting with their mother's social worker and resident. They entered their mother's room as the medical team arrived on rounds. Barely greeting the attending psychiatrist and saying nothing to the mother, the daughters stood sullenly to one side while he spoke with the patient. At one point the mother reached out to caress the nearest daughter, who coldly moved out of reach. The two daughters asked no questions of the team and offered no comfort to their mother. Subsequent history-taking revealed the mother had been living with the daughter who had rejected her touch, and that the mother had delusionally accused that daughter of not caring for her and of stealing from her. This accusation created friction between the two, contributing to the hospitalization.

Parent–child relationships are often best understood in informal settings rather than in the examination room. The depressed mother may neglect a young child in the waiting area, but become harsh and physically controlling if the child becomes overly active or loud. If the child is the patient, parenting skills and the parent–child relationship will likely be observable. Does the young child take advantage of a play area? Is the toddler curious or frightened in response to all the new things to be seen in the waiting area? Is the teen sullen or interactive with the parent? Is the parent comforting?

"Free-field" behaviors

Clinicians mostly examine patients in the privacy of the office or hospital room. These settings are necessary, but restrict observation of some diagnostic and treatment-influencing information better seen when the patient is in a more open, natural setting. A medical team needing to evaluate a hospitalized patient with mania need only stand outside the nurse's station and have a conversation. The acutely ill manic will find them and interrupt.

Students of non-human primate behavior employ this "free-field" strategy when they study apes in the wild.[6] Studies of normal pre-school children interacting with their mothers in their homes,[7] and the assessment of the neural development of toddlers by comparing those at risk for developmental disorder with normal children in a laboratory play area,[8] are other examples. The famous study of Walker and Lewine (1990), successfully predicting from home movies which young children would grow up to be normal or would develop schizophrenia, underscores the importance of free-field observations. Patient 6.1 illustrates what can be missed in the structured examination setting.

Patient 6.1

A 38-year-old man was hospitalized for an exacerbation of chronic manic-depression. His behavior was ameliorated with lithium and olanzapine. After the initial improvement, however, he began to lose weight dramatically, and an occult cancer was suspected. A medical student, however, decided to go to the cafeteria with the patient to watch him eat, and noticed that the patient was unable to choose from all the items simultaneously placed on his food tray, and so he spent the meal looking from one food compartment to another rather than eating. Once his food was offered one dish at a time he ate voraciously, and quickly regained all the lost weight, making unnecessary a costly and inconvenient cancer evaluation.[9]

Age and gender

Seeing a person for the first time immediately elicits recognition of their gender, likely racial background, and approximate age. Age and gender substantially influence diagnostic considerations. Race and ethnicity affect the odds less.

In persons under age 50, for example, depressive illness is a more likely cause of cognitive decline than is dementia. A teen with a movement problem is more likely to have abused drugs or to be catatonic than to have Parkinson's disease. A mother is many times more likely than the father to experience severe depressive illness after the birth of their child.[10] Traumatic brain injury, alcoholism, and illicit drug use are more commonly seen in males; while depressive illness, and eating disorders are more often seen in females. Men are at higher risk for suicide because of their greater access to guns and their greater use of alcohol.

Although the diagnostic conclusions of some clinicians are influenced by the patient's race and ethnicity, these decisions are typically spurious. For example, 139 representative British psychiatrists completed a questionnaire about a clinical vignette of a patient with psychosis. Forms of the vignette were identical except that the gender and race of the patient varied. The psychiatrists deemed the Afro-Caribbean version to be potentially more violent and warranting criminal proceedings. They also judged this version to have a shorter illness duration and needing less antipsychotic agents. The female version was perceived as less violent, less criminal, and also less likely to need an antipsychotic agent. The Afro-Caribbian version was more often said to have a cannabis-induced or an acute reactive psychosis and less often to be schizophrenic, contrary to the claim that schizophrenia is over-diagnosed in this demographic group.[11]

Racial and gender bias in diagnosis, however, is not always found. Psychiatrists in the USA were recruited and randomly assigned to assess one of four video vignettes depicting an elderly simulated patient with a depression.[12] The vignettes were identical except for race (Euro- or African-American) and gender of the patient. Eighty-one percent of the psychiatrists correctly recognized the depression. The patient's race and gender were not associated with diagnosis, other patient characteristics, or treatment recommendations.

The modest effect of race and ethnicity upon diagnostic considerations primarily relates to co-occurring general medical and neurologic conditions associated with a particular racial or ethnic group. For example, sickle cell disease, more common in African- than Euro-Americans, can lead to vascular brain disease and behavior change. Being African-American per se, however, does not increase the risk for severe mood disorder, but being African-American does alter access to health care.[13]

Social behaviors

Every culture fosters culture-specific normative behaviors. In diverse societies, knowing the dominant cultural norms and the typical social behaviors of ethnic groups in populations being served is necessary to provide good care. Social behaviors can enrich or muddy the big picture.

A common ideal in many societies is "good manners" and "common courtesy". These social graces include saying please and thank you, appropriate turn-taking, sharing, waiting in line, and not interrupting others in conversation. Public spitting, nose picking, loud flatulence, nose blowing without a tissue, wiping one's face on one's sleeve are frowned upon in most cultures. Once acquired, social behaviors last a lifetime. The loss of social graces is associated with degenerative brain disease and behavioral disorders such as alcoholism and chronic drug abuse, and schizophrenia.

In Western countries, it is expected that, upon meeting, adult males will shake hands with brief eye contact. In many parts of Asia, hand-shaking is not the rule, and new adult male émigrés to the West reluctantly accommodate the Western standard. Western women in professional situations are increasingly adopting the adult male greeting ritual. In Japan, a simultaneous bow is preferred.

Permitting a visitor to enter a room first, a man holding a door open for a woman, standing when a person enters a room or approaches a seated person in a public setting are still common social graces in the West. These behaviors are also observed in the waiting room area, and when the patient is ushered to the examination room. The standard culture-norm greeting, however, is often altered, depending on the past relationship with the patient, and the patient's present illness acuity. For example,

A 60-year-old professional woman with a severe depressive illness was waiting to be seen by a psychiatric consultant. The physician approached the patient, introduced himself, and extending his hand in greeting. The patient rose and, rather than taking the proffered hand and responding with the customary "hello", immediately apologized for taking the doctor's "valuable time", saying that seeing someone like her was a "waste of the doctor's time".

A 50-year-old physician from the UK was seen for a diagnostic evaluation. He greeted his psychiatrist from India by theatrically raising her hand and kissing it. The patient had long history of manic-depression and had recently stopped taking his medication.

Aspects of general appearance

Level of arousal

Normal alertness is recognized when the patient can focus attention and responds to commands and requests promptly within the limits of the patient's physical strength and understanding of the instructions. Ambient room noise and minor activity are not distracting. The patient will not doze during lulls in the examination.

Increased arousal typically elicits increased motor behavior and verbal output. When arousal is mildly increased, the patient is somewhat distractible, restless, and may speak more rapidly than usual. When arousal is moderately increased, the patient appears excited, agitated, and may be hyperactive. Speech is rapid, and thought associations are distracted by ambient room activity. When increased arousal is severe, excitement is extreme, and the patient appears delirious. The patient may move and speak continuously. He may shout, scream, and require restraints to keep from self-injury. General analgesia may be present. Severe distractible speech (rambling), or flight-of-ideas, is observed. Sympathetic nervous system signs can be extreme, and before the development of sedative drugs, such patients were said to have Bell's mania, more than half succumbing to fatal arrhythmias or cardiovascular collapse. The modern term is delirious mania. Such patients will also have catatonic signs that may evolve into malignant catatonia. Increased arousal is associated with anxiety, mania or hypomania, the frontal lobe disinhibited syndrome, and stimulant drug intoxication.

In 1828, George Burrows described manic delirium that is instantly recognizable to an experienced psychiatric hospitalist.

some positive delusion exists; the patient is very loquacious and vociferous, raving incessantly, or with short intervals, during which, perhaps, a transient ray of reason gleams; or he laughs, cries, whistles, shouts, screams, or howls; is restless, full of antics, mischievous, tearing his clothes, and destroying all he can reach; is malicious, swears, prays, perhaps desperately intent on violence to himself or others; is lecherous, obscene, shameless, nasty, and indifferent to the calls of nature.[14]

Decreased arousal, due to metabolic disturbances, sedative–hypnotic, or other sedating drug intoxications is associated with reduced movement and verbal output. When arousal is mildly reduced, the patient looks fatigued and is sluggish. When arousal is moderately reduced, the patient drifts into sleep during lulls in the examination, and focuses on strong stimuli with effort. Responses are slow, speech is rambling, and examination requests are not fully understood or followed. In coma, analgesia is profound. When the reduced arousal is part of a delirium, agitation and fearfulness are commonly observed. When partial complex epilepsy is the cause, automatic motor behavior may be seen. When the reduced arousal represents benign stupor (the patient mute, immobile, and staring), depressive illness and catatonia are considered.

Stupor is also seen with brainstem lesions, infection (e.g. encephalitis lethargica), metabolic disorders, and normal pressure hydrocephalus. In benign and other stuporous states, the patient is persistently unresponsive, and general analgesia is present. When associated with melancholia, the stupor may represent severe psychomotor retardation. Melancholia attonita was the term used by Kahlbaum to describe this syndrome. When the stupor is part of the catatonic syndrome, an IV dose of a benzodiazepine can temporarily relieve the condition.

A dreamy state during which the patient is mobile and may speak and interact to a limited extent is termed oneiroid state, oneirophrenia, or oneiroid syndrome.

It occurs in both manic and depressive episodes, and has been recognized for over two centuries. Such patients appear restless and frightened. Their fears may lead to hiding in small spaces or fleeing into the street. When recovered, they describe a nightmarish experience characterized by derealization, the feeling that the world is unreal, part of a dream, flat and insubstantial. Catatonic features (stereotype, grimacing, posturing, echolalia and echopraxia) are common. Negativism and automatic obedience are almost always present. Sleep–wake cycles are perturbed and fantastic confabulations may be elicited, the patient describing grotesque events and activity outside physical possibility (e.g. a patient said "I remember my skull being removed with pliers"). Sympathetic arousal is substantial, and without appropriate treatment death due to cardiovascular collapse is reported.[15]

Hypersomnia is defined as over nine hours of sleep per day, but such patients may sleep for many more hours daily. They are difficult to arouse, and act as if drunk when awakened. Such sustained drowsiness has been associated with sedative drug intoxication, gross obesity, and low blood oxygen levels (Pickwickian syndrome), disease of the midbrain, the Klein–Levin syndrome (associated with megaphasia and mood disturbances), depressive stupor, and catatonia.[16]

Dissociation

The DSM and ICD recognize four types of dissociative disorder: amnestic, fugue, identity, and depersonalization. There is no support for these constructs as independent disease states, and they are best considered features of other established conditions (e.g. dissociative fugue as a feature of seizure disorder). The reliability and validity of dissociative identity disorder has been questioned.

Dissociative states are seen in non-ill sleep-deprived persons and those with illness (e.g. anxiety disorder, seizure disorder). Because patients commonly describe the experience as dream-like, being befogged, drugged, or "in a daze", a dysfunction in the sleep–wake cycle has been proposed as a pathophysiologic final common pathway. EEG changes during these states are similar to patterns seen in non-REM sleep, but not while dreaming.[17] The subjective experience of dissociative phenomena is also likened to severe "jet lag", where sleep patterns are disrupted. In addition to the association with sleep-like EEG changes, patients that frequently experience dissociation have an increased prevalence of sleep disorder.[18] During the dissociation, the sufferer's level of awareness is disconnected from the activation mechanisms associated with the fear response.[19] Hypothalamic–pituitary–adrenal hyperactivity dysregulation during dissociation is a consistent finding.[20] Functional imaging studies point to right cerebral hemisphere involvement.[21]

Depersonalization and derealization

Dissociative experiences are linked to depersonalization and derealization, and these phenomena can be considered to have a similar pathophysiology. They represent alterations in the normal integration of attention, thinking, emotion and memory, patients experiencing an altered reality so that they feel separated from themselves (dissociated), unreal, or "not themselves" (depersonalization), or that their immediate environment is altered, unnatural, and unreal (derealization).

Depersonalization is the subjective experience of feeling detached from oneself as if an outside observer of one's subjective experiences and actions, while simultaneously maintaining adequate accuracy of perceptions of the immediate environment. Depersonalization also involves estrangement from immediate surroundings. Episodes are unpleasant and typically brief. Depersonalization is identified by the following questions:

"Have you experienced brief episodes when you felt as if you were detached from yourself . . . as if you were watching yourself . . . as if you were floating above yourself more like an observer than the normal you . . . that you were detached from what was happening around you?"

"How often do these episodes occur? How long do they last? Are they vague experiences, or definitely different from the normal you? Does anything trigger them or warn you that one is about to happen?

Derealization is often associated with depersonalization, and is defined as experiencing the immediate environment to be strange, unfamiliar,[22] or unreal. Derealization is identified by the following questions:

"Have you experienced brief episodes when you felt that the world around you was somehow different . . . strange . . . unfamiliar . . . unreal . . . as if you were in a dream but you knew you were awake? When this happens, does the world seem like a cartoon . . . flat . . . dreamlike . . . flimsy, as if things weren't solid?"

"How often do these episodes occur? How long do they last? Are they vague experiences, or clearly different from the way things normally look and feel to you? Does anything trigger them, or warn you that one is about to happen?"

Depersonalization and derealization are symptoms, not disorders, and they do not warrant a special classification category. Depersonalization and derealization are seen in patients with anxiety disorders, early in the initial psychotic episodes of schizophrenia, in patients with chronic mood disorder, in toxic and drug-induced states (particularly hallucinogenic agents), traumatic brain injury, seizure disorder (often with a temporal lobe focus), migraine, vertigo (often associated with a panic attack), and cerebral tumors and vascular disease (often involving the left temporal lobe).[23] Other psychopathology associated with depersonalization and derealization are those classically linked to definable neurologic disease. These included Capgras syndrome, olfactory hallucinations, déjà vu and jamais vu, dysmegalopsia, and autoscopy (or heautoscopy).

Hemidepersonalization refers to the experience that one side of one's body is unreal, odd in shape or color, composed of material other than flesh and bone, or belongs to someone else. It is akin to the passivity delusion of experience of alienation. Hemidepersonalization is associated with contralateral brain disease (usually on the right with the left side of the body perceived to be different), and anosagnosia (non-recognition of illness).[24]

Dissociative amnesia

The concept of psychogenic amnesia has been challenged, and a historical review finding no evidence of such a syndrome before the nineteenth century concluded that it is a cultural, not a natural phenomenon.[25] Psychogenic or dissociative amnesia is said to be precipitated by stress and to involve profound retrograde amnesia. Memory for personal events is said to be more affected than is memory for public events. Autobiographic memory is reported to be substantially impaired.[26] But a recent literature review concluded that: "it may be impossible to distinguish among dissociative, factitious, and malingered amnesia. In addition, elements of each may coexist in the same patient. Suffice it to say that all three conditions are disorders of behavior, not diseases of the brain."[27]

In the neurologic literature the concept of transient global amnesia (TGA) comes closest to the description of dissociative amnesia, and all patients with the complaint of sudden recent memory loss should be presumed to have a neurologic explanation for their memory problems. TGA is defined as abrupt onset, temporary anterograde amnesia without focal neurologic signs. Language, perception and procedural memory are intact.[28] Retrograde amnesia is variably affected.[29] Despite its image as a benign condition, long-term cognitive impairment occurs in verbal fluency, memory for new events, and autobiographical memory.[30] TGA is associated with migraine, epilepsy, and cerebral vascular disease. These etiologies, however, may not be initially clinically obvious and each is associated with altered arousal, encouraging the dissociative amnesia diagnosis.[31]

A recent literature review and presentation of 142 additional patients with TGA prospectively examined over a 10-year period clarifies the syndrome.[32] Two-thirds were women, although in the literature, gender representation is about equal. The majority of attacks occurred between ages 50 and 80. The typical attack lasted about 4h. All of the studied patients underwent careful neurologic examination, and the majority was also assessed with EEG and CT scan. Some had a Doppler scan of their supra-aortic blood vessels. Twenty-five percent of the EEG studies were abnormal, but non-specific. About 8% had abnormalities on CT scan, and only one of 41 Doppler assessments revealed an abnormality.

The lack of a clear association between a defined brain lesion and the amnesia is consistent with other studies. Functional imaging is the most productive laboratory aid for such patients, but this technology was not typically used. When imaging was done in this case series and in other case series, abnormalities in the hippocampus and frontal circuitry are reported. Of the 142 patients, 129 had a possible contributing medical history, including hypertension and migraine. Previous psychiatric disease was present in about 40% of the sample, particularly personality problems. Almost 90% of attacks followed an event considered stressful (e.g. a medical procedure, coitus, family conflict, physical labor, and a period of exhaustion).

Although focal neurologic signs preclude the diagnosis, other symptoms were found, including headache, nausea, and emesis, dizziness, chills or flushes, and severe sudden anxiety. The authors concluded that migraine was the most likely neurologic cause of TGA in younger patients, and personality deviation and stress was a contributing factor in women.

Dissociative fugue

Fugue refers to a sudden loss of all autobiographical memory and sense of personal identity, with a period of wandering for which there is an amnestic gap upon recovery. Documented fugue states last several minutes to a few hours. The most common cause of fugue is seizure disorder or other defined neurologic disease (see Patient 6.2). Mood disorder is the next most likely associated condition, and such patients will often have features of catatonia and the fugue state an example of benign stupor. Dramatic stories of a person suddenly losing all biographical memory, disappearing and returning months or years later with a different identity in a different community are fraudulent.[33] An example of a fugue associated with neurologic disease follows.

Patient 6.2

A middle-aged man found himself in a van by the side of the road nearly 30 miles from his home. He had no memory for how he got there. Although this experience occurred several times yearly, he said nothing about it to his family or to his physicians. Finally, the police saw his van weaving erratically along that county road and when the van stopped, they found the man to be disoriented and making no sense in his responses to questions. His blood alcohol level was zero, and a subsequent urine drug screen was negative. Further evaluation identified a seizure disorder and his traveling as a post-ictal fugue.

Dissociative identity disorder (multiple personality disorder)

The existence of dissociative identity disorder (DID) is controversial. Its psychodynamic understanding is not validated. The notion that DID represents a fluctuation in one of two aspects of the sense of self relies on a few methodologically weak studies.[34] This construct envisions a "core sense of self" (a cerebral representation of one's momentary body state that lacks a sense of past and imagined future) and an "autobiographic sense of self" (long-term memories influenced by environment and disease). When dysfunctional, the latter elicits different autobiographic selves, i.e. DID.[35] In a review of the DID literature, Piper and Merskey[36] concluded that it was not a valid condition and that over the next decade it would have "a steep decline . . . and a gradual fall into near oblivion thereafter". They point out that most such patients fluctuate over time in meeting criteria for DID, and that only 20% have any features meeting criteria at initial evaluation. Diagnostic criteria are vague and over-inclusive so that it can "be defined anyway imaginable". The alleged increase in its prevalence is also artificial, the associated legal proceedings in many such patients hinting at malingering or manipulation of the patient by a treater.

Other studies indicate that some patients with the DID diagnosis have conditions that explain their sudden shifts in temperament, particularly manic-depression.[37] Depression is reported in nearly 90% of such patients,[38] and seizure disorder is found as the source of symptoms in many.[39] Mesulam (1981) reports 12 patients with DID, finding them to have partial complex epilepsy with likely temporal lobe involvement. Devinsky and associates (1989) identified six patients with DID, but could not find them to have active EEG seizures during their dissociative episodes. However, Ahern and colleagues (1993), finding an association between DID and temporal lobe epilepsy, point out that the temperament changes in DID are not dependent on the seizure discharge per se, but are related to dominant versus non-dominant cerebral hemispheric changes in activation. They stress that in documented cases of DID in the neurologic literature two temperament patterns are the rule, not patients with high numbers of "personalities". The patients reporting high numbers of "personalities" are likely the product of therapist influences.

Differences in hemisphere activation as assessed by EEG is reported in patients with the DID diagnosis, but the meaning of these findings is unclear.[40] Hippocampal and amygdala volumes are also reported to be smaller in patients with DID, but these findings are also seen in patients who, like the DID samples studied, experienced sustained substantial stress in childhood.[41]

Patient 6.3 illustrates the needless diagnosis of DID in a patient with migraine and co-occurring seizure disorder.

Patient 6.3

A 36-year-old woman was referred to a consultant with the diagnoses of bipolar mood disorder and identity disorder. She experienced her first

depression at age 8, a second at age 11, and then many episodes of depression and mania afterward. Her depressions were characterized by profound anergia with social isolation, despondency, and apprehension. In later episodes, hallucinated voices encouraged her to kill herself. Her manias were characterized by irritability and grandiosity.

In her late teens she drank alcohol heavily, but after age 20 she rarely drank. She denied all illicit drug use. Her father was an alcoholic. Two of her three brothers were alcoholic. Her mother had manic-depression, as did several members of her father's family. The patient had no significant general medical problem, and never had a head injury. Her development was normal, but her periods were never regular, and she had been taking five-day courses of progesterone every three months for many years to induce them. She showed no other signs of an endocrinopathy or developmental problem.

Since her teens, the patient suffered from migraine, ranging from one to seven monthly. Her headaches often began with scotoma, but at other times with a panoply of sensory experiences. Her headaches began over the right temple and then generalized. Associated nausea and photophobia often incapacitated her for a day or more. Her mother also had migraine.

Beginning in her late teens, the patient began to experience multiple episodes of hallucinosis usually lasting a few minutes. When looking in the mirror in the morning, and occasionally at other times, she sometimes clearly saw that she had a different person's face. Sometimes she experienced great anxiety before seeing the image, but not always. At other times she saw "ghosts", vague shadowy ominous figures walking to and fro in front of her. She also saw "bugs" that sometimes looked "real" and at other times like "sci-fi creatures". The bugs sometimes covered her body. She could feel as well as see them. These experiences were often preceded by headache different from the migraine, sudden anxiety, a feeling as if intoxicated, or intense total body skin discomfort leading her to remove her clothes. Sometimes she fell to the floor for no apparent reason, but only recalled losing consciousness twice. At other times she lost periods of time, usually for several minutes, but she believed one or two lasted for "weeks". Many of her longer memory lapses occurred during an exacerbation of her mood disorder.

Because of her erratic moods her job history was poor. When describing her changing moods, some of her sensory experiences and time losses to an employment counselor, she was advised that she had multiple personality disorder. When she saw this phrase in a note by her psychiatrist she concluded the diagnosis was confirmed. Based on the different faces she saw in the mirror and the frequency of time losses, she estimated that she had 140 different personalities and gave names to those faces in the mirror that recurred.

In addition to antipsychotic medication and lithium for her mood disorder and "psychosis", she had been receiving therapy for her "identity disorder".

Other than having substantial extrapyramidal side effects from rispiridone and mild circumstantiality, the patient was without psychopathology on examination. She seemed to be a mild-mannered, dependent and easily influenced person. Anticonvulsant and adjunct management strategies for seizure disorder were recommended and the patient made a slow recovery over the next several months.

Grooming, hygiene and dress

Although the degree of grooming and hygiene and what a person wears is influenced by social class, and culture, appearance may also reflect personality deviation and brain disease. The histrionic person dresses more flamboyantly and sexually provocatively. The person with antisocial personality disorder may wear the intimidating black leather, metal-studded costume of "the biker". Elaborate tattoos, body piercing and complicated hair design (e.g. the Apache with brightly colored spikes) reflect at a minimum high novelty seeking and non-conformity.[42] Perfectly lacquered finger and toe nails, carefully applied facial make-up, highly styled hair-do, all-year tan take substantial time and effort to accomplish and represent at best vanity and self-absorption. The sloppiness of Oscar Madison and the neatness of Felix Unger, the characters in Neil Simon's *The Odd Couple*, represent their deviant personality traits.[43]

Being reasonably clean and neat is an accepted norm in many societies. A loss of this standard implies disease. When a person no longer adequately self-grooms and cleans despite the means, general medical functioning, and visual acuity to do so, the most likely cause is poor executive functioning and self-monitoring. The disheveled and unclean patient has lost interest or the ability to attend to the task and the recognition of the problem. Severe and chronic mood disorder, brain damage from trauma and illicit drug use, and dementing conditions are common causes. Unilateral grooming and hygiene problems indicate contralateral brain disease. A patient with a right parietal lobe lesion failed to shave the left side of his face. He first denied any asymmetry in his beard. When pressed to explain it, he said "I'm letting my sideburns grow". When shown that only one side of his face was involved he became irritable and uncooperative.

Persons with substantial perseverative behaviors may collect debris and other items, hoarding them on their person – pockets bulging, shopping bags filled to the bursting with useless items. In the 1950s in New York City, the homeless women of that era were called "shopping bag ladies". Playing with, smearing, or ingesting feces (coprophagia) is seen in patients with severe mood disorder, psychosis, dementia, or mental retardation.

Self-decoration that includes tattoos, body piercing, make-up and clothing are acceptable adornments in moderation in Westerners raised after 1960. When excessive and beginning early in life, these choices reflect personality deviation. When they occur for the first time after maturation and are strikingly different from previous appearance, they indicate disease. For example,

A Euro-American physician whose demeanor and appearance had always been that of the stereotypic middle-class Mid West suddenly let his hair grow long and dressed in loose-fitting clothes of African patterns. He lost substantial weight. A year latter his erratic behavior was clearly evident and subsequently he was arrested for using and selling illicit drugs.

Excessive self-decoration has been recognized since the nineteenth century in association with manic-depressive illness. Staid European women overwhelmed by mania are described wearing brightly colored turbans, drapery, beads, and feathers. Manic men are pictured wearing decorative flowers and military paraphernalia. Manic patients continue to excessively self-decorate. Patient 4.3 dressed as Robin Hood is an example. The following vignettes also illustrate.

A middle-aged manic man calling himself "a preacher" was hospitalized for loud public orations and irritability during the height of the summer heat. He spoke rapidly, his words overflowing each other. He was wearing 12 overcoats and several hats.

A middle-aged manic-depressive man dressed himself in a paper suit and hat made from the cartoon section of a Sunday paper. In this garb he loudly and intrusively harangued passers-by in the street. In the hospital, he stood on a chair in the dayroom "addressing" other patients.

An elderly, chronically ill manic-depressive man prowled the hospital grounds wearing a raincoat, every inch of its surface covered with campaign and other novelty buttons. He clinked as he walked and on fair days the sun reflected off his buttons as if they were electrified.

A middle-aged manic-depressive man dressed entirely in black leather, including a black leather helmet, ran down Fifth Avenue in New York City with long kitchen knives attacking sky-scrapers, mimicking Don Quixote attacking windmills.

Sudden changes in culture-specific behaviors in émigrés that cannot be readily explained by efforts at acculturation may also reflect illness.

A 46-year-old timid housewife from India who always spoke to her elder brother-in-law in a soft voice and with downcast eyes, and who covered her hair in deference, when manic abandoned the head cover and started calling her brother-in-law by his first name, a highly unusual interaction for Indians. She also publicly blamed him for her marital failure.

Manic patients often decorate their heads. Men shave one side of their head hair or beard. Women manic patients place their hair in exaggerate styles. They use elaborate make-up schemes with garish colors not typical of their euthymic taste. They wear bedsheets and towels as if togas, or scanty, sexually provocative clothing untypical of their usual dress. The semi-nudity is associated with inappropriate sexual advances to staff and other patients. One manic-depressive physician came to work only in her white coat and high heels. Patients who suddenly remove all their clothes without apparent sexual intent, however, are more likely to be delirious or demented, or in a post-ictal state.

When ill, manic patients cannot give a clear reason for the change in their appearance. They may cite a delusional belief or become irritable and threatening. An early sign of treatment response is the attempt to normalize the decorative changes made during the height of the mania. Manic men who shave one side of their head or beard suddenly shave the other side. When asked about the change toward norm they often respond "It looked silly".

Body size and shape

A person's body build may communicate personality traits and disease. The body builder's exaggerated musculature conveys histrionic traits. The skeletal look of the anorectic is defining. Bulimic and manic-depressive patients tend toward obesity; the latter may also be large-framed and big-boned (endomorphic).[44] The rounded "moon face" and fatty deposit at the base of the neck ("buffalo hump") characterizes Cushing's disease. A wasted musculature and large abdomen suggests chronic alcoholism. Developmental and genetic disorders such as Down's syndrome (short stocky stature, thick neck, wide-spaced eyes with an epicanthic fold), fragile-X syndrome (long, narrow face, prominent ears, other large facial features, velvety skin and large gonads),[45] Marfan's syndrome (long thin skeleton with disproportionately long arm span, and large hands and feet), XYY syndrome (unusually tall man with acne), and many others have been associated with behavioral syndromes. Dysplastic features (disproportionate size of body parts such as limbs too long or short for the torso, small head circumference, ectopic features such as low-set ears and wide-spaced eyes) are associated with developmental problems and behavioral symptoms emerging in childhood.

Examination of the patient's skin is also important. Scars may indicate violence, surgery, self-harm and IV or subcutaneous drug use. Abnormal tanning is associated with Addison's disease. Jaundice is associated with liver dysfunction. Lyme disease, syphilis, and other infectious agents produce tell-tale lesions. Dry skin, brittle nails, and sticky hair suggest depression or hypothyroidism. Palmar erythema, broken nasal blood vessels and rhinophyma, and spider angiomata indicate alcoholism.

Assessing for minor physical anomalies is also revealing. These mostly cosmetic reflections of either a genetic or gestational perturbation are recognized in infancy and are stable over the person's lifetime. Many non-ill persons exhibit one or two. The presence of four or more, however, suggests that an adverse obstetrical event occurred that may have contributed to the present psychopathology.

Table 6.1. Minor physical anomalies

Head

    Abnormal circumference (norm for adult males 21–23 inches; for females 20.5–22.5 inches)

    More than one central hair whorl

    "Electric" hair (remains erect despite combing)

    Low-set ears (entirely below the plane of the pupils)

    Malformed or asymmetrical ears

    Close-set (hypotelorism) or far-set (hypertelorism) eyes

    Abnormal epicanthic folds

    Wide-spaced nares and upper lip furrow hinting of subthreshold cleft lip

    Furrowed tongue

    High arched palate, bifurcated uvula

Hands and feet

    Curved small finger (clinodactyly)

    Single palmar crease

    Wide gap between the first and second toe

    Third toe larger than second toe

    Partial syndactyly of toes

Schizophrenic patients and persons with conduct disorder and violent criminal behavior are found to have such features. Table 6.1 displays the commonly seen minor physical anomalies.[46]

Manner

Manner refers to the general characteristic tenor of the patient's interactions with the examiner. The degree of cooperativeness is noted. Suspiciousness and hostility suggests delusional thinking or lack of candor.[47] Indifference to the examination despite obvious dysfunction suggests apathy or avolition, or denial of illness. Failure to make eye contact is seen in depression, catatonia, and autistic spectrum disorders. Over-eager persistent questions and demands (importunate behavior) is seen in mania and other frontal lobe disinhibited syndromes. When associated with agitation, importunate behavior suggests depressive illness. The process of personality assessment begins by broadly characterizing the patient's temperament (e.g. mild mannered, shy, outgoing).

Gestures, facial expression and body language

As people converse they also communicate non-verbally. Facial expression changes with mood. The norm is modest variability during social interaction. An expressionless face throughout most of an evaluation is abnormal. Reduced facial expression is associated with reduced arousal, catatonia, Parkinsonism, depressive stupor, schizophrenia and frontal lobe apathetic syndromes, and motor aprosodia. The patient with melancholia may have an unwavering gaze, as if staring into an abyss. Patients who are toxic from antipsychotic medication will have a blank, stiffened look, with a greasy skin sheen from sebaceous gland hypersecretion. Manic patients will have increased skin turgor and a wide-eyed animation. Schizophrenics will offer little facial expression and will indifferently shift their attention.

Body language is an aspect of interpersonal communication. When persons converse they assume similar postures as their listeners, and these postural behaviors are considered to have evolved as enhancers of communication and cooperation among primates.[48] Body language also conveys the person's emotional state and aids in the interpretation of facial expression. It is easier for an observer to correctly identify a person's emotional state when facial expression and body language are congruent. For example, a person who paces vigorously, shouts in a language unknown to the observer, and is wide-eyed with clenched jaw and tight fists, is angry. If the same person is laughing rather than shouting, the valence of the person's emotional expression is unclear. Body language can convey happiness, sadness, fear, pain, and anger.[49] The importance of body language as an expression of a patient's emotional state is recognized by dentists, nurses managing pain in patients who are cognitively or verbally impaired, clinicians caring for potentially violent patients, psychotherapists, and assessors of psychopathology.[50]

Intense mood of any valence is a state of heightened arousal, and thus typically associated with increased activity. Anger is also associated with approach behaviors. The angry person stands and assumes the largest posture possible while looking directly at the person who may be the target of aggression. Feet are wide-spaced, hands may be clenched into fists, the upper body may be thrust forward, as is the head and jaw. Manic patients may stand too close to the examiner or prolong eye contact. The fearful person withdraws and will try to appear small, look down and away, and when terrified, tensely huddle. The sad person will slump and also make little eye contact.

Hand gesturing during conversation is linked to speech production as these movements have overlapping neurologic underpinnings. Speech-related gestures vary in intensity across cultures and ethnic groups, but hand gesturing during speech production is universal and occurs even when the speaker knows that others cannot see the gestures (e.g. during a phone call).[51] Congenitally blind persons gesture when speaking with each other.[52] Speech-related hand gestures freeze at the same time speech is disturbed in persons who stutter while non-speech-related hand movements continue normally.[53] Speech gesturing is seen in infants, and is hypothesized as an early step in language development and learning.[54] Adults show laterality differences in speech gesture during conversation, men when listening making increased left-hand gestures, while women show no laterality, a finding consistent with other gender differences in cerebral laterality.[55]

Larger arm movements during speech are hypothesized to facilitate spatial representations in working memory during the conversation and close scrutiny of persons conversing reveals that these larger gestures mimic the shape or spatial idea of what is being discussed.[56] One schizophrenic man with formal thought disorder repeatedly used the neologism "glob" while making a hand movement indicating putting on a glove, thus providing the meaning of his phonemic paraphasia. Such representative hand movements are helpful clues to understanding patients with word-finding difficulties.

A patient who does not gesture during the conversational aspects of the evaluation has dysfunction in the motor system, the language system, or both. Left hemisphere strokes in pure right-handed men are associated with loss of gesture laterality.[57] Manic patients exaggerate their speech gestures, while depressed patients and those with Alzheimer's disease have reduced gesturing.[58]

Summary

The form of the psychopathology of behavioral syndromes is consistent across cultures and, for many syndromes, across centuries. The image of melancholia, mania, neurasthenia, and obsessive–compulsive disorder is recognizable worldwide and from texts from antiquity. The patient's dress, hygiene, manner, and general behaviors are all reflections of brain function as well as culture and subculture, and when deviant, shape differential diagnosis.

NOTES

1 Fish (1967, p. 1).
2 "Odd" does not necessarily mean "bad", just as "deviance" and "abnormal" do not always mean disease. A person with a 150 IQ is statistically deviant on that measure. Professional athletes are deviant in their skills because most persons cannot perform at their level.
3 Mason (2000).
4 Todorov *et al.* (2005).
5 Rapoport *et al.* (1995).
6 Goodall and Van Lawick (1971).
7 Wahler *et al.* (2001).
8 Hempel (1993).
9 Being able to make a decision among choices is an executive function. The famous neurophysiologist, Aleksandr Luria, describes an experiment in which he damaged the frontal

lobes of dogs. When the dogs were hungry he fed them. When he offered them one bowl of food they ate voraciously. When offered two bowls of food they stood at the bowls going first to one then the other, but not eating (Luria, 1963, pp. 89–90).

10 See Taylor and Fink (2006, patient 6.5) for a description of a man who experienced an episode of melancholia following the birth of his first child.

11 Lewis *et al.* (1990).

12 Kales *et al.* (2005).

13 Carrington (2006).

14 Burrows (1976), page 346.

15 Fink and Taylor (2003).

16 Critchley (1962).

17 Giesbrecht *et al.* (2006).

18 Watson (2001).

19 Das *et al.* (2005); Williams *et al.* (2006b).

20 Simeon *et al.* (2007).

21 Markowitsch (1999); Yasuno *et al.* (2000).

22 This definition overlaps with the definition for jamais vu, the false memory that previously encountered people, places or things are unfamiliar.

23 Lambert *et al.* (2002).

24 Critchley (1953).

25 Pope *et al.* (2007).

26 Kopelman (1996).

27 Brandt and Van Gorp (2006).

28 Hodges and Warlow (1990).

29 Ibid.

30 Guillery-Girard *et al.* (2006).

31 Santos *et al.* (2000); Gallassi (2006).

32 Quinette *et al.* (2006).

33 Kopelman (1996).

34 Saxe *et al.* (1992); Reinders *et al.* (2003).

35 Parvizi and Damascio (2001); Reinders *et al.* (2003).

36 Piper (1994); Piper and Merskey (2004).

37 Savitz *et al.* (2004).

38 Coons *et al.* (1988).

39 Mesulam (1981); Devinsky *et al.* (1989); Ahern *et al.* (1993).

40 Flor-Henry *et al.* (1990).

41 Vermetten *et al.* (2006).

42 A study assessing tattoos in a sample of patients presenting to a Minneapolis emergency department found no association between the presence of a tattoo and psychopathology. Of patients under age 35, 35% had a tattoo as did 19% of the staff (Rooks *et al.*, 2000).

43 *The Odd Couple*, Neil Simon, 1965.

44 The classic work of Kretschmer and Sheldon on body type and illness is reviewed and quantified by Parnell (1958).

45 Half of male patients with fragile X are hyperactive as children, all have attentional problems, about 15% have seizure disorder, and many have Autism spectrum disorder (Fein *et al.*, 1996).

46 Ovsiew (1997).

47 Psychiatric patients, however, do not knowingly lie with any greater degree than other patients (Udell, 1994; Rissmiller *et al.*, 1998).

48 Shockley *et al.* (2003).

49 Meeren *et al.* (2005).

50 Freeman (1992); Gabe and Sjoquest (2002); Rapoport *et al.* (1995); Cembrowicz and Shepherd (1992); Herdieckerhoff (1985); De Boucaud (1971).

51 Nishitani *et al.* (2005).

52 Goldin-Meadow (1999).

53 Mayberry and Jacques (2000).

54 Goldin-Meadow and Wagner (2005).

55 Saucier and Elias (2001).

56 Morsella and Krauss (2004); Miller and Franz (2005).

57 Foundas *et al.* (1995).

58 Carlomagno *et al.* (2005).

7

Disturbances of motor function

If the proper study of mankind is man, the proper study of mental illness starts with the description of how he thinks and feels inside – chaos of thought and passion, all confused.[1]

Abnormal movements have been recognized as aspects of behavioral illness for millennia, and all severe psychiatric conditions are associated with changes in motor functioning. Changes can be subtle and non-specific, limited to restlessness that suggests anxiety, or dramatic and diagnostic, such as the classic postures indicating catatonia. Kraepelin and Bleuler both describe choreiform movements of the face and fingers, tremor, dysdiadochokinesia, and ataxia as features of schizophrenia, Kraepelin referring to "a cerebellar form" of dementia praecox.[2] A modern study of 100 patients with the diagnosis of schizophrenia found 98 exhibited motor disturbances *before* the antipsychotic era.[3]

Abnormal movements are often associated with problems in executive and other cognitive processes, and frontal lobe structural and metabolic abnormalities.[4] Intense emotion adversely affects this brain region, and there also is a strong association between motor function and mood.[5] Several investigators consider melancholia a disorder of both mood and motor functioning.[6] The most common associations of motor and mood disturbance are listed in Table 7.1.

Without movement there is no emotional expression, which is recognized only with changes in facial muscle positioning, gestures, body language and vocal inflection. Fear-circuitry and flight/fight processes link fear and anger to motor responses necessary for species survival.[7] The triggering of avoidance or approach behaviors requires the correct processing of facial recognition and the emotional expressions of others.[8]

The motor system, linked to emotional expression, also plays a role in motivated behavior: most basic are drives to seek food, and eating and drinking behaviors.[9] When this system is dysfunctional, as in catatonia and melancholia, patients are avolitional and apathetic, and may starve and become dehydrated. The cerebellum, another component of the motor system, is implicated in the

Table 7.1. Diseases commonly associated with motor and mood disorder

Parkinson's disease	Encephalitis
Huntington's disease	Demyelinating disease
Wilson's disease	Stroke
Alzheimer's disease	Autoimmune disease
Epilepsy	Toxic encephalopathy
Migraine	Endocrinopathies
Traumatic brain injury	Melancholia
Schizophrenia	Mania
Autistic spectrum disorder	

pathogenesis of autistic spectrum disorders and schizophrenia.[10] Both conditions are characterized by abnormal emotional expression, including the movements of emotions (e.g. facial expression, hand gestures), and in the recognition of the emotional valence expressed by others.[11] The examinations of motor and emotion systems are conjoined. Understanding their related psychopathology is essential to diagnosing behavioral syndromes.

Disturbances in activity

Abnormal activity level is common among patients with behavioral illness. Determining what the patient does during a typical day or observing the patient in the waiting area, examining room, or in the common areas of the inpatient unit reveals many of these disturbances.

Hyperactivity

Hyperactive patients exhibit many actions simultaneously or in a short period of time. They rush from one undertaking to the next. Severe hyperactivity appears as frenzy, the patient failing to complete even simple household or personal hygiene tasks. The lack of an apparent goal in the plethora of activity, however, does not delineate syndromes. It is a sign of severity, not of specific pathophysiology. Hyperactivity is the motor equivalent of distractibility and flight-of-ideas (thought associations that jump from topic to topic). It is a classic feature of mania and stimulant drug intoxication.

When severe, hyperactivity is associated with excitement (extreme hyperarousal and intense emotional expression), a state termed manic delirium. Almost all such patients will have catatonic features.[12] A hyperkinetic state is also seen in children with complex partial seizures. This state can be intense, involving frenetic movements of the extremities and trunk. Flailing, kicking, screaming, and shouting occur. Intense fear may be present. Alteration in consciousness is minimal, making recognition challenging, and sufferers can be misdiagnosed as having attention-deficit hyperactivity disorder, conduct disorder, mood disorder, or non-epileptic (pseudo) seizures. A developmental history and video monitored EEG assessment are helpful in recognizing the syndrome.[13] An example of manic delirium follows.

Patient 7.1

A 33-year-old man was brought to an emergency room by the police who found him running through the streets nude on a cold, wintry night. He was yelling at imaginary persons and fought the police, who had to restrain him. Urine drug screen was negative and other laboratory test results were normal.

His rapid-fire speech was of flight-of-ideas and strings of clang associations (associations by sound rather than meaning). His mood was labile, shifting rapidly from euphoria to irritability, to laughing while crying. Any distraction elicited a comment and a new string of associations. When directly questioned (whispering the questions helped to temporarily gain his attention) he automatically repeated the question and then laughed. He required seclusion and restraints, sedation having little effect. When tied into a chair with a bed sheet as an alternative to seclusion he struggled to walk about the unit, the chair on his back, like a snail shell. His constant speech left him hoarse. He refused all food and drink. High doses of sedatives had no effect. ECT was prescribed, and two bilateral ECT on two consecutive days broke the manic delirium. ECT was continued in the usual schedule and he made an uneventful recovery.

Hypoactivity

Hypoactive patients do little. When severe, the patient remains idle for hours, accomplishing little, even the simplest of household or personal hygiene chores. Reduced speech and thought and a paucity of ideas are typically present. Hypoactivity is a feature of avolition and apathy, stupor, depressive illness, and schizophrenia. When due to sedative drug intoxication, alertness is also reduced.

Severe anxiety also elicits immobility, and thus hypoactivity, the patient appearing terrified. Hypoactivity is distinguished from motor retardation (slowing of movement) and stupor (hypoactivity with reduced arousal). All stuporous patients and patients with substantial motor slowing are hypoactive, but not all hypoactive patients are slow in movement and most are not in a stupor.

Agitation

Agitation is increased frequency of non-goal-directed movements as opposed to the increased actions of hyperactivity. Agitation is the motor expression of an intense mood. It can be mild, with restlessness and fidgeting, and picking at bed sheets, or it can be severe, such as constant hand wringing, head and face rubbing, pacing, and frenzy. Agitation is observed in depression and mixed mood syndromes, states of anxiety and excitement, delirium, and drug intoxication.

Agitation and hypoactivity may occur simultaneously in melancholic depression, and combined with reduced interactiveness identifies this depressive illness.[14] Psychomotor disturbance is the most recognized feature in almost all studies that identify melancholia,[15] and is as fundamental to melancholia as are vegetative signs.[16] In a review of factor and cluster analytic studies of depression, Nelson and Charney (1981) concluded that psychomotor change was the clearest and most consistent feature associated with melancholia. Among nine operational definitions of melancholia, Rush and Weisenberger (1994) reported psychomotor retardation to be the single feature common to all. Five of the nine definitions also included agitation.

Akathesia

Akathesia is a state of motor restlessness, the patient unable to sit or be still. Akathesia can be mistaken for anxiety, but sufferers describe a subjective feeling of jitteriness or terrible restlessness of the muscles, rather than apprehension. They say "I can't sit still ... I'm jumping out of my skin". Motor stereotypy is an associated finding, including purposeless self touching, picking at clothing, rocking, and repeatedly shifting position. Patients may continuously retrace their steps, march in place, and sit, then stand, and then sit again. When drug-induced, akathesia occurs early in treatment, and antipsychotic drugs and SSRI are common offenders. When it persists after the offending agent is stopped, it is termed tardive akathesia. Akathesia occurring early in treatment presages future tardive dyskinesia.[17]

Gait problems

The patient's gait reflects general medical health, the presence of musculoskeletal disease, neurologic impairment, and psychiatric disorder. The ability to walk affects treatment outcome and disposition.[18]

Many conditions affect gait. Slowed gait is seen in depressive illness, hypothyroidism, frontal–temporal dementia, and sedative drug intoxication. A jerky, bird-like gait is seen in persons who chronically abuse stimulant drugs. Cerebellar ataxia (unsteady trunk, wide-based gait with leg intentional tremor) is seen in intoxications and destructive disease of the cerebellum. A spastic gait (abnormally stiff and awkward) is seen in myelopathies and upper neuron disease. A wide-based gait suggests peripheral nerve disease or proprioception problems, both often the results of alcoholism. A hesitant gait, as if hit in the chest by a strong wind, is characteristic of Huntington's disease. Small, rapidly increasing steps (festination) with loss of arm swing signals Parkinsonism.[19] A flexed posture of the trunk while walking and decreased arm swing without rigidity are seen in patients with frontal lobe dementias. A gait apraxia, the slipping clutch syndrome, is recognized when a patient with adequate elementary neurologic function has difficulty starting to walk and then does so in bursts of small steps. Many musculoskeletal diseases elicit difficulties in walking.[20]

Disturbances of motor regulation

Difficulty regulating one's movement despite adequate muscle strength is a hallmark of many behavioral syndromes and includes "soft neurologic signs", features of neurologic disturbance, but less localizing than classic aphasias and paralysis.[21] When these features dominate the clinical picture, the evaluation should first focus on the identification of structural brain disease.

Pathological inertia

When adequate limb function is present and the patient understands the task, movement should be started quickly and ended immediately when the task is completed. Failing to promptly start, hesitation and false starts as if to gain momentum, and persisting of movement when no longer appropriate define pathological inertia. Pathological inertia is seen in patients with frontal lobe dementia, Parkinsonism, depressive illness, and schizophrenia. Catalepsy with its prolonged immobility is an extreme form of pathological inertia.

Perseveration and impersistence

Motor perseveration is the unnecessary repetition or continuation of movement or position beyond what is needed and despite injunctions that the movement should stop. Impersistence is the inability to continue a movement or maintain a position until told to stop (15 s). Assessment includes asking the patient to make a fist, keep his eyes closed, and hold his arms out. Motor overflow is also considered with these tasks.

Adventitious motor overflow

Unneeded extra movements that occur during a task are signs of motor dysregulation. A young child sticking the tip of his tongue out while practicing his letters is an example of overflow that usually resolves with maturation.

Choreiform movements, involuntary sudden brief twisting jerks, may occur when a patient is asked to hold his arms out in front, palms down. When pronounced, as in Huntington's disease, the patient may try to disguise the movement by continuing it as a voluntary or habitual act such as brushing hair from the forehead. Overflow is also elicited by having the patient walk. Pronounced extension of the fingers (fork hand) or other unnecessary hand postures may be seen. In its severest form, chorea is seen as writhing, dancing movements.

Fine motor problems

Rapid finger tapping requires sustained attention and fine motor control. The patient is asked to tap his index finger as rapidly as possible for 20 s, palm flat on a table or thigh. When motor strength is adequate and arthritis is minimal, 40 or more taps with the preferred hand is an expected performance in persons under 70 years of age. Healthy older persons achieve 30 or more taps in 20 s. As one hand performs, the other, also palm down on a thigh or table, is watched for overflow. Drumming one's fingers in sequence from little to index finger combines finger tapping with motor sequencing. Patients with chronic behavioral conditions commonly have problems with finger tapping and motor sequencing. Poor performance is a sign of basal ganglia disease, hypothyroidism, and depressive illness.[22]

Motor sequencing difficulty

The completion of a task requires a sequence of movements. Skilled sequences (e.g. suturing) are over-learned. The ability to create novel motor sequences is necessary in learning new tasks, and is tested by asking the patient to perform a simple continuous movement. Motor strength must be adequate and the patient must understand the task. The patient is instructed to use one palm, a thigh or table top as the surface and then to rapidly place the other hand in a fist on that surface, raise it, come back down with the side of the opened hand, raise it, and come back down with the palm on the surface. The sequence of fist, hand edge, palm is repeated five times with each hand. Abnormal performance includes slow, awkward and hesitant movement, out of sequence movements, repeating a movement (perseveration), and combining movements (e.g. hitting the surface with the hand edge as the fingers flex into a weak fist). Patients with depressive illness will have problems with sequencing that resolve with episode remission. Sequencing problems persist in patients with chronic psychotic disorders and disease in the frontal lobes.

Catatonia[23]

Catatonia is a syndrome of motor dysregulation. Variations of catatonia range from patients with a few features to those whose catatonia dominates the clinical picture. Many conditions elicit catatonia. The most common sources are mood disorder, toxic metabolic and drug-induced states, seizure disorder, disease or trauma to frontal lobe circuits, and psychotic disorders. Why only some patients with these conditions develop catatonia is unclear.[24]

When systematically examined, about 10% of consecutive admissions to acute psychiatric hospitals exhibit two or more catatonic features.[25] Forty percent or more of manic patients meet criteria for catatonia. Many patients with melancholia exhibit several catatonic features. Institutionalized persons with developmental disabilities commonly exhibit catatonic features.

The classic image of catatonia is the Kahlbaum's syndrome, named to honor Karl Ludvig Kahlbaum who first defined catatonia in 1874. The patient is mute, immobile, stares off into space, and is in a prolonged posture (often mundane). But there are many gradations of this picture which can fluctuate with other behaviors, particularly depressive and manic symptoms. So-called "catatonic excitement" is the emergence of an underlying mania and not a unique syndrome.

Catatonia can be profound, presenting with extreme rigidity, the patient frozen in a posture and mute. Fever is common in such patients and can be high. Vital signs fluctuate dangerously. When described in the nineteenth and early twentieth centuries as lethal catatonia, most sufferers died from renal or heart failure. Now termed malignant catatonia, the syndrome responds to proper treatment.

Malignant catatonia is induced by the sudden withdrawal of dopaminergic drugs, or the inappropriate prescription of antipsychotic and related D2 blocking drugs or serotonergic agents. The neuroleptic malignant syndrome (NMS) is indistinguishable from malignant catatonia that occurs for other reasons. Muscle rigidity and other catatonic features are always present. Fever, unstable vital signs, elevated serum creatinine phosphokinase, and a dropping serum iron are common findings. The serotonin syndrome is identical but may also be associated with cramping and diarrhea. NMS and the serotonin syndrome are successfully treated as catatonia.[26] A recent case report illustrates.

Patient 7.2
A 15-year-old girl suffered a 5–25 min period of asphyxia following attempted suicide by hanging. In the ER, a CT scan of the head and neck were considered normal. Blood toxicology was negative, and serum alcohol was not present. On examination she could open her eyes, but not follow a moving target. Muscle tone and tendon reflexes were mildly increased. Plantar stimulation elicited extension, bilaterally. Over the next several days she had several daily 2–15 min episodes of extreme posturing into opisthotonus, hyperextension of the hips and "catatonic posturing of the upper extremities" associated with tachycardia and hypertension. She became diaphoretic, with hyperthermia and tachypnia. A repeat head CT showed generalized sulcal effacement, and an MRI revealed abnormalities in

the left frontal subcortical areas with a fifth cervical vertebral fracture. A repeat MRI demonstrated thalamic and cerebral cortical abnormalities. Serum creatinine phosphokinase was 659 U/L and an EEG showed diffuse slowing without epileptiform activity. Continuous dystonia and chorea developed. Dantroline treatment did not help. After 2 months her symptoms gradually abated. The authors concluded that her condition was malignant catatonia.[27]

Many catatonic patients are simultaneously manic. Sometimes, these patients exhibit echolalia (repeating the examiner's words) and echopraxia (repeating the examiner's movements). Other catatonic features can be demonstrated.

Some manic patients are so excited that they appear to be in frenzy, constantly moving and shouting, never resting or sleeping. They are disoriented. They may confabulate with fantastic stories. Their speech is so rapid and their associations are so jumbled that they cannot be understood. This form of delirious mania was originally termed Bell's mania. These patients are not rigid, and so catatonia can be missed. Associated grimacing, echophenomena, and mannerisms, however, alert the examiner to the presence of catatonia.

Other catatonic patients are in an oneiroid state.[28] They appear frightened and agitated, thrashing, hurting themselves and others. Stereotypy, grimacing, posturing, echolalia and echopraxia are common. Negativism and automatic obedience are almost always present. Fever may develop, and a malignant catatonia may unfold.

Some patients rapidly shift from delirious mania into an oneiroid and akinetic state and back again. When shifts are gradual, periodic catatonia is diagnosed. Periodic catatonia was first metabolically studied by Gjessing, who wrongly concluded it was an expression of fluctuations in nitrogen balance.[29] Such patients experience cycling periods of stupor and excitement, each with catatonic features. Although the original reports described phases that lasted for weeks, rapid shifts also occur, as illustrated by Patient 7.3.

Patient 7.3
Over the course of a weekend, a 47-year-old man became increasingly agitated, excited, and suspicious. He told his wife people were looking at him through their second-storey bedroom window. He stopped sleeping, paced and chattered continuously as he described his "great gifts". Frightened, his wife brought him to an emergency room on Monday morning. There, the patient was agitated, despondent; expressing ideas that he was a bad person and deserved to die.

In the hospital, he was found to be in a stupor, almost mute, staring, with automatic obedience and Gegenhalten. Several hours later he was in bed, unresponsive except to substantial painful stimuli. When so stimulated, he slowly turned to the examiner, and in a slurred voice said "Get thee from me,

Satan". He remained somnolent for several hours, with stable vital signs. He then suddenly jumped out of bed and began tap dancing up and down the unit hallway. When his efforts brought him to the nurses' station, he danced in place and continuously sang, told jokes and commented on anything a staff member did. After several hours in this excitement, he returned to bed and into his stuporous state. This cycle continued for several days. When stuporous he also became cataleptic.

Lithium carbonate was prescribed. The periods of agitated despondency, euphoric excitement, and stupor resolved over the next week and the patient was discharged fully recovered. The patient had never used illicit drugs and rarely ingested alcohol. Other than type II diabetes controlled with diet, his general medical health was good. Hypertensive on admission, his blood pressure normalized without medication in parallel with his resolving mania and catatonia.

Other variations of catatonia have been proposed. Karl Leonhard (1979) formulated a unique classification system based on his understanding of the importance of motor features in delineating psychotic disorders. These states, however, are best seen as catatonic variants and not different illnesses. Cataphasia was characterized by alternating phases of excitement and inhibition, the former similar to delirious mania and the latter like the Kahlbaum syndrome. Parakinetic catatonia referred to excitement with extreme fluctuating mood states and continuous movements throughout the body, such as shaking, shoulder shrugging, facial tics and twitching, odd hand and finger movements, and jerky arm and leg movements. It is a form of delirious mania. In children and teenagers, these motor features of catatonia can be difficult to distinguish from tic disorder.[30] Dysmetria and other cerebellar signs are also described. Kraepelin called this condition manneristic dementia.

Mutism and other catatonic speech disturbances

Verbal unresponsiveness, or mutism, is not always associated with immobility. The neurologic term is aphemia. Many mute patients are ambulatory, but typically slowed in their movements (bradykinesia). Mutism is often incomplete, the patient occasionally uttering a few whispered words, or only speaking to selected persons. This may be misunderstood as feigned, but is a form of negativism (Gegenhalten of speech). When mutism is complete and the patient rigid and immobile, akinetic mutism is diagnosed.[31] The patient may follow the examiner about the room with his eyes, but unlike the locked-in syndrome does not communicate by responding to questions with eye blinks. The face is mask-like, and blinking will not be elicited by glabellar tap.[32]

In speech-prompt catatonia, the patient briefly speaks only when spoken to. The speech is typically hesitant and slow, and may be limited to "I don't know", or with a "yes" or "no" often as contradictory statements. For example, the question "Do you like ice cream?" is answered "I don't know". The question "You do like ice cream, don't you?" is answered "yes". The question "You don't like ice cream, do you?" is answered "no". This is an example of verbal automatic obedience.

Other catatonic patients will respond with non-sequitive answers or seemingly silly answers (Vorbeireden). The question "How many legs does a three-legged stool have?" is answered "Four". The question "What was the color of George Washington's white horse?" is answered "Brown". These responses are forms of verbal negativism. When occurring in an oneiroid state, the condition is termed Ganser's syndrome. Ganser's original patients had many other catatonic features.[33] These patients often act "silly" or in opposition, and are misunderstood as malingerers or histrionic manipulators. It was originally associated with prisoners or persons whose illness appeared to provide for some legal or monetary gain.

Prosectic speech is whispered, mumbled speech that slowly declines in audibility and speed until it stops, like a car running out of gas. Stereotypic speech, Verbigeration, is filled with repetitive phrases and sentences. Repeating the last phrase or word of a sentence with increasing frequency is termed palilalia.

Speech mannerisms are also observed. The patient may speak robotically (like a computer voice), or with an accent inconsistent with the patient's background.[34] Echolalia, a stimulus-bound phenomenon in which the patient constantly repeats some or all of the examiner's utterances,[35] and echopraxia, in which the patient spontaneously copies the examiner's movements or is unable to refrain from copying the examiner's test movements (e.g. raising an arm above the head) despite instruction to the contrary, are seen in manic patients or those with frontal lobe disease and disinhibition.

Stupor

Stupor is extreme unresponsiveness and hypoactivity associated with altered arousal during which the patient fails to respond to questions. When severe, it is associated with immobility and the patient does not withdraw from painful stimuli (generalized analgesia). Stupor may last for hours, days, or longer. The patient in stupor seems unaware of the happenings around him.[36]

Negativism and Gegenhalten

The negativistic patient resists stimulation. Resistance to limb manipulation is with equal and opposite force (Gegenhalten). Attempts to move the patient's head or open his eyes are met with equal resistance. The eyes look away with only the whites showing. Directly facing the patient leads to greater resistance, another form of Gegenhalten. Questioning the patient from the side in a whispered voice reduces negativistic responses.[37]

Some patients do the exact opposite of the instruction. When asked to stand, they sit. When asked to walk, they stop. When asked to face the examiner, they turn away. The same question is answered with opposite responses. An action is stopped at an obviously inappropriate moment (e.g. going to the bathroom when asked but then urinating on the floor or without removing the necessary clothing). The patient uses the back end of a key to open a lock, tries to write with the wrong end of a pen, pours water onto the floor instead of into a cup, and when going to bed, sleeps at the edge of the mattress or with feet on the pillow.[38]

Catalepsy and posturing

Maintaining positions for prolonged periods of time defines catalepsy.[39] This immobility was termed obstruction, and is a variant of pathological inertia. In addition to posturing, the patient may freeze in the middle of a movement, or is unable to start a movement when asked but later performs it. For example, they do not answer the examiner's questions until the examiner is about to leave the room ("The reaction at the last moment").

Catatonic postures can be mundane or strange. A catatonic teenage girl sat immobile for hours in a chair with a writing tablet on her lap, pen in hand and point in contact with the paper and head bent as if deep in thought.[40] Other patients sit with their heads tilted and arms raised as if resting on an imaginary desk. Others stand for hours at attention, saluting, or lying in bed, upper body raised as if on an imaginary pillow (psychological pillow). Some precariously lie on the edge of the bed, squat for hours on the bed or in a hallway, twist their upper body into an almost right angle to their lower body, or sit with arms and legs extended as if falling. Postures may involve only the hands (e.g. the fingers held like a fan in front of the mouth, the hands held as if they were pistols) or the face (e.g. grimacing, puckering the lips, wrinkling of the nose with an exaggerated pouting of the lips, Schnauzkrampf).

Waxy flexibility (Cera flexibilitas)

Cataleptic patients can be moved into different positions, but with difficulty. They offer initial resistance before gradually allowing themselves to be repositioned as if made of softened wax, thus the term waxy flexibility. Waxy flexibility is not observed, it is demonstrated by manipulating the patient's limbs.

Stereotypy

Stereotypy is the automatic repetition of mundane movements such as tapping, gesturing and grooming. Constant head and face rubbing is a common example.

The patient is often unaware of these behaviors. Psychotic patients with stereotypic behaviors can be mistaken as having obsessive–compulsive disorder.[41]

Stereotypic movement disorder has been given a separate category in present classification when its onset is in childhood.[42] Head shaking and banging, rocking, self-biting, picking at skin or body orifices, and hitting oneself are described, often in association with mental retardation. These stereotypes, however, also occur in adults without mental retardation. When the patient exhibits the tendency to make automatic movements seemingly in response to an external stimulus, the term is proskinesis.[43]

Automatic obedience

Automatic obedience is the inability to resist tactile stimulation, despite instructions to the contrary. The patient is encouraged to hold the arm of a chair or the bed sheets tightly and to not let the examiner open the grasp and move the hand. Despite this continued encouragement, the patient submits to the examiner's gentle manipulations.

Mitmachen is observed when there is only mild initial resistance to the examiner's efforts. When the examiner releases the patient's arm it returns to its resting position. Mitgehen is observed when the patient responds to the slightest touch, even to following the examiner about the room (magnet reaction). In another example, the patient is told to keep his arm "limp" as if asleep and let the examiner do "all the work". The patient, however, cannot resist the stimulus of the examiner's manipulations or the light stroking of the hand, and the patient's arm follows the stimulus and can be postured by this technique. When asked, "What is your arm doing up there?" the patient may look at it in bewilderment, saying, "I don't know."

Forced grasp may be elicited by lightly stroking the patient's finger tips, despite repeated instructions not to grasp the examiner's hands. The rigid patient may be lifted from his bed by the finger tips. At other times, the examiner moving the patient's hand in a repeated simple motion (e.g. rotating the wrist while holding the fingers) elicits a perseveration of the movement that continues after the examiner releases the patient's hand.

Ambitendency

Catatonic patients cannot make choices. Competing stimuli requiring opposing actions elicit indecisive movements, hesitancy, or the appearance of being stuck between movements. The examiner offers the patient his hand as if to shake hands, while stating "Don't shake my hand. I don't want you to shake it." Ambitendency is present when the patient extends his hand as if to shake hands, moves his hand back-and-forth unable to complete the movement, or lightly touches the examiner's hand.

Table 7.2. Catatonic mannerisms

Tiptoe walking, skipping, hopping, high-stepping gait[44]

Hand or finger movements, not typically dyskinetic, such as repeatedly touching the extended index finger to the lips as if "shushing", making gun-shooting hand movements, and idiosyncratic hand signals

Inconspicuous repetitive actions, such as making clicking sounds before or after speaking; automatically tapping or touching or handling of objects or body parts; tongue chewing, licking, lip smacking, pouting, teeth clicking

Odd robotic speech like a child learning to read; speaking without common contractions (e.g. "I can not" rather than "I can't"). Using foreign accents not typical of the patient

Rocking, shoulder shrugging, sniffing and wrinkling of the nose, opening eyes wide and then squeezing them shut, grimacing, frowning; continuous irregular movements of the entire musculature including the face, resembling Sydenham's chorea (parakinesia)

Rituals, such as tapping the dishes and eating utensils in a specific order before eating; tapping the buttons before buttoning a shirt

---

Mannerisms

Catatonic patients make odd movements. When asked about these they may become angry or mute. When recovered, some cannot explain the behavior and have only a vague memory of what occurred. Others associate the mannerism to a delusional idea. A young catatonic man said he was trying to balance special fluids in his body when in response to questions he blew three times over his left shoulder before offering a delayed whispered answer.

Catatonic mannerisms look like compulsions, and catatonia should be suspected when a psychotic patient or a patient with mood disorder is also diagnosed as having obsessive–compulsive disorder. Table 7.2 lists the many mannerisms associated with catatonia.

Catatonic cultural variants

Several syndromes linked to specific cultures are better considered variations of catatonia. Ganser's syndrome, detailed above, is reported in Western culture.

Latah, reported in Arcadian Maine but linked to Malaysia, is characterized by echolalia, echopraxia, coprolalia (repetitive use of profanity), and automatic obedience within a manic delirium (shouting, yelling, hitting, jumping, and running). Its association with an excessive startle response and its sporadic nature suggests an infectious etiology or manic-depressive illness.[45]

Amok is a culture-related syndrome associated with south-east Asia, although cases are reported from North America, Britain, and Europe.[46] It is characterized by sudden, frenzied, violent, and often murderous attacks on strangers in public settings with multiple victims. The episode may last hours. Depressive illness or vertigo with visual hallucinations are common prodromes. "Amoks" that are not themselves killed are found in stupor and are amnestic for the attack. Systematic examinations of Amok perpetrators have not been done, but case literature suggests the presence of catatonic features similar to those seen in Latah. Seizure disorder and psychotic mood disorder are possible etiologies.[47] William Hammond offered a nineteenth-century example of Amok that he considered a form of monomania with depression:

> Within a recent period several such cases have occurred in this city [New York], one of which I had the opportunity of investigating. It was that of a Frenchman … who, having for several years been affected with delusions of wrongs and injuries being done to him, and having made several assaults on persons whom he imagined had conspired against him, finally rushed through a crowded street, striking right and left with a pair of carpenter's compasses at every woman he met. Some seven persons were stabbed by him, one of whom died. The only reason he could give me for his conduct was that "the women were talking about him" … the affliction is often transformed into melancholia, and it is then, doubtless, the tendency to suicide is exhibited.[48]

Lycanthropy, associated with eastern European lore of wolf-men, is the combination of catatonia with the delusional belief of being changed into an animal due to the influence of the devil. Delusional memories of eating children, killing domestic animals, having coitus with the devil, and interacting with demons were related by sufferers. Associated manic excitement, or "dancing mania" or tarentism is described. Sufferers acted as if wild animals. Epidemics of the syndrome were reported in eastern Europeans during the sixteenth and seventeenth centuries. Many sufferers were tortured and burnt as witches, accused by their neighbors out of spite or greed.[49] Fink and Taylor describe a man who was found by the New York police scurrying around the streets on all fours, roaring, snapping, and biting at passers-by. In the hospital, the man became mute and immobile with generalized analgesia and automatic obedience. He said later that he thought he was a tiger.[50]

Dyspraxia

Dyspraxia in a patient with a psychiatric syndrome suggests structural brain disease.[51] Dyspraxia is the inability to perform simple motor tasks despite adequate motor strength, the somatosensory guidance of movement, and an understanding of the task to be performed.

Ideo-motor dyspraxia

Ideo-motor dyspraxia is the inability to link the idea of the motor task (ideo) to the movement (motor). The resulting action is incorrect, awkward, or cannot be performed without the patient self-guiding his movements by first speaking each step. The patient is asked to silently demonstrate how to use an imagined key, comb, and hammer. "Hand as object" is an example of ideo-motor dyspraxia, the patient mimicking the object rather than how to hold and use it (e.g. extending the index finger as the key, making a fist to represent the hammer head). The inability to open one's eyelids on command while retaining the ability to spontaneously do so is termed eyelid apraxia, and is associated with Parkinson's disease,[52] frontal lobe lesions, right hemisphere disease, and catatonia.[53]

Kinesthetic dyspraxia

Kinesthetic dyspraxia is the inability to repeat the examiner's simple movements. The patient is asked to mimic hand postures (left and right) such as making a fist, pointing with the index finger, and the "OK" and "stop" signs. The examiner next places one of the patient's hands in a posture out of the patient's view, and asks the patient to make the same posture with the other hand. To accomplish this, the patient's corpus callosum must be functional.

Dressing dyspraxia

Dressing dyspraxia is the inability to dress oneself. It may be observed in the patient's failure to properly dress, or tested by asking the patient to put on a hospital gown.

Construction dyspraxia

Construction dyspraxia is the inability to copy simple geometric shapes (e.g. intersecting pentagons, diamond, square, and mushroom), or to draw the face of a clock from memory, the hands at 2:45.[54]

Abnormal eye movements

Abnormal eye movements are seen in patients with behavioral syndromes. Schizophrenic patients with classic emotional blunting, formal thought disorder and childhood neurodevelopmental and behavioral abnormalities have difficulties with smooth eye pursuit. Jerky movements lagging behind the target are characteristic, and are demonstrated by asking the patient not to move his head while following the examiner's finger.[55] Such movements are also seen in Huntington's and other basal ganglia disease, and in patients with frontal lobe disease.[56] Asking the patient to move his head from side to side while focusing on a stationary target may also reveal subtle ophthalmoplegia.[57]

Abnormal saccades are also reported in patients with manic-depression, schizotypal disorder,[58] and in the first-degree relatives of these patients and those with schizophrenia.[59] Associated poor executive functioning and frontal circuitry abnormalities are noted.[60] Patients with OCD have subtle oculomotor perturbations, and these are associated with poor executive functioning.[61]

Jerky and chaotic eye movements (opsoclonus and ocular flutter) occurring when the eyes are at rest are associated with cerebellar disease. Horizontal and vertical gaze nystagmus are also cerebellar signs. Nystagmus and abducen's nerve (sixth cranial nerve) palsy (the patient cannot look up and laterally) are seen in Wernicke's encephalopathy (an acute delirium most often seen in patients with chronic alcoholism and associated low thiamine levels).

Apraxia of gaze is the inability to move the eyes to the examiner's requests while spontaneous eyes movement is preserved (an aspect of Bailint syndrome).[62] Abnormal gaze is also reported in thalamic, pontine, and brainstem lesions that can best be identified by positron emission tomography (PET), not standard MRI.[63]

Rare syndromes with disturbance in gaze that can elicit the diagnosis of hysteria are the Miller–Fisher syndrome from brainstem involvement (progressive upward, lateral, and downward gaze paralysis with ataxia and areflexia),[64] Parinaud's syndrome from midbrain involvement (intermittent tonic gaze upward or downward deviations),[65] and Claude's syndrome involving the dorsal midbrain (ipsilateral third nerve palsy with horizontal gaze problems and contralateral ataxia).[66]

Movements associated with seizure disorder

Seizure disorder is common, and about 10% of epileptics are hospitalized for psychiatric reasons, while another 20% are regularly treated in psychiatric outpatient settings.[67] Most movement features of seizure disorder are sudden in onset, repetitive, and of short duration (Table 7.3). None is pathognomonic. Myoclonus, for example, is also seen in toxic states, early in the course of Creutzfeldt–Jakob disease, and late in Alzheimer's disease, in several genetic storage disorders, following cerebral anoxia, disease in the central tegmental tract (e.g. infarction, neoplasm, inflammatory), and in disorders of voluntary movement (e.g. Ramsey Hunt syndrome with associated intension tremor, dysarthria, and ataxia). Asterixis differs from myoclonus, and represents a flapping movement of the outstretched arms due to lapse in postural tone, and is seen in toxic states.[68]

Sleep-related abnormal movements

About a third of the general population at any given time suffers from sleep difficulties, and sleep disturbance is a common feature of neuro-psychiatric illness.[69] Melancholic patients have prolonged sleep onset and shortened REM latency.[70] Some seizure disorders typically emerge at night, while some sleep disorders are

Table 7.3. Abnormal movements seen in epilepsy

Dystonia: With generalized seizures, dystonia occurs as a sudden full body spasm (tonic) that may progress to a period of full body myoclonic movement (tonic–clonic or grand mal). In focal seizures, all of the dystonias described below can occur, often at night. These are termed *nocturnal paroxysmal dystonias*, and attacks include tonic and choreoathetoid movements, and oculogyric crisis.[71]

Atonia: Sudden and brief (a few seconds) loss of all motor tone (drop attacks) is a form of generalized epilepsy. In absence seizures (petit mal), tone is maintained but the patient becomes unresponsive and stares for 20–30s. Slow blinking may occur.

Myoclonus: Myoclonus is a sudden, automatic rhythmic or jerky movement, often repetitive. It is associated with focal and generalized seizures (including absence) as well as other neurologic conditions and medication toxicities.[72] In children, myoclonic seizures (typically in the morning) can be mistaken for "clumsiness".

Catalepsy and posturing: All forms of catatonia occur in epilepsy. Ictal posturing is usually of short duration. Post-ictal catalepsy can last for hours. Stereotypy occurs in both these phases of seizure disorder. Hand and arm postures are typical of some frontal lobe seizures.

Speech disorders: Frontal lobe seizures may elicit speech arrest (transient mutism), forced vocalizations and coprolalia, screaming, grunting and mumbling, muttering, and palilalia. These vocalizations are sudden and transient. Brief classic aphasia syndromes occur. The patient is not fully alert.

Automatisms: Automatisms are classic signs of partial complex seizures, but may occur after generalized clonic–tonic seizures as the patient awakens. Automatisms are repetitive behaviors performed in an automatic fashion such as chewing, lip smacking, pedaling and kicking, grimacing, foot stomping, pelvic thrusting and other coital behaviors, and rubbing and scratching of body parts. The patient is not fully responsive.

Complex actions: Aimless walking (or fugue that is typically post-ictal), drinking, urinating and defecating, undressing, and all forms of so-called conversion disorders and hysterias are associated with epilepsy. The patient is not fully responsive during these events.

---

expressed during wakefulness.[73] Not recognizing or ignoring the sleep disorder leads to misdiagnosis, inappropriate treatment, and exacerbation of any co-occurring behavioral syndrome.

The dyssomnias are associated with excessive daytime sleepiness or complaints of insomnia. The parasomnias are associated with behavioral, movement, and sensory disturbances. Some sleep disorders are identified solely by their motor manifestations. Table 7.4 displays the present classification of sleep disorders with associated specific abnormal movements.

Movements associated with the dyssomnias[74]

Periodic limb repetitive flexion movements during non-REM sleep affecting most commonly the legs are involuntary and are seen in persons without disease,

Table 7.4. International classification of sleep disorders

Dyssomnias
Periodic limb movement disorder
Restless leg syndrome
Nocturnal eating and drinking disorder

Parasomnias
Arousal disorders: confusional arousal, sleep walking, sleep terrors
Sleep–wake transition disorders: rhythmic movement disorder,
    sleep starts, nocturnal leg cramps
REM-related parasomnias: sleep paralysis, REM behavior disorder

Other parasomnias
Sleep bruxism, benign neonatal myoclonus

particularly the elderly. Movements are repetitive, occurring at regular intervals. Patients with sleep apnea often have the syndrome. Thirty percent of patients also experience restless leg syndrome.

Restless leg syndrome is exacerbated during inactivity and is worse at night, particularly the first half. It is characterized by leg movements during sleep that may throw the covers from the bed. Patients also experience an urge to move with associated uncomfortable sensations (dysesthesias) such as burning, itching, grabbing, "worms" moving under the skin, and an inner restlessness. Patients try to relieve these sensations by rubbing, stretching, or getting out of bed and standing or walking. A family history of restless leg syndrome is reported in half of sufferers. The syndrome is also associated with narcolepsy, sleep apnea, Huntington's disease, amyotrophic lateral sclerosis, and myelopathies and peripheral neuropathies. Twenty percent of patients with Parkinson's disease have the syndrome. About 80% of patients with restless leg syndrome also have rhythmic movement disorder described below.

A nocturnal eating and drinking disorder has been described. It is a form of sleep automatism. Patients exhibit eating and drinking movements immediately upon waking and may get out of bed and eat compulsively. Other procedural movements such as washing dishes, getting dressed and undressed, and driving a vehicle are reported. Continuous oral–facial automatisms with chewing and swallowing, and lip-smacking are also seen during sleep. Disorganized utterances occur. One to several episodes nightly last a few minutes each, and most patients report experiencing the episodes while "half asleep". Partial or complete amnesia in the morning for the events is common. Some patients will have other dyssomnias or narcolepsy.

Movements associated with the parasomnia

Parasomnias occur during sleep, but are not due to the process responsible for sleep and wakefulness. They are most common in children, and involve the autonomic and motor systems.

Arousal disorders expressed as "confusional" states, sleep walking or somnambulism, and night terrors have no characteristic motor features. Sleep–wake transition disorders occur at the transition between wakefulness and sleep, and between sleep and wakefulness, or between different stages of sleep.

Rhythmic movement disorder (periodic limb movements) is characterized by stereotyped, repetitive movements, typically involving large muscle groups like the head and neck, and occur from just prior to sleep onset into light sleep. They last minutes to hours, and consist of head banging, rolling, side-to-side movements, body rolling, leg banging, leg rolling, humming, or chanting. Patients are usually unresponsive during the events. Severe movements can cause injury. Frequent episodes are associated with daytime sleepiness. Mild forms and most episodes in children are seen in non-ill persons, but severe movements and adult onset episodes are associated with Gilles de la Tourette's syndrome, and other neurologic disease. About 30% will also have restless leg syndrome.

Sleep "starts" (hypnopompic and hypnogogic jerks) are short, non-periodic, intense whole body myoclonic jerks of the large axial muscles or one or two limbs associated with the subjective feeling of falling. Vocalization may accompany the jerk. Sleep jerks occur in normal persons as they fall asleep or awaken, during rapid eye movement sleep, and as hiccoughs. When severe and frequent, sleep myoclonus can elicit insomnia. Although myoclonus as a result of disease can occur alone (essential myoclonus), it is more often associated with other neurologic features.[75]

Nocturnal leg cramps are involuntary strong and painful contractions of the posterior muscles of the lower leg and foot lasting for seconds to minutes that interrupt sleep and that can be relieved by stretching. It may be familial and is most common in women and the elderly. It may have no clinical significance or be associated with hypertension, renal and vascular disease, diabetes, electrolyte disturbances, thyroid disease, Parkinson's disease, and cancers.

Somnambulism – sleep walking – is seen most commonly in children. It usually consists of brief, aimless wandering associated with purposeless repetitive behavior. Any vocalizations are short and monosyllabic. The patient is not fully alert, but injury is unusual. Sleep walking occurs in deep non-REM sleep and thus typically during the first third of the night.

Night terrors also occur in deep sleep early in the night. It is co-morbid with sleep walking. Episodes are brief, usually occur only once nightly, and are characterized by intense, inconsolable fear with signs of heightened sympathetic arousal. Like episodes of sleep walking, the sufferer is amnestic for the event.

Narcolepsy is a non-REM sleep disorder characterized by periods of semi-wakefulness at night with associated hypnogogic and hypnopompic hallucinations (see Chapter 10) and sleep paralysis. Daytime episodes of cataplexy (a sudden loss of tone and collapse that can elicit injury) and overwhelming sleepiness also occur.

REM-related parasomnias occur in the second half of the night and rarely after daytime naps. They include episodes of violent and dramatic motor activity such as talking, yelling, swearing, kicking, punching, and jumping out of bed and running. Bed partners can be hurt. Acute onset conditions are associated with the use of antidepressant medications and cholinergic agents, barbiturates, alcohol, or excessive caffeine. Chronic conditions are idiopathic or associated with Parkinson's disease, Lewy body dementia, and olivo-ponto-cerebellar and multiple system atrophy.

Movements associated with other parasomnias

Sleep bruxism is the forcible grinding, clenching, or tapping of the teeth by rhythmic contractions of the jaw muscles during sleep, sometimes producing audible sounds. It can lead to complaints of jaw and facial pain mistaken for somatization disorder, and the grinding may lead to dental damage. It is common and its cause unknown. Benign neonatal sleep myoclonus occurs during the first few months after birth and is characterized by intervals of repetitive jerks of the distal limbs lasting up to 20s. No associated pathology has been demonstrated. Dystonias can occur during periods of non-REM sleep, particularly during the first third of the night.[76]

Cataplexy and sleep paralysis

Cataplexy and sleep paralysis (transient weakness or inability to move) are features of narcolepsy. Cataplexy occurs during wakefulness and can be triggered by sudden emotion and excitement, the patient suddenly collapsing without loss of consciousness. Sleep paralysis occurs on sleep onset as the patient immediately enters a REM period. It may be associated with hypnogogic and hypnopompic hallucinations. Excessive daytime sleepiness is a typical feature of narcolepsy.[77]

Basal ganglia motor signs

"Extrapyramidal" motor signs are described in never medicated patients with psychosis. In a recent study of never medicated schizophrenics, 35% exhibited dyskinesia, and 15% Parkinsonism. These features are considered part of the disease process and are associated with cognitive impairments.[78]

Resting and postural tremor

Resting and postural tremor results from involuntary dysregulation of opposing muscle groups. Resting tremor is typically fine, worsens with anxiety and increased arousal, and decreases during sleep. Pill-rolling (continuous finger movement as if rolling a pea between one's finger tips) is an extreme form. Unilateral tremor is seen from a contralateral stroke, in the early stages of Parkinson's disease, and in drug-induced tardive dyskinesia. Postural tremor is associated with anxiety, and essential tremor, and when coarse and irregular, encephalopathy.

Postural tremor is a side effect of many psychotropic drugs. Placing a piece of paper between the patient's index and middle fingers while the arm is extended can reveal subtle postural tremor.

Tremor also occurs with orthostasis, unmedicated patients (primary orthostatic tremor) experiencing a rapid tremor and a severe sense of unsteadiness. Walking, sitting, and lying down are unaffected, and the remaining neurological evaluation is unrevealing.[79]

Dystonia

Sudden prolonged muscle spasm characterizes dystonia.[80] Acute dystonias are terribly painful, and when they continue for more than a few hours can lead to muscle breakdown and renal damage from myoglobinuria. Acute dystonias are generalized or focal. Oculogyric crisis, in which the patient is in a pronounced and prolonged total body and head exaggerated extension (opisthotonos), is life-threatening. Respiratory muscles are also in spasm and cannot aid ventilation. Respiratory stridor with cyanosis occurs. Extra-ocular muscles are affected and vision is compromised. Spatial disorientation occurs.

Focal dystonias include blepharospasm, Schnauzkrampf or "snout spasm", the patient's mouth in an exaggerated pucker (also seen in catatonia), torticollis when the sternoclidomastoid muscle is in spasm and the patient's head and neck are twisted as if looking over the shoulder, other segmental dystonias of axial muscle groups, laryngopharyngeal dystonia producing labored and vocally distorted speech, and writer's cramp. Acute dystonia may be induced by antipsychotic drugs and some SSRI agents. Young men and older women with previous neurologic disease are at highest risk.[81] When drug-induced, acute dystonias occur during the first several days of treatment.[82]

Chronic dystonia results in rigidity. Facial expression is masked, eye-blink may be minimal, speech becomes difficult, head and neck movements are stiff and reduced, and the patient walks looking at the floor, chin almost on the chest. Secondary arm movements while walking are reduced as the shoulder girdles are frozen; gait is stiff and shuffling, arms are held stiffly at the sides or in front of the torso as if carrying wood. The patient looks "frozen". Manipulating the patient's limbs is difficult and cog-wheel can be elicited in the elbows and other joints. Writing deteriorates and becomes small (micrographia) and choppy. Monitoring writing assesses the effect of antipsychotic medication on the basal ganglia.

Parkinsonism

Bradykinesia with increased muscle tone, features of rigidity, a resting and postural tremor, a flexed posture, and a shuffling or propulsive gait, define the Parkinson syndrome. Postural difficulties occur, and falls are common. When drug-induced, it occurs early in treatment and rarely after three months of exposure. The syndrome is associated with a greasy sheen (sebaceous gland secretion) when induced by a typical antipsychotic agent.

The "on–off" effect seen in many patients with Parkinson's disease has been attributed to long-term L-DOPA treatment. Following a gradual decline in the drug's effectiveness and rapid dosing adjustments, the on–off phenomenon emerges. The abrupt swings in activity are unrelated to the timing of dosing, occurring many times daily. Transition between states occurs over several minutes, the patient going from "frozen" to a flurry of stereotyped dyskinesia, with flexion–extension leg movements, foot stamping, head turning and hand wringing. Patients sense the change. The "on" state lasts several minutes to hours, with a rapid return to the "off" state that follows on the heels of a return of tremor. Autonomic associated signs are pallor, profuse sweating, palpitations, and extreme lassitude.[83]

Dyskinesia

Dyskinesia is involuntary, repetitive, and sometimes distorted movement of muscle groups, not due to tremor. Dyskinesias include choreoathetoid (writhing) movements of the fingers, head twisting or overextension, shoulder shrugging, oral–buccal puckering and perioral tremor (the "rabbit" syndrome), lip smacking, licking, tongue flicking, chewing, blinking, pelvic thrusting, rocking, weight shifting from one foot to the other. Hemiballismus and myoclonus are other examples.

Unlike other basal ganglia signs, ballismus is typically associated with a specific, usually vascular, lesion in the subthalamic nucleus or its outflow tracts. The movement is a sudden, violent and random flinging of limbs. Hemiballismus is unilateral. Facial and throat movements also occur at these moments. In chronically ill psychotic patients with tardive dyskinesia, the emergence of ballismus can be mistaken for additional antipsychotic drug toxicity and not a new stroke. Pre-ballismus hyperanalgesia of the affected limb, and the associated agitation, altered arousal, and speech difficulties[84] can be misunderstood as psychogenic and not a newly emerging brain vascular disease process.

Athetosis is the continuous movement of a limb due to instability of posture. Athetosis of the arm is a slow, sinuous flexion and extension of the fingers and wrist, the thumb opposed and flexed with variable degrees of forearm pronation and supernation. The foot and neck can be similarly affected.

Some movements, previously considered tics or psychogenic, may be focal forms of athetosis. These include blepharospasm, spasmodic torticollis, oromandibular and orofacial dyskinesia, writers' and other occupational "cramps", and axial dystonia.[85] They also occur in tardive dyskinesia.

Dyskinesia occurs following beta-hemolytic streptococcus infection, particularly in children. Associated mood disorders, obsessive–compulsive disorder, attention deficit hyperactivity disorder, and tic disorder have been described as PANDAS (Pediatric Autoimmune Neuropsychiatric Disorder Associated with Streptococcal infection; see later).[86] Choreoathetoid movements are reported in heavy cocaine users, and, when severe, termed "crack dancing". It occurs with akathesia, Parkinsonism and tremor.[87] It is also reported in association with rapid dosing changes with opioids,[88] and in never-medicated schizophrenic patients.[89]

Tardive dyskinesia (TD)

TD typically results from prolonged exposure to dopaminergic receptor-blocking drugs. The inducing dose is highly individualized, and patients with previous basal ganglia disease are at high risk.[90] TD is associated with general slowing of cognitive function (bradyphrenia), problems in attention, working memory and new learning,[91] and worsening of symptom severity.[92] Diaphragmatic and esophageal muscle involvement can lead to severe breathing and eating difficulties, and aspiration of food. All the dyskinetic movements listed in the previous section occur in TD, but their emergence after weeks or months of exposure to an antipsychotic agent adds the term "tardive". Early signs are vermicular movements of the tongue while on the floor of the mouth and subtle choreoathetoid finger movements in the preferred hand. Later features are protruding, twisting, and curling tongue movements combined with sucking, pouting, and bulging of the cheeks, severe choreoathetoid movements of the extremities, ballistic arm movements, constant shifting of weight, lorodosis, rocking and swaying, pelvic thrusting and rotary movements, grunting, and chest heaving. Inability to stand fully erect, the "Pisa Syndrome", is described. Persistent dystonic movements occur, and sufferers can be left in a twisted posture, like a corkscrew. Meige's syndrome, a cranial dystonia with blepharospasm and oromandibular dystonia, is considered idiopathic, but is also seen as a drug-induced movement disorder. Rapid twitching and pouting movements of the lips is termed the "Rabbit

Syndrome". All antipsychotic agents are associated with drug-induced movement disorder, high-potency typical agents the most likely offenders.[93] Patient 7.4 illustrates a needless case of tardive dyskinesia.

Patient 7.4

A 12-year-old girl was brought by her mother from Texas to a university hospital in another state for ECT. Texas does not permit the administration of ECT to persons less than 16 years of age. The girl had a several-year history of manic-depressive illness without psychosis that had not responded to treatment, forcing her to miss school. Atypical antipsychotics, prescribed because of their alleged mood-stabilizing properties, led to tardive dyskinesia. Her abnormal movements consisted of the Meige's syndrome, repeated blinking and squeezing her eyes shut to blepharospasm and twisting, pouting of her lips, and forward thrusting of her jaw. She also had a vocal dystonia reducing her speech to a halting frog-like croaking. Twelve bilateral ECT resolved her mood disorder and her drug-induced movement disorder and she returned home and to school.

Tic

Tics are sudden involuntary twitches of small muscle groups. Blinking, distortions of the forehead, nose and mouth, teeth tapping, clearing of the throat, and twitching of the shoulders are most common. Vocalizations, clicks, snorts, hisses, shouts and bursts of profanity (coprolalia) are other examples. The tic is often associated with a subjective feeling of needing to move and relief after the movement. Myoclonus is more rhythmic than tic and is not associated with these subjective feelings. Tics and compulsions are the hallmark of Gilles de la Tourette's disease.[94] Tics are also seen in children with attention deficit hyperactivity disorder, all the anxiety disorders, and in some persons with mood disorder.[95]

Compulsions

Compulsions are repetitive, often ritualistic actions commonly driven by obsessions.[96] Sufferers are aware that they are performing a needless or maladaptive task, but cannot resist the urge to act. Checking the household to insure safety, hand washing and showering, and performing tasks in a specific manner and for a specific number of times to ward off an undefined danger are most common. For some patients, the compulsions take on a life of their own, and are experienced as autonomous acts such as sniffing, squinting, touching, tapping, throat clearing, smelling one's hands or objects, foot stamping, pulling out one's hair (trichotillomania), scratching, nail biting, and chewing on one's lips and the inside surface of one's cheeks.

Repetitive ritualistic behaviors like compulsions can be inhibited only briefly. Sufferers are compelled to perform these behaviors, often in a formulaic manner. Repetitive self-mutilating behavior includes cutting, burning, hitting, head banging, and eye gouging. Speech compulsions include automatically repeating words or phrases. Stock words is another speech compulsion. Echolalia and echopraxia occur. Echolalia is also associated with receptive transcortical aphasia, autism, abnormal startle reactions (seen post-encephalitic states), Gilles de la Tourette's syndrome, and catatonia.[97]

Utilization behavior in which the patient compulsively manipulates, takes, or uses objects not his own is reminiscent of the unwanted release of procedural memories. It is associated with echopraxia. The patient sees a pen, takes it and writes with it. The patient sees a bed and lies on it. The patient sees an object in a store and takes it (kleptomania). The patient sees an attractive person and inappropriately touches the person. This exaggerated dependency on environmental cues is associated with a deficit in self-monitoring.

A rare variant of compulsion is abulomania. It was originally described as a paralysis of will without accompanying obsessions in which the sufferer was unable to perform certain actions despite the strong desire to do so and adequate motor and sensory capacity. There was no associated psychosis or acute mood disorder, and no other features suggestive of catatonia or a focal neurologic disruption. Examples are: a notary who could no longer write his signature, despite great effort to do so, raising his hand, making writing movements but unable to put pen to paper; a woman who could carry out all needed minor activities but was immobilized when faced with making a decision that she thought important; and a man who could not make decisions about dressing or undressing and so remained in the same clothes for days unless assisted.[98]

Cerebellar motor signs

The classic motor features of cerebellar disease are ataxia, poor coordination of movements, unstable gait, impaired speech articulation, and difficulties with eye movements and swallowing.

Speech and language problems associated with cerebellar disease, discussed in Chapter 9, include scanning dysarthria with slowing of utterances, irregular rhythm and volume, slurring, intention tremor in the voice, and ataxic respirations.

Many pharmaceuticals affect cerebellar function. Cerebellar dysfunction is also associated with schizophrenia, autism, dyslexia, alcoholism, and multiple sclerosis.[99] Kraepelin recognized a "cerebellar form" of dementia praecox.[100]

Intention tremor

Intention tremor is coarse and is observed by asking the patient to reach for objects. There is no tremor when the limb is at rest. It is seen in cerebellar disease, essential tremor, and exposure to many pharmaceuticals (e.g. caffeine and other stimulants, alcohol, lithium).

Past-pointing (dysmetria)

Past-pointing is difficulty in accurately directly one's hand to grasp an object, missing and going past the object. It can be observed, or tested by asking the patient to touch the examiner's index finger with his index finger, the examiner's finger moving into high, low, left and right positions. The patient touching the examiner's finger and then his own nose is a variation of the test. The heel to shin test is another example.

Dysdiadochokinesia

The inability to perform rapid, alternating movements such as pronation and supernation of one palm against the other (10 trials) defines dysdiadochokinesia. Another test is asking the patient to rapidly touch the tip of his thumb with the tip of each of his fingers in sequence, while his arms are extended, palms up. Mistakes in placement, breaks in movement, jerky irregular movement can occur. Other errors in movement regulation can be observed during this testing.

Asynergy

Asynergy is the inability to smoothly perform simple movement. Jerky, robotic movements occur. Any of the hand tests of movement can be used to observe for asynergy.

Coordination problems

Poor coordination is observed while the patient performs other motor tasks. Movements are awkward and jerky. When severe, ataxia, weaving movements of the head, trunk, and gait is seen. The gait becomes wide-based, turning is difficult and can result in falls, and high-stepping, staggering, and side-to-side lurching occurs. Ataxia is tested by asking the patient to heel-to-toe walk across the examination room with eyes open (tandum gait). Dystaxia is elicited while the patient is standing erect, feet together and eyes open, a slight push to his back causing swaying or staggering.

Procedural memory problems

Declarative memory is memory for facts and events. Memory for skills is termed procedural memory and is a form of implicit memory. The demonstration of knowing the "information" is not declared but demonstrated, and by the demonstration the knowing is implied. Driving a vehicle correctly through city streets from home to work demonstrates implicit knowledge of how to drive a car, the rules of the road, and the route from home to work. Activities of daily living (buttoning shirts and dresses, tying shoelaces, preparing a meal), playing sports (swinging a golf club, serving a tennis ball), performing a skill (playing the piano, typing, knitting, conducting the medical physical examination) are complex movements that must be over-learned to be done efficiently, and must be practiced continually to be fully maintained. The more complex the skill, the more fragile its procedural memory, and the more likely it will be affected by brain disease.[101] It is, however, less affected by aging than other cognitive processes.[102] Conditions associated with disturbed procedural memory include basal ganglia structural disease,[103] cerebellar atrophy,[104] and obsessive–compulsive disorder.[105] Patient 1.1 with carbon monoxide poisoning was misdiagnosed as depressed. The clue to the correct diagnosis of carbon monoxide poisoning was his loss of the motor skills for knitting and playing the guitar.

Conversion, hysteria, and idiopathic abnormal movements ("psychogenic movements")

The mind–body notion is reflected in behavioral syndromes being divided into "organic" (with demonstrated pathology) and "functional" or "psychogenic" (without identified pathology and of assumed psychological origin). The "hysteria" of past eras continues to be given a psychological interpretation, and is conflated into the categories of conversion and psychogenic movement disorder, non-epileptic or "pseudoseizure", and dissociative disorder. The reliability and validity of these categories, however, are challenged, and nervous system pathology is identified in many such patients.[106] Chronic impairment is common, particularly when symptoms are unilateral.[107]

The DSM offers the following examples of conversion symptoms: impaired coordination and balance (astasia–abasia), paralysis or localized weakness, aphonia (a whisper), difficulty swallowing or the sensation of a lump in the throat (globus hystericus), urinary retention, loss of touch or pain sensation, double vision, blindness, deafness, and hallucinations. Although the DSM cautions that the diagnosis of "conversion" should be made only when symptoms do not conform to known anatomical pathways and physiological mechanisms, in practice the attending physician's weak database or bias are the most likely sources of the diagnosis of conversion.[108] The manual demonstrates this limited database by offering stocking-glove anesthesia as an example of a symptom without a neurologic basis,[109] although it is a well described sign of neuropathy.[110]

Many other classic symptoms of hysteria are shown to result from specific disease. At one time, Parkinson's disease, St Vitus' dance, tetanus and eclampsia were considered neurotic disorders.[111] Denial of illness, *la belle indifference*, and hemianesthesia, classic signs of conversion, are associated with thalamic disease. Many non-epileptic fits are in fact partial complex seizures identified by laboratory studies. Anatomically inconsistent pain patterns are often prominent early signs in multiple sclerosis, and astasia–abasia, the "classic" hysterical gait and walking difficulty, is associated with dementia,[112] and midline cerebellar and corpus callosum lesions.[113]

Many examples of motor conversions and psychogenic movement disorder are understood as features of catatonia or specific neurologic disease. Patient 1.7, the 78-year-old woman who was said to have psychogenic "confusion" and catatonia (diagnosed by a university hospital neurology team, and then a psychiatrist), was found to be in non-convulsive status epilepticus. Patient 4.1, the 56-year-old nurse who was said to have a psychogenic movement disorder (diagnosed by a psychiatric resident, his faculty supervisor, a neurologist, and several other psychiatry faculty members), was found to have familial cerebellar–pontine degeneration.

Patient 7.5 also illustrates the value of not assuming symptoms to be "psychogenic" even if they appear associated with so-called primary or secondary gain (psychological or tangible, respectively).[114]

Patient 7.5[115]

A 30-year-old woman was referred to a psychoanalyst by her primary care physician because of neck and head pain of six months' duration keeping her from going to work, and for which no medical cause was determined in a cursory evaluation. She was pain-free most of the time, except when riding the commuter train to work. The train ride took about 25 min, and her pain began shortly after she boarded and worsened as the train approached the terminus and her workplace, forcing her to return home. She had been at the job for about six months, and found it "stressful".

Obtaining a careful history (the story of the illness), the psychoanalyst discovered that by the time the patient boarded the train all the seats were taken and she had to stand on the platform near the car exit, receiving the full energy of the car bouncing over the tracks. He surmised that the car's up and down movement affected a cervical spine abnormality leading to nerve root inflammation and the pain. This was confirmed on CT scan and a neck brace worn during the commute resolved the patient's difficulties.

Patient 7.6 also illustrates the dangers of automatically accepting the patient's symptoms as "psychogenic" if they do not fit the examiner's understanding of neuroanatomy and function.

Patient 7.6

A 28-year-old man came to an emergency room because of left-sided numbness and "loss of feeling" that had progressed over several hours. The man
appeared anxious and said he was under substantial work-related stress.
Examination revealed the numbness ending at the midline contrary to the
anatomic distribution of dermatomes. The findings of the remainder of the
basic neurologic and general medical examination were reported as "normal".
A "psychogenic" disorder was considered, and the patient sent home with
several doses of an anxiolytic and the recommendation to follow-up with his
primary care physician in the next few days. The patient died that night and an
autopsy revealing a ruptured aneurysm that had bled into his right thalamus.

The emergency room physician may also have been swayed by the patient's symptom
being left-sided, because of the long-held notion that unilateral psychogenic movement and somatosensory disorders will be more common on the left because of
influences of the right cerebral hemisphere, the putative site of unconscious processes.
This left bias has been questioned, and a review of 121 studies totaling 1139 patients
considered to have conversion disorder could find no left–right difference.[116]

Many studies reinforce the need for careful consideration of alternative explanations to conversion and psychogenic disorders.[117] Gould *et al.* (1986) reported
30 patients with documented structural nervous system damage who were mistakenly said to have symptoms that were not understood by their treating
clinicians and therefore considered signs of hysteria. *La belle indifference* (a calm
unconcern for the disabling features), introduced by Janet as a pathognomonic
sign of conversion hysteria, was found to be an unreliable feature. Extracts from
the case presentations are instructive.

Patient 7.7

"A 56-year-old woman" experienced "double vision and facial numbness ...
diminished sensation on the right side of her face ... with exact midline split
of the forehead and jaw but the sensory loss spared the nose ... less sensation
of vibration (to a tuning fork) on the right side" and "apparent giveaway
weakness at the left biceps and deltoid." The patient's symptoms were eventually understood as arising from a nasopharyngeal epidermoid carcinoma.

Patient 7.8

A 59-year-old woman with a "history of complaints involving many organ
systems but no medical diagnosis except hypertension" had recent "left-sided
weakness ... She was euphoric ... denying any weakness or numbness.
Examination did not reveal any motor deficit but decreased appreciation of

pinprick ... over the left body and extremities ... sensory loss was patchy with inconsistent borders; she expressed no concern." Her symptoms were eventually understood as arising from a recent infarction of the right parietal and temporal lobes.[118]

Gould and colleagues reported that persons most likely to be misdiagnosed as "hysterical" were women, homosexual men, patients with previous psychiatric diagnoses, and those with a plausible psychological explanation for their condition. The biases in the application of the hysteria label are patent.

Devinsky *et al.* (2001) described 79 patients previously diagnosed with conversion disorder who were then found to have defined brain disease. Sixty patients (76%) had unilateral cerebral abnormalities, of which 85% were structural. Ictal or inter-ictal EEG abnormalities were found in 78% of these patients. A right hemisphere lesion was found in 78% of the patients with a defined abnormality.

A four-year follow-up of children and adolescents with the diagnosis of conversion found the conversion features had fully resolved in 85%, but 35% suffered from mood or anxiety disorder.[119] Among 103 patients with dystonia considered psychogenic or a feature of somatization disorder, most were explained by previous peripheral injury or the presence of other psychiatric conditions. For some patients, no cause, including psychiatric, could be identified.[120]

Motor conversion and pseudoseizure diagnoses are most likely to presage a definitive neurologic diagnosis, and dystonia and chorea are features of disease most often misunderstood and labeled "psychogenic".[121] Among patients said to have psychogenic non-epileptic seizures based on video-EEG monitoring, common features are clonic and exaggerated movements of the extremities, pelvic thrusting, head movements, and tonic posturing of the head, a "trembling" syndrome of all extremities, and an "atonic" condition, the patient falling to the floor as the only feature.[122] As illustrated by Patient 7.9 and other reports,[123] such patients, although reported as having a "psychogenic" condition, often have a seizure disorder.

Patient 7.9
A 22-year-old active-duty military service woman was hospitalized for possible malingering to avoid work responsibilities. Her difficulties were described as "nightmares" during which she was observed by her roommates to get out of bed, scream for several minutes, and then return to sleep. She had similar episodes during the day and these continued in the hospital. She was noted to suddenly stop the activity in which she was engaged, flex both her arms with clenched fists, start screaming and then repeat the phrase "It's okay, it's okay ...". Her arms moved up and down symmetrically as if she were pounding a table.

She looked tense, with clenched teeth and tension in her general musculature. She had several episodes daily, lasting several minutes, and these were
followed by the desire to lie down and sleep. On one occasion she was
incontinent of urine. Although "conversion hysteria" was diagnosed by the
attending psychiatrist, the resident considered seizure disorder likely,
obtained a prolactin blood level 20 min after such an episode which was
four times the patient's baseline and diagnostic of a seizure. Anticonvulsant
treatment resolved the episodes.[124]

The tell-tale signs of pseudo- or non-epileptic seizure are well known. All,
however, are also expressions of true seizures.[125]

In an extensive review, Krem (2004) details many severe neurologic conditions
presenting with features initially eliciting the diagnosis of conversion disorder.
More than 60% of such patients were young women. Common psychiatric
co-morbidities were depression and personality disorder. Among the identified
causes of motor conversion were amyotrophic lateral sclerosis, Guillain–Barré
syndrome, Huntington's disease, intracranial hemorrhage, malignancy, multiple
sclerosis, myasthenia gravis, Parkinson's disease, post-encephalitis syndrome, and
systemic lupus erythematosis.

Mood disorder is another common co-morbidity among patients defined with
a psychogenic movement disorder.[126] Further, just as epilepsy is a common
finding in patients who also have non-epileptic seizures,[127] many patients with
the diagnosis of psychogenic movement disorder also have a movement disorder
secondary to a neuropathologic process.[128]

Diagnostic and treatment considerations alone indicate that if a defined illness
explaining the movement disorder cannot be determined it is best to consider
such patients as having idiopathic movement disorders, not "psychogenic" or
"conversion" disorder.

Psychogenic movement disorder, however, is typically diagnosed when other
causes are not apparent, the movements are inconsistent with the clinician's
understanding of neurologic functioning and disease, and the movements tend to
worsen when the patient is under stress and improve with distraction or placebo.
Idiopathic movement disorder is also commonly associated with sensory symptoms or pain. *La belle indifference* is not a consistent or specific finding. Thalamic
lesions, however, can elicit motor disturbance, sensory symptoms and neglect or
"denial" of dysfunction, and such lesions are not always considered in the evaluation of patients with idiopathic movement disorder.[129] Female patients are more
likely than men to receive the diagnosis. Most patients remain symptomatic for
years, and few consider their condition as primarily psychiatric in origin, despite
many having a psychiatric co-occurring condition.[130]

Specific idiopathic movement disturbance

The many idiopathic movement disturbances are broadly categorized as those where movement is inhibited, such as weakness and paresis without atrophy,[131] and those where an abnormal movement occurs but the etiology is deemed psychological, e.g. "psychogenic" myoclonus,[132] tremor,[133] dystonia (spasmodic, fixed, torticollis, torsion), globus hystericus (difficulty swallowing), and Parkinsonism.[134]

In specialty clinics, conversion dystonia and tremor are the most common (>50%), followed by tic, myclonus and Parkinsonism.[135] Among persons in the general population with a conversion disorder diagnosis, over half have an idiopathic movement problem, commonly weakness and paresis without atrophy.[136] Studies of neurologic patients estimate the diagnosis of conversion disorder between one and 9%.[137]

The pathophysiology of idiopathic movement disturbances

The pathophysiology of idiopathic movement disturbance is unclear. There are three alternative considerations to the psychogenic model. The movement disturbances represent: (1) subtle motor system regulatory dysfunction and is a distinct pathophysiologic disorder, (2) feigned behavior, or (3) features of a primary psychiatric or neurologic condition and do not exist independent of these conditions.

The subtle motor system model proposes that idiopathic movement disturbances are expressions of a subtle but specific abnormal neurologic process. The evidence for this understanding is weak. Neuropsychological studies focus on the right hemisphere, because as the "non-language" hemisphere with arousal and emotional expression and receptive functions it is hypothesized as the site of the dynamic unconscious. A few studies report bi-frontal and non-dominant hemisphere impairment in patients with conversion diagnoses.[138] Others propose a disconnection between sensory processing and awareness,[139] a disconnection between pre-conscious processing of emotion, perception and memory,[140] and a defect in mapping of the body state.[141] The disconnections are presumed functional not structural, resulting in disrupted motor–perceptual coordination leading to neglect and abnormal or non-movement.[142] The preparation to move and the attempt to move fail to activate the sensory motor cortex to properly guide movement.[143] This loss of feedback is also proposed as an explanation for catatonia, a condition that is often misinterpreted as conversion disorder.

Neuroimaging studies consist of small samples and case reports. Patients with motor conversions are reported to exhibit cortical hypometabolism and are unable to properly generate[144] or fully use motor programs[145] because of cortical functioning being disrupted by limbic system over-activation.[146] The disruption is between the brain systems of intention and motor execution and the result is non-movement.[147] The metabolic dysfunction also appears contralateral to the affected limbs.[148] For example, when attempting to move, a patient with left-sided idiopathic paralysis was found to have loss of activation of the right primary motor strip and hypermetabolism in the right orbitofrontal and anterior cingulate cortex.[149] This is not willed inactivity, because voluntary inhibition of limb movement is associated with increased, not decreased, cortical activity.[150]

The factitious/malingering model posits that patients with the conversion diagnoses are feigning illness. In a report of 37 persons identified as having "psychogenic" stance and gait disturbances, video study revealed characteristic signs of factitious impairment, including momentary fluctuations in the abnormality, excessive slowness or hesitation without any associated neurologic or psychiatric explanatory findings, Romberg sway amplitudes that were delayed and subsequently improved by distraction, a "walking on ice" gait with the person taking small steps with fixed ankle joints, and sudden buckling of the knees without falling.[151]

Among patients admitted over a 27-year period to a rehabilitation department, less than 1% ($N=34$) were identified as having "conversion motor paralysis".[152] The investigators identified 4 "malingerers" and the remaining 30 are offered as examples of possible psychogenic movement disorder. Five illustrative vignettes are presented. Two of these were also clearly malingering or exaggerating their symptoms, and a third, a man with a head injury and L1 and L2 vertebral fractures and associated right hemiplegia, stuttering, rage attacks and "confusion", was said to have an "organic brain syndrome" (possibly a seizure disorder). The fourth, a woman who fell, sustaining a C8 injury and peripheral nerve injury followed by left-sided weakness, was also said to have "a genuine organic problem". The fifth patient, a 22-year-old woman who lost consciousness after being hit by a motor vehicle and had posttraumatic amnesia, developed weakness in all limbs and clonus temporarily relieved by traction. Her spastic weakness without sensory or autonomic deficits resolved after a week of rehabilitation. This last vignette is the only one presented that can be seriously considered to have symptoms without an identified adequate neurologic or malingering explanation. Considering the review covered almost three decades of admissions, that less than 1% of the admissions were considered psychogenic, and that most of those patients had explanatory pathology or were malingering, the independence of psychogenic movement disorder is doubtful.

The non-independent model of conversion disorder proposes that such conditions are symptoms that reflect neuropathology or a psychiatric disorder with established validity. This view is consistent with the studies cited previously and numerous case reports.[153] Patient 7.10 describes a man with a movement disorder associated with melancholia.

Patient 7.10

A 50-year-old man was hospitalized for melancholia. He was noted to have jerky neck and shoulder movements more pronounced on his left side that were said to have begun with the emergence of his depressive illness, five years earlier. His wife said "He looked like a fish out of the water . . . His whole body would jerk. His neck, arms, and legs would jerk until he was exhausted."

At that time, the patient was extensively evaluated separately by two neurologists who concluded that the "jerky motor movements" were due to his melancholia. MRI showed periventricular ischemic changes that were unlikely to explain his condition. Various antidepressant drug trials were unsuccessful. A course of 10 BL-ECT then resolved the melancholia and the abnormal movements. A year later, the patient relapsed and his movement disorder returned. A second course of ECT again resolved the melancholia and the "jerky motor movements". The patient remained well for the next two years until the index admission where he again received ECT, again leading to a resolution of the melancholia and movement disorder.

Patient 7.11 illustrates the misidentification of catatonia as a conversion disorder.

Patient 7.11

A 23-year-old woman with a long history of generalized seizure disorder was brought to an emergency room by the police who found her wandering the streets "confused". She was only intermittently responsive to questions. Over the last 4 months she had been to that ER 8 times for a generalized seizure, the last fit 10 days before.

The patient was admitted to the neurology service, where she was found to be slow to answer or to just stare mutely at the examiner. She was said to be oriented to the month and year, to know her mother's name, to follow simple commands and when speaking to be fluent and not dysarthric. She "would not count or say the alphabet". She moved all extremities. She performed the finger–nose-to-finger test without difficulty. She "could not give a good history". Her initial EEG showed generalized slowing and spike and waves in left temporal areas. Repeated EEGs showed improvement over a few days, with the last showing "mild slowing" and a few "bi-frontal sharp waves" consistent with diffuse, mild encephalopathy. The patient, however, was said to "refuse to participate in her care" (meaning she stopped moving) and she stopped communicating. Conversion paresis or malingering was considered and a psychiatrist consulted.

The consultant found the patient to be mostly mute with stereotypy, negativism, automatic obedience, arm rigidity and a mild grasp reflex.

The consultant diagnosed post-ictal catatonia following a period of status epilepticus and prescribed lorazepam. Eight milligrams daily resolved the catatonia and the patient was discharged on a new anticonvulsant drug regime.

Rare motor syndromes mistaken for conversion hysteria

Apraxic agraphia

Apraxic agraphia is a language-related motor disturbance. "Pure" apraxic agraphia is the inability to construct letters in the absence of a disturbance in spelling, reading, or substantial praxis or visual–constructional difficulties.[154] In its mildest form, handwriting is deteriorated but legible. Cursive writing may be lost, the patient reduced to child-like printing. The alignment of the writing may also be askew. Apraxic agraphia is associated with lesions in the left superior parietal lobe[155] Patient 7.12 illustrates.

Patient 7.12[156]

A 78-year-old, right-handed man, referred for a follow-up evaluation of a depression-like syndrome, was in his usual state of health until age 61, when he had what was described as a "transient ischemic attack". The patient said that at that time his speech was not impaired, but he experienced transient weakness in both arms. Since then he noticed that he was unable to write in cursive, but he could print upper and lower case letters. Because the patient had a pacemaker, an MRI could not be done. Functional neuroimaging (SPECT), however, revealed bilateral hypoperfusion of the parietal and occipital lobes. Uptake in the basal ganglia was normal and symmetrical. Carotid Doppler imagery showed no hemodynamically significant carotid arterial stenotic or occlusive disease. The patient was discharged home still unable to write in cursive. At his bank his new signature (Figure 7.1) was accepted and the patient did not feel that his deficit affected his daily living.

Alien hand syndrome

The alien hand syndrome is characterized by the patient not recognizing the actions of one of his hands as self-generated, instead experiencing the hand's actions as autonomous and elicited by an outside agency. The patient may ignore the hand or delusionally conclude it belongs to another. Typically the non-dominant hand is the alien hand. Case literature describes one hand grasping unneeded objects and refusing to release them, constantly groping bedclothes, objects and body parts, and the compulsive manipulation of tools or objects. The

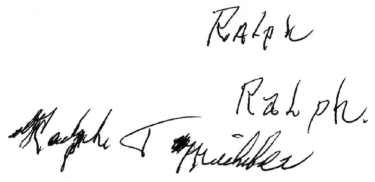

Figure 7.1 The signature of a patient with apraxic agraphia

non-dominant alien hand may be experienced in conflict with the patient's stated purposes, the patient grabbing or slapping the alien (the "bad") hand to prevent an action, angrily shouting at the alien hand, and the alien hand attacking the sufferer. This uncommon delusion of alienation and control is most commonly associated with anterior brain lesions: the anterior corpus callosum, the mesial frontal cortex contralateral to the alien hand, the supplementary motor area, anterior cingulated gyrus, and medial prefrontal cortex of the dominant cerebral hemisphere, or in the thalamus.[157]

Periodic paralysis

Periodic paralysis is a hereditary disorder (usually autosomal dominant) character-ized by episodic muscle weakness associated with abnormal potassium levels (hypo- and hyperkalemia) or sensitivity to changes in serum potassium. Attacks last minutes to days. They are triggered by exercise that is quickly followed by sustained rest, excitement, or cold temperature. Episodes typically begin in prox-imal muscles spreading distally. After several years, permanent weakness occurs.[158]

Startle disease

Startle disease, or recurrent exaggerated startle (a flexed crouch, blinking, and grimacing), represents a group of conditions associated with many etiologies. Startle epilepsy is one form, mostly seen in children with other signs of neurologic disease. Triggered by unexpected stimuli, the startle can progress to a generalized or partial complex seizure.[159]

Stiff person syndrome

Stiff person syndrome is also elicited by sudden tactile or emotional stimuli or startling noises. The sufferer suddenly develops painful spasms of the axial muscles that become "board-like". Spasms can last weeks, although brief spasms are most common. Spasms are reduced during sleep, and motor and sensory functioning appears otherwise normal. An autoimmune process is the likely etiology.[160]

Astasia–abasia

Astasia–abasia is the inability to walk, stand or sit upright without assistance and without any other neuropsychiatric abnormality. When prone or sitting the patient can move his legs. Some patients may walk like the "Scarecrow" in the *Wizard of Oz*, limbs flopping about haphazardly, the patient teetering on falling. When they do fall, the decent is slow and rarely causes injury.

Astasia–abasia has been reported in patients with identifiable illness such as Sjogren's syndrome,[161] the Bailey–Cushing syndrome involving midline cerebellar lesions,[162] and corpus callosum lesions.[163] In a rare follow-up of patients with astasia–abasia, 27 children and adolescents who received the diagnosis between 1965 and 1979 were re-examined from 5 to 22 years later. Most were symptom-free.[164]

Camptocormia

Camptocormia is a forced posture with a forward-bent trunk which appears during standing or sitting, as if the patient had abdominal pain. It was described among soldiers and interpreted as psychogenic or as an effort to avoid responsibility. Recent studies identify it as a segmental dystonia of abdominal muscles associated with several neurologic and psychiatric disorders.[165]

Paroxysmal dyskinesia

Paroxysmal dyskinesia is characterized by episodes of sudden, usually short (less than 30 min and often less than 5 min), painful dyskinesia that may include chorea, athetosis, and ballismus. Orobuccal movements can cause tongue-biting, and leg movements can lead to falls with injury, eliciting the consideration of seizure disorder. Consciousness, however, is maintained. For most patients the cause is unknown, and many are said to have psychogenic movement disorder. Many such patients also have co-occurring behavioral and sensory features such as numbness, paresthesia, electrical sensations, and painful burning. In a study of 46 patients identified as having paroxysmal dyskinesia, no specific cause could be identified in 21. Two others had a family history of paroxysmal dyskinesia, but no other pathology was noted. Among the rest, nine were said to be psychogenic, four had cerebral vascular disease, two multiple sclerosis, two encephalitis, two cerebral trauma, two peripheral trauma, one migraine, and one kernicterus.[166] A study of 20 new patients and a review of 130 case reports concluded that identified causes are more common than previously thought, although still the minority of patients. Multiple sclerosis, cerebral vascular insufficiency, stroke, head trauma, metabolic abnormalities and encephalitis were the most likely defined etiologies.[167] Many such patients, however, have non-specific EEG abnormalities, and a seizure spectrum disorder has been suggested as an underlying factor in these patients.[168]

Conclusion

Almost all psychiatric disease is associated with disturbances in motor functioning. Almost all patients with movement disorder also experience behavioral disturbances. Because the brain's motor system is extensive, many brain diseases impinge on that system, eliciting abnormal motor signs and symptoms. All the motor signs and symptoms detailed above are seen in psychiatric and in neurologic patients, and this common experience illustrates the artificial nature of separating these patient groups as either "neurologic" or "psychiatric". The presence of cerebellar or basal ganglia signs, for example, does not exclude the likelihood that the patient has other features that warrant a psychiatric diagnosis. The presence of the movement disorder increases that likelihood. The presence of depressive illness or psychosis also increases the likelihood that the patient may also have a recognized neurologic disorder. Evaluating the motor functioning of a patient with disturbed behavior thoroughly is essential to diagnosis and treatment. The evaluation of a patient with a movement disorder for the presence of a behavioral disturbance is also necessary for proper diagnosis and treatment.

The identification of co-occurring movement and behavior disorder has diagnostic and treatment implications. The presence of motor features consistent with epilepsy, for example, suggests that if such a patient has a depressive illness or psychotic disorder, that anticonvulsants might be the best treatment options. The presence of catatonic features warns against the rash use of antipsychotic agents. Examining the patient from the three-way view perspective of the motor system (see Chapter 3) may reveal circumscribed disease that radically alters the differential diagnosis (e.g. identifying a right-sided subcortical stroke as the etiology of the psychotic disorder). The presence of motor signs in a person who chronically abuses illicit drugs suggests brain damage that involves higher cognitive functioning and the limits of disposition and behavioral intervention. The emergence of new motor features may reflect an adverse medication effect or the harbinger of a progressive pathophysiology.

NOTES

1 Alexander Pope: *An Essay on Man*, cited in Sims (1995, p. 22).
2 Taylor (1991).
3 Rogers (1985).

4 Executive function refers to prefrontal cortex oversight of cognition. Recognizing problems and opportunities, and developing, carrying out, monitoring, self-correcting, judging the results, and stopping when appropriate are examples of executive function.

5 Saint-Cyr *et al.* (1995).

6 Taylor and Fink (2006).

7 Bracha *et al.* (2005).

8 Volchan *et al.* (2003); Leslie *et al.* (2004).

9 Ono *et al.* (2000).

10 Schutter and van Honk (2005).

11 Williams *et al.* (2006a).

12 Fink and Taylor (2003).

13 Weinstock *et al.* (2003).

14 Parker *et al.* (1993).

15 The extensive studies by Parker and Hadzi-Pavolvic summarized in their monograph *Melancholia: A Disorder of Movement and Mood* (1996) emphasize psychomotor disturbance as the classic sign of the syndrome.

16 Lewis (1934).

17 Braude and Barnes (1983).

18 Rubino (2002).

19 Kaufman (1995).

20 Venna and Sabin (1992).

21 Smith *et al.* (1999).

22 Koroshetz *et al.* (1992).

23 For a detailed presentation of the catatonia literature, see Fink and Taylor (2003).

24 Fink and Taylor (2003, chapter 8); Caroff *et al.* (2004, chapters 16 and 17).

25 A rating scale of catatonic features developed at the State University of New York at Stony Brook can be used to systematically assess patients for both clinical and research purposes (Fink *et al.*, 1993).

26 Fink (1996a,b); Carroll *et al.* (2001); Fink and Taylor (2003).

27 Diesing and Wijdicks (2006). Patient 7.2 illustrates that NMS and malignant catatonia are similar and that NMS need not be associated with exposure to antipsychotics. The appropriate treatment is an initial trial with lorazepam (often in daily doses of 8–20mg) followed by bilateral ECT if needed. This approach typically producing relief from the life-threatening features within a few days and full remission with 12–15 treatments (Fink and Taylor, 2003).

28 See discussion in Chapter 6.

29 Gjessing (1938, 1974).

30 Catatonia in a young patient is associated with the same conditions that are seen in adult patients, with the exception that epilepsy and developmental disorders are more frequent. When the catatonia is the result of a mood disorder, there will likely be a family history of depressive illness (Fink and Taylor, 2003).

31 In addition to catatonia, akinetic mutism is seen in bilateral lesions involving the anterior cingulate gyri and supplemental motor areas. Lorazepam challenge may relieve the syndrome when it is an aspect of catatonia (Fink and Taylor, 2003).

32 Normal persons will initially increase their blink rate and then habituate to the examiner's tapping the glabellar, the striking finger is not in the patient's visual field. An abnormal response is also seen in Parkinson's syndrome.

33 Ganser and Shorter (1965).

34 A young woman who had lived her entire life just outside New York City and who had never spoken a language other than English when manic had periods of excitement during which she spoke with a German accent as if in an old World War II movie. At other times she lay on her bed in a stupor, barely mumbled, and could be put into postures. As the stuporous phases of her illness ended, the German accent reappeared.

35 Echolalia is also associated with transcortical aphasias, autism, Gilles de la Tourette's syndrome, and frontal–temporal dementia.

36 In the nineteenth century, stupor associated with mutism and immobility was said to define melancholia attonita (Taylor and Fink, 2006).

A stuporous, mute, and immobile catatonic patient can be temporarily relieved of the condition with several mg of IV lorazepam. Around the clock lorazepam (8–24 mg daily) can maintain the relief without sedation in many patients. Catatonic patients who do not respond fully to lorazepam will respond fully to bilateral ECT. See Fink and Taylor (2003) for detailed discussions of the treatment of catatonia.

37 A similar technique is often helpful in getting the attention of a manic patient. Rather than trying to outshout the manic patient interrupting his press of speech (an impossible task), the examiner whispers the patient's name. The whisper stands out from the din and draws the patient's attention.

38 Bleuler (1950, p. 215) referred to this as hyperkinetic catatonia or faxen-psychosis.

39 Cataplexy is the sudden and usually brief loss of muscle tone and is associated with narcolepsy (Kobayashi et al., 2002).

40 Her catatonia was remitted by a trial of lorazepam, reaching a maximum effect dose of 24 mg daily.

41 Some manic patients will have classic OCD features (Hantouche et al., 2003).

42 APA (1994, p. 121).

43 Ungvari and Rankin (1990).

44 High-stepping gait or "cock walk", along with other movements, psychosis and cognitive impairment is seen in manganese poisoning. Manganese is use in the manufacture of paints, disinfectants fertilizers, and varnishes (Clayton and Clayton, 1981).

45 Joseph and Saint-Hilaire (1992).

46 Adler et al. (1993).

47 Carr and Tan (1976); Kon (1994); Pal (1997); Martin (1999).

48 Hammond (1883/1973, p. 854).

49 Hammond (1883/1973, pp. 507–14).

50 Fink and Taylor (2003, vignette 2.5, pp. 24–5).

51 Dyspraxia typically reflects parietal lobe disease, but is also seen in disconnection syndromes. A disconnection syndrome is recognized when two associational cortical areas are disconnected from one another by a structural brain lesion. Lesions of the corpus callosum lead to disconnection syndromes. Some patients with Broca's aphasia from stroke will have

a disconnection of their left hand from right frontal associational cortex control, and will show left-hand sympathetic dyspraxia, termed sympathetic because the right hand is paretic or paralyzed (Kolb and Whishaw, 1996, pp. 345–50).

52 Lamberti *et al.* (2002).

53 Ovsiew (1997).

54 Chapter 13 provides a detailed discussion of bedside cognitive testing.

55 Kennard *et al.* (1994).

56 Carter and Zee (1997).

57 Gresty (1977).

58 O'Driscoll *et al.* (1998).

59 Thaker *et al.* (1996).

60 Tien *et al.* (1996); Hutton *et al.* (2004).

61 Tien *et al.* (1992); Gambini *et al.* (1993).

62 Balint syndrome refers to optic ataxia in which visual cues interfere with movement, making the movements imprecise. Directed gaze is impaired. The syndrome is associated with right temporo-parietal–occipital junction lesions (Valenza *et al.*, 2004).

63 Clark and Albers (1995); Kiyosawa *et al.* (1996); Thomke and Hopf (1999).

64 Al-Din *et al.* (1994).

65 Serdaru *et al.* (1982).

66 Fong (2005).

67 Taylor (1999, chapter 10).

68 Ronthal (1992).

69 National Sleep Foundation, Washington D.C. "Sleep in America" poll 2005; Breslau *et al.* (1996).

70 Benca *et al.* (1992).

71 Arroyo *et al.* (2001).

72 Antidepressant drugs also elicit myoclonus (Lemus and Lieberman, 1992).

73 Montagna (2004); Arroyo *et al.* (2001).

74 Montagna (2004); Phillips (2004).

75 Pranzatelli (2003).

76 Demirkiran and Jankovic (1995).

77 Narcolepsy, a heritable disorder, is identified from the presence of DR15 (DR2) and DQ6 (DQ1) human leukocyte antigen testing, low levels of hypocretin-1 in the spinal fluid, and from polysomnograms (Kobayashi *et al.*, 2002).

78 McCreadie *et al.* (2005).

79 Bottin *et al.* (2005).

80 Reduced muscle tone is associated with dementia. Such patients are slack-jawed, stooped, limp-limbed and shuffle when they walk.

81 APA Task Force (1979); the incidence may be as high as 15% (Ballerini *et al.*, 2002).

82 Diphenhyramine, 50mg bolus IV, can quickly relieve most antipsychotic drug-induced acute dystonias. Because the half-life of all antipsychotic drugs is longer than the half-life of diphenhyramine, several days of additional treatment with amantidine or benztropine are needed to prevent recurrence.

83 Saint-Hilaire and Feldman (1992).

84 Shefner (1992).

85 Adams and Salam-Adams (1992).

86 Dale *et al.* (2004).

87 Bartzokis *et al.* (1999); Daras *et al.* (1994).

88 Bonnet *et al.* (1998).

89 Fenn *et al.* (1996).

90 APA Task Force (1979).

91 Wade *et al.* (1987).

92 Tenback *et al.* (2007).

93 Stubner *et al.* (2004).

94 Teive *et al.* (2001). Chapter 12 discusses Gilles de La Tourette's syndrome as a variant of obsessive-compulsive disorder.

95 Kurlan *et al.* (2002).

96 Alsobrook and Pauls (2002).

97 Ford (1989).

98 Hammond (1883/1973, pp. 524–34).

99 Schmahmann (2004); Varambally *et al.* (2006).

100 Taylor (1991); Nopoulos *et al.* (1999); Ichimiya *et al.* (2001).

101 Robertson (2004).

102 Smith *et al.* (2005a).

103 Vakil *et al.* (2004).

104 Hermann *et al.* (2004).

105 Roth *et al.* (2004).

106 Mace and Trimble (1996); Krem (2004); Stone *et al.* (2005), in their extensive review, found 29% misdiagnosis in early studies but only 5% misdiagnosis in more recent reports. Attempts to delineate personality traits that predict non-epileptic seizures have not been successful (Vanderzant *et al.*, 1986).

107 Stone *et al.* (2003).

108 Slater (1965); Slater and Glithero (1965); Critchley (1950); Heilman *et al.* (1985).

109 DSM-IV, p. 453.

110 Duncan (1996).

111 Dubois (1905, pp. 22–6).

112 Venna and Sabin (1992).

113 Pollmann *et al.* (2004).

114 Primary gain is the presumed easing of intra-psychic tension from the behavior while secondary gain is the tangible gain from the behavior. Patient 4.1's cerebellar motor signs were initially considered "psychogenic". Her primary gain was the easing of tension between her dependency and autonomy needs – the disease taking the decision out of her hands. Her secondary gain was the attention she received from her doctors and nurses.

115 Personal communication, Phil Lebowitz, MD.

116 Stone *et al.* (2002).

117 Slater (1965); Merskey and Buhrich (1975); Moene *et al.* (2000).

118 The motor weakness is explained as a combination of two factors. First, right-sided lesions are associated with some neglect that is expressed as "weakness". Second, the bend of the internal capsule carrying crossed motor fibers is in the anterior part of the parietal lobe, and lesions near or in it can cause motor weakness.

119 Pehlivanturk and Unal (2002).

120 Schrag *et al.* (2004).

121 Keane (1989).

122 Groppel *et al.* (2000).

123 Simon *et al.* (2004).

124 Vignette provided by Aida Rjepaj, MD, who was a PGY-2 resident at the time. The patient had partial complex seizures with their origin in frontal brain regions as they were associated with bilateral upper limb movements and forced speech. Of patients with partial complex fits, 40–60% will have elevated prolactin levels as the limbic seizure drives the hypothalamic–pituitary system. The peak level is seen about 20 min after the seizure ends and is cleared within the next 5 min providing a very narrow window of opportunity to obtain this diagnostically useful information (Chen *et al.*, 2005).

125 Green and Devinsky (1992).

126 Factor *et al.* (1995); Stone *et al.* (2004).

127 Kotagal *et al.* (2002). These authors identified a seizure disorder in 34% of patients diagnosed with non-epileptic seizure events. Jedrzejczak *et al.* (1999), in a study of over 1000 patients assessed for possible epilepsy, found 85 (7.8%) to have non-epileptic seizures. Of these, 37 (42%) had epileptic seizures at other times.

128 Kellinghaus *et al.* (2004).

129 Krem (2004).

130 Feinstein *et al.* (2001).

131 Wirthrington and Wynn-Parry (1985).

132 Monday and Jankovic (1993).

133 Fernandez-Alvarez (2005).

134 Fahn (1993).

135 Factor *et al.* (1995); Lang (2006).

136 Wirthrington and Wynn-Parry (1985).

137 Krem (2004).

138 Flor-Henry *et al.* (1981).

139 Mailis-Gagnon *et al.* (2003).

140 Starkstein *et al.* (1992); Dolan (2002).

141 Damasio (2003).

142 Black *et al.* (2004).

143 Marshall *et al.* (1997).

144 Yazici and Kostakoglu (1998); Vuilleumier (2005); Fink *et al.* (2006).

145 Ron (2001).

146 Vuilleumier (2005).

147 Athwal *et al.* (2001).

148 Vuilleumier (2005).

149 Marshall *et al.* (1997).

150 Stippich *et al.* (2006).

151 Lempert *et al.* (1991).

152 Heruti *et al.* (2002).

153 Yazici *et al.* (2004).

154 Baxter and Warrington (1986).

155 Alexander *et al.* (1992); Roeltgen *et al.* (1983).

156 Modified from Popescu and Vaidya (2007).

157 Feinberg *et al.* (1992); Chan and Ross (1997).

158 Brown (1992).

159 Joseph and Saint-Hilaire (1992).

160 Blum and Jankovic (1991).

161 Lafforgue *et al.* (1993).

162 Bailey and Cushing (1925).

163 Laroche *et al.* (1976); Kumral *et al.* (1995).

164 Stickler and Cheung-Patton (1989).

165 Reichel *et al.* (2001).

166 Demirkiran and Jankovic (1995).

167 Blakeley and Jankovic (2002).

168 Hines *et al.* (1995).

8

Disturbances in emotional experience

During that long process, or rather succession of processes, in which the sexual organs of the human female are employed in forming, lodging, expelling, and lastly feeding the offspring, there is no time at which the mind may not become disordered; but there are two periods at which the body is sustaining the effects of labour, the other several months afterwards, when the body is sustaining the effects of nursing. I have repeatedly seen the commencement of mania and of melancholia in women who were in childbed, or who had recovered from their delivery ... Nearly all these cases were instances, not of mania, but of melancholia ... There was an incipient stage in which the mind was wrong, yet right enough to recognize that it was wrong ...[1]

The origin of human "awareness of self" and the recognition of a personal past and future has been attributed to experiencing emotion. Normal emotions are transient and context specific. This awareness leads to recognizing previous emotional experiences of similar valence (e.g. quality of the emotion, such as happy, sad, and angry), that the present emotional experience is self-generated and uniquely personal, and that the emotion will end but there will be others. Past, present, and future are understood subjectively within the context of emotional experience.[2] For millennia, sufferers of a derangement in this emotional life were recognized as separated from the human experience and were said to be maniacal, mad, or delirious.

While all non-ill persons experience sadness, irritability, anger, and happiness, the emotions endured and expressed in depressive illness, mania, and anxiety disorder are subjectively and objectively distinct. This chapter describes the psychopathology of these states.

Terminology of emotional experience

The terminology of emotion is confounded by the blending of expressions of common usage (e.g. feeling), neuroscience (e.g. emotion) and psychology (e.g. affect). Mood can be considered "disordered" and a category of illness, but being in a "bad mood" or "good mood" describes a normal occurrence. Present-day mood disorders were once termed affective disorders. However, mood and affect are considered different aspects of emotional life, and thus the change in terminology implies incorrectly a new understanding of these conditions.

Taber's medical dictionary defines *affect* as "an emotional reaction with an experience", *blunted affect* as "greatly diminished emotional response", and *flat affect* as the "virtual absence of emotional response". *Emotion* is defined as a subjective experience with associated physiological changes: "a passion or sensibility marked by physical changes in the body such as alteration in heart rate and respiratory activity". Also included in the definition of emotion is "a mental state or feeling such as fear, hate, love, anger, grief, or joy, arising as a subjective experience rather than as a conscious mental effort". Emotion is considered "a drive". *Empathy* is the "objective awareness of and insight into the feelings, emotions, and behavior of another", while *feeling* is "the conscious phase of nervous activity". *Mood* is "a pervasive and sustained emotion" with the same examples that were used to illustrate emotion. *Mood disorder* is "any mental disorder that has a disturbance of mood as the predominant feature". Emotion and mood are considered as the same construct, emotion being brief and mood sustained. Affect is also defined as emotion.[3]

Psychopathology texts offer similar imprecise and overlapping terms. Sims, for example,[4] defines feeling as a transient positive or negative reaction to an experience. Affect is "differentiated specific feelings towards an object". Affect is said to be momentary while mood is "a more prolonged emotional state". Emotion is related to "the physiological and psychosomatic concomitants of mood". Sims recognizes the interchangeability of these terms.

The DSM-IV is better organized, but equally confusing. It uses "mood" to characterize emotion throughout the mood disorder section, while in the schizophrenia section "affective flattening", "negative symptoms" and "inappropriate affect" are employed. But what is observed in identifying negative features is the diminution in intensity or the absence of moods or emotional expression. No term is used in the anxiety disorder section other than anxiety, fear, and panic.[5] The psychoanalytic literature further roils terminology by the addition of anhedonia (loss of the ability to experience pleasure), and alexithymia (difficulty expressing and recognizing one's emotional state).

The confusion in terminology reflects the lack of a clear structure for examining, understanding, and organizing the psychopathology of emotion. Overlapping traditional terms are poorly formulated and imprecise. In contrast, the neurobiological literature of emotion offers some guidance in delineating emotional experience. The term most used is *emotion*, and when possible, the perturbations of emotional life are discussed here with this designation.

Table 8.1. Aspects of emotional expression

Intensity: from absent (in apathy, stupor, catatonia, emotional blunting, and motor aprosodia)
   to intense (in rage, panic, despair)

Quality (valence): happy, sad, angry, anxious

Variability: from extremely labile (as in metabolic and manic delirium) to continuous
   expression of a single emotional state for weeks (as in mania) or months (as in melancholia)

Appropriateness: from congruence between the expressed quality and the situation to no
   connection (as in melancholia, mania, panic attack)

Recognition: poor self-recognition is an aspect of denial of illness (anosagnosia);
   poor recognition of the emotional expression of others is receptive aprosodia

---

Disturbances in emotional expression

Table 8.1 displays the aspects of emotional expression considered in the examination.

Disturbances in intensity

Perturbed intensity of emotional expression can be increased as in rage, panic, and euphoria, or substantially decreased as in stupor, apathy, and emotional blunting.

Decreased expression

Emotional blunting (affective flattening or stiffening)

Emotional blunting is the loss of emotional expression in gesture, facial expression, and tone of voice. It is characteristic of schizophrenia and structural frontal lobe disease.[6] Emotional blunting combines the two independent dimensions of volition and emotional expression.[7] The loss of volition without a loss of emotional expression is also seen in patients with chronic manic-depressive illness.[8]

Emotionally blunted persons appear stiff or still, their faces mask-like and their voice monotone. Chronic schizophrenics typically have profound loss of emotional expression. In contrast, patients with severe depressive illness express apprehension and distress unless in a stupor or catatonic state.[9]

Kraepelin emphasized the presence of emotional blunting as characteristic of dementia praecox, stating that patients have "no desire ... no visible effort of the will", being "languid and expressionless ... quite dull, experiencing neither fear nor hope nor desires ... this peculiar and fundamental want of any strong feeling of the impression of life, with unimpaired ability to understand and to remember, is really the diagnostic symptom of the disease before us."[10]

Emotional blunting can be reliably assessed and there are several rating scales that facilitate the evaluation.[11] Table 8.2 displays features common to the scales.

Table 8.2. Emotional blunting

Loss of emotional expression	Avolition
Absent, shallow, incongruous mood	Indifference or unconcern for own
Constricted expression	present situation
Unvarying expression lacking	Indifference or unconcern for own future
modulation	(lacks plans, ambition, desires, drives)
Expressionless face	
Unvarying monotonous voice	

Unlike patients suffering with motor aprosodia (see later), the emotionally blunted patient also loses subjective emotional experience, described as emotional dullness.[12] The patient is indifferent toward family members and other previously close persons. They experience little or no pleasure, grief, joy, satisfaction, or disappointment. They are without sentiment or sympathy, and are indifferent to their circumstances. They may laugh suddenly, but offer no reason for the outburst, and deny any sense of associated joy, an ataxia of feelings.[13] When asked if a prolonged hospital stay would interfere with their plans, they commonly respond "Well, if I have too". When asked what they would do if they won the lottery, their response is often limited to "Put the money in the bank".

The emotional dullness is associated with a loss of social graces, and such patients become rude and ill-mannered, but usually without aggression. When suddenly assaultive, violence is unemotional, and may be related to a delusional idea or a hallucination. Many of the features of emotional blunting reflect deficits in executive functioning.[14]

Motor aprosodia

Motor prosody is the expression of emotion in spoken language, facial expression, gesture and body language. Receptive prosody is the ability to recognize the emotional expression of others. Motor aprosodia is associated with disease in the non-dominant cerebral hemisphere, particularly in frontal circuitry. Motor aprosodia is descriptively identical to the loss of emotional expression described as emotional blunting/flat affect. Motor aprosodia is described in autistic spectrum disorders,[15] schizophrenia,[16] and depression.[17]

Avolition

Avolition is reduced interest and activity associated with an absence of emotion, interest, and concern. Avolition is associated with schizophrenia and frontal lobe disease.[18] Such patients have a paucity of ideas and reduced interests, ignore once-cherished hobbies and skills, are indifferent to their situation, and take little interest in work, interactions with others, or their medical care. When asked what their typical day is like they are at a loss to provide details, their days empty of activity unless prodded by others. Prodding may lead to irritability and angry outbursts.

A schizophrenic patient when asked what he did on a typical day said "I go and get the paper every morning and bring it back to the house (a halfway facility)." When asked what he liked in the paper he said "I don't read it." "What do you do then?" "I sit in the day room." Offering no other details, he said he was not bored and had no desire to do anything else.

Such patients offer no plans beyond the next meal or cigarette. They lack long-range goals, and the plans they mention are unrealistic or never pursued. One young schizophrenic said his hobby was the guitar. When asked what music he liked to play he responded "Well, I don't have the guitar yet. I'm thinking of getting it." Another patient with limited education who had been in the hospital for several years said he wanted to be a doctor. Another chronically hospitalized patient, when asked what his future plans were, said "I'll get an education." He could not elaborate other than saying "English and things." Avolitional patients have a paucity of thoughts and ideas. They cannot elaborate or provide a detailed history of their lives or illness.

Apathy

The apathetic patient appears listless, does little, makes minimal effort on assigned tasks or needed chores, and is indifferent to his situation. Will and initiative are lost. *Abulia* is a synonymous term. The minimal expression of emotion may be distorted. A proposed mechanism is the disruption of emotion-cognition processes so that emotional life no longer drives thinking and the generation of ideas, leading to waning of interests and actions (sometimes referred to as "psychic akinesia"). The inability to generate ideas leads to loss of interest and thus hypoactivity.[19]

Increased emotional expression

Sustained and substantially increased intensity in emotional expression is seen in manic-depressive illness. Brief, but equally intense, emotional expression is seen in panic and phobic disorders, angry outbursts associated with epilepsy, traumatic brain injury, catastrophic reactions of persons with cognitive disorders, delirium, and in some persons with personality disorder, and in association with pathologic crying and emotional incontinence. Manic-depression and anxiety states are described at the end of the chapter.

Disturbances in the quality of emotion

Witzelsucht

Witzelsucht is a happy-go-lucky carelessness and silly facetious humor. *Moria* is a synonymous term. The patient cannot refrain from making light of any situation, makes inane jokes and puns, and can rarely be engaged in a serious conversation. The jocularity, however, is shallow. No other signs associated with hypomania need be present. Witzelsucht is associated with lack of foresight and the ability to plan. It is a sign of frontal circuitry and cerebellar disease, and is an aspect of the frontal lobe disinhibited syndrome.[20]

Pathological laughing and crying, and emotional incontinence

Pathological laughing and crying and emotional incontinence entail the sudden, socially inappropriate and embarrassing release of intense emotion-related motor sequences. Involuntary emotional expression disorder has been offered as an official term.[21] In pathological laughing and crying, there is no or only a mild corresponding subjective experience. The brief paroxysms occur without an apparent motivating stimulus or in response to a stimulus that would not elicit the emotion in the past. The facial expression and associated movements of the emotion are exaggerated, and the quality of the emotion can be typical or may seem feigned. These sudden emotional "release" phenomena are associated with cerebellar–pontine and non-dominant cerebral hemisphere disease.[22] Associated conditions include stroke, dementia, traumatic brain injury, multiple sclerosis, and amyotrophic lateral sclerosis.[23] In emotional incontinence, the observed emotion is congruent in quality but not in the intensity to the subjective experience, which is milder.

Emotional paroxysm is also a sudden and brief expression of an emotion, but the paroxysm is accompanied by the intense corresponding subjective experience. Emotional incontinence and paroxysms are associated with manic-depression, seizure disorder, and brain damage from trauma or chronic hallucinogen drug use.[24]

Disturbances in the variability

The valence of emotional expression normally changes as circumstances change. Constricted emotional expression (also termed constricted affect) is the loss of normal variability. Constricted emotional expression is independent of the quality or intensity of the expressed emotion. The melancholic patient does not vary his/her apprehension and gloom despite reassurances that his/her life circumstances are fine. The agoraphobic patient remains fearful regardless of the reality outside his/her home. The manic patient is irritable, defying placation. The schizophrenic is indifferent, regardless of his circumstances. Lability of emotional expression is experienced in manic-depression. For example:

A manic woman was shouting angrily at the nurses in the nursing station. She abruptly screamed and ran down the inpatient unit's long hallway. The nurses and unit psychiatrist gave chase. The patient darted around the corner of the L-shaped unit. As the pursuers came to the corner, they almost collided with the patient who was standing looking out the large window. She was in tears, sobbing uncontrollably, and saying how sad it was that she was "locked up" on such a sunny day.

A manic, euphoric man stood on a chair in the day room of the inpatient unit declaiming in loud theatrical tones his fantastic accomplishments. Another patient, annoyed at the noise, lightly slapped the orator and told him to be quiet. The orator burst into tears, stepped down, and began relating why he was "no good".

A manic patient was laughing and expounding on his "great ideas" about life. Coming to a sad personal topic, he suddenly burst into tears. The examiner commiserated with the patient, and then said, "But just before, you were so happy and about to tell me a joke". The patient, face still tear-stained, immediately brightened, smiled and began to tell a joke.

Some patients with dementia also exhibit lability in emotional expression.

An elderly woman with Alzheimer's disease was giggling girlishly and flirting with the examiner. Not understanding something she said, he asked her for clarification, upon which she scowled and angrily told him he was "an idiot". She tried unsuccessfully to hit him. He distracted her with a comment about a piano in the room, knowing she had once played piano. She immediately brightened, laughed and moved to the instrument.

Appropriateness of emotion

Normal emotional experience is commonly a response to what is occurring in the immediate surroundings, or to a recollection. The expressed emotion is congruent to the situation. In patients with mania and severe depression, emotional expression may become "stuck" in one valence. The apprehension and despair of the melancholic clouds all thoughts and cannot be relieved, despite the presence of loved ones or attempts at engaging the patient in a previously enjoyable activity. The manic patient rages or declaims euphorically despite his mundane circumstances.

Transient emotions (seconds or a few minutes), usually of great intensity, that are incongruent to the situation are associated with complex partial seizures (sudden intense fear, uncontrollable laughter).[25] Episodes of incongruent fearfulness that last from minutes to a few hours are seen in patients with panic and phobic disorders.

Parathymia

The expression of an emotion that is the exact opposite of what is expected under the circumstances (e.g. laughing at tragic news), or the expression of emotions that appear unnatural, exaggerated or theatrical is termed parathymia. The expression is shallow and flat. Emotional rapport is poor. Bleuler considered this an important sign of schizophrenia.[26] Senseless laughing without mirthfulness is considered a sign of hebephrenia.

Pathological anger

Irritability is associated with several psychiatric syndromes, most commonly depression and mania. Persons with paranoid personality disorder and delusions of persecution are typically angered in response to their view of a hostile world.[27] Patients who have abused chemical inhalants are prone to sudden, potentially lethal violent anger.[28] Pre- and post-ictal aggressiveness is typically not goal-directed. When frustrated or denied a demand, persons with antisocial personality can be lethally and criminally violent.[29] Irritability and anger is also observed in patients following stroke in frontal–temporal brain regions.[30] This irritability is associated with difficulties with speech and language, and mobility.[31]

Recognition of emotion

Subjective awareness of emotion

The subjective awareness of one's emotional state is a human trait. The concept of *alexithymia* (from the Greek *alexis* [no words] and *thymos* [emotion]) was formulated to define a deficit in which the affected person has reduced capacity to experience, identify, verbalize, think about, and fantasize emotion.[32] Overlapping forms have been described.[33] In one, there is an absence of the emotional experience (can't feel it), and consequently the absence of the cognition accompanying emotion (can't describe it or fantasize about it). A second is a deficit in the cognition of emotion, sparing the capacity to experience emotion. A deficit in corpus callosum transfer of non-linguistic information (i.e. the subjective emotional experience) is another formulation.[34] Alexithymia is presumed to be a personality trait,[35] but it is also considered an aspect of emotional blunting, and reported in persons with Parkinson's disease, depression, anxiety disorder, substance abuse, and eating disorder.[36]

Empathy and receptive aprosodia

Empathy is the capacity to experience the emotional state of others by "putting oneself into their shoes". Recognizing the emotion expressed in the other person's face and body language is a prerequisite for empathy. High empathic responses are associated with the tendency to imitate others during social interactions.[37]

Receptive prosody is the capacity to recognize and understand the emotional expression of others. Poor receptive prosody undermines the capacity for empathy, but they are not synonymous constructs. Persons with antisocial personality disorder, for example, recognize the emotional state of other persons, but do not experience their distress.[38]

Strokes in the right basal ganglia and temporal lobe, and the parietal opercu-
lum are associated with poor recognition of the emotions expressed by others.[39]
Poor receptive prosody in patients with schizophrenia is associated with deficits in
the recognition of facial emotion.[40] The deficit is reflected in patients with persecutory delusions concluding that others "look angry" or are about to hurt them.

Examining for disturbances in emotional expression

The emotional state of the patient is recognized in his/her facial expression and
body language. Some patients cry, laugh, threaten, or shakily scan the room wide-
eyed and fearful. Changes in emotion are accompanied by changes in motor
behavior. Severely depressed patients are agitated and perseverative. They pace the
hallway of the inpatient unit. They rock when seated and may perseveratively rub
themselves, excoriating their skin. They may pull or twist their hair. Others are
slowed and in stupor or a catatonia. Manic patients and other patients experiencing substantially increased arousal are hyperactive.

Facial expression varies little in severe depression. The eyes are downcast.
The corners of mouth are lowered. The brow is furrow (Omega sign) and the
folds of the upper eyelid are prominent (Veraguth's folds).

In mania, the eyes are opened wide. Facial skin turgor is heightened. In light-
skinned persons the face is flushed. Depressed patients may smile, but it is a forced
social smile with a widening of the mouth but no crinkling around the eyes.

Anger is reflected in facial expression and body language, with a clenching of
jaws, baring of teeth, tightening of fists, and agitated shouting. Subtler expressions of anger are a tightening of lips, avoiding eye contact, and reduced communication. Anxious persons may over-respond to unexpected sudden noise with
a startle reaction. When severe, the eyes are forcefully closed, lips are tight, head is
bent, shoulders are hunched and knees are drawn up.

The examiner also tries to elicit emotion. Strong emotion is often linked
to family members, reasons for hospitalization, and general health concerns.
Discussing these topics in history-taking probes for strong emotion. Humor,
however, is the best all-purpose probe for testing the patient's ability to express
emotion appropriately. Using humor to assess for the presence of severe depression is invaluable. Patient 8.1 illustrates.

Patient 8.1

**A 55-year-old Scottish woman required a liver transplant. Following the
procedure, she developed a severe infection. Her infection required extended
ICU care and she was intubated and under sedation for several weeks.**

**As she was being weaned from sedation and increasingly aware of her
circumstances, she became tearful and related (by brief whispering efforts**

and writing) her pessimism about her future. She communicated that she was having thoughts of wishing she were dead.

A psychiatry resident diagnosed depression, and as was common practice, recommended low doses of an SSRI for "mild" depression. An attending physician, however, suggested the patient was likely demoralized, was not melancholic, and that no medication was needed.

After introducing himself to the patient he opened the examination by saying he was particularly sorry to find her unable to speak in her normal voice because he "loved a Scottish accent". The patient broke into a big grin, weakly laughed and quipped that she too was sorry she couldn't speak in her normal voice. By the end of the examination it was clear the patient was not suffering from depressive illness. Several follow-up supportive visits resolved lingering psychiatric concerns.

Classic syndromes of disturbed emotion: manic-depression

Melancholia is the core syndrome of manic-depressive illness, and sufferers of manic-depression experience depression more often than forms of mania. The classification of manic-depression and mood disorders is presented in Chapter 16.

Hypomania

In the classic psychopathology literature, hypomania is not simply heightened feelings of optimism or increased energy; it is the expression of disease. A patient described the unfolding of the illness as if "I'm running fast down a steep hill. At first it's fun, exciting, great. I love the feeling. But then I'm running too fast and start to lose control and I'm in danger of falling. Then I'm afraid I won't be able to stop."

Kraepelin noted that at first the hypomanic patient "may appear livelier, even more capable than formerly [producing] witty remarks and fancies, puns, startling comparisons ... Nevertheless even in the slightest degrees of the disorder the following features are characteristic, the lack of inner unity in the course of ideas, the incapacity to carry out consistently a definite series of thoughts, to work out steadily and logically and to set in order given ideas ... Mood is predominantly exalted and cheerful, influenced by the feeling of heightened capacity for work ... Increased busyness is the most striking feature ... he is a stranger to fatigue, his activity goes on day and night; work becomes very easy to him; ideas flow to him ... the tendency to debauchery usually becomes especially fatal to the patients. He begins to get drunk frequently, to gamble foolishly, to frequent brothels."[41]

Acute mania

All criteria for acute mania[42] require the presence of abnormal emotional expression with increased or fluctuating intensity and emotions ranging from giddiness to ecstasy and irritability to rage. Intense emotion colors thinking and the patient is expansive, loudly and dramatically expressing a sense of great self-importance. Outlandish dress and self-decoration occur. Kraepelin offers a photograph of one of his manic patients, corsage in his lapel, smoking a cigar and a pipe simultaneously. He carries a baton with which, we are told, he insists on conducting other patients in song.

When emotional expression is labile, periods of despair, apprehension and tearfulness intermingle with euphoria. These intense "mixed" states are not distinct forms of mania; they *are* mania.

The intense emotion of acute mania is associated with increased arousal that elicits hyperactivity. Flooded with racing, multiple lines of thinking and great energy, the patient rushes from one chore to the next. Anything that catches his eye is immediately attended to. At its height frenzy occurs. Psychosis is present.

The patient's many thoughts are expressed in a torrent of speech. When this pressured speech is substantial, it is difficult to interrupt the patient, who typically becomes angered by attempts to lead him back to the examiner's question or nursing care effort. Such patients are unpleasant and can be dangerous, often requiring temporary seclusion, where the reduced external stimulation modulates their excitement. When emotional expression is mixed, hyperactivity and press of speech yield to periods of psychomotor slowing. When slowing is severe, stupor and catatonia ensue. Table 8.3 displays the psychopathology seen in acute mania. The numbers in parentheses indicate the proportion of acutely hospitalized manic patients found to have the feature.[43] Nearly 50% will also have a history of alcohol abuse. Acute mania is similar in presentation worldwide.[44]

Patient 8.2 is an acute manic patient described by Taylor and Abrams.[45]

Patient 8.2

A 69-year-old woman was brought to the hospital in restraints by the police. She had entered a restaurant, threatened the patrons, and demanded $500 000 from the owner. In a prior similar episode she was said to have paranoid schizophrenia. On admission she was animated and overactive, dressed in a bright, theatrical fashion. Her emotional expression was intense and labile. She was euphoric and irritable, with angry outbursts requiring seclusion. Her speech was rapid, pressured, and circumstantial. She spoke constantly to several hallucinated voices which "provoked" her to speak up for her rights and to claim her "billions". She described the voices as clear, continuous, and coming from two people above her. She believed she was the richest woman in the world, and that there was a plot to harm her. Lithium monotherapy resolved her mania and she remained well for over a year.

Table 8.3. Features of acute mania

Irritability (80%)

Expansiveness (65%)

Euphoria (30–70%)

Emotional lability (70%)

Mixed emotional state with substantial depressive features (25–60%)[46]

Extravagant (25%)[47]

Assaultive or threatening (40%)

Hyperactivity (80–100%)

Intrusive (25%)

Delirious (30%)

Pressured speech (80–100%)

Flight-of-ideas (70%)

Head or body decoration (30%)

Singing or dancing (30%)

Nudity or sexual exposure (20%)

Fecal incontinence or smearing (10%)

Catatonia (20% plus)[48]

Grandiose delusions (50%)

Persecutory delusions (40%)

Auditory hallucinations (50%)

Visual hallucinations (15%)

Olfactory hallucinations (10%)

Experiences of control or alienation (10%)

Suicidal thoughts (5%)

Racing, jumbled, or "too many" thoughts, "out of control" thoughts (80%)

Perseverative ideas about religion (40%), wealth (5%), sexual activities (10%), being
   persecuted or in danger (40%), political concerns (10%)

Hypersexuality (30%)

Reduced sleep time (90%)

Increased alcohol consumption (35%)

Cognitive impairment [distractibility (90%), disorientation (10–30%),
   substantial executive function and memory difficulties (30–50%)]

Acute manic episodes typically emerge rapidly over a few days to several weeks. Psychotic features are commonly expressed and catatonic signs often can be elicited. Kraepelin describes the typical onset:

The beginning of the illness is always fairly sudden; at most headaches, weariness, lack of pleasure in work or a great busyness, irritability, sleeplessness, precede by some days or weeks the outbreak of the more violent manifestations, when a definite state of depression has not, as is very frequent, formed the prelude. The patient rapidly becomes restless, disconnected in their talk, and perpetrate all sorts of curious actions.[49]

John Haslam,[50] recognizing the "stages of mania" more than 170 years before Carlson and Goodwin brought them again to the attention of psychiatry,[51] detailed the unfolding symptoms. This is important for diagnosis, because in its most severe stage mania can be mistaken for a metabolic or toxic delirium or for paranoid schizophrenia, resulting in inappropriate treatments.[52]

On the approach of mania they first become uneasy, are incapable of confining their attention, and neglect any employment to which they have been accustomed; they get little sleep, they are loquacious, and disposed to harangue, and decide promptly and positively upon every subject that may be started. Soon after, they are divested of all restraint in the declaration of their opinions of those, with whom they are acquainted. Their friendships are expressed with fervency and extravagance, their enmities with intolerance and disgust. They now become impatient of contradiction and scorn reproof. For supposed injuries, they are inclined to quarrel and fight with those about them. They have all the appearance of persons inebriated … At length suspicion creeps in upon the mind, they are aware of plots, which had never been contrived, and detect motives that were never entertained. At last the succession of ideas is too rapid to be examined; the mind becomes crowded with thoughts, and confusion ensues. (Haslam, 1809/ 1976, pp. 41–3)

Hammond also recognized that an episode of mania emerged with "a prodro-matic stage" that lasted "several days, or even weeks." Then:

The most prominent symptoms which others observe in a person about to become the subject of acute mania are excessive irritability of temper from very slight causes, a general condition of unreasonableness, suspicions against those he has always esteemed and trusted, and marked changes in his modes of feeling and of expression. His subjective symptoms are pain or uneasiness in the head, vague fears, for which he cannot account, an indisposition to indulge in mental efforts, and often an impossibility of concentrating the attention on any matter requiring any considerable amount of thought, wakefulness, and sleep, when obtained, inquiet and disturbed by morbid dreams.

As the affliction advances to fuller development, these symptoms are all increased in violence, and others make their appearance … His dislike of friends and relations becomes pronounced, and he either treats them with unnatural indifference, or exhibits a degree of active hostility productive of ill feelings and quarrels … From having been economical, he becomes prodigal; from having been temperate and sedate in language, he becomes extravagant and profane; from having held the most moral sentiments, he expresses licentious and obscene views; his ideas are expressed in incoherent language, and often the ideas themselves are illogical and incomprehensible. His handwriting becomes more or less illegible, words are omitted, letters are dropped, he misplaces the date and signature, and introduces phrases which have no relation to the subject … (Hammond, 1883, p. 53)

Delirious (Bell's) mania[53]

Luther Bell first systematically described delirious mania in 1849 as an acute mania with fever and delirium. Kraepelin described delirious mania as an uncommon, rapidly emerging state characterized by extreme excitement, hallucinations and delusions (often fantastic and grandiose), clouding of consciousness, lability of mood with shifts from exaltation to despair to simultaneous moods, and catatonic features including posturing with waxy flexibility, and echolalia and echopraxia. Periods of stupor, excitement, and despondency were followed by a gradual resolution. Kraepelin maintained that the more intense the manic attack the shorter its duration.[54] Delirious mania with its commonly association catatonia has been described repeatedly.[55]

Cyclothymia and the manic-depressive spectrum ("soft bipolar spectrum")

The image of manic-depression is of dramatic episodes of illness interspersed with periods of quiescence. Episodes of mixed symptomatology or of substantial frequency are also recognized. Long-standing, low-grade features, however, were also defined by Kraepelin in the nineteenth century and re-affirmed by Akiskal 80 years later.[56] These "affective temperaments" are the earliest and most subtle expressions of manic-depression and include cyclothymia and traits identified as dysthymic, hyperthymic, and irritable. The various presentations of manic-depression that have been artificially separated into bipolar I, II, rapid cycling, seasonal, and mixed disorders and other low-grade forms constitute a manic-depressive phenotypic spectrum.

Cyclothymia is characterized by gradual and modest mood swings lasting weeks or months. When the mood is elevated, the person is extroverted, outgoing, cheerful, optimistic, impulsive, restless, talkative, and uninhibited. The need for sleep is reduced and appetitive behaviors increase, the latter often leading to interpersonal and social indiscretions. When the mood is depressed, the person is irritable and short-tempered, lethargic and inactive and over-sleeps, taciturn, shy, unsure, pessimistic, and slow in thinking. Table 8.4 displays the behavioral patterns observed in patients with cyclothymia.

Hyperthymia is characterized by continuous overtalkativeness, extroversion, being uninhibited, bombastic, optimistic, restless, meddlesome, vigorous, needing only a few hours of sleep nightly, and cheerfulness to the point of hypomania. Such persons are "hard workers, hard drinkers, and hard players". Dysthymia is characterized by hypersomnolence, brooding, anhedonia, self-blame, passivity, and indecisiveness. The irritable condition is characterized by being hypercritical, brooding, complaining, dysphoric, restless, sarcastic, irritable, and choleric.

In children with manic-depression, episodes are less distinct and sufferers exhibit many spectrum features. Problematic distractibility, rage attacks, and severe

Table 8.4. Behaviors defining cyclothymia[57]

Mood: periods of irritability lasting several days; explosive and aggressive outbursts; grandiose overconfidence followed by periods of low self-esteem and confidence

Cognition: periods of sluggish thinking and poor concentration interspersed with periods of creative, focused and rapid thought

Vegetative symptoms: Hypersomnia alternating with periods of decreased need for sleep; periods of increased food, illicit drug, and alcohol consumption interspersed with periods of abstinence and indifference to such consumption; periods of hypersexuality and promiscuity followed by periods of low or no libido

Activity: Buying sprees and financial extravagance, erratic work efforts from great intensity and productivity to little interest; periods of intense involvement in new often unusual topics followed by periods of profound disillusionment

depression are commonly experienced. During their brief periods of mania, elation, grandiosity, and racing thoughts are reported.[58] Such persons can be misdiagnosed as having borderline personality disorder.[59]

Melancholia

Melancholia is a syndrome that has been recognized for millennia, and a recent review of the mood disorder literature finds it to be the core depression in classification.[60]

Pathological emotional state is always present from the onset and is experienced as unease, inner agitation, irritability, or tearfulness. Some patients initially experience a dulling of emotion. In its severe form, a pervasive and unremitting apprehension and gloom colors all cognitive processes, resulting in a loss of interest, decreased concentration, poor memory, slowed thinking, feelings of failure and low self-worth, and thoughts of suicide. The patient may become terror-stricken and tormented by delusions of guilt or by condemning hallucinated voices, or the hallucinated screams of their "victims". Some cognitive disturbance is always present. The experience is unremitting, and the patient cannot be consoled.

Psychomotor disturbance, either as retardation or agitation, is always present.[61] Retardation varies from a reluctance and hesitation to participate in daily activities, to prolonged inactivity and stupor.[62] Agitation is expressed as restlessness, hand-wringing, and inability to remain still. Patients pace and are in continuous movement progressing to purposeless activity.

Vegetative functions, basic physiologic processes, are severely affected. Sleep is disrupted, appetite and weight lost, sex no longer arouses interest, and the response to stress and chronobiologic functioning are disturbed. The signs of illness are obvious in a loss of weight, unkempt appearance, body odor, and haggard look.

Patients describe these changes as beyond their understanding or control. Neuroendocrine dysfunctions are identified in laboratory studies.[63]

In his memoir, the novelist William Styron describes his illness.[64] After years of alcohol abuse "as a conduit to fantasy and euphoria, and to the enhancement of the imagination", he was suddenly unable to drink without experiencing nausea, "wooziness", and epigastric distress. He first experienced malaise; the shadows of nightfall seemed more somber, the mornings less buoyant. Insomnia and a host of bodily fears followed and everything "slowed down". He became suicidal, explaining that "The pain of severe depression is quite unimaginable to those who have not suffered it, and it kills in many instances because its anguish can no longer be borne."[65] Frightened of these thoughts, he turned to a hospital for asylum where he slowly recovered.

Simple melancholia

Simple melancholia (melancholia simplex) was melancholia without delusions or what was then termed "delirium".[66] It was recognized as a "mental depression" that appeared gradually with the earliest symptom of exaggerated emotional responsiveness that coalesced into fretful unhappiness, silent brooding, loss of mental clarity, and social withdrawal. The patient exaggerates the nature and consequences of his acts and those of others. Inadvertent slights become proof of animosity. Guilt over past indiscretions is re-experienced. Mundane financial concerns become looming disasters. Melancholia progresses into a state of agitation or sluggishness. Concentration becomes difficult. Thoughts may race or be sparse. Everyday chores become overwhelming burdens. A continuous cloud of pessimism envelops all experience.

From the beginning the patient sleeps poorly. Dreams are vivid. Awakenings are frequent and associated with great anxieties, tachycardia and diaphoresis. The morning hours are particularly fitful. Fatigue is constant. Tears and saliva dry up and the patient may experience a constant bitter taste. Appetite is diminished and eating becomes an afterthought. Modest aches and pains become intolerable. Constant complaints elicit repeated and unfruitful medical evaluations and intervention. In women, menstrual function is perturbed. Suicide becomes the solution to ending the experience.

George Man Burrows offers the following descriptions:[67]

From whatever remote cause this affliction proceeds, before any specific hallucination is developed, the patient manifests great susceptibility and nervous agitation, lowness of spirits, and groundless apprehensions; is anxious about trifles, sighs deeply, and perhaps sheds tears. He falls into long reveries, with look fixed on vacuity; neglects all former favourite pursuits, seeks solitude, and shuns intercourse with his nearest and dearest friends ... There is a sense of weight about the stomach, praecordia, and head ... the bowels are disposed to be constipated.

Melancholics are much addicted to biting their nails, picking their fingers, or any pimple or abrasion ... the attending pain is unheeded.

Not to be outdone, Kraepelin describes:

The total absence of energy is very specially conspicuous. The patient lacks the spirit and will-power, like a wheel on a car, which simply runs but in itself has no movement or driving power. He cannot rouse himself, cannot come to any decision, cannot work any longer, does everything the wrong way about, he has to force himself to everything, does not know what to do. A patient declared that he did not know what he wanted, went from one thing to another. The smallest bit of work costs him an un-heard-of effort; even the most everyday arrangements, household work, getting up in the morning, dressing, washing, are only accomplished with the greatest difficulty and in the end indeed are left undone. Work, visits, important letters, business affairs are like a mountain in front of the patient and are just left, because he does not find the power to overcome the opposing inhibitions. If he takes a walk, he remains standing in the house door or at the nearest corner, undecided as to what direction he shall take; he is afraid of every person whom he meets, of every conversation; he becomes shy and retiring, because he cannot any longer look at any one or go among people.[68]

When this state of severe psychomotor retardation worsened, stupor was recognized. When hallucinations and delusions emerged, melancholia gravis was defined. When persecutory delusions were prominent, paranoid melancholia was diagnosed. Fantastic melancholia was identified when hallucinations became intense experiences with visual and auditory phenomena merging into spirits, monsters, body parts, wild beasts, and the devil, and other hallucinatory phenomena (e.g. tastes of soap, excrement; odors of rotting flesh, mildew).

Hammond wrote about the onset of "simple melancholia":

The patient is indisposed to either physical or mental exertion, he shuns the companionship of others, is averse to speaking, frequently remains silent for hours, and if forced to respond to questions put to him does so in the fewest possible words, and without change of countenance ... his conversation is entirely in regard to himself, of his horrible feelings, his despair, his weariness of life, and the unhappy hours he passes, his mind filled with the most dreadful thoughts ... His eyes are scarcely raised to look at those who address him, and the most exciting events do not engage his attention. The pupils are dilated, the brows contracted, the corners of the mouth drawn down, his whole aspect that of a person plunged in the deepest sorrow. (Hammond, 1883, p. 562)

Delirious melancholia

Delirious melancholia is a severe episode characterized by clouding of consciousness, delusions and hallucinations, and catatonic features including mutism, immobility with posturing, and automatic obedience alternating with "anxious resistance". Stupor alternates with restlessness, agitation, and hand-wringing, crying, and begging for forgiveness. The risk of suicide is heightened during this agitation.[69]

Psychotic depression

Psychotic depression has been understood for centuries as a form of melancholia. Kraepelin defined it as melancholia gravis. Systematically collected data support that view and that the treatment of choice for psychotic depression is ECT.[70] Approximately one-third of melancholic patients are psychotic.[71] Psychotic features in melancholia are reported at all ages, although the recognition of psychotic depression increases with age. In some reviews nearly all patients with psychotic depression are melancholic.[72] The congruence or non-congruence of the delusional content does not define the condition.[73] Patient 8.3 had a psychotic melancholia with catatonic features.

Patient 8.3

A 52-year-old woman with a history of manic-depressive illness was hospitalized after experiencing four months of depression with increasing severity and suicidal thoughts. She spent her time in bed or on a sofa, mostly unresponsive. She ate little and never appeared to sleep deeply. When manic, she drank up to a case of beer daily. On the day of hospitalization she was found wandering along a railroad track contemplating jumping in front of a train.

On admission she said her problems were because she hadn't "been keeping up with the news", that "retarded people are smarter than me", that her arms were not "connected correctly to her body" and were not working properly. She believed she had parasites. She said she heard muffled voices enumerating the bad things she had done. She said she emitted a foul odor that was making others sick. On the second day of hospitalization she said patients on the unit were dying because of her odorous poison.

On examination she moved as if drained of energy. She looked frightened and perplexed, and was perspiring heavily. Her muscle tone was normal and she was not tremulous. She said she was anxious and guilt-ridden for harming so many people. She exhibited automatic obedience and her arms could be postured, despite repeated instruction to "be limp and floppy" and to let the examiner "do all the work". She was surprised to find her arm raised and affirmed that she understood she was to be limp. Speaking took great effort. There were long pauses before her responses, which were sparse and limited to her delusional concerns. Her voice was monotone and just above a whisper. If not engaged she sat or lay motionless, staring. After her sixth bilateral ECT she was discharged home and after nine treatments she was fully recovered.

Other examples of the delusions of psychotic depression are:

"A piece of food is stuck in my throat ... I can't swallow."
"I am putting my shit on the walls and it will make people sick."
"My brain waves are killing people."
"My guts are filled with garbage ... they give off a foul odor."
"The devil rapes me every night."
"We have lost all our money and will be thrown out onto the street."

Other examples of the perceptual disturbances experienced by patients with psychotic depression are:

"The voices yell at me, call me 'a whore', 'a bitch' ... dirty things."
"I hear them [my victims] screaming in agony in the street below."
"The voices call me the devil."
"I see a green, bad smelling gas around me ... It makes me sick."
"I see a man who is trying to kill me."

William Hammond described a patient with psychotic depression and from his words the condition is unmistakable.

The individual affected with melancholia with stupor presents a very striking picture. He sits motionless, his hands clasped before him, his head bent forward, his eyes closed or staring vacantly, or fixed upon the floor. His half-opened mouth allows the viscid saliva to drop from his lips. If spoken to, he does not answer or even give any sign that he has heard, and he rarely speaks spontaneously. If he does, he is very apt to utter some irrelevant word or sentence, and may go on repeating it for hours at a time, day after day. His movements are torpid, and rarely spontaneous. If told to rise, he takes no notice of the direction, but if pulled up from his chair, makes only passive resistance, or none at all. His cutaneous sensibility is greatly diminished, both to sensations of touch and pain. His expression is either one of absolute apathy or vacancy, or is indicative of astonishment or terror. The pupils are, as a rule, widely dilated ...

At times tears flow from his eyes, and he exhibits all the evidence of grief; and again he appears to be under the influence of extreme fear. As stated by patients who have recovered from their disease, these and other signs of intense emotional disturbance were due to terrible hallucinations of sight and hearing, of events taking place from which they were powerless to escape. (Hammond, 1883, p. 472)

Melancholia associated with mania

Efforts to distinguish the depressions associated with mania or hypomania from those without such episodes has been unsuccessful.[74] Some reports find "atypical" features of hypersomnia, motor retardation, apathy and leadened paralysis to be characteristic, but most studies find melancholia to be the characteristic depression of manic-depression. Table 8.5 displays the features of depressive episodes observed in the manic-depressive patients reported by Winokur *et al.* (1969, pp. 84–91).

Table 8.5. Symptoms of the melancholia in manic-depression

Distinct quality of mood different from grief (100%)

Irritability (75%)

Anxiety attacks (60%)

Gloomy ruminations (90%)

Abnormal and inappropriate pessimism (100%)

Psychomotor retardation and prolonged latency of response (80%)

Poor concentration or memory (90%)

Diminished speed and clarity of thought (90%)

Guilt (100%)

Hopelessness (50%)

Worthlessness (95%)

Delusions (33%)

Excessive concern for finances (45%)

Fear of losing mind (50%)

Suicidal thoughts (80%)

Suicide attempts (15%)

Insomnia (100%)

Anorexia (95%)

Decreased libido (70%)

Symptoms worse in the morning (60%)

Headache (60%)

Their patients described the experience as "a black cloud or shadow coming over me" or as "a heavy weight on me", and their features are classic for melancholia.[75]

Classic syndromes and features of anxiety

Acute anxiety

Acute anxiety is an adaptive physiologic state associated with flight/fight mechanisms responsive to external threat. In humans it occurs with the subjective experience of fear. The subjective emotion, physiologic signs of sympathetic surge, and the behavioral expression of acute anxiety is the same whether the person is facing real, sudden danger or a phobic situation. Chronically experienced anxiety differs from acute anxiety in its persistence and lower intensity, but it is similar in other behavioral and physiological aspects to acute anxiety, and is the same whether the person is facing real and persistent danger or experiencing constant amorphous unrealistic worry.

Precisely what triggers abnormal acute and chronically experienced anxiety is uncertain, but once triggered, the anxiety cascade is a shared final common pathway. There are no laboratory tests that distinguish normal from abnormally

Table 8.6. Panic attack

Emotion: Apprehension, fear, terror

Flight/fight features: Dilated pupils, exophthalmus, piloerection, increased muscle tone, tachycardia, sweating, vascular shunting away from the periphery and gut to large muscle groups

Nonadaptive features: Tremors, inner shakiness, dry mouth, blurred vision, chest pain or discomfort, palpitations, vascular throbbing, air hunger, feeling of choking, dyspnea, hyperventilation, dizziness and syncope, paresthesia, flushing or chills, weakness, sudden increased bowel motility with abdominal distress or incontinence, nausea

Cognition: Thoughts of impending doom, fear of dying, losing control, going crazy; inability to concentrate; depersonalization and derealization

---

elicited anxiety. Persons with abnormal anxiety, however, are sensitive to blood pH change and agents that accomplish this (e.g. sodium lactate, carbon dioxide) induce panic attacks in patients with anxiety disorder but not in comparison persons.[76]

Panic attack

Although panic disorder has been established as a separate entity within the anxiety disorder category in the DSM and ICD, panic attacks occur in other anxiety disorders as well as in general medical illness (e.g. hyperthyroidism), neurologic conditions (e.g. seizure disorder), and mood disorder (particularly during an episode of melancholia). Recurrent panic attacks without an apparent reason constitute panic disorder.

Panic attacks emerge suddenly without an obvious trigger. The attack develops over several minutes, peaks quickly and lasts for minutes to hours. It is characterized by feelings of intense fear and apprehension, the sufferer commonly believing death is imminent. Arousal is heightened with tachycardia, palpitations, shortness of breath, air hunger, sweating, and trembling. Table 8.6 displays the features of a classic panic attack.

Panic attacks are incapacitating, often leading to an emergency room visit, extensive but unproductive evaluation, and hospitalization. Following an attack the sufferer feels exhausted. Jitteriness typically lingers for several hours to several days.

Specific phobia

A phobia is an unrealistic or exaggerated fear of a specific object (e.g. an animal), place (e.g. a public space), situation (e.g. being in a thunder storm), or activity (e.g. public speaking). Fearing the sight of blood or receiving an injection are other specific phobias. About 12% of the general population has a life-time risk

Table 8.7. Specific phobias

Acarophobia: fear of itching from infestation

Achluophobia: fear of the dark

Aichmophobia: fear of needles or pointed objects

Acrophobia: fear of heights; being on a ladder

Astraphobia: fear of lightning

Anthropophobia: fear of being with a group of people (*Enochlophobia*: fear of crowds)

Aviophobia: fear of flying

Claustrophobia: fear of closed in spaces (elevators, closets, public vehicles)

Gephyrophobia: fear of being on a bridge

Hydrophobia: fear of water

Hemophobia: fear of blood

Monophobia: fear of being alone

Mysophobia: fear of being contaminated

Pyrophobia: fear of fire

Thanatophobia: fear of death or dying

Zoophobia (animal phobia): defined by specific animal (e.g. *Ailurophobia*: fear of cats;
   Arachnophobia: fear of spiders, *Acarophobia/parasitophobia*: fear of bugs, *Cynophobia*: fear of
   dogs or of rabies; *Herpetophobia*: fear of reptiles or "creepy, crawly things")

---

for specific phobia and commonly identify the following phobias: animals, being alone, closed places, heights, storms, water, blood, injuries and injections, flying, elevators (lifts), driving, physical exams, doctors, vomiting.[77] Terms for some phobias are listed in Table 8.7.[78]

Specific phobic disorder is defined as a circumscribed, unrealistic fear. While persons with a specific phobia may be anxiety-free at other times, they are more likely to also have other anxiety disorders and somatoform disorders, and experience non-melancholic depression.[79] About 15% will have more than one phobia.[80]

The phobic fear-response can be mild or severe, the terror-stricken patient attempting to flee the phobic situation. Patients often go to great lengths to avoid the phobic situation. Animal phobias emerge before puberty. While many mild to moderate phobias gradually resolve through repeated exposure, some phobias become chronic, waxing and waning in intensity over decades.[81]

While most phobic patients have co-morbid anxious–fearful personality traits, some late onset phobic conditions are associated with metabolic disorders and toxic states.[82]

Chronic anxiety

Some persons experience continuous anxiety that cannot be attributed to a mood disorder. These patients are said to have Generalized Anxiety Disorder (GAD).

Table 8.8. Common symptoms of chronic anxiety

Apprehension and the constant experience of "feeling tense"	Palpitations
	Dry mouth
Irritability	Nausea
Worry over trifles	Urinary frequency
Poor sleep	Abdominal discomfort and bowel
Muscle tension	movement problems
Tremor	Sweating
Dizziness and syncope	Cold skin

Persons with GAD experience daily, non-specific, or "free-floating" anxiety. The intensity of the daily distress waxes and wanes, but is generally mild to modest, and sufferers are less housebound than persons whose illness has progressed to agoraphobia. Social phobia, although given separate identity in the DSM, is a likely variant of GAD and agoraphobia. Neurasthenia and chronic fatigue syndrome have overlapping clinical features and can also be considered variants of GAD. All experience chronic anxiety (Table 8.8).

Neurasthenia and chronic fatigue syndrome

Neurasthenia as originally understood consisted of long-standing fatigue and weakness, and low-grade anxiety. It was first defined by George Beard in 1869 as a "functional" disorder involving a "weakness in the nerves".[83] Sufferers fatigued easily after minor exertion and experienced panic attacks. The condition worsened under stress.[84] Musculoskeletal and gastrointestinal complaints (e.g. nausea) were reported.[85] Low-grade anxiety with palpitations, shortness of breath, dizziness, and muscle pain were commonly occurring features.

The neurasthenia construct was recently conflated in the chronic fatigue syndrome (CFS), also characterized by chronic fatigue that waxes and wanes, unrelieved by rest.[86] Onset is acute or subacute and is ascribed to follow a viral infection with low-grade fever, sore throat, tender and periodically enlarged lymph nodes, muscle and joint pain, headache, sleep disturbances, anxiety, irritability and weepiness, and visual scotomata and photophobia. Cognitive impairment, particularly in attention and new learning, and work difficulties occur. The features of CFS overlap with those of generalized anxiety disorder. Half or more of patients with CFS are also said to have mild to moderate non-melancholic mood disturbances.[87]

Social phobia, agoraphobia, and generalized anxiety disorder (GAD)

Patients with social phobia or generalized anxiety often find most comfort at home, resulting in a reluctance to leave it and the emergence of agoraphobia.

These conditions are variations of the same syndrome, and overlap with neurasthenia. Persons with these conditions may also experience specific, multiple phobias.

Persons with social phobia are fearful of public speaking, talking on the telephone, and any novelty, including meeting new people. The notion that they are fearful of being scrutinized or judged is unproved. Persons with agoraphobia are fearful of being away from home, particularly in unfamiliar places, and of having a panic attack. Persons with GAD have continuous unspecified anxiety.

Phobic-anxiety-depersonalization syndrome (PAD)

Martin Roth first described a variation of GAD that is characterized by initial episodes of depersonalization, usually following acute stress. As the episodes of depersonalization became less frequent, anxiety becomes more prominent. Dizziness and syncope are often experienced. Episodes of panic also occur. The more severe and frequent the symptoms, the more likely agoraphobia will emerge.[88] PAD is a variant of GAD.

Conclusion

Human emotional expression and its subjective experience represent an evolutionary change from the fight/flight protective function common to many species. The psychopathology of emotional expression and experience reflects deficits in stimulus perception and the generation of emotion and its subjective and observable expression. The distinction between emotional expressions that represent normal adaptive processes from those that are pathological is the clinical challenge.

Prolonged and intense states of emotion are associated with disruption of adrenocortical–hypothalamic pituitary functions and related neurochemical cascades that alter brain structure and function. Persons with melancholia, mania and anxiety disorder have features of an abnormal response to stress. The abnormal emotional states are themselves stress-inducing and elicit further stress-related brain changes. Several general medical and neurologic disorders produce neurochemical changes or involve neuroanatomic lesions in the circuitries subserving emotional experience, also causing abnormal behavior and emotional expression.

NOTES

1 Robert Gooch, lecturer on midwifery and physician to London's Lying-in Hospitals, cited by Hunter and Macalpine (1963), p. 798.

2 Damasio (1999).

3 Thomas (1997).

4 Sims (1995), pp. 273–4.

5 APA (1994).

6 Ross (2000).

7 Berenbaum *et al.* (1987).

8 Jampala *et al.* (1985).

9 Tremeau *et al.* (2005).

10 Kraepelin (1987), p. 22.

11 Abrams and Taylor (1978); Andreasen (1982).

12 Kraepelin (1971), p. 32.

13 Ibid., p. 35.

14 Donohoe and Robertson (2003).

15 McCann and Peppe (2003).

16 Knight and Valner (1993).

17 Tremeau *et al.* (2005).

18 Levy and Dubois (2006).

19 Levy and Dubois (2006); Levy and Czernecki (2006).

20 Starkstein and Robinson (1997).

21 Duda (2007).

22 Parvizi *et al.* (2006).

23 Duda (2007).

24 Kim (2002); Tateno *et al.* (2004).

25 Trimble (2002); Blumer *et al.* (2004).
    The disorders of laughter are associated with lesions in a neuroanatomic circuitry that
    includes the anterior cingulate gyrus, caudal hypothalamus, temporal–amygdala structures,
    and a pontomedullary center.

26 Bleuler (1976), pp. 380–1.

27 Hodgins *et al.* (2003); Volavka (2002).

28 Volavka (2002); Elliot (1984).

29 Blair (2003); Volavka (2002).

30 Blair (2003); Mendez *et al.* (2005).

31 Santos *et al.* (2006).
    Depression post stroke is also common and associated with deficits in memory, visual
    perception and language, resulting from lesions in frontal brain circuitry (Vataja *et al.*,
    2004; Nys *et al.*, 2005).

32 Hendryx *et al.* (1991).

33 Larsen *et al.* (2003).

34 Dewaraja and Sasaki (1990).

35 Farges *et al.* (2004).

36 Van't Wout *et al.* (2007).

37 Bodini *et al.* (2004); the capacity for empathy is thought important in human evolution
    for establishing interpersonal bonding while maintaining awareness of self (Decety and
    Lamm, 2006).

38 Although empathy generally refers to responses to another person's distress, it may also involve positive emotions. Excessive empathy that elicits maladaptive behavior is associated with an inability to regulate emotional responses to the discomfort of others (Lazarus, 1991).

39 Ghika-Scmid and Bogousslavsky (2000).

40 The failure of patients with schizophrenia to activate the right fusiform gyrus when asked to identify facial emotional expressions suggests a deficit in early facial identification (Johnston et al., 2005).

41 Kraepelin (1976), pp. 54–60.

42 Young et al. (1983).

43 Taylor and Abrams (1973, 1975a); Abrams et al. (1979); Winokur et al. (1969); Goodwin and Jamison (1990, chapter 2).

44 Yan et al. (1982).

45 Taylor and Abrams (1973).

46 In addition to mixed states, many manic episodes are preceded by a longer period of depression and end with a period of depression. These depressive periods can be severe, suicide risk is high, and treatment for the depression often needed.

47 Not seen in chronically ill, poor patients who do not have the minimal resources for over-spending.

48 In some samples the prevalence of catatonia is as high as 70%. It is a critical misconception that a catatonic patient must be mute and immobile (Fink and Taylor, 2003).

49 Kraepelin (1976), pp. 61–2.

50 Haslam (1809/1976).

51 Carlson and Goodwin (1973).

52 Abrams et al. (1974); Taylor et al. (1974).

53 *Mania A Potu* was the term for pathological intoxication, an idiosyncratic excitement response to small amounts of alcohol that is no longer considered a valid syndrome. Such patients may have experienced a delirium or delirious mania (Bell, 1849).

54 Kraepelin (1976), pp. 70–4.

55 Fink (1999); Fink and Taylor (2003).

56 Perugi and Akiskal (2005).

57 Akiskal et al. (1977).

58 Stanton et al. (2007).

59 Carlson et al. (2000).

60 Taylor and Fink (2006).

61 Psychomotor change is essential to melancholia in the studies by Parker and Hadzi-Pavlovic (1996), Rush and Weissenberger (1994), and Taylor and Fink (2006).

62 The description of benign stupor by August Hoch (1921) is excellent. He described patients with stupor who were severely depressed, delusional, and often with signs of catatonia. The overlap of catatonia and melancholia is not limited to patients in stupor, and careful examination of patients with melancholia often finds multiple signs of catatonia; among patients with retarded catatonia, other signs of melancholia are often described (Fink and Taylor, 2003).

63 Taylor and Fink (2006).

64 Styron (1990), p. 40.

65 Ibid., p. 33.

66 Hammond (1883/1973), pp. 454–60.

67 Burrows (1976), pp. 353–4.

68 Kraepelin (1976), pp. 77–8.

69 Kraepelin (1976), pp. 95–8.

70 Taylor and Fink (2006).

71 Among referrals for ECT, about 30% of the patients meet criteria for psychotic depression (Mulsant *et al.*, 1997; Petrides *et al.*, 2001), and about 60% are melancholic (Max Fink, personal communication, June 2006).

72 Rush and Weissenburger (1994).

73 Taylor and Fink (2006).

74 Benazzi (2004a,b); Taylor and Fink (2006).

75 The atypical depression construct has not been clearly validated (Benazzi, 2003c). Its reported unique response to MAOI agents is also unclear (Taylor and Fink, 2006).

76 Pitts and McClure (1967). This classic paper in psychiatry demonstrated for the first time the biological nature of neurosis.

77 Becker *et al.* (2007); Iancu *et al.* (2007).

78 www.phobia-fear-release.com/types-of-phobia.html

79 Becker *et al.* (2007).

80 Iancu *et al.* (2007).

81 Marks (1969).

82 Cummings (1985a), p. 170.

83 Shorter (1997), p. 129.

84 Shorter (1992).

85 Stubhaug *et al.* (2005).

86 Shorter (1992).

87 Trimble (2004), pp. 60–3.

88 Roth (1959).

9

Disturbances in speech and language

For every twisted thought there is a twisted molecule.[1]

Abnormalities in speech and language occur in several psychiatric disorders. Although these abnormalities overlap with verbal thinking and memory functions, the speech and language problems identified in schizophrenia and other psychiatric conditions are true language impairments related as much to aphasia as to cognitive dysfunction. Thus, speech and language is examined separately from cognition, and also considers aphasia, as patients with cortical strokes often have initial behavioral changes that may be misinterpreted as emergent psychiatric illness.

The examination relies on the standardized bedside techniques of the neurologist. The focus is on the form of the abnormalities as expressions of disturbances in the mechanisms underlying language. The diagnostic question is whether the patient's language is normal, aphasic from a stroke, seizure, or degenerative brain disease, or consistent with schizophrenia, delirium or manic-depression.

The overall appraisal of the conversation with the patient begins the examination of speech and language. Attention is paid to the patient's turn-taking, spontaneity of speech, speech fluency, articulation, auditory comprehension, ability to repeat words and phrases, word usage, and in what ways the patient's speech deviates from grammatical and syntactic rules. The patient's abilities to read and write are also assessed at this time, because loss of these abilities further demarcates the brain language-based systems involved in the patient's illness. The organization of the patient's utterances is considered. Are they to the point, or circumstantial, or do they stray from the topic as in flight-of-ideas? Is formal thought disorder present?

Aspects of conversational speech

The psychiatric evaluation is a semi-structured conversation between the patient and the examiner. In this conversation there is a give and take. The examiner asks questions or makes comments encouraging the patient to continue or to elaborate. The patient listens and responds, and spontaneously asks questions and makes comments. The examiner listens. This "turn-taking" is part of every normal conversation. Gestures, facial expression, and body language enhance communication. Tone of voice conveys meaning.

Abnormal conversational behavior is associated with behavioral disorders. Patients with substantial psychomotor retardation or a paucity of thoughts will not "take their turns". Manic patients will not easily "give up their turns". Catatonic patients with negativism literally turn away from conversation. Hallucinating patients stop attending to the conversation and listen to the hallucinated voices. Some patients repeatedly return to the same topic regardless of the examiner's focus. Other patients cannot stick to the topic and repeatedly lead the conversation astray to seemingly irrelevant considerations.

Examiners experience thousands of conversations in everyday life and know "a bad one" when they hear it. The challenge is parsing the conversation into its components to determine what makes it "bad" and what are the diagnostic and neurologic implications of the findings. Table 9.1 displays the areas to consider.

Aphasia

Psychiatric illness does not protect a sufferer from other disease and care-givers cannot assume that a recent behavior change is a recurrence and not the expression of new brain pathology. Patient 9.1 illustrates the point

Patient 9.1

A 55-year-old chronic alcoholic man was hospitalized on a psychiatric service because over the previous week he had become "uncooperative" at his nursing home. He no longer followed the facility's rules and was repeatedly found smoking in his room. When confronted he said "I'm a very special person". When forced to comply, he became irritable.

In the hospital, he was alert and cooperative, but did not appear to understand instructions. His interactions were pleasant and he could recognize individual staff members, and use objects appropriately. When shown in pantomime what to do, he could do it. He could dress himself and perform personal toileting tasks. He remembered his way about the unit. He could copy geometric shapes. When told what to do, or when asked a question, his response was typically "I am a very special person". At other times his utterances varied, but all were fluent, short, and well articulated. Pure word deafness from a left temporal lobe stroke was diagnosed and behavioral care strategies recommended rather than pharmacotherapy.[2]

Table 9.1. Aspects of conversational speech

Spontaneity: Comments should occur spontaneously, not only as responses to questions. Lack of spontaneous speech is observed in expressive cortical aphasias and left basal ganglia and thalamic strokes, drug-induced and abnormal metabolic states leading to reduced arousal, some ictal and post-ictal states, depression, catatonia, schizophrenia and other psychotic disorders, states of anxiety and fearfulness, and guardedness due to personality deviation or concern for self-incrimination.

Fluency: Reduced speech output is not synonymous with poor speech fluency. Non-fluent speech is also halting and the patient labors to make utterances, often with poor articulation as in Broca's and transcortical motor aphasias, and some ictal states.[3]

Turn-taking: Comments are made or questions asked and then the speaker stops, awaiting a response. Not taking an appropriate "turn" suggests a lack of spontaneity and the conditions associated with it. Lack of spontaneity may be coupled with a paucity of speech. Not allowing the other person to take a "turn" and monopolizing the conversation is associated with mania and hypomania, stimulant drug intoxication, and the frontal lobe disinhibited syndrome. Speech will be intrusive. Anxious persons and persons with histrionic or narcissistic personality traits also monopolize conversation.

Mutual topic: Constantly straying from the focus or topic is associated with mania and hypomania, stimulant drug intoxication, and the frontal lobe disinhibited syndrome. Repeatedly and inappropriately returning to the same topic (perseveration of theme) is seen in mood disorders, delusional and paranoid personality disorder, and obsessive conditions.

Comprehension: An adequate conversation requires each participant to understand the utterances of the other. When auditory comprehension is poor, the patient may respond with non-sequitive speech.

Making sense: Speech that is not understandable despite adequate articulation indicates an inability to follow grammatical or syntactic rules or a cognitive problem.

Associated behaviors: Facial expression, gestures, and body language convey conversational information. Absent facial expression and gesturing is associated with neurologic disease affecting motor systems, depression, catatonia, and sedative drug intoxications. Exaggerated expression and gesturing is associated with states of excitement, anger, drug intoxication, and histrionic personality traits.

Several aphasia syndromes are recognized (Table 9.2). "Neighborhood" signs, additional features associated with some aphasic conditions, are not always present, but their appearance aids in identifying lesion location. They include paresis and paralysis (Broca's, conduction, global, basal ganglia) and sensory loss (conduction). In Broca's aphasia, left hand ideo-motor apraxia may also be present as the left hand is disconnected from the ideational information of the

Table 9.2. Speech patterns of some classic aphasia syndromes

Aphasia type	Spontaneous speech	Speech fluency	Auditory comprehension	Repetition	Syntax/grammar and word usage
Broca's	Poor and labored, telegraphic, dysarthric, sparse, and monotone	Non-fluent	Reduced, but globally adequate	Poor	Mild word-finding and naming problems
Transcortical motor	Paucity of labored, but not dysarthric, speech	Non-fluent	Adequate for conversation	Adequate or mild problems	Normal, but may have difficulty reading aloud
Wernicke's	Spontaneous, well-articulated, abundant	Fluent	Poor	Poor	Severely paraphasic, agrammatical, poor naming, reading, and writing
Transcortical sensory	Reduced	Fluent	Poor	Adequate	Paraphasic, agrammatical, poor naming, reading, and writing
Conduction	Mild articulation problems	Fluent	Adequate for conversation	Poor	Paraphasic, poor naming
Global	Sparse, monosyllabic	Non-fluent	Poor	Poor	Paraphasic, agrammatical, poor naming, stereotypes

Basal ganglia	Dysarthric, reduced spontaneity and output	Fluent	Adequate for simple questions and commands, otherwise poor	Fair	Mildly paraphasic and agrammatical
Thalamic	Spontaneous, well-articulated, may be logorrheic	Fluent	Adequate for simple questions and commands, otherwise poor	Adequate	Mildly paraphasic and agrammatical
Cerebellar	Scanning, dysarthric, and monitone	Fluent	Adequate for conversation	Adequate	Mildly agrammatical with some naming problems and cognitive slippage; misuse of verb tenses

motor task. Behavioral changes (e.g. agitation, irritability, features of depression) are common early features of many aphasic conditions.[4]

Spontaneity, fluency, syntax, grammar, word usage, and conversational auditory comprehension are assessed by listening to the patient's responses and comments during history gathering. Lapses in grammar and syntax or in word usage are immediately addressed:

"What did you mean when you said …? I didn't get that. What was it you just said?"

"You seem to be having trouble getting words out, true? You seem to be having trouble finding the words you want to say, is that so?"

Word finding and naming are also examined by asking the patient to identify common objects (e.g. keys, a coin, a pen) and then finding named objects in the room: "Can you show me a (phone, lapel or cuff, button, cup)."

Repetition is tested by asking the patient to repeat phrases such as "No, ifs, ands, or buts … Methodist-Episcopal … Massachusetts Avenue."

Auditory comprehension is further tested by observing if the patient can follow the examiner's verbal instructions without non-verbal cues (e.g. nodding or pointing to the object): "I'd like you to take the piece of paper on the desk, fold it in half and then hand it to me", and suggestions "Why don't you take a seat in the blue chair next to my desk?"

Reading and writing

Newly emerged difficulties in reading or writing, or the partial or complete loss of these abilities, reflects brain disease and helps delineate behavioral illness. When asked to read the cover of a bedside magazine, manic patients often embellish with flight-of-ideas. When asked to write a simple sentence they elaborate and give long fanciful writing samples, often in an untypical flowery hand, or with enlarged lettering that fills the page. Patients with chronic limbic disease write copiously, filling notebooks with repetitive, sometimes delusional discourses on religion, science, philosophy, and cosmic events. This *hypergraphia* may be adorned with strange images and designs that the patient insists reveal universal mysteries or other conundrums.[5]

Micrographia, small, choppy lettering, is seen in Parkinsonism. Writing samples are regularly assessed for subtle basal ganglia effects of patients receiving antipsychotic medication. *Dysgraphia*, the loss of the ability to properly construct letters, is seen in the loss of cursive writing. The patient prints as if a child or creates distorted or reversed lettering that cannot be constructed on the horizontal, the writing rotating away from the usual alignment. Dysgraphia is a sign of dominant parietal lobe disease.[6]

Dyslexia, problems with reading, is associated with neurologic disease and is a feature of developmental deviation. Patients with lesions in the dominant angular gyrus of the parietal lobe, for example, may have a disconnection of visual perceptions from language systems. They can write spontaneously, but not read what they have written (alexia without agraphia). When both reading and writing are affected, the patient is said to have visual asymbolia.[7]

Patients with frontal lobe disease may have difficulty reading and understanding complex sentences.

Disturbances of speech articulation

Dysarthria

Dysarthria is abnormal speech articulation. Speech sounds are distorted and speech is typically slow and labored. Dysarthria is characteristic of Broca's aphasia and isolated lesions in the dominant precentral gyrus of the insula, a cortical area between the frontal and temporal lobes. This area is involved in motor speech planning.

Acute dysarthria is associated with oral–buccal dystonia, often from antipsychotic drugs but also from some SSRI agents. When laryngeal muscles are dystonic, speech becomes husky, gravelly, or strained, disrupting the flow of speech and making any utterance difficult. Primary dysarthria is associated with impaired hearing. The slurred speech of alcohol intoxication is a form of dysarthria that represents ataxia of the muscles of speech. Slurring also occurs with basal ganglia disease and pseudobulbar palsy. Increased muscle tone is associated with the former and dysphagia, drooling, and emotional incontinence are associated with the latter. Brainstem lesions cause dysarthric speech that appears "breathless" and nasal. *Scanning speech* is characterized by the over-emphasis of all syllables, stretching out their sounds, and is a sign of cerebellar–pontine disease.

Manneristic speech

Manneristic speech is characteristic of catatonia and basal ganglia disease. Speech mannerisms include using foreign accents inconsistent with one's language or background,[8] robotic and stilted speech, speaking as if a child learning how to read (slow and halting, not using combined verb forms [e.g. "can not" rather than "can't"]), speaking in odd rhythms, falsetto, staccato or nasally, with unexpected stress on some words or syllables, and as if engaged in great oratory (seen in mania).

Stammering and stuttering

In stammering the normal flow of speech is interrupted by pauses and the interjection of repeated words or parts of words. Stammering is associated with tic disorder. Stuttering is difficulty in uttering speech sounds at the beginning of words. Utterances are repetitious, sounds prolonged, and pauses while speaking are common. Stuttering can be primary, occurring in childhood with the development of speech, or as the result of stroke, traumatic brain injury and extrapyramidal disease. In primary stuttering, dysfunction is reported in the left basal ganglia, supplementary motor area and cerebellum, suggesting stuttering is a speech dyscontrol syndrome.[9] Primary speech and language areas are not involved.[10]

Modulation

Normally, speech modulation varies with the emotional content of the conversation. The appropriate linkage facilitates communication. Many behavioral conditions are associated with a disturbance in modulation. Manic patients shout and speak loudly despite being close to the listener. Melancholic patients loudly whine or scream as if being tortured. Catatonic patients whisper and mumble. Manic patients in mixed states affect all of these derangements. Histrionic patients may also speak loudly and dramatically. Patients with anxious–fearful personality traits are often barely audible.

Disturbances of speech production

Pressured speech (logorrhea)

Pressured speech is defined as speaking too much, too often and with too many words. The patient cannot keep silent and speaks without regard for turn-taking. When associated with rapid speech it is a classic sign of mania, but speed and logorrhea also occur independently. Pressured speech is also observed in agitated depression, anxiety states, intoxications, the frontal lobe disinhibited syndrome, and chronic limbic system disease.

Paucity of speech and mutism

The amount of speech is independent of speech fluency. Although patients with non-fluent aphasia have reduced speech output, non-aphasic patients with substantially reduced speech output may speak fluently. This combination is seen in schizophrenia and depressive illness. In patients with schizophrenia, paucity of speech is associated with loss of emotional expression and avolition (i.e. emotional blunting or negative symptoms).[11]

Aphonia is the inability to vocalize. The patient may be mute or speak in a whisper or in a "strangled" voice (*Wurgstimme*). *Dysphonia* is abnormal fluctuations in speech sound levels, or hoarseness without mutism. Both occur in disease of the peripheral speech apparatus, stroke, and catatonia. *Mutism* can be elective, complete or partial and also occurs in depression, sedative drug intoxication, stroke in several brain regions, and conditions that affect arousal.

Thought blocking and speech arrest

Thought blocking is the sudden cessation of speech as if "the plug were pulled from a machine." It is reminiscent of *petit mal* seizures, but in thought blocking the patient appears "stuck" or as if his mind has gone blank, rather than being in an altered state of consciousness. When speech again begins it is often on a different train of thought. When asked "What just happened?", the patient will not know or offer a delusional explanation. When asked "What were we just talking about before?", the patient will not recall the previous train of thought. Unlike patients with seizure disorder, schizophrenics who have thought blocking may recall the experience as thoughts and words suddenly being inaccessible. Thought blocking is one of the classic *first rank symptoms* of Kurt Schneider. However, it occurs in other psychotic disorders, mood disorders and dementia.[12] When speech suddenly stops as a feature of a seizure disorder, it is almost always associated with a dominant frontal lobe focus and is referred to as *speech arrest*.

The sudden cessation of speech described during psychoanalysis or the sudden loss of train of thought in an exhausted or anxious patient is distinguished from thought blocking. These persons do not appear as if without thought and they are aware of the experience. The psychotherapy patient will reluctantly remember the previous train of thought.

Stereotypic speech (Verbigeration, palilalia, and logoclonia)

In perseveration of theme the patient repeatedly returns to the same topic regardless of efforts to change the subject. This "adhesive speech" is associated with melancholia, mania, seizure disorder and in persons with developmental disorder and autistic spectrum conditions.

In *stereotypic speech*, words and phrases are delivered repetitively and automatically, as if speaking was no longer fully under the patient's control. *Verbigeration* is the increasingly rapid repetition of words or phrases usually at the end of a sentence, such as "Doctor when can I leave the hospital? When can I leave, leave, leave …?" Palilalia is the neurologic term for the same phenomenon. In *logoclonia* the last syllable of the last word is repeated, such as "I don't want to go into the hospital, hospital, tal, tal, tal …". Verbigeration, palilalia, and logoclonia are similar phenomena and are not expressions of different pathophysiologies. Verbal stereotypy is most commonly associated with basal ganglia disease and catatonia.

Perseveration of speech

Perseveration of speech is identified when the patient repeats phrases and sentences beyond the point of the conversation. It sometimes appears as a compensation for the inability to think and articulate ideas clearly, and is most commonly associated with degenerative brain disease and mood disorders. It can be mistaken for stereotypy of speech, which is more autonomous with words and phrases uttered automatically. Speech associations by sound (clang speech) are commonly perseverated. An example of perseveration follows:

"I have wondered about why I'm here and so on and so forth. It's a strategic move. My business and so forth and so on . . . I was working in the city, with the food service and that's how I got involved, and so forth and so on . . .".

Disturbances of speech organization

Circumstantial speech

In circumstantial speech associations are linked, but are interspersed with non-essential details and asides. Speech takes a circuitous route before reaching the point. The goal or the main idea of the expressed thoughts is not lost. Circumstantial speech is associated with the early stages of mania, hypomania, personality changes associated with chronic epilepsy and manic-depressive illness,[13] the chronic use of drugs that elicit limbic system sensitization (e.g. cocaine, alcohol), and in the frontal lobe disinhibited syndrome. Fish also associated mild circumstantiality with "dullards who are trying to be impressive, and pedantic obsessional personalities."[14]

Example:

Q: "What happened that you had to be hospitalized last year?"
A: "Well, you know, all that's been going on with my health, and the work at the factory, business has increased enormously since we got the new machines, and then problems that I was having with my wife, and she's got that new job, I wasn't getting enough sleep and sort of slipped, became irritable and needed my meds adjusted."

Flight-of-ideas, tangential speech, and looseness of associations

Flight-of-ideas is speech that jumps from topic to topic. The patient appears distracted by his own associations and ambient stimuli, and may incorporate what is taking place in his immediate surroundings into his speech in a seemingly unrelated string of utterances. When most severe this *word salad* is incomprehensible. It is unhelpful in delineating patients with mania from those with schizophrenia. In *Manic-Depressive Insanity and Paranoia*, Kraepelin described flight-of-ideas:[15]

they [manic patients] are not able to follow systematically a definite train of thought, but will continually jump from one series of ideas to a wholly different one and then let this one drop again immediately. Any question directed to them is at first perhaps answered quite correctly, but with that are associated a great many side remarks which have only a very loose connection, or some not at all, with the original subject (page 13) ... the flight-of-ideas only represents a partial phenomenon of heightened distractibility (page 14).

Fish wrote: "the thoughts follow each other rapidly, there is no general direction of thinking and the connections between successive thoughts appear to be due to chance factors, which can easily be understood" and that the train of thought is determined by "chance relationships, verbal associations of all kinds, such as assonance, alliteration ... clang associations" (page 36).[16]

Flight-of-ideas is also associated with drug intoxications (phencyclidine, ecstasy, cocaine and other stimulants), and the frontal lobe disinhibited syndrome. The more quiet and controlled the situation, i.e. the fewer distractions, the less likely flight-of-ideas will be elicited. Conversing with such patients in inpatient common areas rather than a quiet examination room can stimulate flight-of-ideas.

Example:

Q: "How are you feeling today Mr. Jones?"
A: "The food here is terrible. I've been dieting to keep the red meat out of my body. I'm no commie, but it's like the Berlin wall in here. You're drugging me ... ruining my health, my wealth. I'm gonna buy the hospital, fix social security. I wrote many books on the subject. I've written mysteries and novels. Oh many novels ...".

Because the flight-of-ideas continuously leads the speaker away from the topic, it is sometimes described as *tangential speech*. Because it may incorporate many themes, it is sometimes described as *interpenetration of theme*. Because the flight-of-ideas reflects a distractibility that prevents the patient from focusing on one topic and its salient details, it is associated with speech that includes many topics and details, sometimes described as *over-inclusive thinking*. Tangential speech, interpenetration of theme, and over-inclusive thinking are descriptors that define aspects of flight-of-ideas, not separate forms of speech problems. Some clinicians also infer schizophrenia from these descriptors rather than mood disorder, making diagnostic discrimination unnecessarily difficult.

When the flight-of-ideas is an expression of an excitement state the patient may repeatedly alliterate, clang, pun, speak in a series of proverbs, old saws, and clichés. Echolalia occurs.

Jaspers offers this example of flight-of-ideas:

When a patient was asked if she had changed during the past year, she responded:

"Yes, I was dumb and numb then but not deaf, I know Mrs. Ida Teff, she is dead, probably an appendicitis; I don't know whether she lost her sight, sightless Hesse, His Highness of Hesse, sister Louisa, His Highness of Baden, buried and dead on September the 20th 1907, when I get back, red–gold–red …".[17]

Looseness-of-association is another term linked to the diagnosis of schizophrenia. Bleuler defined it as associations which lose their continuity and are

incorrect, bizarre, and utterly unpredictable: Often thinking stops in the middle of a thought … (blocking) instead of continuing the thought, new ideas crop up which neither the patient nor the observer can bring into any connection with the previous stream of thought.[18]

Bleuler considered associational looseness a fundamental feature of schizophrenia, but his descriptions are also consistent with flight-of-ideas:

Clang-associations receive unusual significance as do indirect associations … the tendency to stereotypy produces an inclination to cling to one idea … blocking … echopraxia … pressure of thoughts … increased flow of ideas[19] … "pressure of thoughts" can continue for years … many patients complain that they think too much, that their ideas chase each other in their heads. They themselves speak of "thought-overflow" … because too much comes to mind at one time.[20]

Bleuler attempted to distinguish flight-of-ideas from looseness of associations by claiming that the associational leaps in flight-of-ideas can usually be understood while in looseness of associations the steps are unintelligible or appear so "bizarre that they would never have entered his [the examiner's] mind."[21] He offers the examples of a patient referring to Brutus as an Italian rather than a Roman, and a patient who in response to the query "Are your thoughts heavy?" said "Yes, iron is heavy." [22] Thus, if the examiner understands the associational leaps the speech is flight-of-ideas, whereas if the examiner cannot understand the leaps, the speech is looseness of associations. This reliance on examiner idiosyncratic abilities, however, insures poor reliability. For example, Bleuler considers the phrase "Blossom time of Horticulture" from a patient as incomprehensible and thus looseness of associations and the patient to be schizophrenic.[23] From an aphasiologist's perspective, however, the phrase can be understood as meaning "springtime" and an out-of-class paraphasia or private word usage (see formal thought disorder below) and has several diagnostic implications.

Bleuler offers the following letter from a patient to his mother as a classic illustration of what he means by looseness of associations. But it best illustrates flight-of-ideas.

Dear Mother: Today I am feeling better than yesterday. I really don't feel much like writing. But I love to write to you. After all, I can tackle it twice. Yesterday, Sunday, I would have been so happy if you and Louise and I could have gone to the park. One has such a lovely view from

Stephan's castle. Actually, it is very lovely in Burgholzli. Louise wrote Burgholzli on her two last letters, I mean to say on the envelopes, no, on the "couverts" which I received. However, I have written Burgholzli in the spot where I put the date. There are also patients in Burgholzli who call it "Holzliburg". Others talk of a factory. One may also regard it as a health resort.

I am writing on paper. The pen which I am using is from a factory called "Perry & Co." The factory is in England. I assume this. Behind the name of Perry & Co. the city of London is inscribed; but not the city. The city of London is in England. I know this from my school days. Then, I always liked geography. My last teacher in that subject was Professor August A. He was a man with black eyes and other sorts too. I have heard it said that snakes have green eyes. All people have eyes. There are some, too, who are blind. These blind people are led about by a boy. It must be very terrible not to be able to see. There are people who can't see and, in addition, can't hear. I know some who hear too much. One can hear too much ..."[24]

Talking-past-the-point (Vorbeireden)

In talking-past-the-point, the patient appears to understand the question, but to be deliberately giving incorrect answers, such as the response "Four" to the question "How many legs does a three-legged stool have?" Vorbeireden is associated with Ganser's Syndrome and other forms of catatonia. Pseudologia fantastica and hysterical pseudodementia are analogous terms, all representing forms of verbal negativism. Ganser's original papers detail the many catatonic features seen in these patients.[25]

Clang associations

Clang associations are linked by the sound of the words more than their meaning. The linkage may seem playful as in hypomania, or driven as in mania and stimulant drug intoxication. Clang associations are often interwoven in flight-of-ideas.

Example:

Q: "Did you go for your MRI Mr. Smith?"
A: "Ha, MRI. It was into the cellar fella. It's a hella a deal. Look in your brain and drain it. A Draino commercial. A TV deal, a feel, a peal. Like a bell. Ha, ha."

Rambling speech

Rambling speech is non-goal-directed, distractible speech. Meaningful connections are lost between phrases and sentences, but the syntax and meaning of the fragments may remain intact. It differs from flight-of-ideas in the degree of jumping from topic to topic (fewer topics but bigger jumps between topics) and in the number of words uttered (less). Rambling speech is the classic speech of delirium and intoxication, and is associated with reduced arousal. It is also seen in patients in delirious mania.

Example:

Q: "Mrs. Brown, where does it hurt?"
A: "I'm away ... She didn't come here ... She didn't see ... It's over there by the tree ... I can't get this water on."

Formal thought disorder (FTD)

The thought disorder literature traditionally blends the concepts of disorders of thinking with disorders of language.[26] FTD, however, is best described and applied to the discrimination of clinical syndromes as a form of aphasia. Once termed *schizaphasia* or *cataphasia* because of its presumed specificity to schizophrenia,[27] FTD is recognized as consistent with the diagnosis of schizophrenia, but not pathognomonic of the condition.[28] When it occurs in schizophrenia, FTD is associated with emotional blunting, frontal lobe executive function problems, poor response to standard pharmacotherapy, long-term chronicity, and similar pathology in relatives.[29]

A historical perspective

Nineteenth and early twentieth century psychopathologists identified FTD by the patient's characteristic speech abnormalities. Later writers assumed that the disordered speech reflected disordered thinking, thus the term "thought disorder".[30] "Thinking disorder" became the clinical euphemism for schizophrenia, as opposed to "mood disorder" as the term for manic-depression. This aspect of the field of psychopathology has never recovered from this error, as investigators vainly search for the specific cognitive process distinguishing the two classes of illness.

The focus on the thinking behind the speech rather than the speech itself adds to the confusion as disparate findings are reported for the same term that is used to mean different things. Some investigators apply validated cognitive tests of various aspects of thinking, while others rely on projective tests with poor reliability and validity, such as the *Rorschach Test*. Still others focus on the lexical aspects of speech rather than the form of speech from an aphasiologist's perspective.[31] The last approach is taken here.

Bleuler considered the thinking behind the speech as basic to his understanding of schizophrenia. Looseness of associations reflected a proposed *autistic* or *dereistic thinking*, the patient's thoughts non-goal-directed, the content fantasy, and the patient associating by sound, alliteration, or non-essential details until the central idea was lost.

Cameron continued the search for the characteristic schizophrenic thinking problem, and used the term *asyndetic thinking* to describe a lack of causal linkage in thinking, the patient uttering clusters of more or less related sequences along with unnecessary information. His descriptions and formulations of *interpenetration of themes* and *over-inclusion*, however, suggest he was observing patients with flight-of-ideas.[32] This focus on "the trees" resulted in missing "the forest". Many present-day clinicians incorrectly continue to see these elements as independent forms of speech assumed associated with schizophrenia, and thus when presented with a patient who has other features of mania, they are compelled to invoke the schizoaffective diagnosis.

Goldstein interpreted schizophrenic speech to reflect *concrete thinking* and an inability to abstract. The patient was said to be unable to generalize, and words ceased to have generic meaning. Goldstein associated concrete thinking with rigidity of thinking and distractibility. The past practice of testing the patient by asking him to interpret a proverb was an attempt to assess for schizophrenic concrete thinking.[33] This idea led to decades of defining as schizophrenic almost any patient who did poorly on proverb testing or gave odd responses to projective psychological tests.[34]

Kurt Schneider also focused on thinking, not speech.[35] *Driveling*, a term still in use, was defined as speech which has the preliminary outline of a complicated thought, but the organization is lost so that all the constituent parts get muddled. *Derailment* was defined as grammatically and syntactically correct speech suddenly interrupted by seemingly unrelated ideas. Schneider's examples, however, are suggestive of flight-of-ideas and not the aphasic-like speech of schizophrenic patients.

"He's been that way forever. I wonder what became of his dog? Some people didn't like him, but I thought he was OK although too Teutonic. I was in Italy with the Gardners at the time. I get seasick, you know!"

Frank Fish championed the idea of negative and positive formal thought disorders, the former similar to the present notion of "negative symptoms" the latter consistent with the definition of FTD used here.[36] These terms are still employed, but positive symptoms has been broadened to included hallucinations and delusions.

Karl Kleist was the first to compare the speech problems of schizophrenics to that of patients with aphasia.[37] He recognized paraphasias (approximate words), agrammatisms (disordered word sequence) and paragrammatisms (normal word sequence but non-sequitive or mixed-up content) in such patients, and used the term *stock word* to denote words that were used repeatedly throughout the speech of schizophrenics as if the stock word had changing meanings. An example of a stock word follows:

"Well, I tried to progress. A progress can vary. Your progress is different from mine. I'm not progressed, but I tried it."

Kleist's separation of thinking problems from speech and language problems has been adopted by many others.[38] Structural and functional brain imaging studies also find abnormalities in traditionally recognized language-related brain structures in patients with FTD defined from this perspective.[39]

FTD as a form of aphasia

The lack of a clear association between the language and cognitive problems of psychotic patients is an important distinction, and is analogous to what is observed in patients with aphasia. Aphasic patients have speech and language problems, but these difficulties result from disruption in the neurologic systems subserving language. Thinking difficulties also occur in aphasic patients and contribute to their overall decline in function and to some of their language deficits, but do not cause the bulk of their language problems.[40] The speech abnormalities of patients with schizophrenia are, however, associated with loss of emotional expression and avolition (i.e. negative symptoms), but not with the presence of hallucinations or delusions (i.e. positive symptoms).[41] FTD is also associated with impaired executive function.[42] The combination of emotional blunting, avolition, and impaired executive functioning as associated findings in patients with FTD is consistent with the prevailing view that schizophrenia is a condition that involves frontal circuitry problems. These problems are bilateral and are also consistent with the neuropsychological findings in patients with schizophrenia.[43] The relationship between FTD and frontal circuitry also suggests a neurologic model for understanding FTD.

Although the speech of schizophrenic patients contains many elements of aphasic speech, it can be distinguished from the speech of aphasic patients with cortical lesions.[44] The speech of schizophrenic patients with FTD, however, is similar to that of patients with left-sided basal ganglia or thalamic strokes, and subcortical aphasia is a model for the "formal thought disorder" of psychiatric patients (Tables 9.3 and 9.4).[45] Similar to patients with FTD, patients with subcortical aphasia have associated apathy and avolition, indifference to their situation, personality change, attentional deficits, poor word generation, and executive function impairment, particularly with working memory, planning and self-monitoring.[46]

The construct of FTD as a form of subcortical aphasia is consistent with present understanding of the neurology of speech. Schizophrenics and psychotic patients with brain dysfunction from illicit drug use exhibit FTD, often associated with motor dysregulation and cerebellar motor signs. Patients with manic-depressive

Table 9.3.[47] Characteristic speech patterns of patients with subcortical aphasia

Initial mutism and non-fluent speech followed by adequate fluency
   but a paucity of speech
Diminished spontaneous speech
Dysarthric speech
Preserved repetition and naming
Phonemic and semantic paraphasia
Preserved auditory comprehension
Word-finding difficulties
Impaired lexical–semantic processing

Table 9.4. Characteristic speech patterns of schizophrenia

Preserved speech fluency despite a paucity of speech
Reduced spontaneous speech
Able to repeat simple words and sentences ("No ifs, ands, or buts")
Adequate auditory comprehension
Adequate use of complex (polysyllabic) words
Mild word-finding problems
Reduced use of nouns (speech seems empty)
Circumloculatory speech
Elliptical and non-sequitive speech
Private word usage (out-of-class semantic paraphasia)
Intermittent use of neologisms, paraphasias, portmanteau words,
   strings of jargon speech, derailed speech, perseveration

syndromes also have speech and language problems, but these are phenomeno-logically distinguished from FTD.[48] One factor analytic study of 170 schizophrenic and 62 manic patients found that the degree of verbal output (high in manics and low in schizophrenics) and the presence or absence of FTD (observed in schizophrenics) captured 44% of variance of the sample, and that using the derived factors in a discriminant function analysis correctly classified 91% of the sample.[49] Manic patients who meet criteria for schizoaffective disorder exhibit some elements of FTD as well as the classic speech of mania, and the presence of FTD in a manic patient is associated with poor long-term outcome.[50] Descriptions follow of the forms of FTD.

Elliptical and non-sequitive speech

Elliptical speech is speech that is fluent and mostly grammatically and syntactically normal, but which skirts the topic rather than getting to the point or straying from it as in flight-of-ideas. The patient with elliptical speech appears to understand what has been asked, but does not directly answer the question. Elliptical speech is vague, contains few nouns and little information.

Example:

Q: "Where were you living when you came into the hospital?"
A: "It was OK there."
Q: "And where is that?"
A: "I lived there without him."
Q: "But where exactly is your place? What's the address?"
A: "I came here from there."

Non-sequitive speech refers to the patient uttering unrelated responses to the examiner's questions or comments. It is observed in schizophrenia and receptive aphasia. Such patients are not aware of the disconnection of their responses. Patients who perseverate a theme may return to their subject rather than the topic at hand, and manic patients may make unrelated statements as part of their flight-of-ideas, but such patients can sometimes recognize their non-sequitive speech and can be briefly brought back to the topic.

Example:

Examiner: "You were telling me about your family ..."
Patient: "The clock tower is near my house."

In- and out-of-class paraphasia (private word usage)

Paraphasia is the imprecise use of words. A *phonemic* or *literal paraphasia* is a misuse of the sound of a word, sometimes creating a new word (neologism), as in "glob" for "glove". A *semantic* or *verbal paraphasia* can be in- or out-of-class, depending on how close it is to the appropriate word or phrase. Semantic paraphasia is more common in cortical than in subcortical aphasia or in schizophrenia. In-class semantic paraphasias are close in general meaning to the correct word and are often understandable substitutes for the correct word, such as "writer" for "pen" or "moving machine" for "automobile". Out-of-class paraphasias are far removed from the correct word or phrase and meaning is often lost. Another term for an out-of-class paraphasia is *private word usage*. Kraepelin used the umbrella term "incoherence" to describe some of the speech problems of his patients with dementia praecox, and illustrates with examples of private word usage:[51]

"A patient said 'Life is a dessert-spoon' ... another 'We are already standing in the spiral under the hammer,' ... and a third 'Death will be awakened by the golden hammer'...". "Dessert-spoon", "spiral under the hammer", and "awakened by the golden hammer" are real words, but used in such an idiosyncratic private way that they lose meaning.

Kraepelin recognized various aphasic-like speech problems in patients with dementia praecox, defining these as *akataphasia*. This speech was described as problems in word-finding, and included derailments, substituted homonyms for the correct words, and misusing words. Kraepelin offered the following examples which today are recognized as paraphasias:

Instead of "under the protection of the police" a patient said he "lived under protected police". Instead of saying that "his fiancée continued to speak to him" a patient said "his fiancée always in speech".[52]

Circumloculatory speech

Circumloculatory speech is identified when the patient refers to an object, event, or person by descriptive terms (e.g. its function or physical characteristics) rather than by its name. Circumloculatory speech is associated with paraphasias and observable difficulties in *word-finding*.

Example:

When describing how he made breakfast, a patient said: "I put the jelly on the burnt bread [semantic paraphasia for toast]. I make it in the . . . you know . . . the metal box with the heating thing" [toaster].

Neologism

Neologisms are new words that do not convey meaning. Some slang words were once new words (e.g. boogie-woogie, jazz, hep, jo), but they now convey meaning. Shakespeare is purported to have created hundreds of new words. Neologisms can be phonemic paraphasias, clang words, or portmanteau words. *Malapropisms* are also new words or misused but without clinical significance. They reflect failed efforts to sound educated and are often humorous as personified by Mrs. Malaprop, a character in Sheridan's play *The Rivals* (1775).

". . . promise to forget this fellow – to illiterate him, I say, quite from your memory." [obliterate]

"I have since laid Sir Anthony's preposition before her;" [proposition]

"I am sorry to say, Sir Anthony, that my affluence over my niece is very small." [influence]

Portmanteau words

A portmanteau is a satchel. It holds many things. A portmanteau word is a neologism constructed from two or more words, such as *parastantial* as a combination of *parallel* and *circumstantial*. In addition to patients with schizophrenia, it is observed in Wernicke's and mixed aphasias and in subcortical aphasia involving dominant basal ganglia and thalamic structures.

Jargon agrammatism or driveling speech

The neurologic term "jargon speech" and the psychiatric term "driveling speech" refer to the same phenomenon. This speech is fluent and associations appear tightly linked and to follow grammatical rules, but the meaning of the speech is lost, as if the patient were speaking a language unfamiliar to the examiner. Driveling speech is similar to the comedic "double-talk", but it is not feigned. When associated with schizophrenia, subcortical aphasia, or chronic illicit-drug-induced psychoses, driveling speech is sporadic and interspersed with understandable utterances, the driveling increasing with the complexity of the conversation, the examiner's persistent questioning, or the patient's anxiety. When associated with Wernicke's or mixed aphasia, driveling is fairly constant, and any understood speech that the patient utters is often non-sequitive.

Example:

Q: "Tell me about your family. What are they like?"
A: "There are three substitutes, one beyond the two. The smaller fidget doesn't get round about, if the peach instructucates."

In this example, the patient's driveling speech includes paraphasias ("substitutes" for children, "beyond" for older, "smaller" for younger). "Fidget" is a descriptor for the youngest child, a boy with attention deficit disorder. "Peach" refers to the boy's teacher (a phonemic paraphasia). "Doesn't get round about" is an out-of-class paraphasic phrase and "instructucates" is a portmanteau word combining instruction and educates. Driveling speech can usually be parsed into elements of aphasia.

Derailment

Derailment refers to the sudden disrupted switch from one line of thought to a new parallel line of thought. Mild derailment, or *cognitive slippage*, is described in patients with schizotypal personality disorder. Severe derailment is observed in patients with schizophrenia, some chronic illicit-drug-induced psychoses, subcortical aphasia, and cerebellar neocortical lesions.

Example:

To the comment: "Your situation at work would be stressful for most people", a patient replied: "The head person [store manager] is often rude and I may not go on vacation." To the question: "How come you switched schools?" a patient replied: "I had a heavy course load. My sister was good at math, but not me."

Sometimes derailment follows blocking: *"They were talking about me in a threatening way . . . I was hospitalized before."*

Schizophrenia

For years, schizophrenia was referred to as a "*thinking disorder*" with characteristic speech and language features. The term delineated it from mood disorders, also recognized as having associated hallucinations and delusions. The distinction was not satisfactory, and schizophrenia remains a problematic construct.

Kraepelin merged early onset dementing conditions, catatonia, hebephrenia, and *dementia paranoides* into dementia praecox based on his acceptance of a tripartite mind concept and that such patients exhibited deficits in all three domains of will, emotion and thinking. Such patients also had a common chronic course.[53] This formulation was vigorously criticized by others, but it was broadened by Eugen Bleuler to included, regardless of course, many patients that were understood to share the proposed three mental deficits.

Excessive numbers of patients, however, satisfied Bleuler's psychological view of the condition's primary and secondary features. To accommodate the resulting heterogeneity and the variability of illness onsets and outcomes, he offered the term schizophrenia, which is now standard usage.[54] But the clinical heterogeneity of the newly formulated schizophrenia was recognized, eliciting attempts to identify subgroups of patients. These efforts resulted in constructs such as schizophreniform, schizoaffective, good and poor prognosis schizophrenia, and positive and negative symptom schizophrenia. None of these proposals defines a valid diagnostic class.[55]

The need to delineate schizophrenia into a more homogeneous population, however, is important. Do all such patients require antipsychotic agents? Do the biological markers associated with the diagnosis pertain to all sufferers, or only to a specific subgroup? Is the proposed genetic vulnerability to the disorder specific to all persons with the diagnosis, a subgroup, or does it reflect a general vulnerability to psychosis?

Recent scholarship has paid scant attention to the above questions, but until the boundaries of schizophrenia are clearly distinguished, scientific effort to answer them will be unsuccessful. The boundaries, however, can be roughly ascertained from the psychopathological literature and studies of the longitudinal pre-psychotic features of the condition.

Delineating schizophrenia

Kraepelin's construct of an early-onset psychotic disorder associated with cognitive impairment and negative symptoms is still recognized clinically.[56] Such patients function poorly in their daily living efforts. Males with emotional blunting and avolition have little interest in sexual activity,[57] and the association between absent sexual activity and schizophrenia in male patients is as strong as that for first-rank symptoms and schizophrenia. The sexual activity of women with schizophrenia is more variable, as are their long-term outcomes. Schizophrenics distinguished by negative features and early-onset are most likely to develop a chronic illness.[58] Such patients, however, are not commonly identified and separately assessed in studies of treatment response and pathophysiology. A delineation of such patients follows.

Characteristic psychopathology

The psychopathology consistently associated with a non-mood disorder psychotic condition that typically emerges in the second or third decade of life are emotional blunting with avolition (also referred to as negative features), and formal thought disorder.[59] These signs are found together in 60–80% of psychotic patients who have no mood disorder or accepted neurologic disease.[60]

Negative features are stable over time, even between exacerbations of psychosis.[61] They reflect deficits in executive functioning,[62] and are associated with years of poor general functioning and chronic, treatment-resistant illness.[63]

Formal thought disorder is also associated with frontal lobe executive function problems, poor response to standard pharmacotherapy, long-term chronicity, and similar pathology in relatives.[64]

In contrast, the phenomena used in present criteria are minimally distinguishing. While auditory hallucinations (hearing sustained voices) and passivity delusions (being controlled by outside forces) are characteristic of the psychotic episodes of schizophrenia,[65] alone these features do not assure the diagnosis.[66] They also do not predict outcome.[67] "Grossly disorganized" behavior and catatonia is also one of the DSM criteria options for the diagnosis. Catatonia, however, is inappropriately linked to schizophrenia in present classifications and while found in some schizophrenics should not be used to define the condition.[68] This was one of Kraepelin's fundamental errors.[69] Defining an illness by the imprecise descriptor "grossly disorganized" further lowers the diagnostic bar, eliciting too many false positive conclusions.[70] The criterion option should be deleted.

Present classifications also offer the schizophrenia subtypes of paranoid, disorganized, catatonic, undifferentiated, and residual. Without first identifying patients by the presence of emotional blunting and formal thought disorder, these sobriquets do not distinguish schizophrenia from other conditions with psychotic features by treatment response, biological correlates, or family illness pattern. Many patients with manic-depression are paranoid, catatonic and behaviorally disorganized, but few are emotionally blunted, avolitional, and exhibit FTD.[71]

Associated features

A review of the numerous studies of the pathophysiology of schizophrenia is beyond the scope of this book. The neurology of hallucinations and delusions is discussed in Chapter 3. In addition, there are neuromotor, cognitive and morpho-logic abnormalities that are consistent but not pathognomonic of schizophrenia that can be identified on examination.

Both basal ganglia and cerebellar motor signs are described by Kraepelin who discussed a "cerebellar form" of dementia praecox,[72] and cerebellar volume loss is reported in patients with schizophrenia associated with negative features.[73] Cerebellar and motor "soft signs" are reported in never-medicated schizophrenic patients.[74] Cerebral cortical and subcortical abnormalities in structure and meta-bolic function are also reported,[75] and basal ganglia signs are seen in unmedicated schizophrenics.[76] The abnormalities are associated with the negative features of the condition.[77] Schizophrenics also exhibit problems with smooth eye move-ment pursuit of objects, a difficulty linked to frontal circuitry disease.[78] The problems are found early in the condition.[79]

While dementia is not the inevitable outcome of schizophrenia, cognitive prob-lems are recognized early in the condition. The deficits, even when mild, involve many cognitive processes, executive functioning the most dramatically affected. The deficits are associated with negative features and formal thought disorder, but not with hallucinations and delusions.[80] Some researchers propose cognitive deficits to be a diagnostic criterion for schizophrenia, but while most sufferers have cogni-tive problems consistent with frontal circuitry dysfunction, these are not specific.[81]

Structural anomalies of body parts (e.g. clinodactyly, small head circumfer-ence, ectopic eyes, ears and nares) are reported to be more common in schizo-phrenic patients. These are reflections of a genetic or gestational perturbation, are recognized in infancy, and are stable over a lifetime. Many non-ill persons exhibit one or two, while schizophrenic patients and persons with conduct disorder and violent criminal behavior are found to have more.[82]

Pre-psychotic features

Over 40 years of research has demonstrated that schizophrenia is not merely a series of characteristic psychotic episodes. Children who later in life experience psychotic episodes characterized by emotional blunting with avolition and formal thought disorder are found to have abnormal emotional expression, inappropri-ate social interactions, cognitive inflexibility, and neuromotor problems. Sub-stantial genetic and intrauterine factors (e.g. maternal malnutrition, influenza) contribute to the condition. The more substantial is the evidence of these factors, the more severe are the childhood abnormalities and the later psychoses.[83] These findings, particularly seen in children with a mother with schizophrenia, are considered by many researchers to support the idea that schizophrenia is a developmental disorder.[84]

Table 9.5. The defining features of schizophrenia

Loss of emotional expression (monotone, no facial expression, reduced gestures)

Avolition (no interests or plans, reduced interactions, apathy)

Indifference to present situation

Formal thought disorder

Executive function and other cognitive deficits (poor sustained attention and working memory, cognitive inflexibility, new learning problems, problems in reasoning, planning and self-monitoring)

Motor disturbances (poor sequential and fine hand movement, stereotypy, poor coordination, past-pointing, dystonia, dyspraxia, poor eye tracking)

Delusions of passivity

Complete auditory hallucinations

Childhood features of cognitive, emotion, and neuromotor problems

Schizophrenia spectrum conditions

Traditionally, schizoid personality has been considered a pre-psychotic feature of schizophrenia and the low levels of emotional expression and volition associated with the schizoid construct are consistent with the pre-psychotic features previously described. Patients with schizoid personality are also reported to be awkward in their movements.[85] Schizoid behaviors are best considered early and mild expressions of schizophrenia.

Schizotypal and avoidant personality are also proposed as part of a schizophrenia spectrum. Both are associated with low emotional expression and reduced volition. Schizotypal personality is also associated with perceptual and cognitive disturbances. The risks for these conditions are also reported to be elevated in the first-degree relatives of patients with schizophrenia.[86] While schizotypal behaviors are best considered low-level signs of illness, avoidant behavior is heterogeneous and encompasses patients with schizoid and other pre-psychotic behaviors as well as others with anxious–fearful personality traits.

Table 9.5 displays the features of schizophrenia that best define the syndrome.

Conclusions

The speech and language functioning of a patient, if understood from a neurologic perspective, is diagnostically discriminating, and indicates prognosis. Present classification reduces this entire chapter to two terms: "disorganized" to indicate a psychotic disorder, and "flight-of-ideas" to indicate mania. A paucity of speech is further recognized as associated with schizophrenia and a press of speech with mania. This rudimentary structure fails many patients and encourages poor treatment choices. Table 9.6 offers a more refined approach.

Table 9.6. Speech and language features of psychiatric patients

Feature	Schizophrenia	Mania	Melancholia	Catatonia	Frontal dementia	Delirium
Spontaneity	●	●●●	●	●	● Avolitional syndrome ●●● Disinhibited syndrome	●
Fluency	●●	●●●	● With retardation ●● With agitation	●	●● Both syndromes	●
Reduced turn-taking	●●	●●●	●●	●●●	● Both syndromes	●●
Verbal output	Low	High	Low with retardation High with agitation	○ With mutism	Low with avolitional syndrome ●●● With disinhibited syndrome	Variable
Modulation	Low	High	Low	Low	Normal	Variable
Poor articulation	●	○	○	○	○	○
Mannerisms	●●	●	○	●●●	○	○
Stereotypes and perseverations	●	○	●	●●●	● Both syndromes	○

Circumstantial	•••	○	○	••• Disinhibited syndrome	○
Flight-of-ideas	•••	○	○	• Disinhibited syndrome	○
Talking past the point	•	○	•	○	○
Clanging	•••	○	○	• Disinhibited syndrome	○
Rambling	•	○	○	○	•••
FTD	••	○	•	○ (Unless an aspect of progressive aphasia)	•

○ Absent; • infrequent; •• common; ••• characteristic.

NOTES

1 This quote is widely attributed to Ralph Gerard, a noted mid-twentieth-century neuro-physiologist, but its exact citation has not been established.

2 Patient 1.5 also illustrates a patient whose stroke and associated aphasia was attributed to her manic-depressive illness.

3 Fluency of speech and fluency of ideas are different. The former is a speech function, the latter is a cognitive function.

4 Damasio and Damasio (2000).

5 Hypergraphia, circumstantiality, hyposexuality, and pseudo-profundity (a superficial, stereotypic interest in science or philosophy) comprise the "Psychomotor Quartet" associated with chronic limbic system disease (Bear and Fedio, 1977; Mungas, 1982).

6 Dysgraphia in Asian writers in the vertical has similar characteristics (Yin *et al.*, 2005) as does dysgraphia of specialized script such as in stenography (Miceli *et al.*, 1997).

7 Berthier *et al.* (1988).

8 Foreign accent syndrome has also been associated with lesions in the dominant frontal lobe (Berthier *et al.*, 1991).

9 Mertz and Ostergaard (2006).

10 Ludlow and Loucks (2003).

11 Bowie *et al.* (2004).

12 Taylor (1972); Abrams and Taylor (1973).

13 Bleuler (1976), pages 102–7.

14 Fish (1967), page 37.

15 Kraepelin (1976).

16 Fish (1967).

17 Jaspers (1963), page 209.

18 Bleuler (1950), page 9.

19 Bleuler (1950), page 14.

20 Bleuler (1950), page 32.

21 Bleuler (1976), page 710.

22 Bleuler (1976), pages 374–5.

23 Bleuler (1976), page 376.

24 Bleuler (1950), page 17.

25 Fink and Taylor (2003).

26 Caplan *et al.* (2000); Goldstein *et al.* (2003); Vaever *et al.* (2005).

27 Schizaphasia was considered associated with excitement, while cataphasia was thought to be associated with reduced speech (Leonhard, 1979, p. 1103).

28 Landre and Taylor (1995).

29 Faber *et al.* (1983); Jampala *et al.* (1989); Caplan *et al.* (2000); Goldstein *et al.* (2003); Vaever *et al.* (2005); Lesson *et al.* (2005).

30 Others use the term formal thought disorder to mean abnormal thinking as interpreted from the Rorschach test (Meloy, 1984) or as measured by specific cognitive assessment (Harrow *et al.*, 2003).

31 Faber and Reichstein (1981).

32 Cameron (1947).

33 Goldstein (1944/1964).

34 Andreasen (1977).

35 Schneider (1942).

36 Fish (1968), pages 46–7.

37 Kleist (1914).

38 See references above by Taylor and associates. However, many investigators have found that schizophrenic patients with speech and language problems also have cognitive difficulties (Arbelle *et al.*, 1997; Rodriguez-Ferrera *et al.*, 2001; Kerns and Berenbaum, 2002; Harrow *et al.*, 2003). But the evidence that this association is causal is weak. For example, schizophrenic patients with formal thought disorder make semantic errors on tests of language functioning, but these errors are unrelated to general intelligence (Oh *et al.*, 2002). Schizophrenic patients identified as having the characteristic speech abnormalities of the illness have been shown to have aphasic-like speech, to do poorly on tests used to assess aphasia, and have deficits in general thinking ability. The thinking deficits and disturbed thought content are not correlated with the language problems, but the language disorder is associated with attentional difficulties. Others have associated the speech disorders in schizophrenia with negative symptoms (Peralta *et al.*, 1992; Taylor *et al.*, 1994).

39 Shenton *et al.* (2001); Kasai *et al.* (2003a,b).

40 Damasio and Damasio (2000).

41 Landre *et al.* (1992).

42 Kerns and Berenbaum (2002).

43 Taylor *et al.* (1981); Taylor and Abrams (1984); Goldstein *et al.* (1999); Mitchell and Crow (2005).

44 Faber *et al.* (1983).

45 Crosson (1985); Crosson and Hughes (1987).

46 Radanovic *et al.* (2003); Carrera and Bogousslavsky (2006); De Witte *et al.* (2006).

47 Kuljic-Obradovic (2003); Radanovic and Scaff (2003). Some studies find different impairment patterns associated with different subcortical structures. A combination of striato-capsular and thalamic dysfunction best fits the FTD pattern.

48 Jampala *et al.* (1989); Cuesta and Peralta (1993).

49 Taylor *et al.* (1994).

50 Jampala *et al.* (1989); Wilcox (1992).

51 Kraepelin (1971), page 56.

52 Kraepelin (1971), page 70.

53 Chapter 2 reviews the evolution of Kraepelin's thinking.

54 Also see Chapter 2.

55 Chapter 2 provides a discussion of these constructs and Chapter 16 offers a reformulation of the psychotic disorders class.

56 Bellino *et al.* (2004).

57 Fan *et al.* (2007).

58 Lasser *et al.* (2007).

59 Details are discussed above.

60 Abrams and Taylor (1978); Andreasen (1982); Taylor (1972, 1981, 1991); Taylor and Abrams (1978); Andreasen *et al.* (1990); Taylor *et al.* (1994).

61 Amador *et al.* (1999).

62 Donohoe and Robertson (2003).

63 Lasser *et al.* (2007).

64 Faber *et al.* (1983); Jampala *et al.* (1989); Caplan *et al.* (2000); Goldstein *et al.* (2003); Vaever *et al.* (2005); Lesson *et al.* (2005).

65 Chapter 10 provides a discussion of hallucinations and Chapter 11 of delusions. Evidence for the diagnostic importance of these features is found in Abrams and Taylor (1973, 1981, 1983); Taylor (1981); Taylor and Amir (1994).

66 Peralta and Cuesta (1999); Chapter 16 provides a discussion of the problems with the diagnostic criteria for schizophrenia.

67 Thorup *et al.* (2007).

68 Fink and Taylor (2003); also see Chapter 16.

69 See Chapters 2 and 7.

70 DSM-IV-TR, page 312.

71 Abrams and Taylor (1976a,b, 1981, 1983); Abrams *et al.* (1974); Taylor and Abrams (1975b); Taylor *et al.* (1974, 1975, 1994).

72 Taylor (1991).

73 Nopoulos *et al.* (1999); Ichimiya *et al.* (2001).

74 Varambally *et al.* (2006).

75 Flashman and Green (2004).

76 McCreadie *et al.* (2005).

77 Sanfilipo *et al.* (2000).

78 Hutton *et al.* (2004).

79 Keedy *et al.* (2006).

80 Taylor and Abrams (1984); Donohoe and Robertson (2003); Bowie *et al.* (2004, 2005).

81 Lewis (2004).

82 Ovsiew (1997).

83 Erlenmeyer-Kimling and Cornblatt (1984); Walker and Lewine (1990); Fish *et al.* (1992); McClellan and McCurry (1998); Hans *et al.* (1999).

84 McClellan and McCurry (1998); Weinberger (1987).

85 Bleuler (1950); Kraepelin (1971).

86 Asarnow *et al.* (2001); Fogelson *et al.* (2007).

10

Perceptual disturbances

For decades psychiatry has been struggling for a new orientation but can obviously not find it, the diversity of opinions in psychiatry today being greater than ever. Kraepelin's teachings have been rejected, but whenever nosological questions are raised, his dichotomy of the endogenous psychoses reappears . . . While the related neurological discipline recognized hundreds of endogenous diseases and continues to describe more, psychiatry perceives only two.[1]

Perceptual aberrations are common features of psychiatric and neurologic illness. Non-ill persons also experience occasional perceptual disturbances, but the presence of frequent or intense aberrations indicates serious nervous system disease.

Perceptual disturbances occur in all sensory modalities. They include misinterpretations and distortions of environmental stimuli, as well as self-generated hallucinations. The pathogenesis of these phenomena is largely unknown, but disturbances in specific sensory modalities have diagnostic implications. The diagnostic challenge presented by the patient exhibiting perceptual disturbances is to distinguish a primary psychiatric syndrome from one associated with more specific brain disease.[2] Psychosensory features described below, for example, are associated with seizure disorder, migraine, chronic hallucinogenic drug use and manic-depressive illness. Extracampine hallucinations, perceptions outside the possible sensory field, and autoscopy, the hallucination of self, are also associated with seizure disorder and limbic system dysfunction. Although auditory hallucinations of sustained voices are not pathognomonic of schizophrenia, their presence increases the probability of that diagnosis. Frequently experienced visual illusions suggest schizotypal disorder. Olfactory and gustatory hallucinations also suggest limbic system dysfunction. Visual hallucinations are most commonly associated with disease within the visual system and with delirium.

Perceptual distortions

Perceptual distortions are alterations in the perception of external stimuli. Distortions occur in all sensory modalities, and the more frequent, intense, and multimodal the distortions, the more likely the patient will have an identifiable neurologic disease.

Hyperesthesia and hypoesthesia

These phenomena are distortions of stimulus intensity. In hyperesthesia the stimulus appears more intense (e.g. a dim light appears "glaring"). In hypoesthesia, the stimulus appears diminished. Hyperesthesia is associated with disorders of emotion, drug intoxications, migraine, and histrionic personality traits.[3]

In somatosensory hypoesthesia the patient experiences "numbness". In visual and auditory hypoesthesia, colors appear "washed-out" and sounds are dulled, muffled or perceived as coming from a distance. Hypoesthesia occurs in severe depressive illness and many neurologic disorders.[4]

Synesthesia

Synesthesia is the stimulation of one sensory modality eliciting a perception in a different sensory modality, as in "seeing a sound". It is associated with toxic states, and is considered the classic perceptual disturbance of LSD intoxication.

Dysmegalopsia

Dysmegalopsia is a distortion of the size of objects and body parts. In *micropsia* objects appear smaller, farther away or retreating into the distance. In *macropsia* or *megalopsia*, objects appear larger or closer. Images are perceived to fluctuate from large (like a zoom lens) to small (as if looking through the wrong end of a telescope). Dysmegalopsia occurs in seizure disorders, chronic manic-depressive illness, retinal disease, and disorders of accommodation and convergence. When associated with left-sided spatial neglect of the left side of the body and environment, it indicates right parietal lobe disease.[5] Memory for shapes, the location of objects and direction are also impaired in such patients.[6]

In retinal swelling the image falls on a smaller part of the retina than usual, eliciting micropsia. Retinal scarring with retraction elicits macropsia, but also visual distortions or *metamorphopsia*. Dysmegalopsia also occurs in anticholinergic delirium and degenerative brain disease affecting the visual associational cortex.[7]

Dysmorphopsia

Dysmorphopsia is the visual distortion of shape and is associated with dysmegalopsia. Objects or body parts appear twisted and bent as if viewed through a glass of water, or as distorted in Fun House mirrors.[8]

Color spectrum distortions

Toxic states and degenerative disease of the visual associational cortex are associated with change in color perception. In degenerative brain disease objects and people seem darker than in fact. In digitalis toxicity, green hues predominate. In caffeinism, blue or yellow hues predominate. In migraine, colors may fade and the environment appears gray.[9]

Illusions

Illusions are false perceptions or misinterpretations of environmental stimuli. They arise from a lack of perceptual clarity resulting from diminished or ambiguous stimuli or from perceptual distortion due to intense emotion. Non-ill persons experience illusions. "Seeing" a "face" or other recognizable images in a cloud is illusory when the experience is intense (a *pareidolic* illusion). Non-ill persons also experience illusions when clarity is diminished as at night and when anxiety is heightened as when walking down a dark street and perceiving a swaying bush behind a tree as a crouching figure.

Delirium and manic-depressive illness are conditions that diminish perceptual clarity and elicit illusions. In delirium, innocent gestures by hospital personnel may appear threatening. Depressive delusions distort the interpretation of sounds and gestures as dangerous or as confirmation of misdeeds. Manic patients perceive car horns as heavenly trumpets and interpret adoration or jealousy in the faces of passers-by. Patients exhibiting persecutory delusions and experiences of self-reference detect conspiracies in the innocent gestures and conversations of persons who are nearby. Patients with schizotypal illness misperceive objects in their peripheral visual field as scurrying animals, supernatural creatures, or body parts.

Auditory illusions usually involve mishearing speech, the distortion often shaped by the person's emotional state. Tactile illusions are rare and typically relate to temperature, the weight of objects, or the character of surfaces. Gustatory and olfactory illusions are also rare and vaguely unpleasant.[10]

Fantastic illusions are perceived extraordinary modifications of the environment. The psychopathologist Frank Fish refers to a patient of Griesinger's who looked in the mirror and saw his head as that of a pig. Fish describes his own patient who during an examination saw Fish's head change into a rabbit's head. The patient also expressed fantastic confabulations.[11] *Muller–Lyer illusions* refer to perceptions that do not agree with the physical stimulus (e.g. Fish's patient). Fantastic illusions are forms of misidentification, and when present suggest right cerebral hemisphere disease.

Psychosensory phenomena

Psychosensory phenomena differ from other perceptual disturbances in that they are *brief* (rarely longer than a minute), *intense and paroxysmal*, and *repetitive*.

Table 10.1. Psychosensory phenomena

SENSORY

Dysmorphopsia: Distortions in shape

Dysmegalopsia: Distortions in size

Gustatory hallucinations: Experiencing odd (metal), unpleasant (blood), or illogical (death) tastes

Macroacusia and microacusia: Illusions of sound intensity

Olfactory hallucinations: Smelling odd (intensely sweet flowers), unpleasant (burning rubber), or illogical odors (death)

Tactile (haptic) hallucinations: Somatosensory experiences (feeling electricity or insects on one's body, sensations of being hit, poked, or pushed)

Visceral hallucinations: Empty or cold gastric feelings, warmth about the head or body; feeling internal foreign objects; a body part composed of alien matter (wood in a limb, chemical fluids coursing through the body)

Complex formed visual hallucinations (autoscopic and panoramic hallucinations): Perceiving two- or three-dimensional images as if scenes in a move. An image of oneself is termed autoscopic

COGNITIVE

Experiences of false familiarity

Déjà vu: Intense false feeling of "I've seen it before". Differs from the commonly experienced similar phenomenon by its increased frequency, intensity, and conviction. Similar experiences are "knowing" what will happen (*déjà vécu*) or what will be said or heard next (*déjà entendu*)[12]

Experiences of false unfamiliarity

Jamais vu: Non-recognition of familiar objects, sounds, and familiar persons' voices (*jamais entendu*), or events and places (*jamais vécu*)

Forced thinking: Intrusive and repetitive thoughts that are often upsetting in content and attributed to external sources

Thought withdrawal: Sudden removal of thought, the "mind" experienced as "going blank", attributed to external influences

EMOTIONAL FEATURES

Emotional incontinence: Emotional expression of unintended laughing or weeping, unrelated to or an exaggeration of the subjective experience

Paroxysmal and transient euphoria or sadness: Elation or despondency without an immediate obvious cause

Fear: Most common emotional psychosensory experience

Rage: Commonly non-goal-directed

Erotic: Unexpected sexual climax (rare)

They involve all senses, emotions, memory and cognition. They accompany complex partial seizures, manic-depressive illness, migraine, and hallucinogenic drug use. They are also features of epilepsy spectrum disorder, a seizure-related syndrome with the perceptual changes characteristic of partial complex epilepsy but without stereotyped spells.[13] In patients with complex partial seizures, specific psychosensory features facilitate the identification of the seizure focus. In manic-depressive illness psychosensory phenomena are signs of severity and emerging chronicity,[14] but do not predict response to anticonvulsant rather than lithium therapy.[15] Psychosensory phenomena include sensory (autonomic perturbations, dissociation), emotion (incontinence), memory (false familiarity and unfamiliarity), and perceptual distortions and hallucinations (Table 10.1).

Hallucinations

Esquirol defined hallucinations as perceptions without an object. Jaspers defined hallucinations as false perceptions which are not sensory distortions or misinterpretations, but which occur at the same time as real perceptions.

Pseudo-hallucinations

Pseudo-hallucination is a misnomer. It is a hallucination that is experienced as unreal. It is vivid but circumscribed from other accurate perceptions. Pseudo-hallucinations tend to localize to a part of the body or a point in near-by space. They differ from "mental images", which are recognized as subjective and not vivid. Pseudo-hallucinations are associated with identifiable neurologic disease more than with the primary psychotic disorders.[16] Patient 10.1 illustrates.

Patient 10.1

An 85-year-old man with long-standing cardiovascular disease had a flu-like syndrome that lasted about a week. Toward the end of this discomfort, he awoke one morning to the sound of a radio playing popular music from his youth. The music was clear and fully recognizable, but the patient knew that the radio was not "on" and that he was "hearing things". He had no other psychopathology. Brain imaging identified a new right-sided temporal–parietal ischemic lesion. Over the next several weeks the hallucination gradually resolved without psychotropic medication.

Hypnogogic and hypnopompic hallucinations

Hypnogogic hallucinations occur as the person is falling asleep. Hypnopompic hallucinations occur as the patient is awakening. These phenomena are not vivid and are experienced as distinct from dreams. Visual experiences are the most common and include seeing shapes, figures, and scenes. Auditory experiences include music, brief voices (e.g. one's name being called) and environmental sounds (e.g. a dog barking). In non-ill persons they are associated with periods of sleep deprivation. When frequent, they suggest narcolepsy.[17]

Extracampine hallucinations

An extracampine hallucination is a false perception outside the limits of the normal sensory field (e.g. hearing plotters in another country). Extracampine hallucinations are associated with manic-depressive illness, seizure disorder, illicit drug use, and delirium.[18]

Elementary hallucinations

Elementary hallucinations are unformed. Flashes of light, undefined shapes and patterns, and non-specific sounds such as buzzing, whirring, and clanking are examples. These phenomena are associated with toxic states and migraine. Migraine scotomata include false perceptions of moving lights, zigzag lines, stars, shimmering lights like the sun's reflection off a body of water, and a gray or dark fog. Hallucinations of well-defined geometric shapes are associated with cocaine intoxication.[19]

Functional hallucinations

A functional hallucination is elicited by an environmental stimulus in the same sensory modality. A particular pitch (e.g. the whine of a rusty faucet turned on) can trigger a hallucinated voice. A wallpaper pattern can change into the heads of demons or other false visual perceptions. Both the triggering stimulus and the hallucination are perceived. Functional hallucinations are associated with delirium and toxic states, seizure disorder, and focal brain vascular disease.[20] A *reflex hallucination* is a form of synesthesia, the stimulus triggering the hallucination in another sensory modality. For example, a patient hears footsteps and then hallucinates lurking figures in the corner of the room.

Palinacousis (auditory perseveration) and *palinopsia* (visual perseveration) are rare forms of functional hallucinations. Palinacousis is the hearing of words, sounds, and fragments of sentences continuously for minutes to hours after the stimulus is removed.[21] Palinopsia is seeing images continuously for minutes to hours after the visual stimulus is removed. The phenomena are associated with temporal and occipital lobe dysfunction. Palinopsia is associated with LSD use.[22] It is also reported in patients taking paroxetine, mirtazepine, and nefazodone, and this rare side-effect must be differentiated from endogenous psychosis.[23]

Experiential hallucinations

Experiential hallucinations were first described by the neurosurgeon Wilder Penfield, who elicited them by stimulating various parts of the exposed cerebral cortex, particularly the temporal lobe, of his patients prior to neurosurgery. Penfield likened them to vivid memories.[24] Experiencing a telephone conversation with a friend, a frightening situation, or a snippet of a family gathering are examples.

Panoramic hallucinations

Panoramic hallucinations are similar to experiential hallucinations. In panoramic hallucinations the patient sees animated scenes as if watching a film strip. Panoramic and experiential hallucinations are associated with psychosensory epilepsy, particularly with a temporal lobe focus, and delirium. The "flashbacks" of PTSD, when validated, are likely experiential hallucinations that include vivid memory in all sensory fields.[25]

Lilliputian and Brobdignagian hallucinations

Lilliputian hallucinations are visual hallucinations of small objects or creatures. Seeing tiny blue men and small bowls of fruit are examples. These phenomena are associated with delirium, particularly delirium tremens, and persons with Lewy body dementia, migraine, seizure disorder, and schizophrenia.[26] Brobdignagian hallucinations, visual hallucinations of gigantic objects or creatures, are also associated with delirium and dementia.[27]

Peduncular hallucinations

Peduncular hallucinations are cartoon-like visual hallucinations without depth. They are typically colorful and non-threatening images of animals or people. They occur in full wakefulness and last a few seconds or minutes, and rarely for hours or days. Sleep disturbances co-occur. Peduncular hallucinations are associated with vascular and white matter lesions in the rostral brainstem or projection sites in the basal ganglia, pulvinar, or medial and posterior thalamic nuclei.[28]

Autoscopic hallucinations[29]

Autoscopy is the hallucination of one's own image. Other terms are *phantom mirror-image, heautoscopy,* and *reduplicative hallucination.* The image is usually perceived slightly to one side and can be vague or vivid. Kinesthetic and somatic sensations are reported with the vision. Autoscopy is associated with seizure disorder, focal disease of the parietal–occipital cortex and toxic states. An extreme version of autoscopy is the *Doppelgänger* phenomenon, the patient seeing his "double" and elaborating the hallucination with an explanatory delusional story. *Anosagnosia,* denial of illness, occurs. One patient arrested for disturbing the peace by throwing garbage on local church steps on Sundays and spitting and cursing at parishioners, insisted that the culprit was his twin brother whom he frequently saw in his house. The patient, an only child, was also avolitional, had reduced emotional expression and elements of formal thought disorder, and was diagnosed as schizophrenic.

Tactile hallucinations

Tactile hallucinations are experienced as emanating from inside the body (haptic) or from the skin. The patient with parietal lobe disease may experience a body part in his abdomen and may feel it move. A falsely perceived limb may be experienced ectopically or as an extra limb (e.g. a third arm).[30] This differs from the *phantom limb* phenomenon following amputation which results from continued afferent stimulation of the sensory homunculus corresponding to the amputated limb.[31]

Patients with parietal lobe seizure foci experience electric shocks as auras. Parietal lobe strokes are associated with the false perception that a limb is not of flesh and blood but is made of wood or metal, or is a body part of a another person or an animal.[32] These *experiences of alienation* were considered pathognomonic ("first rank") of schizophrenia by the psychopathologist Kurt Schneider when no specific brain disease could be detected.

Some seizures begin with a perception of emptiness and cold in the abdomen that pushes upward into the chest. Patients with frontal lobe seizure foci experience an aura of heat over their upper body or head.[33] Chronic stimulant use is associated with hallucinated insects crawling on or under the skin (cocaine bugs). Such *formication hallucinations*[34] elicit intense scratching, resulting in scarring excoriations. The experience also accompanies alcohol withdrawal and toxic states.

Paresthesia, a tingling pins-and-needles sensation, may be a hallucinated experience, but is most commonly due to peripheral nerve compression or disease. It is also experienced during panic attacks from hyperventilation.[35]

Some psychotic patients describe elaborate tactile hallucinations of sexual assault or electric or magnetic forces controlling their body, forcing them to perform actions against their will. One patient felt tingling over his body that made him continuously sweep the inpatient unit. Others describe a wind or a hand that pushes or pokes, making them move a certain way. Kurt Schneider considered these *experiences of control* to also be first rank when specific brain disease could not be detected.

Secondary delusional ideas are often associated with tactile hallucinations. A catatonic patient experienced the perception of alien fluids coursing through his blood vessels and related his stereotypy as efforts to balance the flow. A schizophrenic man felt his brain being physically manipulated and recognized it as a persecuting force at work.

Gustatory and olfactory hallucinations

Sudden, intense, and brief gustatory or olfactory hallucinations are classic signs of psychosensory epilepsy. These perceptions are unpleasant: foul or metallic tastes, the odor of rotting flesh, feces, burning rubber, or a cloying sweetness. Gustatory and olfactory hallucinations are also experienced at the onset of some migraine headaches.[36]

Sustained hallucinations of taste and smell are reported in manic-depressive illness and psychotic disorders. The depressed patient experiences a foul odor emanating from his body that he "knows" sickens others, or he smells the lethal disease his doctors are denying he has or the rotting garbage in his bowels. He smells the poisons that are being pumped into his room or sprayed on his furniture. He tastes ashes and bitterness, metal and blood. The schizophrenic smells poison and the by-products of imagined sexual assault.

Rarely, peripheral nerve disease elicits a hallucination. *Phantosmia* is the brief (seconds) sensing of a vague odor without the scent being present. Phantosmia can begin following sniffing or sneezing, and is associated with damage to peripheral neurons that inhibit or stimulate olfaction. It is also experienced following trigeminal nerve excitation inducing excitation in brain areas regulating olfaction, contralateral frontal, insular and temporal regions.[37] *Phantageusia* is a sudden, vague taste without the presence of the substance normally causing the sensation.[38]

Phonemes (voices)

Carl Wernicke, the German neurologist, introduced the term "phoneme" in 1900 to mean hallucinated voices. Phonemes are the commonest form of hallucinations among patients with manic-depressive illness or schizophrenia. Hallucinated voices vary in intensity from vague whispers or muffled utterances, as if coming through a thin wall, to sustained, clear voices perceived as originating from a source external to the patient's sense of self. Voices are also perceived as originating from body parts (e.g. the abdomen), imagined implants (e.g. transmitters in a tooth filling, or in the brain), electronic devices (e.g. TV sets and radios) and near-by locations (e.g. heating ducts, the street in front of the patient's house).

Experiencing constant, mostly low-intensity phonemes without substantial deterioration in functioning, personality, and emotional expression defines *phonemic paraphrenia*. The paraphrenias, a concept still found useful in Europe, are discussed with other delusional syndromes in Chapter 11.

The content of hallucinated voices is not diagnostic and the most common voices are angry and abusive. Rarely, the voices are comforting. Some content, however, is diagnostically suggestive. Patients with psychotic depression hear voices calling them "evil . . . damned . . . whores . . . blasphemers . . . and degenerate", and encourage suicide. One patient heard the tortured screams of the victims of his "brain waves" coming from outside his home. Another heard devils and angels arguing over her evil actions and the need for her to die. Both these patients fully recovered with a course of bilateral ECT. Patients with mania hear "God's voice" or angels. Patients with psychosis associated with frontal lobe disease experience fantastic hallucinations of extraterrestrial transmissions and the sounds of machinery controlling the planets and stars.

Phonemes are assessed for their specific features:

Clarity: "Do you hear whispers or muffled voices as if they are coming from another room? Can you hear them as clearly as you hear my voice now?"

Perceived source: "Where does the voice come from?"

Constancy: "Do you hear only a few words here and there, or is the voice constantly bothering you?"

Pattern and frequency: "Is there a particular time of the day when the voices are at their worst? Do you only hear them after something else happens? Do you hear them all day long? Do you hear them every day? Are you hearing them now?"

Musical hallucinations

Musical hallucinations are experienced as vivid familiar tunes, instruments and lyrics. The most common cause is acquired deafness.[39] Other causes include stroke, epilepsy and neoplasm. When associated with seizure disorder, musical hallucinations have an experiential element not reported in deaf patients (i.e. a sense of remembering the hearing of the music in a particular setting as well as hearing the sounds).[40] They are uncommon in degenerative brain disease. Temporal lobe and brain stem lesions are the commonest associations.[41] Lesions in both cerebral hemispheres are reported, but most commonly on the right.[42]

Musical hallucinations are also reported in patients with depressive illness, obsessive–compulsive disorder, alcoholism, and schizophrenia. Commonest among patients with OCD, it is unclear whether the experience is a true hallucination or vivid mental activity as lyrics are experienced more so than musical sounds.[43] Affected patient are typically middle-aged or older. In one large series, most were women.[44]

First rank symptoms (FRS)

Kurt Schneider catalogued symptoms he believed pathognomonic of schizophrenia in the absence of evidence of coarse neurologic disease.[45] The DSM permits the diagnosis of schizophrenia with the presence of one of these phenomena and no other features if there is also a decline in daily functioning.

FRS occur in patients with manic-depressive illness, delirium or intoxication, dementia, seizure disorder, and stroke. They are not exclusive to schizophrenia.[46] Delusions in this category are covered in Chapter 11.

Complete auditory hallucinations

Sustained hallucinated voices, clearly heard and perceived as originating outside the patient's sense of self, are the most common FRS. They are the classic phoneme.

Secondary delusional ideas that "explain" or elaborate upon the hallucination are common.

Voices commenting and conversing are given separate status in some classifications, but the distinction is in content, not form, and of little clinical significance. Phonemes constantly heard, comment on the patient's actions, feelings, thoughts, and experiences. Sometimes two or more voices converse about the patient. Typically, the voice or voices are hostile, commanding acts of violence or self-harm. The number of voices, their gender and identity have no diagnostic implications, other than the more like a memory the experience seems, the more likely it represents temporal–limbic disease.

Thought echo (écho de la pensée)

Thought echo is the experience of hearing one's thoughts repeated aloud by some outside source, as if an echo. A variation is the experience of hearing voices that are saying what the patient is about to think or say (*Gedankenlautwerden*). Thought echo is typically revealed by the patient's delusional statements such as "Everyone knows what I'm thinking." The examiner's response to such a statement and other delusional statements is always "How do you know that?" The question can be "sugar-coated" by sympathetic comments such as "That must be upsetting."

The details of the experience are ascertained by questions such as: "Do you mean that you hear your thoughts repeated aloud to you as if listening to a radio? If I were standing next to you, could I also hear them?"

Some patients are very specific: "I have the feeling, as if someone beside me said out loud what I think . . . As soon as the thought is in my head, they know it too . . . When I think anything I hear it immediately . . . everyone can read my thoughts . . . When [I] read the newspapers, others hear it."[47]

Further examination techniques

Patients who experience perceptual disturbances may not report the experiences for fear of being labeled "crazy". The examination for these features is facilitated by framing questions within the context of other symptoms. For example:

"When people are as depressed as you are, they sometimes experience odd or disturbing things. Does that happen to you? Do you ever hear other people talking about you?"

"Depression often makes the world seem different. Have you noticed anything like that . . . Does food taste odd . . . do you smell disturbing odors . . . do people look at you in odd ways . . .?"

Once the perceptual disturbance is identified, its contextual "story" is delineated. Frequency, fluctuations in intensity, triggers, and the pattern of the experience are detailed. Such information distinguishes patients with epilepsy, schizophrenia, migraine, sleep disorder and many other conditions.

Alterations in somatosensory experience

Alterations in somatosensory experience are common features of many disorders. Patients with thalamic strokes experience increased pain perception, even to stimuli not considered noxious. Patients with depressive illness report increased pain perception that encourages delusions of hidden illness or persecution. Chronic pain syndromes are common co-occurring conditions among psychiatric patients.[48]

Somatoform disturbances

For the diagnosis of somatoform disorder, present classifications require multiple symptoms without a clear medical explanation in multiple organ systems. The construct is based on unproven etiologic and pathophysiologic assumptions, and the sobriquet *Briquet's syndrome*, in honor of Pierre Briquet who first defined the syndrome, is preferred by some.[49] Among the 10 symptom groupings originally offered by Feighner *et al.* (1972), many are classic descriptors of conversion and hysteria (e.g. lump in throat, aphonia, anesthesia, trouble walking), and others are consistent with a mood disorder (e.g. depressed feelings, anorexia, thinking about dying, suicide). The associated histrionic personality traits seen in such patients further undermine the validity of somatoform disorder as a distinct disease.

The recommended assessment for somatoform disorder includes a careful review of systems, a detailed sensory and motor examination, and the reliance on *Waddell's signs.*[50] Patients with migraine, when between headaches, also meet the Waddell criterion of hypersensitivity to stimuli.[51]

Common concerns of patients given the somatoform diagnosis are dyspnea, palpitation, chest pain, dizziness, headache, fatigue and weakness, anxiety, abdominal discomfort, constipation, back and joint pain, memory loss and depression. Women patients also report menstrual difficulties.[52] There is a familial association between the somatoform diagnosis and antisocial personality, with somatoform features expressed mostly in female and antisocial personality mostly in male family members.[53] The presence of somatoform features is associated with intolerance to and exaggeration of treatment side effects.[54]

Pain

Allodynia
Allodynia is pain elicited by a stimulus which typically does not provoke pain (e.g. the light stroking of the skin or the feel of a soft cloth). For this reason, patients with fibromyalgia are unable to wear tight clothes or rough fabrics.

Hyperalgesia

Hyperalgesia is the increased response to painful stimuli. Patients with fibro-myalgia report "pressure points" that are extremely painful to moderate pressure, and these "points of tenderness" are offered as a diagnostic criterion for the condition. Associated features include chronic fatigue, joint stiffness, poor sleep, feelings of cold or numbness in the extremities, and reticular skin discoloration.[55]

Analgesia

Analgesia, the absence of pain to normally painful stimuli, is associated with some strokes, stuporous states, toxic metabolic states, depressive illness, and catatonia.

Dysesthesia

Dysesthesia, or causalgia, is an unpleasant sensation that occurs spontaneously or is evoked by typically non-noxious stimuli. When associated with peripheral nerve disease, the experienced is of burning, numbness, tingling, paresthesia, and weakness in the distal parts of the limbs that assumes a stocking-glove pattern eliciting the misdiagnosis of conversion.[56]

Central pain

Central pain is associated with a lesion or dysfunction anywhere in the pain pathways. About 90% of patients with central pain have had a stroke, but only 7% of these patients experience the pain contralateral to the stroke. Other causes include tumor, hemorrhage, and multiple sclerosis. About 85% of patients with central pain experience constant pain while the remainder experience daily but intermittent pain. These patients experience a spectrum of sensations including burning (59%), aching (30%), pricking (30%) or stabbing (26%). Allodynia, dysesthesia and paresthesia are also reported.[57] As the lesion in central pain may be quite small and the clinical findings subtle, physicians and family members may misunderstand the patient's experience as manipulative, histrionic, or psychogenic.

"Psychogenic pain"

Psychogenic pain is defined by the limits of the clinician's knowledge, the patient experiencing chronic pain without identified explanatory tissue pathology. Many patients with chronic pain, however, have changes in the neurologic structures subserving pain sensation. Many also have co-occurring depressive illness or anxiety disorder that impact pain pathways.[58] Alcoholism, illicit drug abuse, and personality disorders enhance the expression of chronic pain.[59] Efforts to distinguish the determinants of the chronic pain of patients with co-occurring psychiatric illness from the pain of those without such conditions have been unproductive. The resolution of the co-occurring psychiatric condition ameliorates the pain, but does not fully resolve it.[60]

Chronic pain can be understood as an expression of neuronal plasticity at the levels of the nociceptor neurons, spinal cord, and brain. Faced with repeated stimuli from an injury, the brain compensates by adjusting its responses to it. At some point the adjustment is sustained even if the injury resolves.[61] The patient is not histrionic or malingering, rather a form of long-term learning has taken place.

The underlying process in plasticity initially involves nociceptor and spinal cord microglia sensitization. This is reported in inflammatory disease, diabetes and injury.[62] Long-term potentiation of dorsal horn neurons occurs, and underlies such experiences as tactile allodynia and sensory hyperalgesia.[63] "On" and "off" cells in the rostral ventromedial medulla that modulate the transmission of pain become "stuck" in the "on" position leading to further sensitization.[64] Pain-specific thalamic nuclei then become sensitized, effecting the cortical perception of pain.[65] Anterior cingulate cortex metabolism increases in response to painful stimulation and thalamic input.[66] The somatosensory cortex reorganizes to accommodate the increased input, highlighting the sensitization of involved body areas.[67] Thus, what appears to be chronic pain of psychological origin is more likely the result of CNS sensitization leading to hypersensitivity. A co-occurring intense emotional state as part of a mood or anxiety disorder exacerbates pain hypersensitivity, but the resolution of the emotional state may not resolve the chronic pain.

Perceptual disturbances associated with migraine

Although migraine is classified as a headache disorder, it is a complex syndrome that also includes perceptual, autonomic and other neurologic disturbances. The perceptual features of migraine may be misunderstood as conversion disorder or hysteria, malingering, or as part of borderline personality disorder resulting in the sufferer being denied appropriate treatment. Patients with cluster headache are so fearful of future attacks that they may threaten suicide to avoid the painful experiences. This risk is high when headache control is poor and the threat misinterpreted as manipulative. Patients with migraine are also most likely to experience severe but treatable headache after ECT.

The psychopathology of migraine is similar to that of seizure disorder, and the two conditions co-occur in patients and their first-degree relatives.[68] In migraine the visual phenomena are commonly experienced in the peripheral visual field, while in seizure disorder perceptual symptoms are experienced centrally.[69] Sixty percent of migraineurs report a *prodrome* of several minutes, hours or days that include non-melancholic depression, irritability, fatigue, drowsiness, sluggishness, photo- and phono phobia, hyperosmia, neck stiffness, feeling cold, feeling thirsty, a change in appetite, and abdominal distress.

About 20% of migraine sufferers report an *aura* of minutes to an hour that immediately precedes the headache. Auras include visual phenomena such as scintillations, fortification spectra (or teichopsia of arcs of scintillating light that form a herringbone or zigzag pattern or geometric shape in one visual field), photopsia (light flashes),[70] and scotoma.

Somatosensory phenomena include numbness or tingling, usually unilateral. Dysarthria, vertigo,[71] tinnitus, loss of hearing, double vision, bilateral paresthesia and decreased level of consciousness occur with basilar-type auras.[72] Other phenomena include transient hemiparesis and aphasia (reduced speech production without dysarthria or impaired comprehension, both with associated paraphasia), depersonalization and derealization, and illusions that objects and persons are split or fractured into two or more parts.[73] Also reported is the *Alice in Wonderland syndrome* (a somesthetic aura) of paroxysmal perceptual distortions of one's body, particularly of the head and arms, and the perception that objects are substantially smaller than in reality. The experience is accompanied by depersonalization and derealization.[74] Complex visual hallucinations are reported in children with migraine.[75] Lilliputian hallucinations occur in basilar migraine.[76]

The *classic migraine headache* begins unilaterally and is throbbing. Tension headache is a migraine variant. Migraine headaches occur at any time but are most commonly experienced upon morning awakening. The pain lasts from several hours to days, gradually peaks and then subsides. Nausea and anorexia, vomiting, and intolerance to sensory stimuli occur. Sufferers seek a dark, quiet room to lie down. Other features include blurred vision, nasal stuffiness, light-headedness, feeling faint, abdominal cramps and diarrhea, polyuria, facial pallor, hot or cold sensations, sweating, localized scalp, face, or periorbital edema, scalp tenderness, temporal vein and artery prominence, and neck stiffness. Concentration and sustained attention are impaired.

The migraine *postdrome* occurs gradually and is characterized by fatigue, irritability, apathy, poor concentration, scalp tenderness, and moodiness that last for hours or days. Attacks longer than three days are termed *status migrainus*.

The sensory experiences of migraine occur independently of headache and may last days or longer. The features may be misconstrued as conversion, dissociative neurosis, or somatoform disorder. Migrainous vertigo includes spontaneous attacks, positional vertigo, and chronic dizziness and imbalance that is mistaken for astasia abasia.[77] Despite its name, transient monocular vision loss from retinal migraine, which typically lasts several hours and is most often seen in women of childbearing age, may become a permanent disability.[78] Migraine with aura but no headache is an exclusive pattern in about 5% of migraineurs, and many sufferers with headaches early in the illness course go on to have fewer headaches while the auras continue.[79] These recurrent transient episodes without obvious neurologic disease lead to the conclusion that they are psychogenic.[80] The misunderstanding of such phenomena is illustrated by Patient 10.2.

Patient 10.2

A 56-year-old woman, well-known to a university hospital inpatient service for having made many suicide attempts and for episodes of self-cutting, was re-admitted for worsening thoughts of self-harm. Previous diagnoses included depressive illness, manic-depression, schizophrenia, borderline personality disorder, conversion disorder, seizure disorder, migraine, diabetes, and hypothyroidism.

The patient was living in a group home. Her ex-husband was dead, her relationship with her grown daughter was stormy, and she was unable to fully care for herself because of chronic loss of visual acuity leaving her with the perception of shadows and movement only, as if in a darkened room or dense fog. No medical explanation for her visual loss was seriously entertained as the traditional neurologic examination was deemed normal and, as her physicians said: "She is able to feed and dress herself". The index hospitalization was precipitated by her daughter's announcement that she and her family were moving out of state, and that the patient was not to join them.

On admission, the patient was wearing dark sunglasses and used a walking cane to ambulate. She was in no distress. Other than mild psychomotor slowing, she had no features of depressive illness. She was obese. She said she was experiencing auditory and visual hallucinations, but that these were chronic. In the past she had auditory hallucinations commanding her to kill herself. Her cognition was said to be "intact", although no serious assessment was done.

On the unit she was said to "split" the staff, being very fond of some and nasty to others. Her treatment over many brief hospitalizations included various psychotherapy programs. Her present medications included low-dose valproic acid (100 mg twice daily) and sumatriptin (25 mg as needed). Past medications included antipsychotics, antidepressants, and mood stabilizers.

A consultant noted that the patient had suffered a traumatic brain injury at age seven when she was kicked by a horse, and that for several years afterward experienced several types of seizures. The patient said she still occasionally had seizures (from her description, partial complex with a frontal lobe focus). Since her head injury she also suffered from weekly migraine attacks, her latest the week before admission. An MRI showed mild diffuse cortical atrophy. There was no record that she had ever received an EEG at the university hospital.

Although no further evaluation was done by the inpatient team, the consultant recommended a visual field examination as migraine may lead to persistent visual acuity loss that is experienced as "a fog"[81] and migraine may follow mild traumatic brain injury.[82] An outpatient visual field examination revealed acuity loss in the 12 and 16 Hz frequencies, a finding reported in migraineurs and one that can last up to 75 days after a headache.[83] Despite this finding, the patient continued her previous treatments for borderline personality disorder and conversion, and returned to her group home.

Summary

Perceptual disturbances commonly occur in patients with psychiatric and neurologic diagnoses. Specific neurologic disease is more likely when (1) a hallucination occurs without other psychopathology and the patient recognizes it as a symptom of illness or is not troubled by it; (2) multiple hallucinations in multiple sensory modalities are experienced; (3) the perceptual disturbances are sudden, brief, or occur at a specific time of the day; (4) a musical hallucination is experienced; (5) illusions and other perceptual distortions or psychosensory features predominated the clinical image; (6) recurrent transient visual hallucinations predominate;[84] (7) kaleidoscopic hallucinations of shifting geometric colored patterns or visual fragments occur;[85] (8) the perceptual disturbance occurs with an alteration in arousal, awareness, or with repetitive motor features, and (9) the patient has a history of traumatic brain injury, seizure disorder, or migraine.

NOTES

1 Leonhard 1979, pages XV–XVI.
2 Braun *et al.* (2003).
3 Goadsby (2005).
4 Yamamoto *et al.* (1993); Mailis-Gagnon *et al.* (2003); Calabrese (2004).
5 Nachev and Husain (2006).
6 Husain *et al.* (2001).
7 Kolmel (1993).
8 Ibid.
9 Ovanesov (1998).
10 McAbee *et al.* (2000); Hayashi (2004).
11 Fish (1967), page 18.
12 These phenomena are commonly associated with temporal lobe disease and disruption of recognition memory (Spatt, 2002).
13 Atre Vaidya and Taylor (1997); Roberts *et al.* (1992).
14 Atre Vaidya and Taylor (1997); Atre Vaidya *et al.* (1998).
15 Ali *et al.* (1997).
16 Van der Zwaard and Polak (2001).
17 Dauvilliers *et al.* (2003).
18 Sato and Berrios (2003).
19 Manford and Andermann (1998).

20 Manford and Andermann (1998), Norton and Corbett (2000).

21 Malone and Leiman (1983).

22 Gaillard and Borruat (2003).

23 Norton and Corbett (2000).

24 Penfield and Perot (1963).

25 Sierra and Berrios (1999).

26 Hendrickson and Adityanjee (1996); Takaoka and Takata (1999); Podell and Robinson (2001).

27 Cummings and Mega (2003).

28 Taylor *et al.* (2005); Serra Catafau *et al.* (1992); McKee *et al.* (1990).

29 Manford *et al.* (1996); Tadokoro *et al.* (2006).

30 Cutting (1989).

31 Ohayon (2000); Cutting (1989).

32 Critchley (1953).

33 Bancaud and Talairach (1992).

34 The term derives from the family name for ants, or Formicidae. The delusions extending from these hallucinations are referred to as *zoopathy.*

35 Schulz-Stubner (2004).

36 Fuller and Guiloff (1987); Morrison (1990).

37 Leopold (2002).

38 Ibid.

39 Stewart *et al.* (2006).

40 Ibid.

41 Berrios (1991); Evers and Ellger (2004); Stewart *et al.* (2006).

42 Berrios (1991).

43 Hermesh *et al.* (2004).

44 Evers and Ellger (2004).

45 Schneider (1959).

46 Abrams and Taylor (1973); Taylor (1972, 1981); Rosse *et al.* (1994); Peralta and Cuesta (1999).

47 Kraepelin (1971), page 12.

48 Mergl *et al.* (2007).

49 Trimble (2004).

50 These include: (1) over-reaction to painful stimuli, (2) widespread and superficial tenderness without anatomic clarity, (3) symptoms elicited by manipulation of unrelated muscle groups or body structures, (4) anatomically contradictory motor function (the patient cannot straight-leg raise in one position but can in another), and (5) lower limb sensory or motor loss that does not correspond to any nerve root distribution (Trimble, 2004, p. 52).

51 Weissman-Fogel *et al.* (2003).

52 Woodruff *et al.* (1974), page 64.

53 Woodruff *et al.* (1974), discussion on pages 69–70, references pages 72–4.

54 Fink (2007).

55 Henriksson (2003).

56 Klein and Greenfield (1999).

57 Gonzales (1995).

58 Covington (2000).

59 Fishbain *et al.* (1986); Polatin *et al.* (1993).

60 Binzer *et al.* (2003).

61 Katz and Rothenberg (2005).

62 Lundeberg and Ekholm (2002); Narita *et al.* (2006).

63 Ma and Woolf (1996).

64 Fields *et al.* (1995).

65 Craig *et al.* (1994).

66 Ibid.

67 Huse *et al.* (2001).

68 Eriksen *et al.* (2004).

69 Ibid.

70 Photopsia is a fairly common symptom in ophthalmologic practice (Amos, 1999). In addition to migraine, it is seen in digitalis toxicity that can be associated with auditory hallucinations and delusions (Gorelick *et al.*, 1978), and as a side effect of atypical anti-psychotic agents (Hazra *et al.*, 2006).

71 Vertiginous migraine may occur without headache and last for days (Neuhauser *et al.*, 2001).

72 Kozubski (2005).

73 Podell and Robinson (2000).

74 Podell *et al.* (2002).

75 Romanos (2004).

76 Podell and Robinson (2001).

77 Lempert and von Brevern (2005).

78 Grosberg *et al.* (2005); *Hysterical amblyopia* is the outdated term for such visual loss.

79 Eriksen *et al.* (2004).

80 Kunkel (2005).

81 Foroozan and Buono (2003).

82 Mihalik *et al.* (2005).

83 McKendrick *et al.* (2000); other prolonged visual difficulties, from both cortical and precortical visual pathways are identified in migraineurs (McKendrick *et al.*, 2001).

84 Weber *et al.* (2005); seen in younger children with migraine or seizure disorder.

85 Winslow *et al.* (2006); associated with toxic states and subcortical brain lesions.

11

Delusions and abnormal thought content

Nevertheless, I am convinced that the only method by which we shall attain an insight into the mysterious phenomena of unsound mind, is to keep ever before us the fact that disorder of the mind means disorder of the brain, and that the latter is an organ liable to disease and disturbance, like other organs of the body, to be investigated by the same methods, and subject to the same laws. In speaking of the pathology of insanity, I have endeavored to keep this in view.[1]

The standard definition of delusion is: *A false notion inconsistent with the person's background that is held with great conviction despite clear evidence to the contrary.* The definition does not characterize the delusional process, only the end result.

Like delusions, obsessions and over-valued ideas are also false notions held with great conviction despite evidence to the contrary. They also result from faulty conclusions, but the connection between the evidence and the conclusion makes better sense. Germs can be dangerous and extraterrestrial life may exist, but a life consumed by these notions is maladaptive. What descriptively defines a delusion is the greater leap from the evidence to the idea (e.g. "my poor cell phone service means my neighbors are aiming electronic beams at my house"), or the lack of any reasonable understanding of how the conclusion was reached (e.g. "they are aiming the electronic beam because the neighbor's new dog has brown spots"). Karl Jaspers considered the lack of understandability of how the patient reached the false conclusion to be the defining factor of a delusional idea.[2]

The content of the delusional idea can be mundane (e.g. my spouse is unfaithful) or fantastic (e.g. "my spouse is an alien here to conquer the earth"). Compared to obsessions and over-valued ideas, delusional ideas are more often culturally or class deviant (e.g. the stockbroker believes a witch inhabits his computer), or overtly strange (e.g. the patient is convinced he is dead). Delusional ideas also reflect a psychopathological process that distinguishes them from obsessions and over-valued ideas.

Sources of delusional development

Like perceptual dysfunctions that may arise from disease anywhere along the sensory pathways, the pathophysiology of delusions may begin at any level of the nervous system that ultimately leads to an articulated conclusion of thought. While the neuropathology of the process is unclear, the progression to the delusional conclusion is distinguishable.

Perceptual disturbance

Delusions that arise from other psychopathology are defined as secondary delusions. The delusional process begins with the sufferer perceiving the immediate environment in such a way that the delusional conclusion is inescapable. Hollywood offers examples of this in films about the supernatural and extraterrestrials. The images on the screen are compelling, and the audience is frightened. The false images trigger a physiological flight/fight response over-riding cortical modulation of the sham. The experience is emotional, not initially cognitive as audience members are fully aware of the subterfuge.

Persons in other settings experiencing equally powerful but false perceptions of their immediate environment (i.e. hallucinations or perceptual distortions) will also be frightened. Intense and prolonged false perceptions over-ride cortical modulation and, despite the protestations of others, the experience elicits false conclusions based on "I saw it with my own eyes". The delusional process unfolds, the false perception eliciting a strong emotional response compromising judgment and self-assessment, which in turn results in a false but inescapable delusional conclusion. The false perception, however, need not be as dramatic as film images. The initiating perceptual disturbance needs to only be sufficient to trigger an emotional response strong enough to overcome judgment, accepting the false interpretation of the experience: "it's real and dangerous" rather than "I'm hallucinating". This mechanism has been proposed to explain the delusions in persons with schizophrenia.[3] Capgras, Fregoli, and delusions of misidentification (see below for definitions) can also be understood as reflecting an initial problem with perception.

The idea that subtle perceptual disturbances underlie delusional formation is supported by studies that report that delusions are not always directly linked to cognitive disturbance.[4] Patients with schizophrenia, the most common diagnostic class studied, also have subtle perceptual problems associated with delusions. Deficits in processing the Gestalt of stimuli (e.g. shape, size, identity of the object),[5] and lateralized abnormal perceptual experiences[6] in patients with schizophrenia are particularly relevant because these visual perceptual problems are similar to those seen in patients with right cerebral hemisphere disease and associated delusional symptoms.[7]

Intense emotion

If perceptual processing is intact, a secondary delusion may still develop if the person's self-monitoring ability is overwhelmed by intense and prolonged emotion, the delusional content taking on the valence of the abnormal emotional state. Delusions associated with depressive illness and manic states are examples. Delusional patients with right cerebral hemisphere disease have associated visual–perceptual disturbances and intense disturbances of emotion.[8] Strong emotional states compromise assessment of the validity of the statements of others[9] and alter memory function with recall bias toward memories with the same emotional valence.[10] The identification of emotionally salient stimuli related to persecutory beliefs is associated with amygdala and anterior insula activation for threat and adverse response.[11] The abnormal emotional state evokes abnormal memories and compromises judgment. The memory bias reinforces the abnormal emotional state. The compromised judgment confirms the validity of the abnormal memory and emotional experience, leading to the delusional idea. Delusional memories are reported to be rated as perceptually and somatosensory richer than memories of actual events.[12]

Faulty thinking and self-monitoring

If perceptual processes and emotional expression are intact, a delusion may still emerge if thinking is faulty and self-monitoring is compromised. These delusions are characterized as primary. The delusions associated with cognitive disorders are examples. Compromised thinking is commonly associated with these delusional ideas. Patients with delusions "jump to conclusions" and tend not to change the conclusions in the "face of evidence" for emotionally neutral content.[13]

Memory disturbance

Delusions also occur when perceptual processing is normal but the memory of what is being perceived is faulty or not fully accessible. The continuous mismatch is first disturbing, then frightening and, compromising judgment, leads to the delusional conclusion.

Unlike non-ill persons, delusional patients are reported to be unable to suppress non-relevant experiences. The experiences are incorporated into their thought process and become part of their memory for the experience, distorting its accuracy. They quickly attach importance to the irrelevant pieces of memory which become intrusive. For example, a person with such a memory bias sees a garbage truck in front of his neighbor's house, but his memory of previous trucks is altered, eliciting the consideration that the truck he sees is different and the difference important. He sees his neighbor talking to the truck driver and gives

Table 11.1. Differential diagnostic considerations of the different sources of delusional development

Source of disturbance	Conditions to consider
Perception	*Temporal–limbic disease* (seizure disorder, traumatic brain injury, hallucinogenic drug use, schizophrenia and schizotypal disorders) Thalamic and parietal lobe disease and related syndromes of misidentification (injury, stroke)
Emotion	*Mood disorders, temporal–limbic disease*
Self-monitoring	*Prefrontal cortex disease or dysfunction*
Thinking	*Posterior non-dominant disease or dysfunction* Prefrontal cortex disease or dysfunction
Memory	*Alzheimer's disease* *Frontal–temporal dementia*
All phases	*Alcohol-related dementias* *Delirium and encephalopathy*

further salience to the meeting. Does the conversation relate to him? Memories about plots, neighbors, and garbage trucks (often used by Hollywood as sinister images) become connected and a delusional idea forms.[14]

The above understanding of the development of a delusional idea shapes the examination and emphasizes that delusional content is not diagnostically critical. Each aspect of the delusional process is assessed as each is impacted by different diseases (Table 11.1).

Examination of the sources of a delusion

When a patient expresses ideas that may be delusional, the examiner immediately expresses concerned interest and asks "How do you know this? Tell me how you figured this out?" Some delusional patients respond "I just know" or "I feel it to be so". Others offer proof that may reveal the source leading to the false idea. These are systematically assessed.

(1) Does the patient have perceptual aberrations explaining his beliefs? Perceptual distortions and illusions are considered, as is the assessment of thalamic integration problems.

> "Do the things you see or hear seem out of sync, like a movie where the sound and picture aren't quite together? Are you experiencing any difficulty with your balance or coordination? Do you experience pins and needles in you hands and feet? Do parts of your body feel numb or overly sensitive? Do they seem different from the way they should?"

"Have you noticed anything unusual/unsettling/frightening about your neighborhood . . .
your neighbors . . . the physical appearances of your family members? Does everything
and everybody look and sound the same to you? When you look in a mirror, do you look
and sound the same as always?"

(2) Is the patient in a sustained and intense abnormal emotional state that
explains his beliefs? The examination of emotions guides this aspect of the
delusional process.
(3) Have the patient's self-monitoring and other executive functions been compromised? Queries about the patient's recognition of symptoms and illness
(i.e. does the patient exhibit denial of illness, anosagnosia), and self-assessment
of his performance on motor and cognitive tasks are considered.
(4) Does the patient have a primary problem in thinking or memory that accounts
for his false ideas? Cognitive assessment addresses this concern and is discussed
in Chapter 13.

Forms of delusions

Delusions that derive from an abnormal emotional state or that are based on
perceptual aberrations are characterized as *secondary delusions*. Delusions
emerging de novo from arbitrary conclusions or that are suddenly fully formed
are characterized as "primary". Primary delusions were thought associated with
schizophrenia while secondary delusions were considered associated with manic-
depression. The DSM employs this old viewpoint by defining schizophrenia with
"bizarre" delusions that are primary in their form. Both primary and secondary
delusions, however, occur in many of the same conditions.

Present classification also defines delusions by their content. However, because
both primary and secondary delusions derive from faulty thinking and inadequate self-assessment, differing content is of less diagnostic significance than the
fact that the patient is delusional. Nevertheless, delusions of illness (hypochondriacal delusions), poverty, sin, and nihilism (termed *Cotard syndrome*) are
associated with melancholia.[15] Delusions of grandeur, great wealth, power, status
or ability suggest mania.[16] Delusional jealousy (*Othello syndrome*) is seen in
dementing conditions and seizure disorder.[17] Delusions of familiar persons being
impostors (*Capgras syndrome*) or that one has a double (*Doppelgänger*) suggest a
definable neurologic process. Delusions that unfamiliar persons are celebrities or
persons from the patient's life (*Fregoli syndrome*) also suggest a definable neurologic process.[18] Patient 1.4, the woman with a right-sided stroke, believed her
daughter looked and acted differently and was an alien. She had Capgras syndrome.[19] A man with vascular dementia and depressive illness with Capgras

syndrome thought his wife was a dangerous imposter, because he perceived that she no longer had a southern USA accent. A woman with end-stage renal disease thought one of her nurses was the housekeeper on the old *Brady Bunch* TV show. A manic-depressive man thought a fellow patient was Charlton Heston, the actor, and that another patient, a man, was Marilyn Monroe. Delusions of infestation by micro-organisms, hair, insects, dust or parasites (*Ekbom's syndrome*) is typically associated with tactile and visual hallucinations and identifiable neurologic disease.

But *delusions of persecution* are the most common and are as frequent in mood disorders as in schizophrenia.[20] Patients with degenerative brain disease also exhibit persecutory delusions.[21] *Paranoid* delusions reflect persecutory content. The content involves government plots, spouse or neighbor cabals, being spied upon by various nefarious agencies, infidelities, and imminent attack by unknown forces.

Delusional mood

Delusional mood, or *delusional atmosphere*, is a state of unease during which the immediate environment feels strange, threatening or ominously changed. The sufferer is apprehensive, puzzled and at times bewildered, but "senses" that "something odd is going on". Delusional moods emerge in the early phase of a psychotic episode and may persist for weeks before fully formed delusions evolve.

Idea of reference

Ideas of reference often emerge from a delusional mood. Ideas of reference are typically based on biased perceptions that encourage a morbid self-reference. A passer-by's cough, an ad in the newspaper, a cloud in the sky are perceived as being odd and then thought to have specific meaning for the patient. The actions of others are understood as directed at the patient. They are being watched or talked about; a public event assumes personal ominous significance. Ideas of reference are common and occur in many different psychotic disorders.

Autochthonous idea and primordial delusion

A suddenly experienced, fully formed idea immediately accepted as true and important, despite being unlikely or impossible, is labeled autochthonous.[22] *Primordial delusion* is a synonymous term.[23]

The American neuropsychiatrist, William Hammond, describes a man who while eating breakfast, suddenly realized that his wife had "endeavored to render him impotent, in order that a condition of forced faithfulness might be induced". As he walked the streets, the man experienced ideas of reference about passers-by and their awareness of his situation. He developed the delusion that his testicles had disappeared and that he had been castrated by the Pope, so that he would be put into the choir at St Peter's Basilica.[24]

Delusional perception

Delusional perception is one of Kurt Schneider's first rank symptoms. It is a delusion derived from a presumed accurate perception that is then given personal significance, without an understandable connection between the delusional idea and the perception. For example, a patient sees two new flower pots on a neighbor's window sill and concludes that he will be killed in his sleep that night. Recent multivariate studies of delusions separate Schneider's passivity delusions (control, thought withdrawal, and insertion) from other forms and links then to a poor long-term prognosis.[25]

Some primary delusions differ from delusional perceptions in that the evidence the patient offers to account for the delusional idea is understandable. For example, the patient concludes that he will be killed in his sleep because he has noticed the same new automobile parked on his street for the past several days, then he sees a man on the street who looked like a person who shouted at him on the highway, and then he hears noises in the house suggestive of persons sneaking about.

Dereistic thinking is thinking based on "feelings" rather than logic.[26] It is the thinking that permits myths or folktales to be accepted, e.g. the idea that the mammalian Easter Bunny lays colored eggs. It underlies delusional perceptions, such as the patient seeing an empty coffee cup on the conference room table as the "proof" that the plot to kill him continues. He "knows" it without understanding how he knows.

Passivity delusions

Experience of control and alienation are defined as passivity delusions because the sufferer feels helpless during the experience, either being controlled by an outside force or inhabited by another person's thoughts.

Experience of control entails some outside force or agency experienced as controlling the sufferer's emotions, thinking or movements, forcing compliance. One patient was forced to say and do things by "people watching" him through the walls of the hospital as if they were "one-way" mirrors. Another insisted a teacher was giving her hidden signals forcing her to assume certain postures. Patients rarely can describe the consequences of resisting.

Experience of alienation is the experience that someone else's thoughts are in one's mind, or that a body part is not one's own but belongs to another person or animal, or is made of other than human tissue. One patient insisted others could erase his mind (thought withdrawal) and then fill his head with their thoughts.

Table 11.2. Misidentification delusions

Phenomena	Description
Capgras	A relative, spouse or familiar person is believed replaced by a similar-looking impostor (most common form)
Reverse Capgras	The patient believes others think he is an imposter (rare)
Fregoli	Unfamiliar persons are thought to be well-known to the patient
Reverse Fregoli	The patient believes that he looks like a famous person
Intermetamorphosis	Familiar persons are believed to be swapping identities while maintaining the same appearance
Doppelgänger/subjective doubles	The belief that one has a double who carries out independent actions
Mirrored self-misidentification	The belief that one's reflection is of another person
Reduplicative paramnesia	A familiar person, place, object or body part is believed duplicated (e.g. the patient thinks his real home has been moved and that he is living in an identical-looking home; a paralyzed arm has a duplicate attached nearby that is fully functional)
Delusional companions	Inanimate objects are believed to be living companions (when transient this is normal in childhood; always abnormal in an adult)
Clonal pluralization of self	The belief that there are multiple versions of oneself

He was also compelled to act on the thoughts. Sufferers typically have secondary delusions that elaborates their passivity experiences, such as being poisoned, exposed to radiation or some electronic device, being hypnotized or possessed.

Misidentification delusions

Several misidentification syndromes are described (Table 11.2).[27] Capgras, Fregoli and reduplicative paramnesia are the most common and best studied.

Capgras syndrome

First described in 1923, more than 50% of patients with this delusion have identifiable neurologic disease.[28] Vascular lesions from stroke and micro-vascular disease, traumatic brain injury, and degenerative brain disease are frequent causes. Several different lesion locations are reported, most commonly right sided and cortical.[29] Non-specific EEG changes and visual–spatial and visual–memory deficits are also described.

Capgras delusions may arise because of selective deficits of faces, processing opposite of what is seen in *prosopagnosia*. In *prosopagnosia*, patients are unable to identify the face but show some emotional responses to familiar faces. In Capgras syndrome, the patient recognizes the face, but the emotional information identifying the face is unavailable and the patient is unable to connect the face to the identity, eliciting the belief that the person is not familiar.[30] The following vignette illustrates.

Patient 11.1

After a traumatic brain injury to the right parietal area, a 30-year-old man claimed that his parents were imposters when he was looking at them, but not when speaking to them on the telephone. Unlike non-ill persons, the patient's skin conductance responses to photographs of familiar people, including his parents, were not greater than his responses to photographs of unfamiliar people. The patient also had difficulty judging gaze direction. When presented with a sequence of photographs of the same model's face looking in different directions, the patient asserted that they were "different women who looked just like each other".[31]

Fregoli syndrome

First described in 1927 by Courbon and Fail and named after a famous Italian impersonator and mimic Leopoldo Fregoli,[32] this delusion is characterized by the notion that familiar persons are disguised as famous people, or that an ordinary stranger is in fact a famous person. A variant is the delusion of having "a double" or Doppelganger.[33] The Greek neurologist, Christodoulou offers the following examples:

A man claimed that his aunt was his mother (who had died when the patient was 11 years old).

A man claimed that an aunt whom he strongly disliked had been transformed into his mother in order to harm him.

A woman believed her lover acquired the physical characteristics of various persons she knew, including her father.

A man believed that a neighbor's daughter was in fact a Greek girl with whom he was secretly in love, and that his dead brother was not dead but appeared in various "reincarnations", his brother "hiding inside other persons but detectable".

A man believed his teacher could transform himself into various known persons.

A man believed a colleague had acquired the appearance of his brother in order to harm him.

Each patient's Fregoli syndrome was associated with a contributing neurologic disease,[34] particularly right-sided.[35] Christodoulou, reviewing all published case reports, also found an association between misidentification delusions and features of seizure disorder (e.g. depersonalization and derealization, and abnormal EEG).[36]

Cotard syndrome

Nihilistic delusions are beliefs of "being dead" or having "no brain, nerves, chest or entrails, and" being "just skin and bone". Identified in the late nineteenth century,[37] it is reported among manic-depressive patients[38] and in patients after brain injury.[39] An analysis of 100 published cases found 89% of the patients to be depressed, the others suffering from various brain disorders.[40] Delusions of nihilism are also reported in persons with migraine and brain neoplasms.[41] The most common nihilistic delusion concerned the body (86%), existence (69%), and immortality (55%). Co-occurring anxiety, guilt, and hypochondriacal delusions were frequent. The appearance of delusions of negation even in the presence of a mood disorder syndrome does not preclude the possibility that the condition is the result of structural brain disease.

Delusional disorder (monomania)

An older term for delusional disorder is *monomania*. Etienne Esquirol, a leading French psychiatrist of the early nineteenth century, delineated the condition and described erotomania or *Clerambault's syndrome*, the delusion that one's love for another person is reciprocated.[42] Hammond offered the definition: *A perversion of the intellect characterized by the existence of delusions limited to a single subject or to a small class of subjects.*[43] Monomania, like delusional disorder, was understood as emerging in the third decade of life or later, and was neither a mood disorder nor hebephrenia. Prognosis was intermediate, but the illness was considered chronic.[44]

Although delusional disorder is presently classified as an independent psychotic condition, its range of psychopathology suggests substantial heterogeneity. Old classifications considered two forms: those that involved delusions focused on a single subject or class (present-day delusional disorder), and those that were expressed in a single intense and prolonged emotional state of either depression or exaltation (now conflated into mood disorders). Hammond referred to them as *intellectual insanities.*[45]

Delusional disorder almost always begins with a prodrome in which "evidence" mounts. One patient with erotomania, for example, erroneously thought he saw the same woman over several weeks in several different places: at work, at a hospital, and in the street near his apartment house. These and related experiences eventually coalesced into the delusion that the woman at work was in love with him and that their families were secretly arranging a marriage for them.

Erotomania, erotic delusions and delusions of jealousy

About 20–25% of patients with erotomania have associated general medical (e.g. HIV, hypertension, alcoholism) or neurologic disorder (e.g. hemorrhage, seizure disorder, and traumatic brain injury). Also reported are schizophrenia (35%), mood disorders (22.5%) and other psychiatric disorders (10%).[46] While right-sided temporal or parietal lobe lesions are the most common sites reported, left temporal lobe lesions are also associated with erotomania.[47]

Delusions of jealousy are associated with cognitive executive function difficulties.[48] The frequency of these delusions in patients with schizophrenia and mood disorder is less than 3% and 0.1%, respectively.

Delusional disorder with grandiose delusions

This combination of features was defined as *monomania with exaltation*. General paresis was the common cause in the nineteenth century, the delusion of being Napoleon the stereotype. It remains an indicator of frontal lobe circuitry disease. Other features of frontal lobe dysfunction will be present if identifiable pathophysiology is present (see Patient 11.2). Unlike the typical manic episode that blossoms within a few days or weeks, delusional disorder with grandiose delusions develops gradually with circumscribed ideas of self-importance, superior accomplishments, bodily perfections, and the attention of others becoming more pronounced and then coalescing into a single delusional conclusion. Despite the grandiose delusion, the sufferer initially continues his usual activities and may go unnoticed by the casual observer. Theatrical speech or manner may occur. Hallucinations and illusions are experienced, but do not dominate the picture.[49] Initial good humor, jocularity, and exaltation are characteristic, but as the illness progresses the sufferer becomes more intense in his actions, persistent in his demands and irritable if frustrated. These behaviors alert the authorities and may force hospitalization.

Patient 11.2

A man in his twenties became convinced that he was someone special. He concluded that his parents must have adopted him and that he was related to a famous family whose name sounded similar to his. He claimed that he owned their large corporation. At first elated, he became irritable when the corporate managers refused to acknowledge him. He stalked the family and was arrested, and then hospitalized.

Other than his delusional conviction and Witzelsucht he showed no psychopathology. Cognitive assessment suggested an executive function decline. Brain imaging identified normal pressure hydrocephalus, which was relieved by surgical shunting. The delusional syndrome resolved. The patient, however, was a periodic marijuana user and periods of heavy use were followed by a return of his symptoms.

The older literature also recognized *monomania with depression*. At present, such conditions are considered as schizoaffective disorder, delusional disorder with depressive content, or psychotic depression. The disorder was characterized by a fixed delusion with melancholic-like content that influenced the sufferer's actions (e.g. apprehension of impending catastrophe eliciting the patient to take evasive actions when in public to avoid being followed, or barricading himself in his home). The actions were described as circumscribed and other functions initially were undisturbed. Sufferers were not incapacitated. As the condition progressed, ideas of reference emerged. Hallucinations and illusions occurred but were not prominent. Delusions of persecution also developed. Patient 11.3 illustrates the diagnostic ambiguity of this syndrome.

Patient 11.3

A 40-year-old woman was hospitalized because of her family's concerns. For much of the past year she had been convinced that her husband was unfaithful and was trying to poison her. She saw evidence in unfamiliar automobiles driving past her home, strange odors emanating from the furniture, and her possessions being "replaced" by similar but "different" ones. Despite these ideas, she continued to adequately perform her family and household responsibilities. When she expressed thoughts of suicide her family brought her to the hospital.

The patient was neither manic nor depressed. Her emotional expression was restricted, but she became irritable if her convictions were challenged. She had no movement disorder. Her speech and language were normal. She had no discernable cognitive impairment. Her general medical health was good and her neurologic assessment normal. Twenty years earlier she had suffered a postpartum psychotic depression that was incapacitating and which lasted the better part of a year, resolving gradually without treatment.

Bilateral ECT was prescribed for the index condition and after 12 treatments the delusional syndrome fully resolved. Maintenance ECT kept her well for the next six months, after which she was lost to follow-up.

Patient 11.3 illustrates the advantage of applying *Sutton's law* and the *Rule of Parsimony* to the diagnostic process when the *duck principle* fails (see Chapter 5). The patient's index presentation was ambiguous (failed duck principle), but the postpartum depression 20 years earlier suggested that the present episode reflected the same pathophysiology (the rule of parsimony). Psychotic depression is also much more common than delusional disorder (Sutton's law).

Paranoia

In its original usage, the term *paranoid* included delusions of grandeur. Kahlbaum introduced it in 1863 to replace the older term *Verrucktheit*. Paranoia referred to an "insanity essentially affecting intellectual activity".

Paranoia and delusions of persecution are synonymous in modern usage. In lay terms it has also come to mean suspiciousness or prone to seeing conspiracies in everyday human affairs. Originally, paranoia referred to a disorder of intellect leading to a fixed false belief, the patient normal in other respects. There were no associated "negative" symptoms or hallucinations, and personality was spared. Kraepelin conflated the syndrome into his dementia praecox construct, but many writers continued to recognize a circumscribed delusional disorder tending to occur in early mid-life without deterioration in other behavioral domains. This view is reflected in the terms: paranoid reaction and paranoid personality (DSM-I), paranoid states and involutional paranoid state or paraphrenia (DSM-II), paranoid disorders, folie à deux (DSM-III) and delusional disorder (DSM-IV).[50]

Paraphrenia

The paraphrenias are syndromes no longer recognized in classification and are subsumed in the delusional disorders category. Their presence suggests definable neurologic disease. If they differ from delusional disorder, it is only in their less structured delusional story. Paraphrenias are of acute onset, occur in late adult life, and are typically associated with intense emotional expression. Prognosis relative to schizophrenia is good, and sufferers continue their daily activities and employment as long as the intensity of the symptoms remains low.

Paraphrenias were classified by the predominating psychopathology (*affect-laden* with rapid intense mood swings, *hypochondriacal* with delusions of organ disease, *incoherent* with a delirious picture, *expansive* with grandiose delusions, and *fantastic* with confabulatory delusions of experiences outside physical possibility). The validity of these designations has not been adequately studied, and they likely represent several different illnesses.[51]

Two forms, however, are usefully separated from delusional disorder. *Phonemic paraphrenia* with continuous voices that gradually wax and wane is discussed in Chapter 10.[52] *Late paraphrenia* ("paranoid states of the elderly") is a delusional syndrome occurring after age 60. Deafness, visual impairment and general medical disability are common co-occurring conditions. It is often a harbinger of dementia. It is also seen in older men, previously abusers of alcohol, who become increasingly suspicious and irritable, accusing wives of infidelity, family members of stealing, and neighbors and local government of various infringements.[53]

Delusional memories

Paramnesia

Paramnesia is false memories derived from illusions in association with intense emotion. Past events become distorted by the present emotional state or associated delusions. When the patient is convinced of the validity of the clearly false memories, the term is *retrospective falsification* or *delusional memory*. The schizophrenic "remembers" the implanting of the transmitter in his brain. The melancholic "remembers" past sins. The manic "remembers" being an infant in a palace or great estate. Pseudo-memories can be described in great detail.

Reduplicative paramnesia is the belief that present surroundings are false and represent a duplication of the real place. It is also a misidentification syndrome. Patient 1.4 believed her neighborhood was not real but a duplication fabricated by aliens.

State-dependent memory is the recall of events or learned material only when the person is in the same drug or medication-induced state under which the event was experienced or the material learned. Patients with psychosis or severe mood disorder experience this phenomenon and, when well, will not recall dramatic experiences that occurred when ill. When ill again, the memories are again accessible and recalled.[54] Patient 11.4, when depressed or euthymic, could not recall events that occurred during manic periods.

Patient 11.4

During morning rounds, a 44-year-old manic man was examined. Every day after the initial examination, the patient sought out, greeted the examiner, and chatted with him for several minutes. After some months out of the hospital, the same patient was re-admitted for an episode of depression. Seeing the examiner, he made no effort to engage in conversation and did not remember their meeting. Later that year, the patient was again re-admitted, this time in a manic episode. As soon as the examiner entered the unit, the patient rushed to greet him, saying he was the doctor that "knew what was going on".

Retrospective falsification

Pseudo-memories are delusional falsifications of memory in which memory engrams are distorted by illness and are offered by the patient as "proof" for his present beliefs. One patient vividly described a childhood trip to the dentist, during which a transmitter was placed in his skull that now was the conduit for his "voices" and the efforts to control his thoughts. Another described in detail the inside of a flying saucer that he had invented many years before. Once the patient recovers, the memory distortions also resolve.

Memory hallucinations

Chronically ill patients may recall hallucinatory experiences as if they were real events. Bleuler used the term *retroactive*.[55] Patients describe nightly rapes in their hospital room, persons yelling at them from outside their homes, and FBI agents ransacking their apartment.

Déjà vu, jamais vu, and similar phenomena

These phenomena reflect an error in matching what is being experienced with recollections. Each is a false memory. *Déjà vu* is the experience of false familiarity: "I have been here before" or "I have seen this before". Many non-ill persons have fleeting and vague déjà vu experiences. Frequent, intrusive, and intense experiences of false familiarity reflect illness. *Jamais vu* is the experience of false unfamiliarity: "I have never done this" or "I have never been here before". It is not commonly reported in non-ill persons. *Déjà vécu* is the feeling that a novel experiencing has been experienced before. *Déjà entendu* is the experience of hearing familiar sounds and voices as novel. These phenomena, when chronic and persistent, are associated with limbic system disease or seizure disorder, use of hallucinogenic agents, and in manic-depressive illness. When jamais vu is frequently experienced, it is a harbinger of dementia.[56]

Confabulation and fantastic confabulation

In most instances, confabulation is an attempt to cover memory gaps. The false information is mundane. The patient who confabulates is influenced by suggestions of what transpired earlier in the day or the night before. Although classically associated with Korsakoff's syndrome, confabulation need not be present in that dementia. It also occurs in other amnestic states, and its presence may be influenced by personality traits.[57]

Fantastic confabulation is a sign of substantial frontal lobe disease. Such patients animatedly engage in the telling of clearly false tales that can go beyond nature's rules. Patients relate their experiences in outer space, flying like a bird, and inside machinery that fills the center of the earth or surrounds it. These fantastic confabulations are often intermingled with other false grandiose memories of great accomplishment.[58]

Pseudologia fantastica

Like fantastic confabulation, these are clearly false statements. *Vorbeireden* and talking-past-the-point are other terms. The phenomenon was initially considered a sign of hysteria and the *Ganser syndrome*, but it is mostly associated with catatonia.[59] Such patients believe the false statements, despite their obvious silliness. For example, to the question, "What color was George Washington's white horse?" the patient with Ganser's syndrome might immediately and with conviction respond "Brown".

Folie à deux (folie communiquée, folie imposée, folie induite, shared delusional disorder)

The French neurologists Ernest-Charles Lasegue and Jean Pierre Falret in 1877 first described a phenomenon of "psychological contagion" as mutually induced false ideas formed by two or more people.[60] William Hammond refers to the phenomenon as *La folie simultanée*, restricted to two or more members of the same family becoming ill at the same time, and not a psychological phenomenon.[61] Case literature finds males and females equally affected, with the duos comprised of married couples, siblings (often monozygotic twins), and mother–child dyads. Common co-conditions are dementia, depressive illness and mental retardation.[62] Although the occurrence is commonly in isolated dyads with one member said to be dominant and the other submissive and suggestible, the conditions reported as folie à deux typically have substantial heritability. Assortative mating in couples with mental illness is also well documented, and these factors may account for co-delusions.[63] In one report both parties to a Doppelganger delusion had evidence of cerebral dysfunction.[64]

Over-valued ideas

Over-valued ideas are beliefs that are plausible, may contain a "kernel of truth", and may be accepted by others. The ideas, however, intrude into the foreground of thought at the expense of other considerations. The sufferer pursues the idea despite the quest leading to interpersonal and financial difficulties, and does not perceive the idea as unusual (conceded by some delusional patients), or as incorrect (understood by obsessional patients). Once established, over-valued ideas persist indefinitely.

The source of over-valued ideas was classically considered a remembrance of an emotional experience, but there is no evidence for this interpretation. Patients with over-valued ideas, however, have strong emotions about them. Eugen Bleuler considered them to be exaggerations of personality traits that could become delusional. In such instances, *monomania* was diagnosed.[65]

Obsessions (or compulsive notions) and ruminations[66]

Obsessions are ideas which continually intrude into the patient's thinking with or without external stimulation. The content is often recognized by the patient as incorrect, except in states of intense emotion. The thoughts are perceived as self-generated, not imposed by an external source. While obsessions occur primarily in obsessive–compulsive spectrum conditions, they are also observed in patients with melancholia, mania, and to a lesser extent in schizophrenia.

Ruminations are similar to obsessions. They are repeatedly experienced and are felt to be less intrusive. The sufferer occasionally recognizes the content as false or exaggerated. Ruminations are linked to abnormal emotion, the valence typically reflected in the content of the thoughts. Persistent ruminations are typical of melancholia.

Non-delusional abnormal thought content

Suicidal thoughts

Recurrent suicidal ideas indicate psychopathology. The most common cause of suicidal thought is mood disorder, and 50–70% of persons who kill themselves are depressed at the time of suicide. Melancholic patients are most likely to kill themselves.[67] Suicidal thoughts are also expressed by persons with personality and substance abuse disorders. Sixty-four percent of persons said to have borderline personality disorder attempt suicide at least once.[68] Transient suicidal thoughts are seen in states of intoxication and are also expressed by patients with severe general medical illness associated with chronic dysfunction or pain. Suicidal thoughts are associated with sadness, despondency, overwhelming apprehension, or anger toward another person. While many studies delineate the risk factors and circumstances of suicide attempts and completed suicides, similar attention is not given to suicidal thoughts.

Reported prevalence rates for suicidal thoughts vary across studies and geographic region. In Asian countries, lifetime suicidal thought is reported in 6–8% of the population. In one Norwegian study, the prevalence was found to be 40%. Suicide is the third leading cause of death among adolescents in the USA. In one study, almost one in five adolescents reported serious consideration of suicide in the prior year.[69] Some suicidal behavior is shaped by cultural pressures.[70]

Not everyone who experiences a suicidal thought attempts suicide, but the presence of suicidal thoughts increases the risk of suicide. A thorough behavioral evaluation always includes suicide risk assessment, and patients are asked directly about self-destructive thoughts and actions. Chapter 5 details the examination for suicide risk.

Homicidal thoughts

Homicide and aggressive behavior is better studied than are isolated homicidal thoughts. The lifetime population prevalence of homicidal thought is unknown, but homicidal ideas do not always translate into murder. Persons engaged in repeated illicit drug use, or who are alcoholics, psychotic, have a traumatic brain injury, or antisocial personality disorder are most likely to harm others. Assessment of risk of violence is presented in Chapter 5.

Culturally deviant ideas

Some thoughts and behaviors that appear deviant in the abstract are not considered psychopathology when they are culturally consistent. *Harakiri* and *Kamikaze* were suicidal behaviors acceptable in World War II Japan and are still admired in some segments of Japanese culture. During the Viet Nam War, Buddhist monks immolated themselves to protest the policies of the American-backed South Vietnamese government. Suicide killing in support of Islam is accepted among some Islamists. In ancient India, some women committed suicide or *Sati* following their husband's death. In Africa, genital mutilation of young women is still practiced. In the USA on any football day, the stands are filled with colorfully body-painted and be-wigged screaming young men half naked even in the worst weather. These behaviors are understood as unusual, but not as illness by the respective cultures.

In the psychiatric evaluation, deviant culturally related behavior is elicited during the focus on family relations, hobbies and interests, typical daily activities, and social and interpersonal relationships. Whether the behavior represents illness is based on the form of the ideas or emotions that elicit the behavior.

Summary

Delusions are associated with many psychiatric, general medical and neurologic disorders. No form is pathognomonic and most often the delusion is a sign of severity, not specific pathophysiology. Isolated delusions occurring without associated psychopathology, however, are most often found within a general medical or definable neurologic illness. Isolated simple persecutory delusions (e.g. "the nurse is trying to kill me") are associated with degenerative brain disease. Isolated elaborate persecutory delusional stories are associated with encephalopathy and temporal lobe involvement.[71]

Certain delusional content suggests diagnosis[72] and involvement of specific brain areas.[73] Delusions of jealousy are rare in schizophrenia and are frequent in alcoholics. Alcohol-induced psychosis is a likely diagnosis in a middle-aged psychotic patient with delusional jealousy and full affect. Delusions of passivity are more frequent in schizophrenia than in mood disorder, while nihilistic delusions occur more frequently in manic-depression. Misidentification delusions point toward right cerebral hemisphere disease.

NOTES

1 From the preface to the first edition (cited in the 1886 third edition) of G. Fielding
  Blandford's monograph of his lectures on insanity which he gave at the medical school at
  St George's Hospital, London.
2 Jaspers (1963), pages 103–7.
3 Uhlhass and Mishara (2007).
4 Langdon and Coltheart (2000).
5 Goodarzi *et al.* (2000).
6 Persaud and Cutting (1991).
7 Persaud and Cutting (1991); Vaina *et al.* (2002).
8 Vaina *et al.* (2002).
9 Rossell *et al.* (1998).
10 Hamann *et al.* (1999).
11 Calder *et al.* (2001).
12 Freeman and Garety (2003).
13 Garety and Hemsley (1994); Garety and Freeman (1999).
14 Nathaniel-James and Frith (1996).
15 Taylor and Fink (2006); Cotard syndrome is also seen in lesions of the non-dominant
   parietal lobe and adjacent thalamic structures (Critchley, 1953; Gardner-Thorpe and Pern,
   2004). Jules Cotard, a Parisian neurologist, first described *délire des negations*, the unshak-
   able belief that one's body or body parts are lost or that one is dead (Pearn and Gardner-
   Thorpe, 2002).
16 Taylor and Abrams (1973), Abrams and Taylor (1981).
17 In Shakespeare's play, Othello has a seizure disorder; also see Richardson *et al.* (1991) and
   Malloy and Richardson (1994).
18 Butler (2000).
19 Poor facial recognition, or *prosopagnosia*, is considered to account for many cases of
   Capgras syndrome (Ellis *et al.*, 1997).
20 Gutierrez-Lobos *et al.* (2001); Suhail K (2003).
21 Cummings (1985b); Gutierrez-Lobos *et al.* (2001); Cook *et al.* (2003).
22 The concept of an autochthonous delusion was first formulated by Wernicke (1906).
23 Bleuler (1976), page 91.
24 Hammond (1883/1973), page 341; similar to Koru that is considered a culture-bound
   phenomenon but which illustrates that brain disease is a human condition not a cultural
   trapping.
25 Kimhy *et al.* (2005).
26 Bleuler (1976), pages 45–6.
27 Cutting (1991).
28 Capgras and Reboul-Lachaux (1923).
29 Forstl *et al.* (1991); Malloy and Richardson (1994); Bourget and Whitehurst (2004).
30 Ellis *et al.* (1997); Halligan and Davis (2001).

31 Hirstein and Ramchandran (1997).

32 Courbon and Fail (1927).

33 de Pauw *et al.* (1987).

34 Christodoulou (1976).

35 Edelstyn and Oyebode (1999).

36 Christodoulou (1991).

37 Pearn and Gardner-Thorpe (2002).

38 Fink and Taylor (2003), chapter 2.

39 Young *et al.* (1994).

40 Berrios and Luque (1995).

41 Gardner-Thorpe and Pearn (2004).

42 Shorter (2005), page 99.

43 Hammond (1883/1973), page 328.

44 During most of the last quarter of the nineteenth century, no classification identified dementia praecox. Hebephrenia was the psychosis of youth. Monomania was always separated from hebephrenia.

45 Hammond (1883/1973), page 328.

46 el Gaddal (1989); Anderson *et al.* (1998); Kelly (2005).

47 Wijeratne *et al.* (1997); Kelly (2005).

48 Soyka *et al.* (1991).

49 Despite little supporting evidence, for the diagnosis of delusional disorder, the DSM-IV requires that the content of the hallucination be similar to the content of the delusion. Thus, if a person who believes she is being poisoned also has hallucinations, they should be consistent with poison, e.g. smelling the odor of the poison or hear voices discussing the poisoning.

50 Shorter (2005), pages 206–11.

51 Fish (1962), pages 69–76; Holden (1987).

52 Holden (1987).

53 Howard *et al.* (1994).

54 Quraishi and Frangou (2002).

55 Bleuler (1976), page 65.

56 Fischer *et al.* (1995); Joseph (1999).

57 Gundogar and Demicrci (2006).

58 Kopelman (1996).

59 Also see Fink and Taylor (2003).

60 Lasegue and Falret (1877).

61 Hammond (1883/1973), page 515. One of us (MAT) has on three occasions had two members of the same nuclear family admitted to a psychiatric inpatient unit within days of each other. In one instance, a mother and daughter with different last names had not spoken to each other for several years.

62 Silveira and Seeman (1995); Kashiwase and Kato (1997); Patel *et al.* (2004).

63 Reif and Pfuhlmann (2004).

64 Christodoulou *et al.* (1995).

65 Bleuler (1976), page 87.

66 Chapter 12 provides a detailed discussion of obsessive–compulsive behavior.

67 Taylor and Fink (2006), chapter 7.

68 Soloff *et al.* (1994).

69 Kennedy *et al.* (2004).

70 *Sati* is an act of ritual suicide reported on the Indian subcontinent, especially among Hindus, for several centuries. Although legally banned, these acts still occur in modern India. There is little evidence to suggest, however, that women who commit *Sati* suffer from a recognized psychiatric illness. Cultural factors and gender role expectations play a significant role in the act and its consequences (Bhugra, 2005).

71 Cummings (1985a,b).

72 Soyka *et al.* (1991).

73 Rao and Lyketsos (1998).

12

Obsessive–compulsive behaviors

It is not our business, it is not in our power, to explain psychologically the origin and nature of any of [the] depraved instincts [manifested in typical cases of insanity] ... it is sufficient to establish their existence as facts of observation, and to set forth the pathological conditions under which they are produced; they are facts of pathology, which should be observed and classified like other phenomena of disease ... The explanation, when it comes, will come not from the mental, but from the physical side – from the study of the neuroses, not from the analysis of the psychosis.[1]

Obsessions are unrealistic, often odd ideas that derive from arbitrary conclusions. When the obsessive ideas are particularly odd (e.g. "I feel like debris in the street might be alive and I collect them just to be on the safe side"), they can be mistaken for delusions and the distinction may become clear only in the context of other psychopathology (e.g. the patient is also hallucinating or expresses other clearly delusional ideas, or is an excessive hand-washer with many rituals). When obsessions involve overwhelming concerns about health or contamination, they can be confused with depressive ruminations. Obsessions can also be viewed as subtle forms of procedural memory gone awry, as ideas of potential danger and other content (e.g. compulsive swearing or coprolalia) spontaneously emerge into awareness. Compulsions are more obvious abnormalities in motor regulation, but persons with OCD also exhibit tics, echolalia, grimacing, and many repetitive movements. Obsessive–compulsive disorder (OCD) and related conditions are therefore expressions of motor (speech and other actions), thinking, memory, and cognitive dysregulation. This multi-domain association is reflected in the examination for OCD and related conditions which can begin when the evaluation is focused on motor, emotion, thinking or thought content. As no one domain lays claim to OCD, we place it in a separate chapter.

The OCD spectrum[2]

The OCD spectrum concept illustrates one of the problems with present psychiatric classification. While most researchers and specialists recognize the association between the classic OCD syndrome and its variants, the DSM and ICD place OCD in the anxiety disorders category and the recognized OCD variants in other categories.

The decision to place OCD in the anxiety disorders category was based primarily on the idea that obsessions lead to anxiety and associated avoidance behaviors (phobic-like), while compulsions reduce anxiety.[3] Anxiety, however, is a non-specific phenomenon and most conditions listed in the DSM Axis I and the ICD equivalent could be classified as an anxiety disorder by the criterion of the presence of substantial anxiety. The recognized OCD variants were placed into different categories based on a narrow focus on one aspect of the condition (e.g. tics), or on the predominant content of the condition (e.g. hair pulling, not eating), and not on the form of symptoms: *uncontrollable repetitive thoughts and actions.*

The phenomenology, demographics, neurobiology, and treatment evidence that define OCD, however, characterize it as a separate class from the other conditions in the anxiety disorder category. The data show that the classic OCD syndrome has substantial similarity to tic disorder, body dysmorphic disorders, and most of the present impulse control disorders, such as trichotillomania.[4] Anorexia nervosa and some of the paraphilias are also best classified in the OCD category. Pathological gambling, now in the impulse control class, appears to represent a heterogeneous category, but some of these persons also have OCD features warranting placement in the OCD class.[5] Kleptomania and pathological gambling appear to be co-occurring. Non-melancholic depression is also reported in patients with OCD and its spectrum, but is not part of the OCD pathophysiology.[6]

The OCD spectrum is seen as several descriptive clusters.[7] A *somatic* grouping includes body image, body concerns and weight disorders, hypochondriasis, body dysmorphic disorder, anorexia nervosa, and binge eating.[8] An *impulse* grouping includes pathological gambling, some paraphilias, trichotillomania, kleptomania, and some forms of self-injury.[9] A *repetitive movement* grouping includes Gilles de La Tourette's syndrome and Syndenham's chorea.[10] Table 12.1 displays the OCD spectrum conditions. Support for the spectrum is detailed in Chapter 16.

Increasing numbers of conditions are proposed for the OCD spectrum. Some of these have substantial validation (see below), others assumed to be co-morbid with OCD are unlikely to share the same pathophysiology. Mood disorder is an example.

Patients with depressive illness often ruminate and have repetitive, sometimes stereotypic behavior. These behaviors, however, are understood to result from the influence of the intense mood state on frontal circuitry regulation of motor and cognition function. The repetitive behaviors resolve with the successful treatment of the depression.[11]

Table 12.1. Obsessive–compulsive spectrum

The classic syndrome: overwhelming hand washing, checking, ordering, praying, counting, silently repeating words, ritualizing, and repeating actions

Impulse control disorders: hoarding, trichotillomania, kleptomania, pyromania, pathological gambling, self-injury and self-mutilation (some patients, and including skin picking and nail biting), hypersexuality

Gilles de La Tourette's syndrome

Pediatric autoimmune neuropsychiatric disorder associated with Streptococcus infection (PANDAS)

Anorexia nervosa

Body dysmorphic disorder (and compulsive grooming)

Hypochondriasis

Paraphilia: exhibitionism, fetishism, transvestic fetishism, frotteurism, voyeurism, compulsive masturbation, bestiality

Chronic posttraumatic stress disorder (some patients)

Manic-depression has also been linked to classic OCD[12] based on problematic data such as those collected by the National Institute of Mental Health (NIMH) ambitious Epidemiologic Catchment Area Study.[13] Using a psychopathologically simplistic structured interview administered by inexperienced examiners, the rates of illness obtained in this study and the degree of reported co-morbidity would lead to the conclusion that half the population of the USA was psychiatrically ill during their lifetime, and many also suffer from several conditions simultaneously.[14]

The classic OCD syndrome

Obsessions are recurrent, intrusive, and intense unwanted thoughts or impulses that are irresistible. They are experienced as unpleasant, autonomous from the sufferer, and senseless even if they have "a grain of truth" (washing hands to rid them of germs). In contrast, delusions and over-valued ideas are experienced as making sense. Compulsions are repetitive, ritualistic actions, often but not always driven by obsessive thoughts. Compulsions are also experienced as autonomous, as if the actions had "a life of their own".

The idea that obsessions and compulsions are associated with fears of danger and are attempts to ward off that danger focus on the content of these phenomena, not their form, and needlessly invokes psychoanalytic theory. The form of obsessions and compulsions is, respectively, that of forced thinking and the uncontrolled release of associated procedural memories. Patients with OCD spend hours daily overwhelmed by their hand washing (to the point of skin abrasions) and their repeated checking to see if doors are locked, windows are shut, stovetops are unlit, and lights are turned off. They are compelled to place objects into special alignment to "straighten-up" the table settings, items on the desk top, furniture in the room, and pictures on the wall. They automatically utter prayers without thought, count the number of incidental things they see (ceiling tiles, lines in the wall paper, chairs in the room, i.e. *arithmomania*), and silently repeat trivial words or phrases. They are compelled to perform certain acts or touch certain objects in a specific way for a specified number of times (opening and closing locks, tapping the table setting objects in a specific order for a specific number of times). When the act is completed, they are seized by doubt, and must repeat the ritual again and again.[15] The overwhelming impulse to ask perpetual questions, seeking explanations for the most mundane circumstance (*folie du pourquoi*) and the fear of uttering certain words (*onomatomania*) are rare compulsions. Factor analytic studies of persons with OCD identify contamination/washing, symmetry/ordering/hoarding, and checking as common themes in adult and child sufferers.[16]

Hoarding

In 15–20% of patients with OCD, the most prominent early feature of the illness is hoarding.[17] Useless objects, debris and unneeded purchases are amassed despite the awareness that the piles of old newspapers, stuffed trash bags, appliances, and everyday objects serve no purpose and are consuming the sufferer's living space, often leaving only narrow pathways to various parts of the house or apartment. Patients with chronic manic-depression similarly hoard. Some manic-depressive patients use these items to decorate themselves or stuff materials into their noses and ears.[18]

"Impulse control disorders" that are OCD variants[19]

Impulsivity is a personality trait that also occurs following traumatic brain injury to frontal brain regions.[20] Most of the conditions listed in the DSM impulse control disorder category, however, are best understood as compulsive behavior associated with OCD.[21] Trichotillomania, kleptomania, and pathological gambling are compulsions. Obsessions do not define these behaviors, but many patients with these compulsions have other OCD features. Associated anxiety occurs when the compulsion is actively inhibited. Some authors consider these conditions linked to addictive behaviors such as alcohol and substance abuse,[22] but alcoholics and abusers of illicit drugs do not have a greater risk for OCD or anxious–fearful personality traits.

Trichotillomania is the compulsion to twirl and pull at one's hair and can lead to spotty baldness. It is associated with chewing, biting, licking and eating the hair.[23] *Kleptomania* is the compulsion to steal unneeded objects. *Pyromania* is the obsessive fascination with fire and the compulsion to set and watch objects burn.

Pathological gambling is a heterogeneous category. Some persons who exhibit this behavior can be seen as suffering from OCD. Pathological gambling characterized by obsessive thinking about gambling that leads to repeated excessive gambling often results in bankruptcy and family disintegration.

Self-injury and self-mutilation is associated with several conditions. In the elderly, it is an uncommon finding associated with neurodegenerative disease.[24] Among adolescents, it is associated with mood disorder and environmental instability.[25] It is an all too common finding in persons with developmental disorders, and when stereotypic may indicate catatonia.[26] Chronic heavy-use of cocaine is associated with severe self-injury.[27] Psychotic patients also may inflict terrible damage on themselves, but these are isolated acts rather than repetitive.[28]

Self-injury and self-mutilation is also associated with personality disorder diagnoses and cultural expectations.[29] Several African and Middle Eastern societies traditionally mutilate the skin (e.g. tattoos, skin scarring) and anatomic structures (e.g. nasal septum, external genitalia). In Western society many puncture their earlobes and pierce other body parts to self-decorate. Counter-cultures also extensively tattoo.[30]

When the self-mutilating behavior is not perceived as painful it is termed *pain asymboly* (or *asymbolia*). Pain insensitivity differs from the generalized analgesia seen in benign stupor and catatonia. In these conditions noxious stimuli are perceived as painful, but only when intense.

A disconnection between sensory and limbic processes is proposed to explain pain insensitivity, the patient perceiving the stimulus but having no associated sensory–emotion experience.[31] Pain asymboly is reported with insula lesions (either hemisphere), parietal lobe or thalamic disease,[32] and in patients with schizophrenia[33] and their relatives.[34] One chronically ill schizophrenic patient without apparent discomfort pushed metal screws into his shin bones to ward off dangerous radiation.

Self-injurious behavior characterized by compulsions to repeatedly self-cut, burn, scratch, nail and finger bite, cheek and lip bite or inflect other self-injury without the desire to die are within the OCD spectrum and are responsive to treatments for OCD.[35] The most common expression is ritualistic cutting, the skin usually slashed in symmetric straight lines avoiding areas with vital tendons and blood vessels. Upper and inner aspects of the thighs and inner forearms are commonly cut.

Self-mutilating behavior associated with OCD is perceived by the patient as unwanted, embarrassing, and as a sign of illness. When scarring results, these behaviors can result in the misdiagnosis of borderline personality disorder.

When genital mutilation (e.g. "amputee fetish")[36] or limb amputation (e.g. "body integrity identity disorder")[37] occur, patients may be misdiagnosed as psychotic. The case literature of these extreme forms of self-mutilation, however, is superficial and there is little evidence presented in the published reports that a careful differential diagnosis was considered.

OCD and psychosis

Many patients with the DSM diagnosis of schizophrenia are reported to have one or more OCD features, and about 10% are reported to meet DSM criteria for OCD. Such patients are also reported to have additional features of anxiety disorder.[38] An association between schizotypal and OCD behaviors has also been reported.[39] The co-occurrence is explained by data implicating frontal lobe dysfunction in both conditions. In schizophrenia dorsolateral prefrontal cortex (DLPC) dysfunction is reported, while in OCD ventro-medial prefrontal cortex (VMPC) dysfunction is recognized.[40] In patients with both features, overlapping brain involvement is suggested. Functional MRI studies done in patients with schizophrenia with OCD features report reduced activation in prefrontal areas.[41]

The reported relationship between OCD and psychosis, however, is weak. Severe obsessions and compulsive rituals can be misunderstood as signs of a psychotic disorder, interpreted to be delusions, stereotypes or catatonic mannerisms, leading to the incorrect diagnosis of schizophrenia. Patients with OCD are more likely to recognize their behavior and to understand it as abnormal. Psychotic patients often deny illness (*anosagnosia*), or are unaware of some of their symptoms or consider some necessary.

The simplistic use of DSM-based checklists to identify psychopathology also encourages over diagnosis of co-occurrence. Schizophrenic patients reported to have OCD are said to be less emotionally blunted and to have more depressive features than those without OCD. They experience more compulsions than obsessions.[42] The pattern suggests that many of the "OCD" features observed in these psychotic patients are catatonic features and not OCD, and the patients to be manic-depressive. Discrete episodes of obsessions and compulsions are also likely atypical presentations of mood disorder and may respond to electroconvulsive therapy.[43] There are also several reports suggesting an association between atypical antipsychotics, especially clozapine, and the development of "obsessive–compulsive symptoms" in psychotic patients.[44] Drug-induced movement disorder is a well-known adverse effect of antipsychotic agents.

There is, however, some association between OCD features and manic-depression.[45] Patients with OCD and associated manic-depression are reported, and these patients exhibit an increased prevalence of mood disorder in their first-degree relatives and an OCD course reported to begin earlier in life,[46] and that is more episodic and less severe than OCD patients without co-occurring manic-depression.[47] Childhood onset OCD is also associated with early onset mood disorder.[48] The pattern suggests the manic-depression dominates the clinical picture.[49] Patients with manic-depression, however, do not have an increased risk for the OCD spectrum, although they do binge eat (see below).

The early emergence of OCD is also associated with PANDAS (see below), developmental disorders, and chromosomal aberrations (fragile-X).[50] When the mania and OCD both are of late onset, secondary etiology such right-basal ganglia stroke and stimulant abuse is found.[51]

Secondary OCD (other than PANDAS) typically emerges later in life than the primary form. Secondary OCD is associated with Sydenham's chorea, Parkinson's and Huntington's diseases, and basal ganglia stroke.[52]

Gilles de La Tourette's syndrome (GTS[53])

In 1885, Georges Gilles de La Tourette described the syndrome named for him as "a nervous affliction" expressed as lack of motor coordination with associated echophenomena.[54] GTS is now understood to be characterized by obsessions and compulsions, tic disorder, and behavioral and sleep disturbances. Half of GTS patients have classic OCD features.[55]

Tics are sudden, involuntary movements that can only be suppressed temporarily and only with difficulty. Tics of the eyes and head are the most frequent initial feature (about 50% of sufferers). They do not disappear during sleep. Simple tics evolve into shrugging and neck twisting and then semi-purposeful sniffing, squinting, touching, hitting or striking, jumping or foot stamping, head banging, lip biting, eye gouging, smelling of hands and objects, twirling, squatting and deep knee bending, and repeated retracing of one's steps. A third of patients sustain substantial injury from these actions. Most will also have uncomfortable sensory experiences of the face, head, neck, and extremities, termed *sensory tics*. These are temporarily relieved by performing a movement in the related body area.

Tic disorders phenomenologically lie on a continuum. Fifteen to 20% of primary school children experience transitory tics problems, most commonly prolonged blinking and other facial movements, and nose rubbing. Transitory episodes of a few weeks or months of vocalizations such as excessive throat clearing are less common. Repeated licking of the hands or touching the genitalia is reported. For some children these tic episodes persist for years. Others progress to the full GTS.

Forced vocalizations are the first sign of illness in one-third of patients and consist of repeated throat-clearing, clicking, teeth tapping and then the utterance of words and short phrases. Grunting, coughing, barking, snorting, hissing, propulsive unintelligible sounds and screaming occur. *Coprolalia*, uncontrollable paroxysms of profanity, affects a third of patients. Echolalia and echopraxia occur in one-third of patients.[56]

Behavioral disturbances including hyperactivity and attentional and other cognitive problems, school and social difficulties, classroom disruption, fighting, temper tantrums, and mood swings are reported in half of GTS sufferers. The pattern may lead to the mistaken diagnosis of manic-depression. A small proportion of GTS patients meet criteria for antisocial personality disorder, exhibit sexually inappropriate behavior (e.g. compulsively groping or commenting), are aggressive and assaultive, and cruel to animals and peers. Phobias occur in 20% of GTS patients.

Sleep disturbances are common in patients with GTS, and include initial insomnia, talking during sleep, nightmares and night terrors, somnambulism (sleep walking), and bruxism (teeth grinding). Up to a third are enuretic.

Pediatric autoimmune neuropsychiatric disorder associated with Streptococcus infection (PANDAS)[57]

Beta-hemolytic streptococcal A infection may be associated in the following two months with the rapid emergence of PANDAS, particularly in patients who early on in the infection develop chorea or tics. Boys aged 6–7 years, often with a family history of autoimmune disease (e.g. Grave's disease, rheumatoid arthritis) are most often affected. Symptoms include GTS features, Sydenham's chorea, squirming and fidgeting that can be mistaken for ADHD, anorexia nervosa, and mood disturbances. High levels of antineuronal antibodies leading to striatal inflammation and the MRI finding of enlarged striatal volumes confirm the diagnosis. While most patients fully recover, some become chronically ill, as illustrated by Patient 12.1.

Patient 12.1

A 17-year-old boy with a history of Asperger's syndrome and migraine was psychiatrically hospitalized because of worsening OCD symptoms and the development of catatonia. He recently stopped eating, losing 15 lbs in the two weeks prior to admission. He spent hours ritually touching certain objects in a certain sequence. He stood for long periods staring. He stopped doing his school work and engaging in his interests. He complained of his migraine headaches worsening during this period.

On admission, his muscle tone was increased and he could be postured, briefly retaining the new position. He exhibited automatic obedience and Gegenhalten. His speech was minimal, prosectic and he had echolalia. Lorazepam did not relieve his catatonia. He received 19 bilateral ECT which did relieve the catatonia, and he was discharged on valproic acid and alprazolam.[58]

He was re-hospitalized four months later, now age 18 years, again for catatonia and an exacerbation of repetitive behaviors including repeatedly getting in and out of bed, repeatedly putting his sunglasses on and off and then on a precise spot on the table, signing his name and repeatedly retracing his signature, and walking in circles. He refused being touched, describing the experience as a shock or tingling. He rubbed his head repeatedly. His movements were slow and stiff, and his ritual counting and re-arranging of objects resulted in his taking hours to dress, wash, and eat. He exhibited echolalia. He said he was "depressed" and exhibited minimal emotional expression. He denied hallucinations and had no delusions. A lorazepam challenged had no effect on his symptoms. The family refused further ECT which they said made him cognitively worse without sustained improvement. Low-dose antidepressants and antipsychotics were continued in his outpatient management.[59]

Because of previous strep throat infections and associated mild choreiform movements, an evaluation was undertaken for PANDAS. A lumber puncture before admission revealed elevated IgG protein, strep O titer was 1:1000 and ASO titer was 249, both high. A PET study showed reduced bilateral temporal lobe metabolism. He had a low red cell count (4.2) and a low hematocrit (37.9). Repeat titers showed a high ASA titer of 270. He was begun on a combination of amoxicillin and clavulanate which led to substantial but not full relief, permitting him to return to school.

Eating disorders

Eating disorders are given a separate category in classifications based on a shared problem with eating or body weight that dominates the clinical picture. This determining factor, however, delineates a heterogeneous patient group. Anorexia nervosa best fits within the OCD spectrum, although some patients have a delusional disorder. Bulimia nervosa is commonly associated with manic-depression.

Anorexia nervosa

William Gull offered the first clear presentation of patients with anorexia nervosa in 1868. In an 1874 address to London's Clinical Society he described two patients and presented woodcuts of their features during the illness and after recovery. His note about one follows.[60]

Miss B., aet. 18, was brought to me Oct. 8, 1868, as a case of latent tubercle ... The extreme emaciated look ... much greater indeed than occurs for the most part in tubercular cases where patients are still going about, impressed me at once with the probability that I should find no visceral disease. Pulse 50, Resp.16. Physical examination of the chest and abdomen discovered nothing abnormal. All the viscera were apparently healthy. Notwithstanding the great emaciation and apparent weakness, there was a peculiar restlessness, difficult, I was informed to control. The mother added, "She is never tired". Amenorrhoea since Christmas 1866.

The prevalence of classic OCD in patients with anorexia is many fold higher than population estimates, and in the more severe forms of anorexia as many as 40% of sufferers also have OCD.[61] About 25% of patients with bulimia have co-morbid OCD and many others have OCD features, but many have a picture of manic-depression.[62] The presence of OCD traits in childhood is a risk factor for the development of anorexia nervosa in later life,[63] and the natural history of anorexia often begins with the emergence of features of body dysmorphic disorder.[64]

Patients with anorexia nervosa who have sustained substantial weight loss are unmistakable in appearance, evoking images of Nazi concentration camp survivors. They are skeletal. They move slowly, their fluidity of movement lost and energy sapped. In light-skinned patients, the skin is gray and dry. Head hair is dry, broken and drained of color.

Patients with anorexia nervosa have an intense fear of gaining weight or becoming fat even though underweight. They deny the seriousness of their weight loss. Most anorexic patients have a disturbed body image. They perceive themselves to be fat despite a cachetic appearance. For diagnosis, the DSM requires a refusal to maintain at least 85% body weight for age and height and absence of three menstrual cycles (a clear gender bias). About 10% of patients with anorexia nervosa are male, and the incidence is estimated to be increasing, particularly in male athletes, models, and actors. In adolescent male patients, stunted growth is a presenting symptom.[65] Males with anorexia nervosa have temperaments similar to those of women with anorexia nervosa.[66] Subtyping into restricting or binge eating/purging groups is not meaningful.

Patients with anorexia nervosa often have associated brain gray and white matter volume loss during the ill state that partially normalizes with recovery.[67] Some of these abnormalities and associated cognitive problems may, however, persist, eliciting concerns of an early-onset dementia. The observed parietal lobe dysfunction may explain their altered body image.[68]

Bulimia nervosa

While the evidence is strong that anorexia nervosa is a variant of OCD,[69] the nature of bulimia nervosa is less clear.[70] Although best fitting an association with manic-depression, it is discussed here to minimize redundancy.

Unlike the patient with anorexia, the patient with bulimia nervosa is not underweight and rather than having personality traits associated with OCD (e.g. perfectionism, reduced expression of emotion), patients with bulimia exhibit chronic problems with regulation of emotion.[71]

Patients with bulimia nervosa have recurrent episodes of binge eating followed by inappropriate efforts to counter weight gain. Excessive consumption of large amounts of high-caloric sweet and fattening foods may be triggered by stress. Subsequent purging includes vomiting, the use of laxatives, and excessive exercise. Sufferers report feeling ashamed and guilty, triggering efforts to treat depression. Those inducing self-vomiting may have dental caries and periodontal disease. Esophageal or gastric rupture may occur. Hand calluses, perioral dermatitis and swollen parotid glands are associated signs of purging. When purging is severe, paresthesia and seizures occur.

Patients who both binge and purge often have co-occurring manic-depression, illicit drug abuse, or anxiety disorder.[72] Among the many studies that have examined for the presence of eating problems in patients with manic-depression, the vast majority report an increased prevalence of binge eating,[73] but these studies offer no evidence for an increased prevalence of OCD spectrum conditions. Among the studies that have assessed the prevalence of manic-depression in patients with eating disorders, the findings are inconsistent and unconvincing.[74] Thus, while patients with manic-depression binge eat, particularly when hypomanic, they do not exhibit the obsessive–compulsive behaviors that are characteristic of the OCD spectrum, and such binging is best considered and treated as a symptom of the mood disorder.[75]

Secondary eating disorders

Binging occurring without other psychiatric illness suggests a circumscribed disturbance of brain areas regulating eating behaviors.[76] A review of all published reports to 2005 of patients over age seven with eating disorders thought to be the result of brain damage identified 54 patients. Body image concerns, obsessions, binge eating, and aggressiveness were associated features. Twenty-three had hypothalamic or third ventricle disease, and all but one of these was a primary tumor. Seven others had primary tumors in the brain stem or fourth ventricle. Thirteen had a cerebral hemisphere lesion, all frontal–temporal and most of these right-sided. Epilepsy was seen in 12 patients.[77]

Body dysmorphic disorder (BDD)

Eating disorders are commonly seen in persons who are said to have body dysmorphic disorder, and body dysmorphic disorder is commonly seen in persons with eating disorders. In persons with both phenomena, the preoccupation with body size and shape precedes the eating disorder.[78] Body dysmorphic disorder is a symptom, not a disease. *Dysmorphophobia* refers to an intense subjective dissatisfaction with one's body shape or form. In addition to weight and overall appearance, body parts of concern include the nose and other facial structures, stomach, hair, teeth, buttocks and hips, and thighs and legs. Most sufferers will also exhibit repetitive self-injurious behavior including skin picking and excessive grooming. About 25% make a suicide attempt.[79]

The classification of body dysmorphic disorder among the somatoform disorders is not supported by evidence. A better term is *body dysmorphic ideas.* The preoccupation with imagined or slight defects in appearance is content, not form. In half of such patients, the preoccupation is delusional and mood or psychotic disorder the likely illness. Patients with a body dysmorphic delusion are also more likely to have abused illicit drugs than those whose preoccupation is due to other causes.[80] In rare instances, an over-valued idea takes the form of a desire to have a healthy limb amputated (*apotemnophilia*) and in pretending to be an amputee. Associated sexual arousal is not necessarily present in such patients.[81]

Many patients with body dysmorphic ideas have many other associated obsessive–compulsive features,[82] and the preoccupation with body image is seen as obsessive rumination.[83] Sufferers also exhibit many repetitive, behaviors such as mirror checking, excessive measuring and touching of body parts, and excessive tanning.[84]

About one-third of persons with body dysmorphic preoccupations also have co-occurring social phobia and many anxious–fearful personality traits.[85] Some have associated eating disorder.[86] In Japan, body dysmorphic ideas are seen as a phobic disorder, the content being anxiety over the perceived deformity of one's body part.[87]

The thalamus and parietal lobes are commonly involved in BDD associated with structural brain disease. Patients experience body parts as being the wrong size, shape, color, weight, or composition (e.g. made of wood rather than flesh and bone).[88] *Phantom limb* and *phantom breast* is commonly associated with surgical amputation of these body parts and result from both continued peripheral nerve afferentation and a preserved sensory cortex schema for the body part.

Hypochondriasis

Hypochondriasis is a symptom not a syndrome.[89] Its present-day definition refers to a persistent preoccupation with exaggerated concerns about one's health.[90] The patient is preoccupied with bodily sensations, is phobic for disease, and is convinced of ill-health. Minor body sensations and ailments are considered ominous and the patient repeatedly seeks medical attention.

Hypochondriasis occurs in persons with anxious–fearful and negative affect temperament traits, obsessive–compulsive disorder, and depressive illness. When severe, hypochondriasis can represent the content of the ruminations and delusions typical of psychotic depression.[91] When an aspect of OCD, hypochondriasis often involves a single focus: the potential dire consequences of a minor body imperfection (*dysmorphophobia*), itchy and dry skin being the result of infestation (*Ekbom's syndrome*), or disease in a specific organ.

Hypochondriasis is associated with compulsions such as checking body parts for changes that might reflect disease (e.g. checking lymph nodes for swelling).[92] Patients also seek repeated reassurance from physicians and others that their fear is unfounded.[93]

Compulsive sexual behaviors

Deviant sexual behavior is reported in persons who have no recognizable illness and in persons with neurologic and psychiatric conditions. Present classification reflects social decisions more than science. For example, violent sexual offenses are treated as criminal acts and there is no DSM/ICD diagnosis for these, but many such persons have neurologic disease (often traumatic brain injury) that may to some degree account for their actions.[94] Homosexuality and bisexuality are also not medical diagnoses and were voted expunged from classification by the American Psychiatric membership, but *before* the weight of evidence indicated that they are biological variants observed in many species.[95] Sexual deviance is also placed in several classes in the DSM, and the paraphilias are delineated as if they represent a specific disorder with common determinants, but there is little scientific support for such homogeneity. Compulsive sexual deviations are considered here.

Most persons reported to exhibit sexually deviant behavior are male.[96] Compulsive sexual behavior is reported in about 5% of the general population.[97] Sexual deviations that are OCD variants are characterized by co-occurring compulsive behaviors, and deviant sexual obsessions and compulsions are both commonly present.[98] In one study of 36 persons with compulsive sexual behaviors, 60% also exhibited other OCD variants including kleptomania, compulsive buying, pathological gambling, trichotillomania, pyromania and compulsive exercise.[99] In another study, in addition to other compulsive behaviors the patients had an increased prevalence of anxiety disorder, depression (most likely non-melancholic) and anxious–fearful personality traits.[100]

Definitions of compulsive sexual behavior vary, but can be condensed to: *repetitive sexual acts and intrusive sexual thoughts that are experienced as having a life of their own*, the person feeling compelled or driven to think and perform the act. Lack of control is more important in the definition than the presence of distress or any reduction in anxiety when the act is performed.[101] Compulsive sexual behavior includes: compulsive searching for multiple partners (*Don Juanism, satyriasis*, and *nymphomania*), fixation on an unobtainable partner, compulsive masturbation, and compulsive sexual activity with a partner. Paraphilia is diagnosed when the compulsive act is considered criminal (e.g. exhibitionism, pedophilia, voyeurism ["Peeping Tom"], and frotteurism [rubbing against a non-consenting person]) or elicits substantial distress in the person or the partner (e.g. because of fetishism, transvestic fetishism [cross-dressing], voyeurism, compulsive masturbation, dependence on pornography, and bestiality).[102] The subjective experiences of such patients before, during and after the sexual compulsive behavior are similar to those with more classic OCD, and also include distress at the loss of control. The use of illicit drugs and alcohol at the time of the behavior is common.[103]

Obsessive–compulsive personality

The place for obsessive–compulsive personality in classification is uncertain. The association with OCD is modest, while the linkage to other Axis II conditions is weak. Overall, the evidence indicates it can be considered a mild form of OCD and part of the OCD spectrum. Obsessive–compulsive personality traits are reported to commonly precede OCD and OCD spectrum conditions, and these traits are also common in the relatives of patients with OCD and OCD spectrum conditions.[104]

Much of the uncertain findings stems from the delineation of obsessive–compulsive personality by psychoanalytic rather than by empirically derived descriptors and the application of descriptors categorically rather than as trait dimensions.[105] "*Anal character type*" and the ICD *anankastic personality disorder* are terms reflecting the theoretical pedigree of obsessive–compulsive personality.

Common descriptors of DSM and ICD (anankastic) obsessive–compulsive personality are: preoccupation with details (rules, lists, order, and schedules), excessive conscientiousness, rigidity and stubbornness, and being overly controlling.

NOTES

1 Henry Maudsley (1874) cited by M.J. Clark in Scull (1981), page 271.
2 Yaryura-Tobias and Neziroglu (1997).
3 Tynes *et al.* (1990).
4 Bartz and Hollander (2006).
5 Dannon *et al.* (2006).
6 Dannon *et al.* (2004a,b).
7 Hollander *et al.* (2005); Lochner *et al.* (2005a).
8 They also propose a "depersonalization disorder" which does not fit the data.
9 Compulsive shopping and Internet usage are also being considered as variants of this cluster.
10 Autism is also being considered for this category.

11 Taylor and Fink (2006).

12 Chen and Dilsaver (1995).

13 Regier *et al.* (1984).

14 Paul McHugh: Overestimating mental illness in America, in A Nation of Crazy People? *The Weekly Standard*, Volume 10, Issue 39, June 27, 2005.

15 Visual–spatial memory is impaired and the sufferer cannot fully access the episodic memory of the recently completed action, thus finding it necessary to repeat it (Zielinski *et al.*, 1991).

16 Leckman *et al.* (2007).

17 Lochner *et al.* (2005b).

18 Kraepelin (1976), page 65.

19 Intermittent explosive disorder is not included here and is not an illness. It is a features of several conditions (e.g. antisocial personality, traumatic brain injury, manic-depression, epilepsy) and does not warrant a separate diagnostic category (Dell'Osso *et al.*, 2006).

20 Chapter 14 provides a discussion of trait behavior and Chapter 15 the effects of brain injury on personality.

21 Grant and Potenza (2006a).

22 Holden (2001), Grant *et al.* (2006).

23 Yaryura-Tobias and Neziroglu (1997), pages 208–9.

24 Parks and Feldman (2006).

25 Lloyd-Richardson *et al.* (2007).

26 Osman and Loschen (1992). Examples are the Prader–Willi syndrome (a deletion of paternal genetic material from chromosome 15), which is defined by self-mutilation, hypotonicity, mental retardation, small gonads and hands and feet. Sufferers have other OCD features. The Lesch–Nyhan syndrome, an error in purine metabolism from an X-linked genetic error, is recognized by mental retardation, choreoathetosis, and mutilating finger and oral mucosal biting (Yaryura-Tobias and Neziroglu, 1997, pp. 204–7).

27 Karila *et al.*, 2007

28 One of us (MAT) has seen two patients with psychosis as part of a manic-depressive illness who injured their eyes. One patient enucleated his left eye in response to delusional ideas. Another jammed a ballpoint pen into each eye socket in an effort to stop visual hallucinations. The patient was blinded, but the hallucinations continued.

29 Simeon *et al.*, 1992

30 Yaryura-Tobias and Neziroglu (1997, p. 201); Yaryura-Tobias *et al.* (1995).

31 Berthier *et al.* (1988).

32 Berthier *et al.* (1988); Masson *et al.* (1991).

33 Singh *et al.* (2006).

34 Hooley and Delgado (2001).

35 Primeau and Fontaine (1987); Yaryura-Tobias *et al.* (1995).

36 Wise and Kalyanam (2000); Stunell *et al.* (2006).

37 Sorene *et al.* (2006).

38 Kayahan *et al.* (2005).

39 Insel and Akiskal (1986).

40 Cavallaro *et al.* (2003).

41 Levine *et al.* (1998).

42 de Haan *et al.* (2005); Stamouli and Lykouras (2006); Ma *et al.* (2007).

43 Swartz and Shen (1999).

44 de Haan *et al.* (2002); Ma *et al.* (2007).

45 Chen and Dilsaver (1995); Perugi *et al.* (2001).

46 Masi *et al.* (2004).

47 Perugi *et al.* (2002); Zutshi *et al.* (2007).

48 Riddle (1998); Sanchez *et al.* (1999).

49 Perugi *et al.* (1997).

50 Asbahr *et al.* (1998); Wang *et al.* (2003); Geller (2006).

51 Robinson and Starkstein (1989).

52 Yaryura-Tobias and Neziroglu (1991).

53 Shapero *et al.* (1988); Sandor (1993); Fahn (1993).

54 de La Tourette (1885).

55 George *et al.* (1993); Teive *et al.* (2001).

56 Although echophenomena are also classic signs of catatonia, clinically distinguishing catatonia from GTS is not difficult. The common experience of features, however, is consistent with the relationship between these conditions and basal ganglia dysfunction.

57 Asbahr *et al.* (1998); Murphy *et al.* (2006).

58 Because catatonia has been associated with an imbalance in GABA (too little A or too much B), the prescription of valproic acid (a strong GABA-B agonist) is risky and can result in a relapse of the catatonia. If a mood-stabilizing agent is required, carbamazepine (having more GABA-A than GABA-B activity) or lithium carbonate are better choices (Fink and Taylor, 2003).

59 Antipsychotic agents can also exacerbate catatonia and elicit the malignant form of the condition (Fink and Taylor, 2003).

60 Thompson (1987), pages 25–47.

61 Speranza *et al.* (2001); Kaye *et al.* (2004).

62 Matsunaga *et al.* (1999); Albert *et al.* (2001).

63 Anderluh *et al.* (2003).

64 Rabe-Jablonska and Sobow Tomasz (2000).

65 Modan-Moses *et al.* (2003).

66 Fassino *et al.* (2001).

67 Frank *et al.* (2004); Wagner *et al.* (2006).

68 Katzman *et al.* (2001).

69 Steiger and Bruce (2007).

70 Angst (1998); Wittchen *et al.* (2003).

71 Wonderlich *et al.* (2007); Steiger and Bruce (2007).

72 O'Brien and Vincent (2003).

73 McElroy *et al.* (2006).

74 Ibid.

75 Ibid.

76 Steiger and Bruce (2007).

77 Uher and Treasure (2002).

78 Grant *et al.* (2002); Ruffolo *et al.* (2006).

79 Phillips *et al.* (2005, 2006).

80 Ibid.

81 Braam *et al.* (2006).

82 Frare *et al.* (2004).

83 Grant and Phillips (2005).

84 Rabe-Jablonska and Sobow Tomasz (2000); Phillips and Kaye (2007).

85 Coles *et al.* (2006).

86 Ruffolo *et al.* (2006).

87 Suzuki *et al.* (2003).

88 Critchley (1950). Cummings (1988) offers terms for specific abnormal perceptions of body parts. These are *hyperschemazia* (larger and heavier), *hyposchemazia* (wasted or light), *aschemazia* (missing), *hemisomatognosia* (one half of the body is felt to be missing), and *paraschemazia* (distorted, twisted or ectopic).

89 Creed and Barsky (2004).

90 The original meaning of hypochondriasis referred to depressive illness with predominant symptoms below the rib cage.

91 Fallon *et al.* (2000); Abramowitz (2005); Fink *et al.* (2004); Ferguson (2004). Ferguson, using the Five Factor Model of personality, found an association between hypochondriasis and low conscientiousness and low emotional stability. Chapter 14 provides a discussion of the dimensional view of personality.

92 Abramowitz and Braddock (2006).

93 Ibid.

94 Langevin (2006) reports that almost 50% of male sexual offenders had previous and substantial traumatic brain injury. Briken *et al.* (2005) found about one-third of sexual murderers to have substantial evidence of brain abnormality. Persons who engage in incest are more likely to also abuse illicit drugs and alcohol (Firestone *et al.*, 2005).

95 DSM III 1980.

96 Black *et al.* (1997).

97 Coleman (1992).

98 Krueger and Kaplan (2001).

99 Black *et al.* (1997).

100 Raymond *et al.* (2003).

101 Anthony and Hollander (1992).

102 Coleman (1992).

103 Black *et al.* (1997).

104 Fineberg *et al.* (2007); Phillips and Kaye (2007).

105 Fineberg *et al.* (2007); see Chapter 14 for a discussion of dimensional personality traits, Chapter 15 for a description of obsessive–compulsive personality, and Chapter 16 for the evidence indicating it is best considered a mild form of OCD rather than an Axis II condition.

13

Cognitive testing and the psychopathology of cognitive dysfunction

The mistake of deriving all phenomena from one principle may occur in somatic and physiological (materialistic) as well as in philosophical and psychological concepts; for instance, when all psychic phenomena are reduced to the single scheme of the reflex process, it is no more a lasting contribution to science than when the philosophical schools deduce this from the principle of identity or that of polarity, etc. The psychic phenomena have first to be viewed and compiled quite without prejudice, like individual phenomena in other sciences, and only when substantial material comes to be available in at least a somewhat different form and in greater abundance than hitherto will it be possible to attempt causal or physiological and anatomical substantiation.[1]

Patients with behavior-altering brain disease often experience cognitive difficulties, and the assessment of their cognitive functioning is essential in their diagnosis and management. Patients with melancholic depression, for example, have profound cognitive difficulties which resolve with successful treatment. If improperly treated, however, their cognitive deficits persist and result in chronic poor functioning. Moderate cognitive difficulty in a patient with melancholia is also an independent risk factor for suicide.[2] Patients with schizophrenia have persistent cognitive problems in working memory, fluency of ideas, and executive function that influence long-term decisions on placement and socialization rehabilitation.[3] Patients with anxiety disorders and obsessive–compulsive syndromes have cognitive difficulties in working memory and visual–spatial function undermining treatment compliance.[4]

Different patterns of cognitive decline are recognized and point to specific disease processes. In the early phases of Alzheimer's disease, visual and episodic memory are affected. In Pick's disease and primary frontal lobe degeneration, problems with executive functioning are early features.[5] Persons with basal ganglia disease have deficits in working and procedural memory and visual–spatial functions.[6]

Several classic psychopathologic phenomena are also associated with specific cognitive deficits. *Capgras syndrome*, the delusion of familiar persons being impostors, is associated with poor facial recognition (*prosopagnosia*) and non-dominant temporal lobe lesions.[7] The delusional experiences of alienation and control are associated with non-dominant parietal lobe lesions and cognitive deficits in spatial recognition and motor–perceptual functioning.[8]

Substantial substance abuse can cause chronic executive function and non-verbal cognitive decline that affects disposition planning.[9] The temporary cognitive dysfunction associated with the acute course of ECT is monitored to help determine the frequency of treatments and termination of treatment.[10]

Integrating cognition and psychopathology

All behavior has a cognitive component and integrating cognitive and behavioral assessments provides the most thorough evaluation of the patient's strengths and weaknesses, information needed for diagnosis and in disposition planning. Like the rest of the behavioral evaluation, cognitive testing begins the moment the examiner sees the patient. Whatever the patient does, part of that behavior reflects a cognitive process and reveals something about the patient's cognition. The following vignette illustrates.

Patient 13.1

On greeting a 55-year-old patient in the waiting area and escorting her to his office, a psychiatrist noted that the patient, from a bordering state, came alone. As he usually did, he asked the patient if she had any difficulty finding her way to the hospital and waiting area. She had not. He asked if she had driven herself. She had. He asked if the referring physician had explained the reason for the consultation and that he would be sending a report to the referring physician. The patient said it had all been explained. As they entered the office, the consultant said without pointing, "Have a seat in the uncomfortable looking gray chair". She smiled good-humoredly and complied appropriately.

In the brief "chat" while walking to the office, the consultant learned a great deal about the patient's cognition and neurologic functioning. He noted that she was alert, neatly and cleanly dressed, and had appropriate greeting behavior. She was oriented to the point of being able to come to the correct place on the correct date and at the right time for her appointment. Her conversational speech appeared normal. She was not obviously aphasic. She was not acutely ill or in acute distress. Her movements and gait appeared normal during the walk to the office. She had demonstrated the ability to follow directions from her home to the medical center and then find the consultant's office, requiring negotiating a complicated route. By driving herself, she had also demonstrated the implicit memories of knowing the rules of the road and the driving of an automobile. By sitting in the gray chair, she demonstrated language comprehension and likely no visual agnosia. By genuinely smiling at the consultant's lame but deliberate attempt at humor, she demonstrated some emotional reactivity.

The usefulness of the information gathered in the brief exchange was clinically relevant. The patient was referred for an evaluation of a "treatment-resistant" depressive illness, and 10–15% of such patients are misdiagnosed as depressed when in fact they have another condition that is not responsive to antidepressant treatment. Apathetic syndromes from structural brain disease are commonly misinterpreted as depression, but this consideration seemed unlikely from the consultant's brief initial assessment.[11] Further examination found the patient to have an atypical depressive condition. She had never been treated with a mono-amine oxidase inhibitor, and that drug class was recommended.

The big cognitive picture

Each domain of the behavioral examination begins with an overview. That image guides the gathering of the details. Establishing the big picture can be done quickly. Is the patient alert? Is the patient having difficulty relating the story of the illness or biographical information? Does the patient understand the examiner's comments and requests? Behavior is the most sensitive expression of brain function. Patient 13.2 illustrates.

Patient 13.2

A 58-year-old man was hospitalized because he was becoming increasingly irritable toward his wife, threatening her on one occasion. He also made vague comments about harming himself.

The patient had been a successful business man and an energetic person who "worked hard and played hard" until six years earlier, when he began to lose interest in his work and other activities. For the two years prior to admission he spent most of his time at home doing little and offering unconvincing reasons for his inactivity. He seemed unconcerned about the change in his behavior, becoming irritated only when excessively prodded by his family who now considered him "lazy" and "resting" on his past success.

A consultant was asked to evaluate the patient for dementia and early-onset Alzheimer's disease. The consultant met the treatment team at the unit. The patient had been admitted late Monday afternoon and it was now Wednesday morning. When the entourage entered the patient's room, the patient recognized his outpatient geriatric psychiatrist and greeted her by name. He recognized his resident, but did not recall her name. He remembered that he was to be seen by a consultant and greeted him, shaking his hand while offering a social smile.

The consultant suggested the group move to a larger room and asked the patient if he knew the room with "the piano" and could he lead the group to it. The inpatient unit was shaped like an H, with the patient's room at the bottom of the lower left section and the piano room in the top of the upper right section. With a perfectly normal, smooth gait the patient led the team out of his room. He immediately turned to his left, walked to the transept, turned right, crossed to the other hallway, turned left and walked to the piano room where he pointed to the piano. As the team was getting settled to observe the consultant's "bedside" cognitive testing, he turned to the patient's geriatric psychiatrist and whispered, "Well, I've just completed most of my evaluation. The patient does not have Alzheimer's disease." Further assessment was consistent with the clinical interpretation and indicated the patient had modest impairment on tasks associated with frontal lobe disease. Functional imaging confirmed mild primary frontal lobe atrophy without evidence of vascular disease.

Patient 13.2 had been in slow decline for six years. Although there is an early-onset form of Alzheimer's disease it is virulent, associated with a strong family history for the illness, and about 30% of sufferers will have associated increased muscle tone or rigidity. Alzheimer's disease typically begins with problems in visual–spatial functioning and new learning. Patient 13.2's facial recognition of his physicians, learning the unit's floor plan and being able to easily negotiate its configuration, remembering where the piano was, and being able to lead the team to the correct room with a smooth gait, eliminated Alzheimer's disease from serious consideration.[12] Accomplishing all that while still maintaining social graces further indicated that Patient 13.2's cognitive decline associated with his apathetic syndrome was likely to be modest. Functional imaging, other history and examination findings also demonstrated that the apathy was not due to vascular disease or depressive illness.

Many behaviors signal specific cognitive difficulties and their presence shape the choice of standardized tasks. Table 13.1 displays the more common of signature behaviors. Along with the assessment for patterns of abnormal motor features, bedside cognitive testing helps identify the circumscribed brain lesions that may underlie the behavioral syndrome.

Principles of bedside cognitive assessment

Reasons for assessment

Table 13.2 displays reasons for cognitive assessment. Relying on screening batteries such as *The Mini Mental State Examination* (MMSE) is of modest utility only

Table 13.1. Behaviors suggesting cognitive problems[13]

Behavior	Likely associated cognitive problem(s)
Avolition and apathy	Poor executive functioning; poor abstract thinking and verbal reasoning
Loss of social graces and coarsening of personality	Poor executive functioning and self-monitoring
Loss of motor skills (e.g. typing, playing a musical instrument)	Poor working memory, recall, and visual–spatial memory
Forgetting to remember (e.g. failing to turn off the oven or to deliver a message)	Poor working memory
"Poor historian"	Poor recall and poor executive function, or loss of long-term memory storage
Getting lost in familiar places	Poor visual–spatial perception; poor visual memory
Having several "fender benders"	Poor visual–spatial perception
Not recognizing familiar people	Poor facial recognition and visual–spatial memory
Episode of melancholia or mania	Poor working memory; recall distorted by quality of mood
Obsessive–compulsive disorder	Poor working memory and visual–spatial memory
Schizophrenia	Poor executive functioning, abstract thinking, verbal and visual reasoning
Chronic mood disorder	Poor working memory and new learning, and ability to organize and relate a sequential history

Table 13.2. Reasons for bedside cognitive assessment

To confirm or reject differential diagnostic possibilities

To obtain specific assessment of the patient's cognitive strengths and weaknesses to shape treatment and disposition plans

To obtain a baseline and then re-examinations to follow the illness progression or to monitor treatments

because such instruments are designed for a general purpose rather than to define specific dysfunction. Knowing a number of bedside tasks that can be applied as needed for one or more of the purposes shown in Table 13.2 permits the gathering of more specific information, helps resolve differential diagnostic questions, and shapes treatment plans. Patient 13.3 illustrates the value of assessing the patient's cognitive strengths *and* weaknesses.

Patient 13.3

A 20-year-old student was hospitalized with an acute psychosis secondary to illicit hallucinogen drug intoxication. He had a long history of such use as well as the abuse of other types of drugs.

His psychosis quickly resolved and he was seen by the unit's staff as an intelligent, highly verbal, pleasant person whose major problem was his substance abuse. A disposition plan centered on psychotherapy was proposed.

The unit psychiatrist, however, noted that in brief conversations about topics the patient had studied in school, the patient's comprehension appeared limited and his thinking vague. A WAIS revealed the patient's full-scale IQ to be 88, although his vocabulary indicated a much higher pre-illness score.[14] The patient's test performance made it likely that he would have been unable to successfully participate in the proposed psychotherapy program that relied on high-level comprehension and abstract thinking. A more modest disposition was then planned that included the recognition that the patient had suffered brain damage from his drug use.

Cognitive assessment is also used to monitor treatment. For example, as a depressive illness resolves in a geriatric patient cognition should improve; if not, dementia is considered. Cognitive assessment is regularly done throughout the acute course of ECT to determine the presence and degree of anterograde amnesia and the best frequency of treatments (twice or three times weekly). Cognitive testing is repeated after the treatment course to determine when the anterograde amnestic process has resolved and the patient can continue normal responsibilities.

Assessment methods

Table 13.3 displays guidelines for cognitive assessment.

Cognitive assessment must be done systematically and precisely so the results are reproducible. Instructions should be clearly stated and the assessment setting non-distracting. The goal is to obtain the patient's best performance. Encouragement is often needed, particularly for depressed patients and those with apathetic syndromes. Knowing the patient's capacity encourages the best prognostic plans.

When psychomotor retardation is substantial or the patient has significant peripheral handicaps, timed tests are still done, but the patient is permitted to proceed past the time limit to see if the function being assessed is adequate to complete the task. Aphasic patients are mostly assessed with non-verbal tasks. The patient's education and abilities in the language of the test are considered in the choice of tasks and their interpretation. One of us successfully treated an

Table 13.3. Guidelines for cognitive assessment

The goal of assessment is the patient's best performance

Choice of tasks should be based on the purpose of the assessment; one group of tests does not "fit all" patients

Each task should be administered consistently and with precise instructions

Arousal and concentration should always be assessed first to determine if further assessment is possible and will be valid

Peripheral neurologic and muscular–skeletal function (e.g. paresis, arthritis) determines what tasks can be done

Patients with aphasia or language skills other than the language of the assessment require special procedures

---

Asian woman for psychotic depression and Parkinson's disease who was left in bed for several years following a neurologist's incorrect diagnosis of Parkinson's dementia that was erroneously confirmed by neuropsychological testing administered in English, her second language.

The patient's general neurologic function is also determined prior to cognitive assessment as most bedside cognitive tests require the patient to have adequate peripheral neurologic and somatosensory functioning (e.g. visual and auditory acuity, somatosensory acuity). For patients with compromised peripheral function, assessment is limited and requires greater reliance on behavioral cues.

An assessment of arousal and concentration are also always done before other cognitive tests, as most cognitive functions are dependent on arousal and concentration.

Test selection is based on the purpose of the assessment. To be performed well, almost all tests require adequate function in several cognitive areas, so tests typically "overlap" in what they are assessing and provide information beyond the specific intent of the test. For example, animal naming (see below) is a timed test that assesses fluency of ideas. It also requires a "plan" for proceeding in an efficient manner from one group of animals to the next. However, this required executive functioning is not the specific target of the test but is evaluated while the patient performs the task. A manic patient with compromised executive function might be able to haphazardly and rapidly rattle off a sufficient number of animal names to "pass" the test, but the executive function problems will be obvious.

Selecting and using cognitive tests also requires working knowledge of neuropsychological functions and the relationships among functions and behavior. A discussion of these relationships is beyond this text, and so the cognitive testing presented here is within the framework of common clinical challenges.[15]

Segues into specific assessment

The reason for cognitive assessment is to help alleviate the patient's problems, not the examiner's. Thus introductions such as "I need to ask you questions you may find silly" have no place in the evaluation. More helpful opening comments are:

"You were telling me about the problems you've been having with (concentration, memory, thinking, etc.). How troublesome are they? For example, have you …?"

"With all the things that have been happening to you, have they affected your (concentration, memory, thinking, etc.)?"

"Are the problems with your (concentration, memory, thinking, etc.) the kind where you get confused about the date or the day of the week?"

"Is your concentration difficulty the type where when you are reading or watching TV you realize you really aren't paying attention or you don't remember what you've just read or seen?"

"Let me check your concentration, just to be sure. What I would like you to do for me is …". Testing concentration follows.

"Let me check your memory and thinking a bit …". The rest of the formal cognitive examination follows.

Assessing for general brain "power": IQ

The patient's present general intelligence influences the response to illness, and the acceptance of treatments and behavioral strategies in long-term management. Signs of cognitive decline also provide needed information. Although performance on standard IQ tests is influenced by education, aspects of such batteries are used at the bedside in assessing general intelligence. Unless impacted by injury or disease, general intelligence remains fairly constant over adult life.

Previous levels of employment functioning and present vocabulary and word usage are associated with pre-morbid IQ. For example, a college professor with hepatic encephalopathy was able to name only 8 animals in one minute (15 or more is normal). His choices of "Aardvark" and "hippopotamus", however, were consistent with his past high level of function. A construction worker with a high school education performed poorly on frontal lobe tasks while he was in an acute mania, but despite his frequent periods of flight-of-ideas, he correctly used such words as "persistent", "theology", and "transient", indicating a pre-morbid IQ level beyond his schooling, and a potential strength to rely on during his long-term care.

Present intellectual functioning is assessed with many of the bedside tests described below. In addition to the actual level of performance, general intelligence level is suggested by the speed at which the patient grasps the instructions and the efficiency with which the patient performs the task.

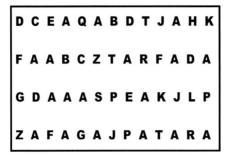

Figure 13.1 The auditory A test

Assessing for delirium

Delirium is a common concern when a patient with general medical or neurologic disease exhibits an acute behavioral change.[16] Although many deliria are characterized by substantial anxiety and agitation and some by delusions and frightening hallucinations in multiple sensory modalities, many delirious patients only appear sleepy, hesitant or unsure of themselves. They have trouble focusing attention and responding promptly. Their thoughts wander and their speech appears vacant. Few have characteristic features that identify the cause of the delirium.[17]

Delirium is suspected when the patient exhibits (1) unexplained failure to participate in or to understand treatment efforts, (2) unexplained fluctuations in behavior (particularly in emotional expression and arousal), (3) newly emerged agitation, (4) newly experienced hallucinations, (5) unexplained failure to remember recent events, and (6) unexplained lack of focused attention.

All delirious processes are associated with altered arousal. Other than the patient's behavior, the most sensitive assessments of arousal require the patient to perform continuously for a minute or more. Figure 13.1 displays an auditory letter cancellation test that serves this purpose.

The patient is asked to listen as the examiner reads aloud the letters in a monotone at the rate of a letter per second. The patient is instructed to signal (e.g. tap with a pen, raise a finger) whenever the letter "A" is said. The "A" is randomly distributed and cannot be predicted. Other letters can be transposed for "A" and so practice effects are avoided and the test can be repeated with the same patient. Not responding when hearing "A" is an error of omission and is often present when arousal is reduced and the patient is not able to focus attention. Responding to a letter other than "A" is an error of commission and is often present when arousal is heightened and the patient is distractible. Five or more errors of any kind indicates poor attention and is consistent with a delirious state and conditions that elicit distractibility (e.g. mania). Asking the patient to say the days of the week backwards is a cruder measure of attention.

Assessing for dementia

Dementia is rare in persons under age 65 but the incidence increases substantially in persons over age 70. As many as 40% of persons between the ages of 80 and 90 years have cognitive impairments in the dementia range.[18] Not all elderly persons, however, are demented, and many who are cognitively impaired have a reversible condition associated with depression or medication toxicity.[19]

Dementia is diagnosed when the patient exhibits substantial cognitive impairment with significant memory difficulties despite minimal deficits in arousal. Once the dementia syndrome is recognized, the next step is to determine the pattern of the dementing process. Once the pattern is delineated, ideology may be established.

Identifying the dementia syndrome

Persons who are in the severe stage of a dementing process are not difficult to recognize as their cognitive impairments are substantial and widespread. Although in a state of normal arousal, they will score below 20 and typically below 15 on the MMSE.[20] It is much more difficult, however, to recognize the early stages of degenerative brain disease and the "pre-clinical" phase of such conditions.

The pre-clinical phase in dementing processes is termed MCI (mild cognitive impairment). Once identified, over the next 4 years, persons with MCI decline further, 10–15% becoming clinically demented each year.[21] Recognizing MCI can lead to early intervention that may delay the progression of the illness, and several bedside tests are sensitive to MCI and the early stages of dementia.

Most dementing processes interfere with working memory, new learning, memory storage, and thinking. The tests below tap those functions and almost all normal persons of all ages perform them within the age-corrected range.[22] Early in the MCI stage, the patient may be able to successfully complete the tests but will require extra time as efficiency is reduced. More than expected errors will occur in persons who previously were high functioning. New learning and recall will be mildly affected. The auditory A test is done first to establish adequate concentration to continue.

Digit span: The patient is asked to immediately repeat a series of numbers, the first number series forward and the next series backwards. Numbers backwards is most sensitive to problems with working memory and normal persons under 55 years of age should recall a minimum of 7 backwards. Normal persons over 70 should recall a minimum of 5 backwards. Asking the patient to say the days of the week or the months of the year backwards is a less sensitive version of this task because those items are over-learned and are easy to remember forward, while digit span offers novel information.[23]

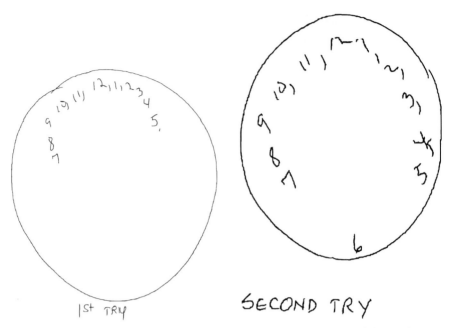

Figure 13.2 Clock drawing in a manic-depressive patient who developed dementia

Clock drawing: Asking the patient to draw the face of a clock from memory taps recall and perceptual–motor coordination and is sensitive to temporal–parietal dysfunction, an early feature of Alzheimer's disease. In some versions the clock's shape (a circle) is provided. The patient is asked to place the clock's hands at 2:45 to also assess for spatial neglect, with such patients often neglecting the left side of space (see Figure 13.2). Asking the patient to judge the quality of his effort assesses frontal lobe executive function. Some patients place all the left-side numbers on the right side of the clock (see Figure 13.3).[24]

The patient's inability to draw the face of the clock correctly on the first try suggests poor planning consistent with frontal circuitry dysfunction. His improvement on the second try suggests that he has no spatial deficit (Figure 13.2).

Copying and recalling shapes: Copying shapes and then recalling them taps perceptual–motor coordination and visual memory. Almost any five simple shapes are acceptable. Figure 13.4 shows some examples. After the effort to copy the shapes, the patient is asked to immediately reproduce them from memory. After this effort the five figures are reviewed and followed by a delayed recall effort toward the end of the testing session.

Similarities and their recall: The understanding of the most fundamental common denominator between two things assesses abstract thinking and is a subtest of the WAIS. Recall of the word pairs assesses verbal memory. Almost any five pairs of increasing difficulty can be used such as orange–banana, North–West,

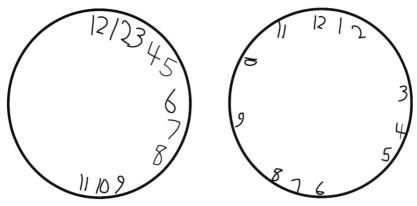

Figure 13.3 Clock drawing indicating left-sided spatial neglect

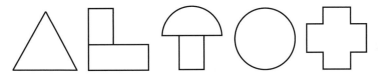

Figure 13.4 Shapes to copy
After: Mesulam, M-M. (1985). *Principles of Behavioral Neurology.* Philadelphia: FA Davis.

airplane–bicycle, axe–saw, fly–tree. Errors range from recognizing a common attribute of the items rather than their common category (e.g. "they have wheels" for airplane–bicycle) to being unable to offer an answer. Three of the five pairs should be recalled after a 10 minute delay. Cuing can be used to distinguish patients who can acquire new information but have difficulty recalling it from those who cannot acquire the information. Cuing statements for the pairs are their similarity. For the items above, the patient is cued with: fruit, directions, transport, tools, and living things.

Verbal absurdities: Understanding verbal absurdities requires reasoning. The patient is asked to consider if there is anything wrong with the following statement, and if so what that might be:

"A man had the flu twice. The first time he died, but the second time he recovered."

"The railroad company discovered that in train accidents the first and the last cars of the train are usually the most damaged. So, to save money they are now going to send trains out of the station without the first and last cars."

These statements seem ridiculously obvious to the novice examiner, but experienced clinicians know the poignancy of watching a PhD or CEO offer a concrete answer such as "Well, you don't need the last car, but you need the first one to pull the train."

Table 13.4. Behavioral warning signs of frontal–temporal dementia

Increasing disinterest and reduced engagement in hobbies

Decreasing efficiency noted in work and household routines not explained by disease or injury

Any personality change (e.g. becoming uncharacteristically unreliable, hedonistic, overly critical)

Altered emotional expression (e.g. moodiness, irritability, apathetic)

Deterioration in personal hygiene, eating habits, social graces and manners

Forgetting to remember (e.g. missing appointments, not doing a chore)

Assessing for frontal–temporal dementia

Frontal–temporal dementia is increasingly recognized. It is associated with many conditions including chronic alcoholism, microvascular disease, HIV/AIDS, and Lewy body disease.[26] Frontal–temporal dementia is characterized by behavioral change in emotional expression and personality, abnormal motor function, and cognitive decline, particularly in executive function.

Behavior change is commonly the earliest sign of frontal–temporal dementia. Personality alterations occur, the patient becoming disinhibited or apathetic, depending on which frontal area is affected first. Socially inappropriate behaviors emerge (e.g. sexual touching of self or others, seductiveness, blunt commentary, use of profanity). Attention to grooming and hygiene is reduced. Tact and table manners deteriorate. Suspiciousness and irritability occur. Efficiency is reduced and a decline in planning ability leads to employment and interpersonal difficulties. Atypical mood symptoms occur and may be misconstrued as depressive illness or hypomania. Behavioral warning signs of frontal–temporal dementia are listed in Table 13.4.

Motor signs are almost always found in patients with frontal–temporal dementia. Prefrontal cortex disease is associated with motor regulatory problems. Basal ganglia disease is associated with mood and working memory problems and classic basal ganglia motor signs. Disease in both regions elicits catatonic features. Thalamic lesions are associated with mood and perceptual changes. Left basal ganglia and thalamic lesions are associated with speech and language problems. White matter disease is associated with bradykinesia and bradyphrenia.

Cognitive deficits associated with frontal circuitry dysfunction occur early in the illness progression of frontal–temporal dementia, and include decline in working memory, new learning, thinking and reasoning, and executive functioning.

The *auditory "A" test* may show errors of commission suggestive of distractibility. *Digit span* performance may be mildly impaired. Performance on *similarities* will decline as the difficulty of the task increases. *Recall of similarities* will be below expectations, but may improve with cueing or by recognition of the just worked on similarities when they are embedded in lists of novel choices. The patient may understand the *verbal absurdity* of the "man with the flu" but may give a concrete answer to the train statement.

Fluency of ideas and problem solving abilities deteriorate in frontal–temporal dementia. Idea fluency is assessed with the *animal naming test.* The patient is asked to name as many animals as he can. The time cut-off is one minute. Normal persons with at least a high school education can name 15 or more animals. Ten or more is acceptable for persons over 80 years of age. Perseverative animal names are counted only once, thus dog, poodle, retriever gains only one point, as does white horse, black horse, and pinto. The most efficient strategy is to begin with the first animal that comes to mind and staying with that category of animal until recall slows and then quickly switching to another category until that too seems exhausted, then switching again, and so on. Executive function and cognitive flexibility must be adequate to perform the task well.

Problem solving is another assessment of thinking impacted by frontal circuitry disease. It is assessed by asking the patient to solve the following:

"If I had three apples and you had four more than I, how many would you have?"

"If you had 18 books and wanted to place them on two different book shelves so that one shelf had twice as many books as the other, how many would be on each shelf?"

Patients with a frontal–temporal dementia perform adequately on perceptual–motor tasks. Early on in the course of illness, memory disturbances will respond to cueing and recognition. Praxis is normal. An example follows.[27]

Patient 13.4

A 70-year-old man experienced decreased functioning over a two-year period. He was becoming more forgetful, had trouble keeping the family accounts, and was distressed that he could no longer remember the names of close friends. His wife observed him urinating in the sink and when challenged, he said that it was to "save water". He purchased several hundred nut trees without good reason, poured several boxes of detergent into the washing machine at one time, wandered in his conversation and became irritable and stamped his foot in anger when challenged. Irritability alternated with inappropriate jocularity. Unlike his past behavior, he was openly amorous toward his wife. He had paraphasic speech, echophenomena, and motor aprosodia. He became gluttonous, incontinent of urine and feces and unable to care for himself. His visual and verbal memory, however, were initially normal. Reading ability was preserved. Brain imaging revealed frontal atrophy.

Table 13.5. Behavioral warning signs of Alzheimer's disease

Conversational word-finding difficulties

Increasing reliance on circumloculatory speech

Losing train of conversational thought and not remembering
  what point was trying to be made

Mixing memory details

Forgetting directions to familiar places

Confusing geographic direction

Frequent "fender-benders"

Misidentifying persons and faces

Forgetting to remember and increasing reliance on "to do" lists

Forgetting the purpose of a task once it is begun

Subtle personality changes, e.g. loss of motivation

Assessing for early Alzheimer's disease

The early signs of Alzheimer's disease include a decline in visual–spatial functioning and memory. Behavioral warning signs of Alzheimer's disease are listed in Table 13.5. Their frequency and intensity distinguishes them from similar behavior seen in normal older persons.[28]

Visual–spatial function is assessed by asking the patient to copy shapes, and testing for body and spatial orientation, and praxis. Both visual and verbal memory is also assessed in the evaluation for Alzheimer's disease.

Body and spatial orientation: Patients with pervasive parietal lobe disease have difficulty with the perception of space and their body orientation within three-dimensional space. When the non-dominant parietal lobe is affected they neglect the left side of space and their body. Men fail to shave on the left side, men and women fail to comb the left side of the head. They may crash into objects on their left and may fall, injuring themselves as they "lose" the location of their left limbs. They are unaware of the deficit, exhibit *anosagnosia*, and offer feeble excuses when pressured to explain the problem. Some patients deny their left-sided paralysis, and offer excuses such as "I sprained by arm ... I'm tired today". Clock drawing and copying of geometric shapes also reveal left spatial neglect.[29]

Topographic orientation: Patients with visual–spatial problems have difficulty orienting themselves to direction, such as correctly answering the question, "If North were directly behind you, were would East be?" To successfully point to their left, the patient must be able to have a representation of a map in their visual memory and then be able to rotate the map from its usually "read" position were North is "up" and East is to the right.

Right/left orientation: In addition to accurately perceiving the left and right sides of the body, the person without brain disease can coordinate motor performance with the perception. This is tested by asking the patient to place his hand on a body part that requires crossing the midline with such questions as, "Place your left hand on your right ear . . . place your right hand on your left elbow." Persons with dominant parietal lobe disease have difficulty with this task.[30]

Praxis: Praxis is tested by asking the patient to do simple motor tasks (see Chapter 7). Patients with dominant frontal–parietal disease will have difficulties with these efforts.

Copying geometric shapes (see above) is used to assess visual–motor coordination.

Verbal and visual memory is assessed by asking the patient to recall some aspect of a previously performed task, such as recalling the geometric shapes previously copied and the objects considered in similarities. Recalling the types of tests in the evaluation assesses memory for events, or episodic memory.

Assessing for amnestic syndromes

Amnestic syndromes are defined as a memory disturbance associated with substantial decline from previous social or occupational functioning. New learning or recall of previously learned information is impaired. The disturbance does not occur exclusively during a delirium or a dementia, and persists beyond the usual duration of states of intoxication or withdrawal.

Memory, however, is not a single process easily assessed by one screening test. The MMSE does not test visual memory. Its three-word immediate and five-minute recall item is a perfunctory assessment of verbal new learning and recall. It is also insensitive to the different patterns of impairment seen in the different dementias. Patients with Alzheimer's dementia have deficits in new learning, whereas those with subcortical dementia have difficulty in retrieving information previously learned.[31] Small but strategically located lesions can cause problems in one aspect of memory but not others. Transient global amnesia is discussed in Chapter 6 as a reflection of several acute neurologic conditions of short duration. When an amnestic syndrome is suspected, all the stages of memory are assessed. A structured assessment is time-consuming and requires expertise.[32]

It is also important to define the characteristics of the emergence of memory deficits. Amnesia due to stroke occurs suddenly. Amnesia from degenerative diseases emerges slowly. Table 13.6 displays the pattern of emergence of the amnestic disorders.[33]

Table 13.6. Patterns of onset of amnestic disorders

Onset	Disorders
Sudden	Amnestic strokes
	Diencephalic or inferomedial temporal traumatic lesions
	Spontaneous subarachnoid hemorrhage
	Carbon monoxide poisoning and hypoxia
	Post-surgical amnesia
Subacute	Acute and chronic depression and mania are associated with substantial deficits in frontal circuitry-related cognitive functions
	Wernicke–Korsakoff's syndrome
	Post-infection
	Posttraumatic stress disorder and other anxiety disorders are associated with problems in working memory, sustained attention and new learning
	Parkinson's disease
Slow	Alzheimer's disease
	Pick's disease
	Prion disease

Working memory

Working memory is a sensory perception[34] or a thought that is "held" for about 30 seconds while the person decides what to do with that information. Working memory requires adequate attention. A common example of working memory is asking for a phone number and "holding" the number long enough to go to the phone and press in the numbers.

Working memory is assessed by digit span and similar tests. Attention is always assessed before testing for working memory. Working memory is always assessed before proceeding with other memory assessments, all of which are dependent on adequate attention and working memory. Many psychiatric disturbances affect working memory, including melancholia, mania, psychosis, and toxic states.

Declarative memory

Declarative memory is the process in which information is learned deliberately and the learning explicitly demonstrated through recall of the information. It has two forms: semantic and episodic memory.

Semantic memory is verbally based, detailed public information, the knowledge of which can be explicitly demonstrated, such as naming all the countries in South America, or the 12 pairs of cranial nerves.[35] Semantic memory is often assessed by testing the patient's fund of information. This information is greatly influenced by education, and includes such things as naming the presidents or prime ministers of the country, capital cities, and prominent geographic places and their relationships. The new learning of semantic information is assessed by asking the patient to learn and later recall several items.[36] Recalling the items in the similarities test is used for this purpose.

Episodic (autobiographical) memory is memory for information known only to a person being tested and to "others who were there at the time". Examples include a particular birthday party and a first date. Episodic memory can be assessed by asking the patient at the end of the testing procedures to describe the tasks that were asked and other events that occurred during the evaluation. History-taking also assesses the patient's episodic memory.

Anterograde and retrograde amnesia

When episodic and semantic memories are poorly acquired or retrieved, new learning is impaired. The patient is said to have anterograde amnesia. Mild to severe anterograde amnesia occurs after closed head injuries. The longer the period of anterograde amnesia following the injury, the more likely there will be problems later in life (e.g. seizures, behavioral syndromes).[37] The patient appears unsure and interacts as if some recent events did not occur, or they are unable to recall recent event-related information. Subjectively patient's describe feeling "fuzzy headed" and as if "in a fog".

Delayed recall of rehearsed verbal (similarities) and visual information (shapes) is one test for anterograde amnesia. Anterograde amnesia is associated with lesions involving the temporal lobes and the diencephalon. Occipital lobe lesions are also associated with visual anterograde amnesia.[38] During a course of ECT about half of patients experience temporary anterograde amnesia that resolves in 2–6 weeks following the last treatment.[39]

Retrograde amnesia refers to the loss of previously acquired information. Most amnestic syndromes are defined by substantial retrograde amnesia.

Meta-memory

Meta-memory is the subjective judgment about one's own memory capabilities. It is influenced by the present state of emotion. Patients who are depressed subjectively experience their performance to be worse than in fact, while those in mania or with the frontal lobe disinhibited syndrome experience their performance to be better than in fact. Patients with temporal lobe epilepsy overestimate their memory capacities and their self-monitoring is less accurate for verbal or non-verbal recall depending on the side of the seizure focus.[40]

Procedural memory

Procedural memory is information and motor-related skills that are learned through repeated exposure and practice, such as riding a bicycle and performing the medical physical examination. Unlike declarative memory, the acquisition of procedural memory cannot be demonstrated by describing what is done, but only by performing the procedure. The carrying out of the task or procedure demonstrates the learning, thus procedural memory is implicit memory. Procedural memory is assessed by asking the patient to demonstrate previously learned skills.

Free recall

Free recall is remembering spontaneously without cues. Free recall is demonstrated when the patient relates his past hospitalizations and treatments without undue prompting. Free recall is influenced by the state of emotion. Being sad is associated with the spontaneous recollection of unhappy experiences, while being happy is associated with the recall of happy events.[41]

Recognition

Recognition is remembering from cues. Examples are the patient remembering a past medication only when the examiner mentions it, recalling rehearsed items only when the examiner gives the patient several choices, and identifying the items on the similarities test only when the examiner provides the category (e.g. "They were tools" to cue the similarity hammer–chainsaw). Persons with cortical dementias such as in the early stages of Alzheimer's disease have impaired free recall and recognition. Cueing does not help. Persons with subcortical dementias such as in Binswanger's disease (subcortical ischemic disease) or Parkinson's disease have impaired free recall but adequate recognition with cueing.

Assessing for cerebral hemisphere disease

Patients with traumatic brain injury, stroke, space-occupying lesions, and seizure disorder often have circumscribed lesions and corresponding cognitive dysfunction. Bedside tests of left cerebral hemisphere functioning are displayed in Table 13.7. They reflect the substantial language functioning of the left hemisphere.

Table 13.8 displays bedside cognitive tests of right cerebral hemisphere functioning.[42]

Distinguishing cortical from subcortical disease[43]

There are characteristically different behavioral changes associated with cortical and subcortical disease. The region of dysfunction shapes differential diagnosis.

Table 13.7. Bedside left cerebral hemisphere cognitive tests

Tests of the right hand for motor regulation
Ideo-motor praxis
Right/left orientation
Assessment for speech and lexical language including reading
   and writing
Calculations
Finger gnosis
Verbal problem-solving (3 plus 4 apples, 18 books)
Abstract thinking (similarities)
Fluency of ideas (animal naming)
Verbal reasoning (absurdities)
Right hand stereognosia
Right hand graphesthesia

Table 13.8. Bedside right cerebral hemisphere cognitive tests

Motor and receptive prosody
Tests of motor regulation of the left hand
Copying shapes
Visual memory
Assessing for left-side spatial neglect
Facial recognition
Left hand stereognosia
Left hand graphesthesia

Cortical disease is more often associated with aphasia, agnosia, and apraxia, and thinking problems. Subcortical disease is more often associated with bradykinesia and bradyphrenia. Using the motor system to circumscribe the disease process is particularly helpful in differentiating cortical from subcortical disease. In addition to bradykinesia, subcortical disease is more likely associated with basal ganglia or cerebellar features. Thalamic disease is associated with problems with proprioception and somatosensory function.

Summary

Behavior change is the most subtle expression of brain function and dysfunction, and all behavior has a cognitive component. Understanding the neurologic implications of specific forms of psychopathology therefore facilitates the cognitive examination. Common considerations in cognitive assessment are delirium, frontal dementia versus Alzheimer's disease, amnestic syndromes, subcortical versus cortical disease, and left versus right cerebral hemisphere disease.

Many classic psychiatric syndromes are associated with cognitive difficulties and some syndromes are delineated by the presence of cognitive impairment (e.g. melancholia versus non-melancholic depression). Cognitive assessment is therefore part of a thorough behavioral evaluation and is not limited to those patients suspected of having a brain lesion. Cognitive assessment is important for diagnosis, estimating prognosis, treatment planning, and the monitoring of treatments.

NOTES

1 Kahlbaum (1874/1973), page 4.
2 Taylor and Fink (2006).
3 Bowie *et al.* (2004); Sapara *et al.* (2007).
4 Purcell *et al.* (1998); Chamberlain *et al.* (2007).
5 Duara *et al.* (1999).
6 Fielding *et al.* (2006); Chang *et al.* (2007).
7 Feinberg and Roane (2005).
8 Critchley (1953); Maruff *et al.* (2005); Ishii *et al.* (2006).
9 Gouzoulis-Mayfrank *et al.* (2000); Cunha *et al.* (2004); Reay *et al.* (2006).
10 APA (2001).
11 Taylor and Fink (2006), chapters 6 and 12.
12 Tippett and Sergio (2006).
13 See previous chapters for discussions of the specific associations of psychopathology and cognitive dysfunction.
14 The WAIS (The Wechsler Adult Intelligence Scale) was one of the earliest psychological test batteries used as a cognitive assessment instrument rather than as a measure of IQ only. The age-corrected norm is about 100. Patient 13.3 was seen by one of us many years ago. Today, several bedside tests would have revealed his deficits as clearly as did the WAIS.
15 For further reading about cognitive testing and neuropsychological concepts that underlie testing, see Taylor (1999, chapters 1 and 4), Kolb and Whishaw (1996), and Lezak *et al.* (2004).
16 Gillis and MacDonald (2006).
17 There are exceptions. Anticholinergic intoxication is characterized by dry skin and mucosa, a facial flush, dilated pupils, tachycardia, and low-grade fever. Wernicke's encephalopathy is characterized by nystagmus, ophthalmoplegia, and peripheral neuropathy. Delirium tremens is characterized by a coarse bilateral tremor and often the patient has other signs of chronic alcoholism.
18 Amieva *et al.* (2004); Helmer *et al.* (2006).
19 Draper (1991).
20 Lopez *et al.* (2005).

21 Amieva *et al.* (2004).

22 See Lezak *et al.* (2004) for discussions of these and other cognitive tests.

23 The digit symbol substitution test from the WAIS is another test sensitive to early cognitive decline. It requires the patient to draw a symbol from an array that corresponds to a number in the box below each number. The test is timed and very sensitive to problems with new learning. It is usually administered as part of a broader neuropsychological test battery.

24 Lepore *et al.* (2004).

25 Mesulam (2000).

26 McKhann *et al.* (2001); Lopez-Pousa *et al.* (2002); Burn (2006).

27 Graff-Radford *et al.* (1995).

28 Strokes in the angular gyrus of the dominant parietal lobe are associated with some aphasic speech, problems with reading and writing, poor understanding of complex sentences and constructional problems that can elicit the misdiagnosis of Alzheimer's disease. Patients with the angular gyrus syndrome have better memory functioning, and visual–spatial function is better preserved than in Alzheimer's disease (Cummings, 1985a, p. 29; Lepore *et al.*, 2004).

29 Critchley (1953); Luria (1973, chapter 5); Kirshner and Lavin (2006).

30 Right/left disorientation when associated with dyscalculia (poor calculation ability), dysgraphia (poor construction of writing), and finger agnosia (being unable to identify one's fingers when interlaced) form the Gertsmann's syndrome that has been linked to lesions in the angular gyrus of the left parietal lobe (Roeltgen *et al.*, 1983).

31 Libon *et al.* (2001); Graham *et al.* (2004). While many studies report distinguishing cognitive problems between patients with Alzheimer's disease and those with subcortical dementias, some do not (Arango-Lasprilla *et al.*, 2006).

32 The Wechsler Memory scale batteries are the most commonly used formal memory tests. The batteries include verbal and non-verbal measures of spontaneous recall of newly learned material and the ability to recognize previously presented material. Other tests used include the Rey Auditory Verbal Learning Test, Benton's Visual Retention test and the California Verbal Learning Test (see Lezak *et al.*, 2004).

33 Lezak *et al.* (2004).

34 Miyashita (2004).

35 Semantic memory is subserved by the *hippocampus, parahippocampus, entorhinal cortex and perirhinal cortex* (Miyashita, 2004).

36 Rizzo *et al.* (2002); Snowden *et al.* (2004).

37 Feinstein *et al.* (2002); Drake *et al.* (2006).

38 Squire and Zola (1997).

39 Abrams (2002).

40 Prevey *et al.* (1988).

41 Surguladze *et al.* (2005).

42 Ibid.

43 Meyer *et al.* (1996); Loeb and Meyer (1996).

14

Personality

People wished to reduce to calculus even the art of healing; the human body, this so complicated machine, was treated by our medical algebraists as if it were the simplest machine and the easiest to analyze.[1]

Each person has a unique personality, but personality types are recognized and provide clinically useful information. Will the patient comply with treatments? Does the patient have the perseverance to continue rehabilitation? Is the patient likely to respond positively to the therapist's praise? Will the patient take advice? Some behaviors (e.g. alcohol, tobacco and illicit drug use, adopting a healthy lifestyle, engaging in "safe" sexual practices) are predicted from the patient's personality. These concerns affect patient care and are relevant to all patients. This chapter outlines the history leading to the present understanding of normal personality, and details personality structure and how to assess for it.

Theories of personality

For much of the history of psychiatry, the humoral theory of illness and personality dominated Western medical thinking and society's views of what "made people tick". This construct prevailed until the nineteenth century when it was replaced by phrenology. However, humoral constructs remain with us as descriptors of personality (e.g. sanguine, choleric, and phlegmatic).

Phrenology and body type

Franz Joseph Gall was an early proponent of the idea that cognitive processes reflected function in specific brain regions. He proposed that as brain structures developed they influenced the developing skull and facial features, and that an examination of the external aspects of the head would reveal the brain's localized differences and thus functions, including temperament. Gall's *phrenology* dominated nineteenth-century European thought about personality.[2] Kretschmer and

Sheldon's empirical efforts (among many others) to relate body type to illness and temperature (particularly Janet's constructs of *extraversion* and *introversion*) were outgrowths of phrenology.[3] Their construct was that personality, like body type, was the result of maturational processes. This idea foreshadowed present understanding of personality.

Psychopathic constitutions

Nineteenth-century efforts at objective description of personality were inconsistent. The term "moral insanity" mixed constructs of disease and trait, initially meaning mood disorder and then antisocial personality.[4] The prevailing view was that deviant personality traits reflected a constitutional (i.e. biological) deficit.

Ernst von Feuchtersleben introduced the term *psychopathy* in 1845 to mean a constitutionally disordered personality *without* psychosis. Julius Ludwig August Koch elaborated this concept of *psychopathic inferiorities* in 1888, indicating a constitutional degeneration (the source of the word "degenerate") that expressed itself not as psychosis but as various trait behaviors, such as a lack of forcefulness, being weak-willed, and shy. Koch considered persons with these conditions at risk for psychiatric illness. Pierre Janet added hysterical personality as a predisposition to hysteria and neurosis in 1893.

In 1896, Bleuler opined about the "born criminal" and "pathological liars and swindlers". In 1915, his list of abnormal personality types included excitable, irresolute, hedonistic, eccentric, liars and swindlers, "enemies of society" (antisocial personality), and the quarrelsome. Kraepelin presented his classification of psychopathic personalities in the 1904 seventh edition of his textbook. Kraepelin also considered these conditions to be trait deviations.[5]

In the twentieth century, Kurt Schneider offered a descriptive classification of personality disorders which he defined in the modern sense of maladaptive trait behavior causing the patient or others to suffer. He considered personality and personality disorder to reflect individual "constitution", the result of biological maturation modified by environment. Schneider used the terms "psychopathy" and "psychopath" as generic terms for personality disorder. His efforts were based on extensive clinical experience rather than empirical study.[6] Schneider's topology influenced German and British clinicians for decades until replaced by the ICD-10 formulation.

Psychoanalytic theory

Sigmund Freud offered another view of personality with three major components interacting unconsciously in a dynamic tension, thus "the dynamic unconscious". The *id* represented inborn immutable instinctive drives seeking expression without regard for reality. The *ego* represented mechanisms of adaptation to reality.

The *superego* represented internalized social prohibitions modulating the instinctive impulses. The ego was also hypothesized as an arbitrator between the id and superego. Too much id or superego, or too fragile an ego, was said to cause personality deviation and, when extreme, neurosis or even psychosis. The balance or imbalance evolved over several psychosexual stages in childhood. Psychoanalysis was envisioned as the process that would reveal the patient's id, ego and superego relationships and the reasons for them. Through an understanding of interactions with the therapist that mirrored the patient's relationships with parental figures (transference), the patient would gain emotional insight and subsequent personality change. Freud's contemporaries such as Jung and Adler,[7] and the "neo-Freudians" such as Karen Horney, Harry Stack Sullivan, Erich Fromm, and Erik Erikson spread psychoanalytic notions, but did not influence psychiatric classification.

In 1909, Freud gave a series of lectures at Clark University in Worcester, Massachusetts, introducing psychoanalysis to the USA. No individual in the twentieth century had a greater influence on American psychiatry and culture. For the next 50 years, psychoanalytic thought dominated psychiatric research and treatment in the USA, and psychoanalysts dominated training programs. From the end of WWII until the 1970s, almost all academic chairs in psychiatry were fully trained psychoanalysts. Despite few current psychiatrists in the USA considering themselves psychoanalysts, the psychoanalytic movement still influences accreditation guidelines for psychiatric residency training programs and DSM and ICD formulations.

Pop culture, literature, the visual and performing arts also consistently present a psychoanalytic view of reality and of human nature. Modern actors "analyze" their "character" searching for "motivations" for the character's actions, a direct link to Freudian theory. Shakespeare, by contrast, indicates no interest in his characters' motivations, yet he is first among Western playwrights and is said to have "invented" by demonstration the modern person. Elizabethan actors played parts not characters.[8]

Learning theory and biology

The most serious early challenge to the Freudian view of human nature came from learning theorists, who proposed that much of human behavior, including abnormal behavior, was learned and therefore could be unlearned.[9] They documented the poor efficacy of psychoanalytic-based treatments,[10] and offered classical and operant conditioning paradigms as processes underlying phobias and other neurotic disorders.[11] Behavior therapy, based on learning theories, was quickly shown to be effective for phobias, and in the late 1970s, after years of acrimonious debate, became the standard treatment for those conditions.[12] The introduction of cognitive behavior therapy further narrowed the perceived indications for psychoanalysis.[13]

Early empirical studies of personality structure

None of the old theories of personality, however, with the exception of Kretchmer's work on body type, was empirically derived, and none was predictive of co-occurring psychiatric illness, course, or treatment response. Empirical study of personality development only became practical with the development of factor analysis, a statistical method permitting a search for patterns of data within a large database. The inquiry began with the recruitment of large samples of non-ill persons who were questioned about their habitual responses and feelings in varying circumstances. The responses were subjected to factor analysis, and the factors that emerged (patterns of behavior) were used to develop new questionnaires. The process was expanded, repeated in different age groups, in both genders, and in populations worldwide.[14] Pioneers in this approach included Francis Galton, Cyril Burt, Lloyd Thurstone, Raymond Cattell,[15] and Gordon Allport. In parallel to this work, the Minnesota Multiphasic Personality Inventory (MMPI) was developed for clinical use and was widely adopted. However, it mixes illness categories such as depression and psychosis with scales for hysteria and other traits.[16]

Early intelligence testing also evolved by similar methodology. In the early 1900s, Alfred Binet was the first to systematically employ such measures. The work of Lewis Terman at Stanford University revised Binet's scale as the Stanford–Binet intelligence test that is still in use.

An extension of the empirical study of normal personality was the work of Tyrer and Alexander, who used cluster analytic techniques to examine the natural groupings of persons with personality trait deviation. Unlike the later DSM formulations, they focused on psychopathology that could be observed, rather than on the social and interpersonal consequences of abnormal behavior.[17] Their work influenced British psychiatrists, but is little known in the USA.

Recent study of personality

Statistical modeling studies of personality continue to refine the image of personality structure.[18] The factors that have emerged are interpreted within the conceptual framework that personality traits, like other behavior, are a product of the brain and have biological meaning. Studies focus on the heritability of traits and the neurologic structures and functions that underlie traits. Personality traits are also studied using physiologic and other biologic measures.[19] Although there are no complete animal models of personality, researchers compare human trait behavior to the highly heritable trait behaviors of laboratory animals. Gray proposed three fundamental behavioral traits: *behavioral activation, behavioral maintenance,* and *behavioral inhibition* as tendencies to react in specific situations.[20]

Several specific neural networks subserving the broad personality traits are proposed. These networks roughly follow the distribution within frontal–limbic structures of the major neurotransmitter systems dopamine, norepinephrine, and serotonin. Behavior inhibition is said to be mediated by serotonin, behavioral activation by dopamine, and behavioral maintenance by norepinephrine.[21]

These traits are found in many species, including humans and are strongly and independently inheritable. Cloninger *et al.* (1993) further developed the concept and proposed the temperament dimensions of *novelty seeking, harm avoidance* and *reward dependence.* A centerpiece of this work is the application of behavioral genetics to personality structure and to individual differences in personality traits.

Behavioral genetic investigators use large samples that permit analysis of small but meaningful individual differences and complex multiple interactions that further clarify trait patterns.[22] Twin pairs, some reared together and other reared apart, are assessed for personality trait similarities and differences. Adopted children are examined to see if they are more like their biological parents and siblings or more like their adoptive parents. Cross-fostering studies also examine the similarities and differences among the foster and biological children in families. Genetic models test the results of the family and twin studies, and gene mapping assesses likely candidate genes.[23] Traits considered to have high heritability are examined for neurochemical and neuroanatomic relationships.[24]

Despite the gains made in understanding personality as a grouping of temperaments that are dimensional, psychiatric classifications continues to formulate personality disorder as categorical. If the person meets a set of criteria the diagnosis is confirmed. If the person does not meet criteria, personality disorder is not diagnosed. Based on the ideas of Theodore Millon, DSM-III and subsequent iterations offered three major categories, *odd–eccentric, dramatic–histrionic,* and *anxious–fearful,* arranged from most to the least severe. Additional revisions added *organic personality disorder* and personality changes secondary to an identifiable cause. In the DSM-IV, this was changed to *personality changes due to a general medical condition.*

However, despite severe criticism of this formulation[25] (also see below), present and proposed DSM and ICD iterations adhere to the categorical notion of Axis II and the inclusion of the problematic conditions (e.g. odd–eccentric types) more from inertia than a lack of understanding.[26]

Present-day image of normal personality

Personality is a pattern of stable, highly heritable, habitual tendencies to respond to specific circumstances, particularly those involving reward or non-reward. The tendencies predict how a person will respond most of the time when confronted with a new situation (novelty), praise, affection, monetary compensation (rewards), and punishment, criticism, or disappointment (non-reward). The pattern is individually characteristic and is formed during the person's formative years and then changes little, except when altered by traumatic brain injury or disease (stroke, epilepsy, chronic mood disorder, degenerative brain disease, and chronic illicit drug use).[27]

Personality patterns are composed of quantified trait dimensions. The dimensions have low and high poles, indicating the strength of expression. These "higher-order" dimensions are in turn composed of a number of "lower-order" subtraits, accounting for the many subtle differences among individuals.[28] A person can have a score anywhere on a dimension, most persons scoring in the middle or normal range for that trait. Low and high scores are by definition abnormal, reflecting deviation from the norm, not pathology. A score on one trait does not predict scores on other traits. Persons with several abnormal traits are defined as having abnormal personalities.

Deviance, however, does not imply disease or dysfunction. Firefighters and police officers score very high (i.e. abnormal or deviant) on dimensions that measure exploratory behaviors in novel situations, traits needed to do their jobs. Similarly, missionaries and relief workers are abnormally high on dimensions of sentimentality and cooperativeness.[29]

Personality structure refers to the big traits and their component subtraits. This structure is shared by all humans as are other body structures, such as the human face and hand. Males and females have the same basic "floor plan", and personality traits are normally distributed in both genders. Women, however, tend to score higher on traits that measure cooperativeness and the tendency to maintain behaviors that elicit external reward.[30]

The number of personality traits and subtraits delineated by research groups varies, but there is substantial overlap on subtraits and unanimity on the hierarchical big picture. Eysenck introduced the dimensional construct of personality to psychiatric diagnosis over 40 years ago, defining *neuroticism, extraversion,* and *psychoticism.*[31] The traditional factor analytic studies of personality generated "The 5-factor model" that describes neuroticism, extraversion, openness to experience, agreeableness, and conscientiousness.[32] Cloninger and colleagues offer a combination of temperaments and character traits. The temperaments are harm avoidance, novelty seeking, reward dependence, and persistence. The character traits are self-directedness, cooperativeness, and self-transcendence.[33] Siever and Davis and colleagues define four dimensions: emotional dysregulation, dissocial behavior, anxiety/inhibition, and compulsivity.[34] Bedside testing for personality simplifies this array of overlapping views of trait dimensions.

The neural systems for emotion and personality overlap and personality traits modulate emotional expression, but emotional expression is also independent of

Table 14.1. Behavioral traits with high heritability

Aggressiveness	Nurturance
Altruism	Persistence
Assertiveness	Physicality
Constraint	Reward dependence
Empathy	Social closeness
Harm avoidance	Sociability
Impulsivity	Traditionalism
Leadership	Wellbeing
Novelty seeking	

personality, and normal persons with dramatically different personalities still express the same range of emotions. Intelligence also modestly interacts with personality, the higher a person's intelligence the lower is the person's score on personality measures of conformity.[35]

Temperament traits have high heritability (about 50%) and each has a putative neuroanatomic and neurochemical substrate. Two types of gene–environment interactions are proposed.[36]

Shared environmental refers to common experience. Shared environment that is considered culturally and interpersonally typical has only a weak affect on individual differences in personality development. This includes mostly pre-school, parent-related experiences. Shared environment, however, plays more of a role when conditions are pathological, e.g. an abusive or chronically ill parent.[37]

Non-shared environmental experience substantially impacts trait development. The impact can be on the phenotypic trait expression or directly on genes by influencing transcription factors. Examples of non-shared environmental influences include intrauterine events, illness-related childhood experiences, playground, school and peer influences, viral infection, and illicit drug use. Individual differences are explained by the astronomically high possibilities of the combined strengths of expression of each trait, each the result of gene expression and unique experience.[38]

Table 14.1 displays some of the more easily recognized traits with high heritability.

Examining for personality traits

Personality traits are long-standing behaviors. Questions that will accurately elicit traits need to reflect the continuity of these behaviors. The patient needs to understand that the examiner is asking about the patient's *typical, most-of-the-time, everyday self when not ill.* Obtaining information from the patient's perspective and what others might think can provide a picture of the temperament pattern. For patients with chronic illness, the task is more difficult and may only succeed with information from family members. Using collateral information is standard in the assessment of children and adolescents and for patients with cognitive difficulties, and should not be thought a burden when assessing the patient's personality.

Because personality traits represent tendencies to behave in *circumstances of reward* (e.g. praise, affection, money, and position), or *non-reward* (e.g. criticism, coldness, and non-recognition), these kinds of situations become the focus of questions, rather than the social consequences of the behavior. Asking a person who grew up in a gang-infested urban area about fighting and using a weapon may not provide a reliable measure of how aggressive they are. Learning about the patient's response to meeting new persons will reveal more about their temperament than just determining the number of their friends. More specific temperament questions also focus on the person's tendency to be irritable, impulsive, and physical. Three broadly defined behavior areas frame the examination.

Behavioral inhibition. The tendency toward behavioral inhibition with avoidance of situations that are novel, unrewarding or socially difficult is associated with shyness and anxious–fearfulness (cluster C in Axis II of the DSM). Substantial tendencies toward behavioral inhibition also associates with low assertiveness, low impulsivity, low physicality and wellbeing, and high constraint and harm avoidance. It is assessed with questions such as:

"Do you think you're a nervous person? Are you high-strung?"

"Are you the kind of person who worries a lot … who usually worries about all the things that can go wrong with a plan or activity?"

"Are you an overly cautious person? Do you think about things too much rather than acting? Are you a timid or shy person?"

"Do others think of you as a nervous/shy/worrying/cautious person?"

"Do you prefer activities that are quiet with little physical activity? Do you get tired easily?"

Behavioral activation. The tendency toward behavioral approach and action is associated with high risk-taking, novelty seeking, assertiveness and aggressiveness, leadership, sociability and being physical. It also associates with low constraint and harm avoidance. Persons in the DSM Axis II cluster B category tend to be high on behavioral activation. It is assessed with questions such as:

"Are you the kind of a person who always likes to be busy … to be doing new and exciting activities, even if there is some risk?"

"Are you a high-energy, enthusiastic person?"

"Are you the kind of person who acts first and thinks about it afterward?"

"Are you quick-tempered and excitable? Do others think of you as an impulsive, excitable, risk-taking person?"

Table 14.2. High and low behavioral traits

Temperament dimension	High tendency	Low tendency
Behavioral inhibition	Anxious, worried, cautious, restrained, pessimistic, low-energy, shy, timid, fearful, full of doubt	Unrestrained, optimistic, confident, risk-taking, carefree, energetic, bold and vigorous, daring, undaunted
Behavioral activation	Impulsive, exploratory and curious, fickle, extravagant, disorderly, excitable, quick-tempered, easily bored, enthusiastic and exuberant	Orderly, reflective, loyal, frugal, rigid and regimented, slow-tempered, stoical, reserved, unenthusiastic, tolerant
Behavioral maintenance	Warm, good-hearted, loving, sensitive, dedicated, attached, industrious and diligent	Cold, detached, unfriendly, insensitive, indifferent, independent, lazy, easily deterred

Behavioral maintenance. Behavioral maintenance is the tendency to continue behaviors that are rewarded. The type of rewards to which the person is sensitive predicts associated traits. Thus some persons with a strong tendency toward behavioral maintenance will also be high on altruism, empathy, social closeness and nurturance. Others will be high on persistence. Persons said to have dependent or avoidant personality disorder tend to be high on behavioral maintenance. Behavioral maintenance is assessed with questions such as:

"Do you think of yourself as a friendly person … sensitive … unselfish … a good friend?"

"Do you prefer to be with people or do you prefer being alone? Do you prefer to work on your own or with a group of co-workers?"

"Are you sentimental?"

"Are you a hard worker? Do you give up easily or do you stick to the job, even after others want to give up?"

"Do other people think you're stubborn … reliable … cooperative?"

Table 14.2 displays descriptors of persons who are high or low on behavioral inhibition, activation, and maintenance. When the strength of the trait, high or low, is substantially distanced from the norm, dysfunction and distress is likely and the person will meet criteria for personality disorder. Persons high on behavioral inhibition appear similar to those labeled "anxious–fearful". Those high on behavioral activation and low on behavioral maintenance appear similar to persons with placed in the dramatic–emotional DSM category.

Deviance without psychopathology

Deviance indicates behaviors and characteristics that are not exhibited by the majority of the population. It does not automatically denote psychopathology. While psychopathology is always deviant, not all deviance is psychopathology. A *Vegan* has deviant eating behavior because the majority of persons are omnivorous. In contrast, an individual who does not eat meat and other animal products because he believes that all meat products are contaminated as part of a government conspiracy is likely delusional, and his deviant eating behavior indicates psychopathology.

In diverse societies, distinguishing deviance reflecting non-pathological variability from deviance reflecting illness is challenging. Many deviant sexual behaviors, for example, reflect obsessive–compulsive disorder and other illnesses. Many are non-pathological variants, and some are discussed here.

Gender identity and sexual orientation

Normal human sexual development requires the compatibility between genetic sex (sex chromosomes), gonads (testes or ovaries), genitalia (external and internal sex organs), other secondary sexual characteristics, and the congruent subjective experience of the gender. Gender consists of the identified sex of the person, and the person's gender role behaviors and sexual orientation (hetero- or homosexual).

While gender identity is modestly shaped by family and cultural influences such as rearing practices, peer gender-specific behaviors and individual traits, endogenous-generated developmental hormones elicit the process of sexual differentiation in humans.[39] Gender-specific steroids during the perinatal period, particularly testosterone, are crucial for the dimorphism of sexual behavior (male or female) in adulthood[40] and sexually dimorphic human brain structures develop between 4 and 7 months of gestation.[41]

Subjective gender identity incongruent with the assigned gender based on the appearance of the gentilia or their genetic sex is also under developmental hormonal influences.[42] In partial androgen insensitivity syndromes (a receptor problem), gender identity may be male or female with incongruity eliciting dysphoric states.[43] Persons with complete androgen sensitivity disorder are raised as females and do not exhibit confusion about gender identity.

Homosexuality

About 90% of humans are heterosexual, 1–2% are homosexual, and the rest are somewhere on the spectrum between the two distinct sexual orientations.

Homosexuality is found in humans and many other species.[44] A genetic effect is proposed based on its presence in many species, and in humans the high concordance among twins, increased prevalence in families of homosexual persons, and evidence of matrilineal heritability.[45] Sexually dimorphic brain structures of homosexual persons are less masculinized in male homosexuals.[46] A selective advantage of a "gay" genotype is proposed that parallels the construct of sickle-cell trait versus sickle-cell disease, the heterozygote having some selective advantage (e.g. being more attractive to the opposite gender). Among exclusive homosexuals, kin altruism is the proposed advantage, gay aunts and uncles without offspring providing extra resources to their nieces and nephews.[47]

Homosexuality is not a lifestyle choice, nor is it considered a form of illness by most neuroscientists. Psychoanalytic explanations of homosexuality are discredited. Homosexual persons, however, are at greater risk for sexually transmitted disease.[48] Their suicide rates may also be higher.[49] Studies comparing homosexual and heterosexual drug abusers have found more severe drug abuse, anxiety and risk of suicide in homosexuals.[50] Homosexual men also have increased risk of suicide even without substance abuse.[51] HIV or AIDS status does not significantly increase rates of depression in homosexual men, but homosexual men as a group do experience increased anxiety and depression.[52]

Transsexualism

Transsexuals are persons whose subjective experience of gender identity does not match their assigned gender at birth based on their normal external sexual characteristics. Transsexuals that come to medical attention state that nature has played a terrible trick on them and that they are "trapped" in a body of the other gender. The condition is rare, with the assigned male feeling female the more common situation.[53]

Transsexual persons experience their gender inconsistency early in life. Parents of boys with gender identity disorders report that at a very young age the boys insisting on being treated as girls and being dressed as girls.[54] Twin studies find increased heritability for gender identity disorder.[55] Genetically male transsexuals show a female pattern in sexually dimorphic nuclei of the hypothalamus, indicating an effect occurring during a critical stage of fetal development. Non-transsexual adult males who take estrogen for medical reasons do not show this pattern.[56]

DSM-IV uses the term *gender identity disorder* and requires the individual to exhibit significant distress or impairment in functioning without a concurrent physical intersex condition (see below). Increased anxiety and depression is reported in some transsexual persons and is termed *gender dysphoria*. This usually resolves after successful sexual reassignment surgery. Some patients, however, are reported to have co-occurring psychotic disorder with the transsexualism considered an epiphenomenon of the psychosis.[57] There is no significant increase in illicit drug use or alcohol abuse.[58]

Intersex

Persons identified as "intersex" have ambiguous external sexual characteristics. The condition is defined as a "congenital anomaly of the reproductive and sexual system". Intersex persons are born with external genitalia, internal reproductive organs, and endocrine systems that are deviant. There is no single intersex condition, and the term includes a wide variety of degrees of abnormality. Intersex is not an identity condition and intersex persons are biologically male or female and have a male or female identity.[59]

Normal personality under difficult circumstances

Life is not without difficulties. Death, separation, illness, social adversity, natural disasters are all stressful. Under stress, human behavior changes, sometimes dramatically. Dramatic changes under such circumstances, however, should not automatically be interpreted as deviant or psychopathological. That determination is made in the cultural context of the situation and the person's previous experience and circumstances. Patient 14.1 illustrates.

Patient 14.1

A psychiatry consult was requested by a surgical team to evaluate the capacity of a 56-year-old man to "refuse" care. The patient, a cancer survivor, was re-hospitalized because of fever of unknown origin, and after several days of extensive testing a complicated biopsy was recommended. The patient, demoralized and fatigued by the days of fever and testing, initially agreed, but asked his surgeons for a day or two advanced notification to "prepare" himself. On each of the previous three days when he asked if the biopsy was scheduled, he was told "not yet". Then without notification, on a Monday morning, an aide with a stretcher came to the patient's room to bring him to the biopsy suite. The patient, distraught and angry, refused. The psychiatric evaluation found him to be behaviorally and cognitively normal.

Bereavement

Normal bereavement and melancholia share some features (e.g. sadness, poor sleeping and appetite). Melancholia, however, is characterized by an abnormal emotional state that has a "life of its own" and a subjective quality that differs from the sadness following the death of a loved one. Motor, cognitive, and vegetative signs also define melancholia. Abnormal bereavement as defined in present classification is melancholic depression, transcends culture, and is a poor term that confuses illness with normal mourning behavior.

Normal bereavement is best understood within the context of the sufferer's family and culture. Cultural rituals, religious and family beliefs associated with death and dying, and the person's family role (e.g. dependent, head-of-household) shape normal bereavement. The circumstances of the death also affect the bereaved (e.g. suicide is less acceptable than accidental death). Patient 14.2 illustrates.

Patient 14.2

A 22-year-old Asian-American college student committed suicide by jumping from a third floor balcony. He had seen a college counselor for depression, who had recommended treatment. When the patient related his sadness to his family, however, he was told to work hard and pray. Immediately before his death, he asked his roommate to have lunch with him, but the roommate said he was busy and unable to go. After his death, the family refused to admit that he had committed suicide and erroneously maintained that his roommate and best friend had accidentally killed him by pushing him off the balcony.

Bereavement is worsened when the death is unexpected, random (e.g. in drive-by shootings), or involves other deaths (e.g. school shooting). The death of a long-time spouse has adverse social network consequences as well as being a personal loss. The death of a spouse may elicit greater sorrow than the death of a friend. The death of a parent is more traumatic for young children and adolescents than it is for adult children.[60] The death of one's child elicits a greater mourning than the death of a parent.[61]

Bereavement also varies in intensity and in associated behaviors across cultures, but is stereotypic within cultures. In Northern Europe, stoicism is the norm. The Irish typically throw a party where the participants often cry and laugh simultaneously. Telling humorous stories is in fashion at public memorials. In the Middle East, mourners scream, beat their chests, tear their hair, and collapse. Political and religious cults demand rapturous behavior in response to the death of their leaders.

Cultures vary in their display rules and have varying degrees of tolerance for expressing grief.[62] For example, a comparison of grief symptoms in Spanish and US men and women found that although both groups perceived loss of a loved one similarly, persons in the USA reported a more negative impact of bereavement, feeling more sense of loss, anger, loneliness, confusion, and guilt. Spaniards were more likely to accept mortality.[63]

Terminal illness

Patients during the terminal phase of illness experience anxiety and sadness. Cancer patients are the most studied. They, as other patients when terminally ill, also have concerns about family, friends, their body image, pain, finances, and how they will die. They may express guilt about a low mood and sadness, their anxiety and being slowed down and being unable to work and earn.[64] They may appear depressed, but demoralization is most likely, followed by depressive-like syndromes due to paraneoplastic disease and malnutrition. Consultant psychiatrists are often asked to see such patients to prescribe antidepressants and anxiolytics as if the behaviors were always signs of pathology. Patient 8.1, the Scottish woman who awoke weeks after her surgery to find her life dramatically altered, only needed "cheering up". Another example of demoralization follows.

Patient 14.3
A 49-year-old woman with incapacitating COPD was hospitalized for fever and a possible lung tumor. At baseline she was mildly anxious and demoralized. A bronchoscopy was advised, but in the discussion of potential problems from the procedure, the patient was told that her pulmonary status was so poor that the procedure might precipitate the need for intubation and that should that occur she might never be off a respirator. That possibility led to her refusal, even after being told that she might die in her present state. A psychiatry consultant was asked to evaluate her capacity.[65]

The patient, in bed and receiving nasal oxygen, was found to be alert, anxious, and tearful. She denied depression or being suicidal, but declared her life was already too restricted and the risk of permanently being on a respirator to be overwhelming: "The only thing left to me is talking to my children." Although she had some cognitive problems (e.g. poor animal naming and delayed recall), she understood the procedure, why it was recommended, her present state of health, and the possible consequences if the bronchoscopy was not done and no further treatments prescribed. The psychiatry consultant considered her to have the capacity to make the decision and recommended counseling, which the patient readily accepted.

Divorce

In societies in which divorce is highly stigmatized, more shame and guilt is experienced by divorcing couples. In male-dominated cultures the consequences are greater for women. Societies where divorce is more accepted, persons experience relief or anger depending on the conditions under which the divorce is taking place.

Divorced couples experience signs and symptoms similar to bereavement. The conflict between parents, loss of daily contact with one parent, and disruption of routines and place of residence associated with divorce affect children, who also experience signs and symptoms similar to bereavement. Children of divorced parents, depending on their age, exhibit sadness and aggressiveness, and transient academic difficulties.[66] Unless persistent, these behaviors do not indicate psychopathology.

Natural disaster

Acute stress reactions are common in persons who have been in a natural disaster (e.g. flood, tornado, and hurricane). These reactions are characterized by anxiety, sadness, and sleep disturbances, tremulousness, feeling of "shock" and numbness, and health-related complaints.[67]

Typically, symptoms abate within a month and for most such persons community support is all that is needed. The symptoms should not be considered psychopathology, as most persons under severe stress experience them and in most persons the symptoms resolve. Only a small proportion of persons with acute stress-related features develop chronic psychopathology following natural disasters.[68] The most salient risk factor for chronic PTSD is previous psychiatric illness. Other risk factors are female gender and the intensity of the subjective response to the acute trauma.[69]

Body injury

Painful and disfiguring body injury from accident, assault, and medical procedures also elicit acute stress responses characterized by sleep disturbance, anxiety, and sadness.[70] In children conduct problems and cognitive difficulties also occur.[71] A third to a half of burn victims experience a disabling stress response, particularly if the face is involved. Persons with pre-burn depressive illness or abnormal personality traits of low behavioral activation and high behavioral inhibition are at increased risk.[72]

Sexual trauma

Sexual traumas in childhood and adulthood have similar outcomes.[73] Sexual trauma in childhood is associated with subsequent depressive illness, eating and chronic anxiety disorder, substance abuse, and lability of emotional expression, impulsivity, and self-injury that elicits the diagnosis of borderline personality. Likely contributing factors rarely considered in studies of such patients are the high heritability of the behaviors and the effects of chronic trauma and substance abuse on the maturation of brain systems subserving the behaviors.[74] Assessment by standardized personality scales finds women who experienced childhood sexual trauma to be high on traits of behavioral inhibition and low on behavioral activation.[75] Chronic PTSD, non-melancholic depression, and to a lesser extent eating disorder may follow rape in adulthood.[76]

Combat, torture, and terrorist attack

Severe stress elicits a stress response in normal persons. A third to 50% of victims experience persistent symptoms up to 18 months post-trauma.[77] Alcoholism is common among combat veterans with persistent stress response symptoms, and this may contribute to the smaller hippocampal volumes reported in these persons.[78] Dissociative experiences during and immediately after the trauma are associated with intense panic during the event,[79] and may predict chronic symptoms, as does previous psychiatric illness,[80] persistent memory difficulties,[81] and brain injury from the event.[82]

Summary

Normal personality represents a complex interaction between maturational environment factors (e.g. parental care, nutrition and general medical health, unique experience early in life) and substantial genetic influences (e.g. multiple small genes with an additive effect[83]) that lead to characteristic individualized response patterns. The maturation process mostly occurs during the first two decades of life, and after that personality changes little.

Personality represents a pattern of behavioral traits that are dimensional and there is no precise cut-off point for a low or high trait. Personality traits are also hierarchical. Several broad, more easily described traits (e.g. behavioral inhibition) are each composed of a number of more behaviorally refined traits (e.g. restraint, pessimism). The refined traits are used as descriptors in the examination of personality.

NOTES

1 Phillippe Pinel, appointed in 1793 as the director of the Bicêtre, Paris' asylum for the insane, is famous for his reforms and humane treatment of the mentally ill, literally releasing them from their chains. He cited this quote from a well-known encyclopedist of that era in a 1791 monograph (Pinel, 1791) decrying the knee-jerk responses to the mentally ill. It could easily apply to the diagnostic approach of present classifications.

   Pinel introduced the procedure of daily rounds and careful note taking. He may have been the first physician caring for the mentally ill to require psychiatric case histories and the keeping of hospital records.

2 Kolb and Whishaw (1996), pages 6–8.

3 Kretschmer (1925); Sheldon and Stevens (1942). Sheldon's ectomorph (lanky and fragile) was associated with low energy, schizoid traits and schizophrenia. His endomorph (round and soft) was associated with good humor and manic-depressive illness. Mesomorphs (muscular) were associated with antisocial personality.

4 Prichard (1833).

5 Shorter (2005), pages 213–14.

6 Schneider (1950; 1959, pp. 15–28).

7 Jung espoused the notion of a "collective unconscious", a pattern of inborn predispositions common to all persons that derive from an ancestral source. The collective unconscious shaped all behavior via ancestral memories or "archetypes". Adler considered a universal striving to compensate for basic inferiority feelings (the "inferiority complex") as the source of future behavior. Both eventually split with Freud professionally and personally.

8 Ackroyd (2005); Bloom (1998).

9 Pavlov (1941); Skinner (1948).

10 Eysenck (1964).

11 Eysenck and Rachman (1965).

12 Wolpe (1958); Yates (1970).

13 Hawton *et al.* (1989).

14 Factor analysis is one of several statistical modeling methods. Others include cluster analysis, latent class analysis and topological analysis. The mathematics is designed to access large amounts of data to extract meaningful patterns of data from "noise". If a pattern emerges (in factor analysis the pattern is referred to as a factor) its existence can be repeatedly tested in different samples until the image of the pattern is clarified. If a pattern is clearly identified the likelihood of it being present by chance is slim and its presence indicates an underlying process explaining it exists. The factor can then be validated by seeing if it predicts important variables.

15 Catell's relatively short temperament assessment scale is still in use.

16 Humphrey and Dahlstrom (1995). The original MMPI was developed at the University of Minnesota Hospitals and first published in 1942. The original authors of the MMPI were Starke R. Hathaway, PhD, and J.C. McKinley, MD. The current standardized version for adults 18 and over, the MMPI-2, was released in 1989, with a subsequent revision of certain test elements in early 2001. The MMPI-2 consists of 567 true or false questions, and takes several hours to complete. There is a short form of the test that comprises the first 370 items on the long-form MMPI-2.

17 Tyrer and Alexander (1979).

18 Costa and McCrae (1985, 1992); Costa and Widiger (1994); Cloninger *et al.* (1994).

19 Barret *et al.* (1995).

20 Gray and McNaughton (2000).

21 Cloninger (1991); Cloninger *et al.* (1993); O'Gorman *et al.* (2006).

22 The Virginia Family Study has recruited over 30 000 participants. The Colorado adoption project is studying close to 500 families. The Swedish twin registry has close to 13 000 twin pairs.

23 Ploman and Bergeman (1991).

24 Cloninger (1991).

25 Bornstein (1998); Widiger and Samuel (2005).

26 At the *American Psychopathological Association Annual Meeting* (1994) devoted to data detailing the dimensional nature of personality, representatives for the DSM committee on

Axis II admitted the inconsistencies between the data and the plans for future DSM versions, but stated changes would be too difficult (personal observation of both authors).

27 Roberts *et al.* (2006); Caspi *et al.* (2005).

28 Clark (2005).

29 Cloninger *et al.* (1993); Svrakic *et al.* (1993).

30 Cloninger *et al.* (1994).

31 Eysenck (1985).

32 Costa and McCrae (1992).

33 Cloninger *et al.* (1993); Svrakic *et al.* (1993).

34 Silver and Davis (1991); Livesley *et al.* (1998).

35 Allen and Levine (1968); Eisenman *et al.* (1968); Kirkcaldy and Siefen (1991).

36 Torgersen (2005).

37 Scarr and McCartney (1983).

38 Ploman and Bergeman (1991); Cloninger (1991). The great variability of trait expressions and the stability of these traits in the individual offered a great selective advantage for evolving humans. The individual variability within a small hominid group provided substantial flexibility of response to nature's challenges. The constancy of personality once formed offered intra-group stability.

39 Nordeen and Yahr (1982); Meston *et al.* (2000); Korach (1994).

40 Nordeen and Yahr (1982); Cohen-Bendhahan *et al.* (2005); Wilhelm *et al.* (2007).

41 Allen *et al.* (2002, 2003). Structures identified are the preoptic area, suprachiasmatic nucleus, the interstitial nuclei of the hypothalamus, the bed nucleus of the stria terminalis, and the anterior commissure.

42 Cohen-Bendhahan *et al.* (2005).

43 Diamond and Watson (2004); Deeb *et al.* (2005).

44 Marine birds and sheep are well-studied examples (Perkins *et al.*, 1995).

45 Pillard and Weinrich (1986); Hamer *et al.* (1993).

46 LeVay (1991); Allen and Gorski (1992); Swaab *et al.* (1992; 1995). The studies apply to homosexual males. Homosexual men have a smaller third interstitial nucleus of anterior hypothalamus (LeVay, 1991), a larger anterior commissure (Allen and Gorski, 1992), a larger suprachiasmic nucleus, and a smaller bed nucleus of the stria terminalis in the hypothalamus (Zhou *et al.*, 1995).

47 Also seen in several bird species; Kendler *et al.* (2000); Camperio-Ciani *et al.* (2004); Gavrilets and Rice (2006).

48 Truong *et al.* (2006); Read *et al.* (2007).

49 Lester (2006).

50 Friedman (1999); Fitzpatrick *et al.* (2005); Cochran and Cauce (2006).

51 Friedman (1999).

52 Rabkin *et al.* (1997).

53 à Campo *et al.* (2003).

54 Cohen-Kettenis and Gooren (1999).

55 Coolidge *et al.* (2002).

56 Zhou *et al.* (1995).

57 Ibid.

58 Bower (2001).

59 Nordeen and Yahr (1982); Cohen-Bendhahan *et al.* (2005).

60 Lindstrom (2002); Middleton *et al.* (1998).

61 Barash (1979).

62 Clements *et al.* (2003).

63 Catlin (2001).

64 Chaturvedi (1994). In this study, cancer patients with additional psychiatric diagnoses more often reported concern for physical health, sadness, anxiety, future, work or occupation and being slowed down, rather than for cancer pain, interpersonal relationships, marital relationship, socialization or body image (Addington-Hall and McCarthy, 1995).

65 There is no legal or ethical requirement that capacity be determined by a psychiatrist, only a physician not directly involved in the patient's care.

66 Amato (1994).

67 Foa *et al.* (2006).

68 Nixon *et al.* (2004).

69 Yehuda (2004); Foa *et al.* (2006).

70 Richter *et al.* (2006); Acierno *et al.* (2007).

71 Caffo and Belaise (2003).

72 Van Loey and Van Son (2003).

73 Molnar *et al.* (2001); Thompson *et al.* (2003).

74 Wonderlich *et al.* (2001a).

75 Talbot *et al.* (2000).

76 Faravelli *et al.* (2004).

77 Van Loey and Van Son (2003); Jehel *et al.* (2001).

78 Bremner *et al.* (1995); Woodward *et al.* (2006).

79 Bryant and Panasetis (2005).

80 North *et al.* (1999).

81 Bremner *et al.* (1993).

82 Bradley and Tawfig (2006).

83 Keller *et al.* (2005).

15

Abnormal trait behaviors: personality disorder

Abnormal personality implies deviation from some notion we have of average personality. The criterion for normality represents an average not a standard. Abnormal personalities merge without any sharp dividing line into what is commonly described as normal.[1]

Abnormal personality is a distortion of normal personality traits. It derives from similar influences as normal personality, maturing in a similar fashion as do other physical attributes (e.g. height, body shape). Unless resulting from brain trauma or disease, abnormal personality is not associated with identifiable neuropathology. Thus personality disorder has substantial heritability (about 50–60%), with non-shared environmental factors having an important influence on expression.[2]

Traits are dimensional, not categorical. There are no absolute cut-off points, for example, for a small or large nose, a short or tall stature, or low or high strength of a personality trait. The "average" person is in the median range for most traits.[3]

An abnormal trait is a statistical deviation from the average and does not necessarily indicate disease or dysfunction. Almost all professional basketball players are abnormal (deviant) in height. What is considered "very tall" or "very short", however, is relative to the average height of the population from which tall and short are judged. The European of average height is considered by most Southeastern Asians to be tall. Deviant personality traits are also relative to what is understood as "normal". The cultural anthropologist Ruth Benedict described cultures in which heightened suspiciousness, theft and lying were considered laudable.[4]

Social and cultural norms evolved under the influence of the expected norms of temperament. Thus, persons with abnormal temperaments will often have inter-personal difficulties conflicting with these norms.[5] Because personality changes little once formed, the problems elicited by the abnormal temperament traits recur often.

The descriptors of abnormal temperaments and the problems they elicit are used to classify personality disorders. The DSM and the ICD recognize the present-day understanding of personality in their brief introductory discussions

Table 15.1. Problems with "Axis II"

Problem	Consequences
Diagnostic unreliability	Personality disorder diagnoses have poor reliability in general clinical practice[6] leading to false positive diagnoses (e.g. patients with low-grade manic-depression incorrectly identified as having borderline personality disorder). False negative conclusions occur when maladaptive traits go unrecognized.
Excessive co-occurrence	Many patients simultaneously meet criteria for several personality disorders, eliciting diagnostic confusion and poor treatment.[7]
Heterogeneity within personalities	Patients who share the same personality disorder diagnosis can be dissimilar in trait behavior. Tarred with the same brush, they receive similar prescriptions and prognoses but require different treatment approaches (e.g. antisocial personality is based on social consequences not observable behavior; a cold-blooded psychopath and an illicit drug user receive the same label and societal response).[8]
Unstable and arbitrary boundaries	Stability over time varies and the NOS designation is the most frequently used diagnosis in clinical practice.[9]
Mixing deviance from illness with deviance from trait	Patients with Cluster A diagnoses have low-grade illnesses, not deviant trait behavior. The prognostic and treatment implications are substantial and prevention strategies and treatments are not considered.

to personality disorders, but then explicitly ignore the dimensional construct in the formulation and details of the personality disorder axes.

The problems with present personality disorder classifications

The problems with the present classification of personality disorders are fundamental and cannot be fixed with cosmetic change. The structure is at variance with the science.[10] Table 15.1 summarizes the problems in the DSM Axis II.

False positive and negative diagnosis

Using the categorical structure to classify personality disorders rather than a dimensional construct is a fundamental error generating many of the difficulties associated with the present system.[11] In categorical grouping, if the patient has a certain number of problems he is identified as having that personality disorder. If he has one less problem he does not have the personality disorder. This "you either have it or not" system misleads clinicians, particularly when the patient's behaviors are not prototypical,[12] and results in false negative (Patient 15.1) and false positive (Patient 15.2) conclusions.

Patient 15.1

A senior business executive was being treated for a non-melancholic depression that began after he was asked to resign from his position because of difficulties with upper management. The patient had long-standing interpersonal problems. Superficially charming, he often manipulated the affections of others to obtain what he wanted, withdrawing his attention when he found others no longer useful. Friends and colleagues eventually avoided him. He said "everything is fair in business", and if people were "stupid" that was not his fault. He frequently asked his subordinates to manipulate the books to cheat his vendors. He believed "you are guilty only if you get caught and the law is for stupid people". He was the only child of wealthy parents. He went to an Ivy League school, joined a fraternity, and according to him was a typical "frat boy" who drank heavily though under age, used illicit drugs, vandalized neighbor's homes, and frequented prostitutes, bragging that he was never caught. He married a family friend because "it was good for the business"; however, over the years he had several extra-marital affairs for which he showed no remorse.

Patient 15.1 exhibits the classic features of antisocial personality: manipulating others, disregard for the law and ethical considerations, and lack of remorse. Coming from a wealthy background, however, he avoided some of the situations included in the DSM criteria such as "repeated physical fights or assaults", "use of aliases", "reckless disregard for safety of self or others", "evidence of conduct disorder with onset before age 16 years". These criteria overly stress behaviors most likely seen in persons from low socio-economic backgrounds.[13]

Patient 15.2

A 56-year-old divorced man was hospitalized with the diagnosis of borderline personality disorder. The index hospitalization and his several previous admissions followed multiple self-inflicted superficial cuts to his arm. Although he endorsed feeling depressed, he denied suicidal thoughts and had not attempted suicide. He had a long history of interpersonal difficulties including problems with women friends and problems in his marriage. He said his wife thought he was too "needy". He would become extremely angry if she did not agree to his demands. For the past 10 years he drank alcohol excessively.

On the inpatient unit, the patient was agitated and anxious. He did not want to be left alone in his room and needed constant reassurance and direction from nursing staff. His slept and ate poorly. He was apprehensive and his mood non-reactive. Until 10 years before, his "personality problems" occurred episodically and always in association with a disturbed mood. He had a strong family history of depressive illness and suicide. In early hospitalizations he was treated with psychotherapy alone, while in later admissions haloperidol and fluphenazine were prescribed.

In the index hospitalization, the patient's difficulties during the previous 10 years, including alcohol abuse, were considered expressions of a mood disorder, rather than deviations in trait behavior. He received bilateral ECT and had a full remission.

Diagnostic instability

DSM and ICD personality disorder diagnoses are unstable. A person may meet criteria one year, not the next, and meet criteria again a few years later.[14] Patients "fluctuate" in and out of the diagnostic categories over time. Deviant dimensional personality traits are more stable.[15] A study of four different personality disorders for fixed and changeable criteria found that certain behaviors are prevalent and fixed while others are not common and are changeable. Among patients with schizotypal and paranoid personality disorders, thought content and unusual experiences were most prevalent and least changeable over time, while constricted affect was uncommon and varied in its presence over time, suggesting the criteria for these categories are a combination of traits and illness behavior.[16]

Diagnoses within specific clusters are also indistinct, and about 40% of persons who receive one personality disorder diagnosis also meet criteria for a second, whereas studies of the patterns of dimensional traits find that a person has only one pattern that changes little over a lifetime.[17] A person who receives a diagnosis of narcissistic personality disorder, for example, may also meet the criteria for histrionic personality disorder.[18] A patient who is diagnosed as borderline personality disorder when depressed may receive a diagnosis of histrionic personality disorder when no longer depressed.[19] Using a dimensional system to assess personality typically elicits stable diagnoses over repeated examinations.[20]

The categorical criteria are also poorly drafted, mixing characteristic behaviors with the non-specific consequences of many behaviors. The borderline patient, for example, is said to be impulsive with affective instability and to have a history of poor interpersonal relationships. While the association may be causal, poor interpersonal relationships have many causes.

Present classification of personality disorders

The defining construct for the personality disorders is "marked deviation" (not operationally defined) that affects impulse control, interpersonal functioning,

Table 15.2. Cluster A observable behaviors

Paranoid	Schizoid	Schizotypal
Emotional range restricted	Reduced emotional expression	Reduced emotional
Irritability	Does not express warm feelings	expression
Hypervigilant and	or tenderness	Low-grade
detail-focused	Poor rapport	suspiciousness
Low-grade suspiciousness;	Indifferent	Ideas of reference
mistrustful	Low sex drive	Illusions and perceptual
Bears grudges for real and	Prefers to be alone	distortions
imagined slights		Circumstantial, low
Fearful of attack or infidelity		content speech
Preoccupied with concerns		Culturally deviant beliefs

affectivity, or "ways of perceiving and interpreting self, other people, and events" and which are long-standing, stable, and maladaptive. No behavior included in the criteria is pathogonomonic, but patterns of behavior are characteristic.

Present classification offers 10 personality disorders in 3 categories arranged by severity, with odd–eccentric personality disorders (Cluster A) the most severe, followed by dramatic–emotional (Cluster B) and then anxious–fearful personality disorders (Cluster C). The severity continuum is not clinically meaningful.

The categorical criteria descriptors for the personality disorders mix past consequences of behavioral problems with behavior that can be assessed in the behavioral examination. The latter are detailed below and in Tables 15.2, 15.3, and 15.4.

Cluster A

Cluster A should be eliminated from Axis II. These conditions are likely low-grade states of illness best considered within Axis I.[21] For example, persons with schizotypal personality have common psychopathology, family history illness patterns, cognitive abnormalities and brain volume changes similar to patients with chronic schizophrenia.[22]

The modest heritability found for Cluster A conditions is consistent with the substantial heritability determined for their associated Axis I conditions. The milder forms of an illness found to be more common than the severe forms and to have less heritability.[23] Schizotypal personality, however, is reported to aggregate in the first-degree relatives of persons with schizophrenia and also in the families of persons with mood disorder, suggesting it is a heterogeneous category representing low-grade states of several illnesses.[24]

A common behavioral denominator of Cluster A is reduced expression and restricted range of emotions. Cluster A categories are associated with the psychotic

Table 15.3. Cluster B observable behaviors

Antisocial	Borderline	Histrionic	Narcissistic
Impulsive	Impulsive	Rapid mood shifts	Lack of empathy
Irritable and aggressive	Affective	Exaggerated emotional	Arrogant manner
Cold and callous	instability	expression	Self-absorbed
Lack of remorse	Irritable and	Signs of vanity and	Manipulative
and sympathy	aggressive	self-indulgence	Controlling and
Signs of vanity and	Signs of self-injury	Self-decoration	impressionistic
self-indulgence[25]		Flirtatious	historian
Self-decoration[26]		Impressionistic	
Evasive historian		historian[27]	

disorders, but paranoid personality disorder is also seen in some epileptics, in long-term heavy drinkers, and chronic abusers of inhalants.[28] Schizotypal personality disorder is also seen in some epileptics and in chronic abusers of hallucinogens. Bleuler considered schizoid personality to be an early sign of schizophrenia. It is also associated with autistic spectrum disorders.[29]

Patient 15.3 meets DSM criteria for schizotypal personality disorder.

Patient 15.3

A 34-year-old man worked only several hours weekly in a transitional center of a large community mental health system. He spoke in a soft voice and often about being clairvoyant and seeing scurrying creatures from the corners of his eyes. His speech was vague. He used few nouns and specific content, and it was difficult to follow his train of thought. He had no friends, lived alone, and interacted only with the center staff that he knew. He never experienced any psychotic symptoms, although he was prescribed antipsychotic medication.

Cluster B

Cluster B personality disorders represent two groupings: (1) narcissistic/antisocial/histrionic, and (2) borderline.

The narcissistic/antisocial/histrionic group is characterized by egocentric and excitable behavior, high behavioral activation and low inhibition. The narcissistic personality criteria are mostly interpretive and historical and may not be observed or clearly elicited during the examination.

Histrionic personality disorder has the longest history, described originally as hysterical personality. Such persons were characterized as egocentric, affectively labile, exhibitionistic, dramatic, excitable, emotionally shallow, flirtatious but sexually frigid, dependent, and suggestible.[30] Other authors added impulsive, impressionistic, reckless, and attention-seeking, including self-injurious behavior and "wishing to be ill".[31] The validity of these observations is unclear. The persons described are invariably women and the physicians offering the descriptions mostly men. In dismissing the sexist implications of this demographic, Trimble writes of the descriptors of hysterical personality:

> In its florid form this style is easily recognized (the essence of femininity – hence the feminists' revolt!), but some authors have revealed these trait patterns as identifiable factors using personality questionnaires in population studies.

Antisocial and histrionic personality disorders reflect similar temperament patterns (high novelty seeking/behavioral activation and low harm avoidance/ behavioral inhibition), but expressed differently by gender. Both categories are found in members of the same pedigrees, indicating a familial if not a genetic shared disposition. Both are co-morbid with about 25% of persons with each personality disorder also meeting criteria for the other. Persons placed in these categories are at greater risk for somatization and conversion disorder diagnoses.[32] Cluster B traits are also associated with bulimic symptoms.[33] In the scant reports of serial killers, most meet criteria for antisocial personality.[34]

Borderline personality is a heterogeneous class. Many such persons suffer from an early onset, chronic and less episodic mood disorder. Biologic markers and treatment studies support this view.[35] Other patients with the label have traits of high behavioral activation (*novelty seeking*) and low behavioral inhibition (*harm avoidance*) that encourages taking high risks resulting in brain dysfunction from illicit drug use[36] or traumatic brain injury.[37] These conditions in turn exaggerate their other personality traits of impulsiveness and aggressiveness, resulting in a combination of state and trait behaviors.[38] The end result is that treatments for traits (cognitive and dialectic behavior therapy) are unsuccessfully applied to illness.

The borderline criteria also include psychological interpretations (e.g. avoiding imagined abandonment, alternating idealization and devaluation) and symptoms of illness (e.g. "paranoid ideation or severe dissociative symptoms"). The term is a remnant of psychoanalytic theorizing of a relationship between neurosis and psychosis. It should be eliminated.

Cluster C

Cluster C personality disorders also represent two groupings: avoidant/dependent and obsessive–compulsive. The cluster is associated with the anxiety disorders and non-melancholic depressions.[39] Almost all criteria are the consequences of implied, but never detailed, temperament traits. A common temperament theme

Table 15.4. Cluster C observable behaviors

Avoidant	Dependent	Obsessive–compulsive
Inhibited (low spontaneity in conversation and actions, reduced emotional expression)	Indecisive Unassertive Submissive	Provides overly detailed responses to the examiner's questions; has difficulty providing "yes" or "no" answers to relatively simple questions
Low energy		May be overly formal
"Mild" mannered		Rigid and stubborn; not open to examiner's suggestions
Appears anxious		Reduced emotional expression

for avoidant and dependent personalities is high harm avoidance (behavioral inhibition). While obsessive–compulsive personality also shares high harm avoidance behaviors, it is best considered an expression of illness within the OCD spectrum.

Personality deviations and associated psychopathology

Deviance on several personality dimensions is associated with psychopathology. Dimensions of neuroticism and harm avoidance have been shown to predict non-melancholic depression.[40] Extraversion and novelty seeking are associated with conduct disorder and drug abuse.[41] Table 15.5 displays other associations.

Abnormal personality from illness or injury

"Epileptic" personalities[42]

Up to 60% of patients with epilepsy are reported to exhibit permanent changes in personality after several decades of illness.

The *adhesive* or *viscous* personality is characterized by perseveration, stubbornness, a narrow field of interest and attention, loss of humor (*humorless sobriety*), circumstantial and cliché-filled speech, and a pedantic dry manner. Such patients are plodding and repetitive in their conversations, which are limited to one or two topics that are over-valued and constantly expressed at the slightest opportunity. They seem compelled to begin the conversation, to exhaust the topic regardless of previous iterations, and are reluctant to stop. Nothing is trivial. They lose sight of the "big picture" or the concept of their topic or theme, and focus on minutiae. Every detail must be mulled over. They "stick" to the topic and to the person to whom they are speaking. They are adhesive. They plod through their interactions and thoughts as if embedded in some "viscous" substance.

Table 15.5. Deviant temperament dimensions and psychopathology

Deviant dimension(s)	Associated psychopathology
High activation (high novelty seeking)	Use of stimulants including caffeine, nicotine and illicit drugs; alcohol abuse; conduct disorder in children; somatoform disorders in adults; pathological gambling[43]
High inhibition (high harm avoidance)	Anxiety disorders; non-melancholic depression; abuse of alcohol and anxiolytic drugs; migraine[44]
Low activation (low novelty seeking) and high inhibition (high harm avoidance)	Similar to high harm-avoidance; atopic dermatitis;[45] eating disorder;[46] late-onset alcoholism but no substance abuse[47]
High maintenance (reward dependence) and high inhibition (harm avoidance)	Similar to low novelty seeking and high harm avoidance; victims of abuse

Patients with chronic manic-depressive illness have similar personality changes, but less severe in expression. They too are *circumstantial* and adhesive. Like patients with chronic seizure disorder, they may keep copious notes of their medical treatments and illness experiences. Diaries of repetitive minutiae can take up several bookshelves (*hypergraphia*). Libido is lost and they are said to be *hyposexual.* They may focus attention on esoteric philosophic or theological topics beyond their training and understanding but they are compelled to talk about them (*pseudo-profundity*).[48]

A *paranoid personality* developing late in life has also been reported in persons with chronic limbic system disease. Such persons are moody and irritable, quarrelsome, spiteful, suspicious, and malicious. They hold grudges, vigorously protest mild or imagined slights and become litigious. They can become the "neighborhood cranks". Alcoholism can also elicit these trait changes.

An *emotional personality* is also described in a small number of persons with seizure disorder. The change in personality is characterized by a subjective deepening of all emotions with sustained intense emotional expression. They cry at any sentiment. Witzelsucht occurs. Deep religious beliefs, for the first time, become central to their lives leading to interpersonal difficulties.

Personality change associated with traumatic brain disease

Personality changes are common following moderate to severe traumatic brain injury (TBI), particularly when frontal lobe circuitry is involved. Table 15.6 lists the characteristic personality changes following TBI. In children, TBI elicits personality changes associated with attention deficits and hyperactivity.[49]

Table 15.6. Personality changes after TBI[50]

Lateral orbital prefrontal injury (40%):* Irritability and episodic dyscontrol and unplanned
    violence; tendency toward suspiciousness, emotional lability, restlessness and impulsiveness;
    self-destructive and unrealistic in plans; lacking insight; childishly self-centered, insensitive
    toward others, overly talkative and exuberant

Dorsolateral prefrontal injury (10–30%): Lack of spontaneity and initiative, loss of drive,
    ambition and interests, sluggish, socially isolative, dysphoric

---

Note:
*Numbers in () are incidence figures.

Table 15.7.[51] Features of frontal lobe personality

Irritable, insensitive toward the feelings of others with a loss of social
    graces, neglectful of appearance
Inappropriately jocular, indifferent, placid, minimizes difficulties
Impulsive, unpredictable, impatient, increased rule-breaking, demanding,
    aggressive, "pseudopsychopathic"
Reduced interests, more pleasant and sentimental

Personality change associated with stroke

Like TBI, stroke can result in changes in personality, particularly large or multiple
strokes in anterior brain regions. Changes are the same seen following TBI.[52]

"Frontal lobe" personality

Persons with frontal lobe disease commonly exhibit personality changes characterized by disinhibition or apathy (Table 15.7).[53]

Patient 15.4 had personality changes associated with frontal lobe disease.
He had little evidence of a defined mood disorder and his changed behaviors
were pervasive and persistent, as are personality traits.

Patient 15.4

**A 63-year-old man was being treated at a psychiatric clinic following a
traumatic brain injury. Brain imaging revealed atrophy in his left frontal lobe.**

**During one of the visits, his wife became extremely angry with him and
complained to the psychiatrist that since her husband's injury it had become
intolerable to live with him. A quiet person before the injury, he had become
"a racist". He frequently made socially inappropriate racial comments and
used racial epithets. He also spoke loudly about women's breasts.**

**The patient exhibited no sustained irritability or euphoria. He had no pressure
of speech or evidence of psychosis. His sleep and appetite were normal.**

Personality deviations associated with Parkinson's disease

Parkinson's disease (PD) is a prevalent neurodegenerative disorder that affects millions of persons.[54] Non-motor features of anxiety and depression occur in 30–50% of sufferers,[55] and may precede the motor features by 5–10 years.[56]

Many sufferers of PD also show personality changes that precede the appearance of motor abnormalities. These changes have been recognized since the nineteenth century: patients are described as rigid, stoic, slow-tempered, frugal and orderly. They are reported to exhibit emotional and attitudinal inflexibility, muted emotional expression and a predisposition to depressive illness.[57] It is unclear whether this characteristic personality is independent of the disease process, predisposes the person to PD, or whether it is an early expression of the disease representing subtle basal ganglia dopamine deficiency.[58]

Personality and alcohol and drug use

Personality plays a substantial role in whether a person regularly drinks alcohol or uses brain-altering drugs. The "addictive personality", however, is an over-simplified notion, and different trait patterns are associated with different addiction risks.

"Addictive" personality traits

Persons who abuse and become dependent on alcohol, or who regularly use illicit drugs, often exhibit abnormal personality traits. Early-onset alcohol abuse (during adolescence or shortly afterward) is identified as type II alcoholism. Late-onset alcoholism (onset after age 30) is termed type I alcoholism.[59] Early-onset alcoholics are characterized as outgoing, emotionally labile, curious, impulsive, and risk-taking. They are constantly looking for new, self-pleasing experiences and adventures. They tend to be uncooperative in group activities, having little desire to please others. They have difficulty beginning and completing long-term efforts (e.g. graduating from college) and employment that they do not enjoy.[60] They cannot delay gratification.

Although superficially gregarious, they have difficulty establishing close interpersonal relationships. They have many acquaintances (usually drinking or partying "buddies"), but few if any close friends. Unlike persons who do not abuse alcohol until later in life, the early-onset alcoholic exhibits high behavioral activation and low behavioral inhibition.[61]

In contrast, persons who begin to abuse alcohol later in life are found to be passive and dependent. They have anxious–fearful traits, are sentimental, sensitive, and overly eager to please others.[62] Some have anxiety disorder, and the abuse is an effort to self-medicate. Such persons may also have a partner who abuses alcohol.[63]

Regular users of illicit drugs and other substances (e.g. inhalants) have personality traits similar to early-onset alcoholics, but with more extreme behavioral activation.[64] Their high behavioral activation combined with low behavioral inhibition predispose to impulsivity, aggressiveness and sensation-seeking.[65] The traits are seen as phenotypic markers for drug and alcohol abuse. When found in children, they predict later substance and alcohol abuse.[66] The genetic influences on personality, adverse neurodevelopmental effects from intrauterine exposure to maternal substance use, and adverse early developmental effects from impaired maternal–child interactions contribute to the addiction-predicting childhood traits.[67] Some early-onset cocaine and opiate abusers, however, are found to be *hyperthymic* or *cyclothymic*, indicating that their abuse reflects disturbances in mood rather than trait behavior. They are more likely to have a family history of mood disorder.[68]

Associated psychopathology

Caffeine and nicotine are the addictive drugs of most common regular usage. Heavy caffeine use presents as anxiety and sleep disorder. Features of *caffeinism* include periodic anxiousness and unease, inner tremulousness, fine tremor, stomach upset, visual blurring or seeing colors as washed out or in the blue range. Heavy nicotine use is associated with other addictions and depressive illness. Both caffeine and nicotine are highly addictive and sudden withdrawal elicits headache, irritability, and sluggishness.

Some patients with depressive illness and anxiety disorder abuse alcohol and sedatives. These patients have no deviant personality traits or have high behavioral inhibition. Their abuse is understood as an effort at self-medication.

The use of illicit drugs has acute and chronic behavioral consequences. Toxicity is associated with psychosis and delirium. Chronic exposure is associated with recurrent psychotic disorder, cognitive impairment, and functional decline. The associated psychopathology is presented in the chapters on motor abnormalities, delusions and perceptual disturbances.

Personality change associated with alcoholism and substance abuse

Chronic heavy alcohol use is associated with personality change. The change is typically observed in men over age 50 that have had few other alcohol-related difficulties. These heavy drinkers become increasingly suspicious, sullen, and irritable. They may become the "neighborhood crank" who repeatedly complains about the deficiencies or underhanded dealings of local government or litigates against neighbors "encroaching" on property. The syndrome can evolve into delusions about spouse infidelity, family attempts at stealing wealth, or government "dirty tricks".[69]

Chronic use of illicit drugs is also associated with personality change.[70] Chronic heavy use of *stimulants* leads to executive function deficits, apathy and movement problems. Lack of spontaneity and initiative, loss of drive, ambition and interests, sluggish thinking, and being socially isolative occur. Some patients become irritable and emotionally labile, restless, impulsive, self-destructive and unrealistic in plans, and lack insight. Persons who repeatedly inhale the vapors from volatile industrial liquids can be violent and suspicious. Patients who use hallucinogenic drugs can be avolitional and apathetic.

Malingering and factitious disorder

The separation of malingering from factitious disorder is based on psychological theory without supporting evidence. Patients in both groups feign illness. The malingerer has a clearly identifiable goal, such as avoiding prosecution, obtaining insurance money, and avoiding responsibilities. Malingering is associated with antisocial personality disorder.[71]

The person with factitious disorder is said to have no obvious reason to fake illness, but rather the "psychological need" to be a patient. When pronounced and chronic, it is referred to as *Munchausen's syndrome.* Such patients commonly "hospital-hop", seeking admission for various medical complaints.[72] Parents who fake signs of illness and laboratory tests of their children are said to have factitious disorder "by proxy". Although treated as child abusers, these parents are still said to have a "psychological need" to be in a sick role. An example of a patient with a likely factitious disorder follows.

Patient 15.5
A 12-year-old boy was seen in the emergency room after having a "spell" just prior to going to school. In recent weeks he had other episodes described as fainting spells, aggressive episodes during which he damaged some object and threw things, "dissociative-like" periods during which he appeared sleepy but responsive, spells during which he acted like an infant or young child or insisted on lying on the floor, and times when he referred to himself as "the other Barry [name changed]". During these events he was somewhat verbally interactive and responsive, but on other occasions "the other Barry" carried on elaborate conversations with his parents and younger sibling.

Initially saying that he had no memory for earlier spells, the patient said he remembered the more recent ones. During his spells, his parents were extremely solicitous. Twenty-four hour continuous EEG and video monitoring captured a spell in association with a normal tracing.

No unusual stress events were identified, either at home or at school. He was not found to be depressed or psychotic. His parents described him as a quiet, shy person, a perfectionist and a pessimist. Until the emergency room visit the patient had never been seen by a psychiatrist or psychologist. He did have a long history of allergies, mild asthmatic-like episodes, and multiple complaints including headaches, ear aches, rashes, breathing problems, and URIs resulting in over 30 physician office visits in the previous 3 years. His father accompanied him for most of the visits. No health problem was considered serious and for many visits no pathology was identified. The patient's parents were said to be extremely attentive and involved with the patient's school activities, but the father's work frequently kept him away from home.

The clinical importance of assessing personality

Personality disorders are medical diagnoses, and about 10% of persons meet DSM criteria for personality disorder. These deviant trait patterns are associated with other conditions. For example, 40–60% of individuals with anxiety disorder, non-melancholic depression, eating disorder, and adjustment disorder have a pre-existing personality disorder, complicating treatment.

Personality dimensions also predict the likelihood that a person will use tobacco,[73] abuse alcohol early in life, or use illicit drugs. Such use compromises health and is associated with non-compliance to treatment. The same traits predict high-risk or criminal behaviors.[74]

In addition, all patients and their family members have personalities. The success in educating the patient and family members about the patient's condition and treatments, how the family can help, and how the patient needs to comply with treatment depends on the clinician's ability to influence others. Recognizing the personality traits of the patient and of family members guides that influence.

Summary

Most deviant personality traits reflect variability in maturation. The determinants of deviant personality are similar to those for normal personality. Disease, injury, and toxicity, however, can affect the neural networks subserving personality altering trait behavior. The conditions that elicit such change tend to occur after personality is formed and a substantial personality change after age 35 is almost always the result of brain disease or dysfunction.

The DSM and ICD categorical approach to personality disorder is inconsistent with the modern understanding of personality structure, and requires replacement by the dimensional formulation. The dimensional perspective offers better clinical guidance to diagnosis and patient care. It better predicts associations with states of illness and shapes behavioral interventions.

NOTES

1 Schneider (1959), page 15.
2 Torgersen *et al.* (2000). Patients with schizotypal personality have associated brain structural and functional abnormality in frontal–limbic areas (Koo *et al.*, 2006a, 2006b; Dickey *et al.*, 2007).
3 Commonly defined as within 1.5 standard deviations from the mean.
4 Benedict (1934).
5 Henderson *et al.* (1981) referred to a state of real or perceived deficiency in interpersonal relationships as *anophelia*.
6 Widiger and Samuel (2005). See also Chapter 16.
7 Bornstein (1998).
8 Widiger *et al.* (1988).
9 Verheul and Widiger (2004).
10 Chapter 16 provides proposed changes. Also see Widiger and Samuel (2005).
11 Jablensky (2002); Sprock (2003).
12 Sprock (2003).
13 After a lecture to second-year medical students on personality disorders, several students who had grown up in inner cities told one of us that some of them and many of their friends behaved in a fashion similar to the criteria for ASP, but that "everyone" knew which kids were "really bad".
14 McGlashan *et al.* (2005); Costa (1991); McCrae *et al.* (2001).
15 Hampson and Goldberg (2006); Durbin and Klein (2006).
16 McGlashan *et al.* (2005).
17 McGlashan *et al.* (2005).
18 McGlashan *et al.* (2005); Nurnberg *et al.* (1991).
19 McGlashan *et al.* (2005).
20 McGlashan *et al.* (2005).
21 Siever (1994); Siever and Davis (2004).
22 Siever (1994); Siever and Davis (2004).
23 Kendler *et al.* (2006).
24 Siever (1994); Siever and Davis (2004).
25 Common examples seen in both genders are designer haircuts, and extravagant manicures and pedicures, all-year-round salon tans, and wearing excessive jewelry.
26 Tattoos in both men and women are clearly designed to attract attention.
27 Persons with histrionic or narcissistic personalities are inexact in relating their history. Description of symptoms is vague, the pain is "all over", the diarrhea is "always a problem", and the onset is "as long as I can remember".

28 Siever (1994).

29 Tantam (1988).

30 Chodoff and Lyons (1958).

31 Jaspers (1963); Shapero (1965).

32 Lilienfeld *et al.* (1986); Smith *et al.* (1991).

33 Ilkjaer *et al.* (2004).

34 James (1991); Morana *et al.* (2006); Frei *et al.* (2006).

35 Pally (2002).

36 Pelegrin Valero *et al.* (2001); Joyce *et al.* (2003).

37 Pelegrin Valero *et al.* (2001); Joyce *et al.* (2003).

38 Pally (2002); Joyce *et al.* (2003).

39 Dyck *et al.* (2001); Bienvenu and Stein (2003); Brandes and Bienvenu (2006).

40 Smith *et al.* (2005b); Cloninger *et al.* (2006).

41 Khan *et al.* (2005a).

42 Bear and Fedio (1977); Devinsky and Vazquez (1993); Mendez *et al.* (1993a,b).

43 Tavares *et al.* (2005).

44 The connection between migraine and behavioral inhibition is attributed to a common association with pertubations in serotonergic systems (Boz *et al.*, 2004; Abbate-Daga *et al.*, 2007; Sanchez-Roman *et al.*, 2007).

45 Kim *et al.* (2006).

46 Bulik *et al.* (1992); Kleifield *et al.* (1993).

47 Basiaux *et al.* (2001).

48 Mungas (1982).

49 Max *et al.* (2001).

50 McAllister (1992); Silver *et al.* (2004).

51 Malloy *et al.* (1993); Eslinger *et al.* (2004).

52 Greveson *et al.* (1991); Beckson and Cummings (1991).

53 See Chapter 3.

54 Cummings and Mega (2003).

55 Richard and Kurlan (2002); McDonald *et al.* (2003).

56 Askin-Edgar *et al.* (2004).

57 Todes and Lees (1985).

58 Glosser *et al.* (1995). Studies of human and laboratory animals report a relationship between trait behavior and later basal ganglia disease. Twin data in humans finds an association between high behavioral inhibition and low behavioral activation and the reduced use of tobacco. In persons with PD, the association between trait and reduced dopamine uptake is seen in the affected twin only. In laboratory animals, decreased exploratory behavior, likened to low behavioral activation and high behavioral inhibition in humans, is also associated with reduced dopamine uptake and is observed in animals with ablated basal ganglia in animal model studies of early PD.

59 Cloninger *et al.* (1981, 1988a,b); Buydens-Branchey *et al.* (1989).

60 Basiaux *et al.* (2001).

61 Cloninger *et al.* (1988a).

62 Earleywine *et al.* (1992); Le Joyeux and Ada (1997).

63 Cloninger *et al.* (1988a).

64 Cloninger *et al.* (1995); Howard *et al.* (1997).

65 Evren *et al.* (2007).

66 Cloninger *et al.* (1988b).

67 Ibid.

68 Camacho and Akiskal (2005); Moore *et al.* (2005).

69 Miller (1991).

70 Fletcher *et al.* (1996); Bolla *et al.* (1998).

71 Gorman (1982); Gacono *et al.* (1995).

72 Trimble (2004), pages 93–4. MAT saw a patient with Munchausen's syndrome when an intern. On his internal medicine rotation, the 38-year-old man feigned symptoms of a heart attack and was observed tampering with laboratory specimens. The man was unceremoniously discharged. Six months later, MAT was on his emergency room rotation when the same patient was rushed into the ER on a stretcher for what was said to be a possible myocardial infarction. Upon seeing MAT, the patient got up from the stretcher and quickly walked out of the hospital.

73 The use of tobacco was initially advertised as a health-promoting activity, and most adults in the West smoked tobacco until recently. The association between personality traits and use emerges only with the persistent 25% of persons in the USA who are regular users.

74 Johansson *et al.* (2005).

Section 4

Evidence-based classification

16

An evidence-based classification

"There's glory for you!" "I don't know what you mean by 'glory'", Alice said. "I mean, there's a nice knock-down argument for you!" "But 'glory' doesn't mean 'a nice knock-down argument'", Alice objected. "When I use a word", Humpty Dumpty said in a rather scornful tone, "it means just what I choose it to mean – neither more nor less".[1]

The present DSM and ICD classifications are at substantial variance with the validating evidence for many psychiatric conditions. Some categories defined as homogeneous are clearly heterogeneous (e.g. major depression). Some that are best classified together, are separated (e.g. obsessive–compulsive disorder and Gilles de la Tourette's syndrome), while others that should be separated are grouped (e.g. conduct disorder and trichotillomania). Syndromes without validity are included (e.g. schizophreniform disorder), while those with supporting data are not (e.g. frontal lobe syndromes). Catatonia remains linked to schizophrenia despite evidence that it is a syndrome warranting its own category. Personality disorders are presented as if they were discrete syndromes with clear boundaries, despite the evidence that personality represents dimensional behavioral traits of maturational development. There are many more examples.

This chapter considers changes to categories where the data clearly mandate change (Table 16.1). Categories requiring further study include mental retardation, childhood developmental disorders, elimination and eating disorders, attention deficit disorder and anxiety disorder, sleep disorders, and sexual phase dysfunctions.

The proposed changes also do not address the DSM shortlist and the ICD brief description formats. These structures are hopelessly inadequate for complex diagnostic problems. Teachers of psychiatric diagnosis should insist the manuals be applied as the last step in documentation rather than as major guideposts to assessment. Longitudinal features also need to be included beyond the 1–6 months and the 2-week duration requirements for some conditions. This applies particularly to the psychotic disorders.

Table 16.1. Proposed changes to present psychiatric classification

Present classification	Recommended change
Major depression: Treated as if a homogeneous disorder	Divide major depression into melancholia and non-melancholia depressive disorders; place perinatal depression, abnormal bereavement, psychotic depression, and the depression of manic-depressive illness in the melancholia class
Psychotic disorders: Defined as conditions always associated with hallucinations and delusions, yet other categories are also associated with the same features	Eliminate the category, retaining as independent classes the valid conditions presently in it (delusional disorder and schizophrenia)
Schizophrenia spectrum disorders: brief psychotic disorder, schizophrenia, and schizophreniform disorder are placed on an explicit duration and implicit severity continuum Schizophrenia criteria have no conceptual coherence. The diagnosis relies on first rank symptoms and offers no longitudinal criterion. Samples identified by the criteria are heterogeneous	Eliminate brief psychotic disorder and schizophreniform disorder. They have no validity Revise the criteria for schizophrenia on the concept that it is a brain disorder with substantial but unspecified heritability whose expression is increased following gestational and perinatal brain insults and signs that emerge in childhood. Criteria should have greater reliance on negative symptoms and pre-psychotic features
Schizoaffective disorder: Placed in the psychotic disorder category	Delete schizoaffective disorder. It is a heterogeneous class of patients, most having psychotic mood disorder
Shared psychotic disorder: Placed in the psychotic disorders category	Eliminate shared psychotic disorder. It has no validation
Catatonia: Exclusively placed with schizophrenia in the ICD and primarily linked to schizophrenia in the DSM	Catatonia should be classed separately as are delirium and dementia, with modifiers of severity and likely cause
Obsessive–compulsive disorder, Gilles de la Tourette's and tic disorder, several impulsive control disorders, some eating disorders, and body dysmorphic disorder, some paraphilias: Each of these conditions is classified separately as if distinct diseases	Conflate into a separate obsessive–compulsive spectrum disorder category with separate modifiers; add obsessive–compulsive personality to the spectrum
Dissociative disorders: Classified as if a distinct group of specific syndromes	Eliminate the category as these are symptoms not syndromes. The features presently in it are better

Table 16.1. (cont.)

Present classification	Recommended change
	used as modifiers for validated syndromes (e.g. anxiety disorder with depersonalization, post-ictal fugue), or eliminated because of lack of validity (e.g. conversion disorder, identity disorder)
Personality disorders: Divided into three poorly validated groupings that are categorically defined	Eliminate Axis II. The cluster construct has no validity. Apply dimensional criteria as descriptors
	Eliminate *Cluster A* as it groups low-grade forms of illness not maturational deviations. Place schizoid in a schizophrenia spectrum class and paranoid as a mild form of delusional disorder. Classify schizotypal as an independent condition
	Eliminate *Cluster B.* Classify borderline personality disorder as an independent condition, recognizing that it is a heterogeneous class representing low-grade illness (e.g. manic-depression, dysfunction of emotional regulation due to illicit drugs, traumatic brain injury, and other neurologic disease) as well as abnormal trait behavior (e.g. high behavioral activation)
	Define a separate antisocial/narcissistic/histrionic cluster by dimensional criteria (e.g. high behavioral activation and low behavioral inhibition)
	Eliminate *Cluster C.* Define a separate avoidant/dependent cluster by dimensional criteria (e.g. low behavioral activation and high behavioral inhibition)
	Place obsessive–compulsive personality disorder in the OCD spectrum
Add missing but validated syndromes	*Frontal lobe avolitional* and *disinhibited syndromes* should be added to the cognitive disorders category

It is also time to reconsider the use of laboratory tests as diagnostic criteria. Taylor and Fink (2006) recommend sleep studies as an adjunct to verifying diagnostic criteria for melancholia. They endorse measures of hypothalamic–pituitary–adrenal hyperactivity (late afternoon serum cortisol, and the dexamethasone suppression test), and note that the specificity and sensitivity of such measures are similar to those for scalp-recorded EEG in the recognition of seizure disorder. They also recommend the use of a lorazepam challenge test to confirm the diagnosis of catatonia.[2] First and Zimmerman (2006) also recommend all-night sleep EEG as an indicator for depressive illness, and report that such a study correctly classified 82% of a mixed sample of normal persons, persons with primary insomnia, and patients with depression.

Some writers place their hopes on classification by gene identification, i.e. genetic nosology.[3] But attempts to delineate specific diseases by specific genotype are premature as the syndromes of interest are phenotypically ill-defined and likely multifactorial in etiology.[4]

Mood disorders[5]

Since 1980, depressive illness has been defined as the single construct, *major depression*, with variations based on illness duration and severity (e.g. *dysthymia and psychotic depression*). *Abnormal bereavement* and *perinatal depression* are given separate status. Modest depressions associated with personal stress are designated *adjustment disorder*. Persons with only recurrent depressive episodes are classified as *unipolar*. Those who also experience hypomania or mania are said to be *bipolar* and to be suffering from a different illness requiring different treatments.[6]

Clinical presentations and pathophysiology of the unipolar form are considered to be so alike that similar treatments are offered, varying mainly in dosage, numbers of agents, or augmentations. The recommended treatment algorithms are the same for all patients with non-psychotic major depression, and slightly modified for patients with psychotic depression and bipolar depression.

Research and clinical samples of depressed patients selected by list criteria, however, are heterogeneous and account in part for poor treatment outcomes.[7] Predictors of good outcomes with newer antidepressants have not been identified. Similar critiques are offered for the poor outcomes in the STEP-BD study of antimanic agents[8] and the CATIE study of atypical antipsychotics.[9]

Dividing the major depression category into melancholia and non-melancholia depressive disorders is an alternative paradigm to the present classification of mood disorders that fits the evidence better. This approach minimizes intra-sample heterogeneity and encourages more specific treatments and precise research. The division also alters the category's unipolar–bipolar formulation (see below).

While several present categories can be combined in the melancholia construct, non-melancholic depression remains heterogeneous. *Dysthymia* is not a valid entity and likely represents patients with poorly treated depressive illness, depressive disorders that are exaggerations of temperament traits (*depressive personality*), and perhaps other undefined conditions (e.g. some anxiety disorders). The same is true for adjustment disorder, depressive type.[10] Separating these conditions from melancholia facilitates their further delineation.

Melancholia

Recognized for centuries, melancholia was understood to encompass depressive and manic phases as a single disease. Recent classifications degrade the construct with non-specific diagnostic criteria blurring boundaries between melancholia and other conditions that share depressive features, while they exaggerate the delineation of unipolar and bipolar categories.[11]

The poor validity of the present classification of depressive illness is demonstrated in numerous studies. For example, in an examination of co-morbidity in twins and the occurrence of future episodes to externally validate the DSM depression criteria, the number of symptoms (the hallmark of the criteria), their duration, and resulting impairment did not predict the presence of depressive illness in a co-twin or future episodes in the proband.[12] Another study found DSM criteria to have poor agreement with core features of melancholia derived from cluster and similar analytic techniques.[13]

Swelling population prevalence rates from 6 to 8% in the 1960s to over 10% for men and 20% for women today reflect the artificially low threshold for the diagnosis of major depression.[14] One Swedish study reports rates of almost 27% for men and a staggering 45% for women, but only 8 men and 9 women of over 2000 subjects were identified as having a "serious" depressive illness.[15] The inflation of depression base rates has profound and adverse effects on genetic research and healthcare policy.

Syndrome delineation

The melancholia syndrome is confirmed by over 70 multivariate analyses of patient and community samples of depressed persons. The studies find sample heterogeneity with a melancholia group most clearly delineated. About half of hospitalized depressed patients are identified as melancholic. The few studies that do not report sample heterogeneity and a recognizable melancholia syndrome have been challenged and re-interpreted.[16]

The defined syndrome is characterized by three symptom clusters, *all* present early in an episode. An *abnormal emotional state* is always present and is dominated by unremitting apprehension and overwhelming gloom. Unlike non-melancholic depressive disorders, the abnormal emotional state has a life of its own and is not reactive to pleasurable circumstances. *Psychomotor disturbance* is always present. Motor functions and cognitive activity are slowed and stupor and catatonia may occur. Other patients with melancholia are agitated, restless, and perseverative in their ruminations and actions. *Disturbances in vegetative body functions* are always present. Patients lose their appetites and weight, sleep little, and lose interest in sex and family activities. The disturbances impair recall and concentration and sufferers are unable to work efficiently. Self-care is abandoned. Thoughts are pre-occupied by despondency, death and considerations of self-harm. Delusions become prominent with thoughts of illness, guilt, worthlessness and danger overwhelming their actions. The DSM shortlist of "melancholic features" does not capture the melancholia syndrome.

Laboratory verification

The clinical features of melancholia mimic features of acute and chronic stress, and melancholia is considered a process eliciting an abnormal stress response.[17] Afternoon serum cortisol levels and the dexamethasone suppression test (DST) assess this abnormal response, and when melancholia is defined by its three symptom clusters rather than the shortlist DSM approach, 70% of patients have a positive test (i.e. non-suppression of serum cortisol following a challenge with 1–2 mg of dexamethasone).[18] A meta-analysis of 14 studies found non-suppression to be substantially higher in psychotic depressed patients (64%) than in non-psychotic patients (36%).[19] Patients with schizophrenia typically do not show abnormal cortisol levels or non-suppression, arguing that high HPA activity is not characteristic of psychosis but of melancholia. Test results normalize with successful treatment, and re-emerged as abnormal when patients relapse. Melancholia is also characterized by sleep abnormalities with a pattern of delayed sleep onset, reduced REM latency and increased REM percent time. These features distinguish melancholia from other disorders of mood.[20]

Pathophysiologic disturbances in persons with depression (e.g. brain metabolic and structural changes) also support the melancholia construct as most of the reports, while not specifically identifying the patients as melancholic, characterize them as severely ill, psychotic, or hospitalized. Half of hospitalized depressed patients and most with psychotic depression will be melancholic. Genetic studies also find the highest heritability in the most severely ill depressed patients.[21]

Treatment validation

The efficacy of ECT and to lesser extent tricyclic antidepressants in remitting melancholic depressive illness supports the diagnosis. About 90% of patients with melancholia who receive a full course of bilateral ECT remit within 3 weeks. In the multi-site collaborative ECT study of continuation ECT versus pharmacotherapy (CORE), bilateral ECT achieved an overall remission rate of 87% among the severely depressed patients who completed treatment, and a 95% rate for the 30%

of patients with psychotic depression.[22] More than 80% of the sample met symptom criteria for melancholia.[23] Successful ECT also reverses the hormone imbalances seen in depressive illness.[24]

Broad pharmacodynamic spectrum antidepressants (e.g. tricyclic agents) are more effective in melancholic than in non-melancholic patients.[25] Lithium moderates abnormal mood and reduces suicidal drive, and is the most effective augmenting agent in the treatment of acute depressive illness, unipolar and bipolar, when the depression is melancholic. It is efficient as continuation therapy for melancholic patients, especially when combined with the tricyclic antidepressant (TCA) nortriptyline.[26]

Although SSRI and similar agents are widely recommended in treatment algorithms as the first agents for major depression, their overall 30–40% remission rates differ only minimally from placebo rates.[27] There is virtually no placebo response among severely depressed patients.

Most of the recent head-to-head drug trials are industry-sponsored and report SSRI and TCA to be equally effective for major depression. But close inspection of these efforts find them misleading, with an advantage for TCA for the hospitalized and more severely ill.[28] A review of 186 randomized control trials found that amitriptyline had a better recovery rate than any of the alternative drugs, although it was less well tolerated.[29] Another meta-analysis found efficacy to favor TCA for hospitalized depressed patients (more likely to be melancholic), but not for other groups.[30] A third meta-analysis found TCA more effective than SSRI in severely depressed and elderly patients, also more likely to be melancholic.[31] Other reports find TCA superior to an SSRI with similar drop out rates and no significant cardiovascular problems with the TCA.[32] Three Danish double-blind randomized controlled antidepressant drug trials that included 292 inpatients, most of whom with melancholia, report clomipramine to be superior to several comparison non-TCA agents.[33]

Melancholic depressive disorder

Once major depression is separated into melancholia and non-melancholia depressive disorders, several present distinctions are best considered severity modifiers of melancholia rather than as separate conditions. This permits the application of the more specific treatments for melancholia.

Psychotic depression

Approximately one-third of melancholic patients are psychotic.[34] Nearly all patients with psychotic depression are melancholic.[35] Psychotic depression and non-psychotic melancholia are not different diseases.[36] Psychotic depression is a severe form of melancholia[37] and psychotic depressed patients have melancholic features similar to non-psychotic melancholic patients.[38]

Like other patients with melancholia, they respond rapidly to ECT.[39]

Mood-incongruence of psychotic thoughts, i.e. the delusional content, is deemed "bizarre" (e.g. delusions of passivity not of guilt or worthlessness) and mood-congruence, i.e. the delusion is considered depressive (e.g. low self-worth, self-blame), do not distinguish subgroups of patients with psychotic depression.[40] Delusions represent the degree of severity, not unique psychopathology. Other than the recognition of psychosis, no measure clearly distinguishes the psychotic and non-psychotic forms of melancholic illness.[41]

Depression with catatonia or stupor

The close association between mood disorders and catatonia is well established.[42] Among newly admitted catatonic patients about 30% are suffering from depressive illness.[43] Like patients with melancholia without catatonic features, depressed patients with catatonic features are more likely to exhibit high cortisol levels that do not suppress when challenged with dexamethasone.[44] Among newly hospitalized depressed patients, about 20% have catatonia.[45] Patients in depressive stupor are indistinguishable from those in stupor with other catatonic features supporting the idea that depressive stupor is a catatonic sign.[46] Prolonged fixed postures (catalepsy) and other catatonic features occur. Hallucinations and delusions are often present.[47]

Perinatal depression

Major depressive illness occurring during pregnancy or in the postpartum period does not differ substantially from depressive illness occurring at other times, and most such patients are likely to be melancholic. Serious depressive illness occurs in about 5% of women during the several months after delivery.[48] Risk factors are similar to those for depressive illness occurring at other times, and include past premenstrual dysphoric disorder, undue psychosocial stress, and a personal or family history of mood disorder.[49] Because postpartum depression is commonly associated with depressive symptoms during pregnancy, pre- and postpartum depressive illness are best considered a single perinatal process.[50]

The psychopathology of severe perinatal depression does not differ from melancholia at other times,[51] although treatment considerations differ.[52] When of psychotic severity, perinatal psychotic depressive illness is also indistinguishable from psychotic depressive illness occurring at other times.[53]

Patients with perinatal depressive illness do not have a unique perinatal illness, they have mood disorder. There is an increased risk of depressive illness among their siblings compared to the siblings of women without depressive illness.[54]

A twin study of parous women reported a heritability of 38% for self-report postpartum depressive symptoms.[55]

A study comparing illness patterns in the first-degree relatives of women with perinatal depression only, perinatal and non-perinatal depressions, and those with manic-depression with no perinatal episodes found over 60% of relatives in all three groups to have a mood disorder and most of these were non-perinatal. The groups did not differ in the prevalence of perinatal episodes.[56] While some studies find that perinatal depression is not related to manic-depression,[57] some find such a relationship.[58]

Follow-up studies from years to decades of patients with perinatal depression find these patients to have long-term courses similar to those of their relatives and other patients with non-perinatal depressive illness: most will have a recurrence of depressive illness and most of these episodes will be non-perinatal.[59] Some studies report these patients have a less severe course than those who only have non-perinatal depression,[60] while other studies report some patients have substantial impairment on follow-up and a manic-depressive course.[61] ECT leads to remission in most such patients within 4 weeks of treatment.[62]

Thus, family studies and follow-up reports are consistent with the psychopathology findings in perinatal depressive illness that these patients do not have a unique form of depression and best fit the model of melancholic illness. They also respond to treatment particularly useful for melancholia. Other than "postpartum blues", a common mild, transient state of weepiness and fatigue, all perinatal depressive illness is best considered melancholic disorder.

Abnormal bereavement

Abnormal bereavement is presented as a specified class of depression, but its operational definitions are consistent with the melancholia construct (psychosis, marked psychomotor impairment, preoccupation with worthlessness and wanting to die, suicide attempt, and failure to regain pre-death social functioning within two months). Although grief may persist for several years and one-third of widowed older persons initially meet DSM criteria for major depression, the common signs of depression rarely last beyond several weeks.[63] Symptoms persisting past one month after the death are associated with continuing mood disorder and echo the classic features of melancholia.[64] Suicide remains a persistent risk.[65] Persons identified as having abnormal bereavement have high cortisol levels and DST non-suppression.[66] This is not the case in those with normal bereavement. For example, among 19 recently widowed persons, while 58% met RDC criteria for depression, only 17% were non-suppressors on the DST.[67] Four weeks following the death of a parent, children and adolescents have normal cortisol functioning. In one study of bereavement, however, 39% were non-suppressors.

These patients had many melancholic features and were suicidal, clinically meeting criteria for melancholia as well as abnormal bereavement.[68] Abnormal bereavement should be eliminated from the classification. The death of a loved one does not elicit a unique depressive illness.

Bipolar and unipolar categories

Syndrome delineation

When depression is divided into melancholia and non-melancholia classes, the distinction between the bipolar and unipolar categories changes. Unipolar disorder becomes non-melancholia depressive disorder. Bipolar disorder is melancholia with associated mania or hypomania. What appears to be recurrent melancholia only and melancholia associated with mania or hypomania are aspects of one disease as formulated by Kraepelin, *manic-depressive illness*. Non-melancholic disorder consists of different depressive illnesses and some anxiety disorders, while melancholic disorder consists of patients all of whom experience melancholic depression and many who also experience mania or hypomania. Others have also reached this conclusion.[69]

The challenges to the present bipolar/unipolar dichotomy are substantial, but the controversy can be resolved with the melancholia/non-melancholia separation. The delineation of manic-depressive illness into unipolar and bipolar distinctions was initially supported by family history studies.[70] The dichotomy was challenged, first in literature reviews and then in prospective studies.[71] Family illness patterns are not clearly dichotomous. The most common mood disorder in the first-degree relatives of patients with bipolar disorder is recurrent depressive illness ("unipolar disorder"). The morbid risk (age-corrected prevalence) for unipolar disorder in the families of the bipolar patients is greater than the morbid risks for unipolar depression in the families of unipolar patients. The risk for manic-depressive illness is modestly elevated in the relatives of patients with recurrent depression.[72] Several investigators concluded that they could not distinguish unipolar and bipolar patients by family data *as long as depression was defined as melancholia*.[73] However, in a large family study, Winokur *et al.* (1995) reported that there was little familial overlap between bipolar and unipolar conditions. But an examination of their data shows that the families of patients with psychotic depression were similar to those of patients with manic-depression. Psychotic depression is melancholia.

Twin studies also show the overlap.[74] In the analysis of 30 monozygotic and 37 dizygotic twin pairs the proband-concordance was higher for monozygotic than for dizygotic twins, with heritability estimated at 89%. In almost 29% of the monozygotic pairs, one twin had both manic and depressive episodes while the other had recurrent depressive illness. Among dizygotic pairs, 13.5% had a mixed concordance. The investigators tested several lability models and concluded that manic-depressive illness was not simply a more severe form of recurrent depressive illness, but that nevertheless the two forms exhibit substantial genetic overlap (about 30%).[75]

In an extensive analysis of the literature of manic-depressive illness, Goodwin and Jamison concluded:[76]

"Taken together, the data suggest that they [unipolar and bipolar] are best considered as two subgroups of manic-depressive illness rather than separate and distinct illnesses. The available data also support a continuum model, with "pure" bipolar illness at one end and unipolar illness at the other. (p. 65)

Since Goodwin and Jamison's review, the unipolar and bipolar dichotomy has been questioned repeatedly. Melancholic depressions associated with mania or hypomania cannot be distinguished from melancholia without the association.[77] Most cross-sectional clinical features do not distinguish a first episode of a recurrent severe depression from the initial depression in a manic-depressive course.[78] Mixed states are common, with manic-like features emerging even in patients with several initial episodes of depression.[79]

Patients initially considered unipolar are commonly re-labeled bipolar.[80] The apparent pure "polar" forms are recurrent and in succeeding episodes 70% of patients initially classified as bipolar experience mostly episodes of depression, while 10–15% of patients with recurrent depressive illness eventually exhibit episodes of mania, and over half show features of mania when depressed.[81] Depression is found to be the predominant and most frequent mood disturbance in bipolar patients, and the depression of bipolar disorder is commonly characterized as psychotic depression, melancholia, depression with severe psychomotor retardation, or atypical depression.

The singularity of manic-depressive illness is described in numerous reports, and the proposed bipolar I, II and III are a continuum.[82] Cassano *et al.* (2004) presented clinical data from 117 patients initially designated as having "remitted recurrent unipolar depression" with 106 said to have bipolar I disorder, and concluded:

Cumulatively our empirical findings support a continuous view of the mood spectrum as a unitary phenomenon that is best understood from a longitudinal perspective. Our data suggest that unipolar disorder and bipolar disorder are not two discrete and dichotomous phenomena but that mood fluctuations – up and down – are common to both conditions.

Laboratory verification

The pattern of neurobiological markers of mania and severe depression are alike and do not delineate recurrent depressive melancholic illness from manic-depression. DST non-suppression[83] and increased cortisol levels[84] are observed with equivalent frequencies in both depressed and manic phases of manic-depression. Hypothalamic–pituitary–thyroid axis dysfunction occurs in both forms, perhaps more so in manic-depressive patients than in patients experiencing only recurrent depression.[85]

Neurochemically, serotonergic and dopaminergic responsiveness appear similar in both forms of illness.[86] Although less consistently observed, both forms have abnormal circadian phase shifts.[87]

Brain structural and metabolic findings are also similar, but the literature on mania is limited.[88] Structural studies report inconsistent findings difficult to reconcile, while metabolic studies are confounded by the inclusion of many medicated patients. When the depressed patients are characterized as moderately to severely ill and thus likely to include many patients with melancholia, overall, the same brain structures are abnormal in mania and depression.[89]

Studies of glucose metabolism report frontal cortex hypometabolism.[90] Increased anterior cingulate and caudate cerebral blood flow is also reported.[91] The few differences reflect opposite patterns of activity. For example, in depressed phases of the illness increased ventral and decreased dorsal prefrontal cortex metabolism is reported in cerebral blood flow and PET investigations. In mania, the pattern is opposite. In studies identifying asymmetrical abnormalities, depression is associated with increased metabolism on the left, while in mania homologous right-sided structures appear less active. Hemispheric instability has been hypothesized to explain these differences and how a patient shifts from depression to mania.[92]

Treatment validation

Lithium's effectiveness in mania and melancholia is additional support for the idea that the present unipolar/bipolar formulation incorrectly merges all forms of depressive illness. Lithium therapy is the most specific and effective treatment for acute mania and is the gold standard for preventing future episodes of mood disturbance. When prescribed continuously for several years, it substantially lowers the risk of suicide in manic-depressives.[93]

Lithium is also effective in patients with recurrent depressive illness who do not experience mania or hypomania. Double-blind placebo-controlled studies of lithium augmentation report substantial benefit, with 50–63% of patients remitting.[94] Melancholic patients benefit at twice the rates of non-melancholic patients. Melancholic patients who suffer recurrent depressions or who have both manic and depressive episodes have similar response rates.[95] Maintenance lithium therapy prevents future depressive episodes, even in patients without a history of mania or hypomania.[96]

Rather than the present separation of mood disorders into bipolar and unipolar groups, a better formulation is: (1) melancholia with or without mania or hypomania, catatonia, or psychosis, and (2) non-melancholia disorders. Abnormal bereavement and perinatal depressive conditions are melancholic depressions and do not warrant separate classification. The delineation of the non-melancholic category awaits further study.

Psychotic disorders

Psychotic disorders are defined by the presence of hallucinations or delusions. Although mood disorders and delirium are frequently accompanied by psychosis, they are separately classified. The distinction of "always" for the psychosis category versus "frequent" for the others is arbitrary and diagnostically imprecise. Classifying by these non-specific features is equivalent to classifying infectious disease by the presence or absence of fever. Latent class analyses of patients with psychosis do not support the present classification, concluding that the present system obscures subtle but meaningfully different illness forms.[97] A psychosis category encourages false positive diagnoses, i.e. a manic or melancholic patient is hallucinating and delusional, and therefore is given one of the psychotic disorder diagnoses. The psychosis category should be eliminated and its valid conditions, i.e. delusional disorder and schizophrenia, independently placed in the classification. The term schizophrenia, however, has less meaning than Kraepelin's dementia praecox. It represents a heterogeneous population most suffering from a chronic psychotic disorder.

The psychosis category's organization is also arbitrary and includes conditions of weak validity. The separation of schizophrenia, schizophreniform and brief psychotic disorder by the duration of their acute psychosis phase (>6 months, <6 but >1, and <1 month) is not valid. A discrete pathophysiology does not end on a certain day and a new one begins. A construct that requires a psychosis beginning on 1 February to be re-diagnosed after 28 days, but the identical condition beginning on 1 March to be re-diagnosed only after 31 days is patently foolish.

The core, commonly shared DSM criterion for schizophrenia (all types), schizophreniform disorder, and schizoaffective disorder is criterion A of the schizophrenia criteria. Two of the following features are required: hallucinations, delusions, disorganized speech, disorganized behavior or catatonia, and negative symptoms. Brief psychotic disorder is defined by a modification of this criterion, one symptom being sufficient and negative symptoms omitted as a choice. One feature alone is also accepted if a delusion is "bizarre" or a hallucination is a sustained voice. This harkens back to the Schneiderian notion of first-rank symptoms, a construct not supported by the data. The use of terminology such as "grossly disorganized" and "bizarre" behavior are vague and over-inclusive, assuring false positive conclusions. The use of catatonia as a criterion disregards the extensive literature on catatonia as a distinct syndrome. From a scientific perspective, catatonia's continued presence in the schizophrenia criteria is unsupportable.

The evidence for schizoaffective disorder as a separate illness from mood disorder with psychosis is unimpressive and the syndrome is best placed in the mood disorders category. There is a clinical adage "If the diagnosis is uncertain and no harm is likely, make the choice with the best prognosis and for which there are better treatments." From this perspective, patients who meet criteria for schizoaffective disorder would best be served if considered a psychotic form of manic-depressive illness rather than a form of schizophrenia with mood features. Shared psychotic disorder has little validation and should be eliminated.

Schizophrenia

The DSM/ICD image of schizophrenia is limited to a few cross-sectional features that can be distorted by idiosyncratic usage of criterion A. Persons who experience only complete auditory hallucinations, or delusions of alienation or control, or catatonic features with any hallucination or delusion meet the criterion. But many other conditions are associated with these features. The division of the syndrome into paranoid, catatonic, disorganized, undifferentiated and residual forms has neither clinical nor research utility.

Identifying schizophrenia by the presence of emotional blunting, however, has repeatedly shown the negative or deficit syndrome to be reliably assessed and stable over time. Patients with these features are likely to have a chronic course, sustained cognitive impairment, and a family history of psychosis.[98] Negative symptoms are the best variable discriminating ICD-10 defined schizophrenics from patients with other psychotic syndromes.[99] Schizophrenic patients, however, cannot be clearly divided into positive and negative symptom subgroups, as most exhibit both types of features.[100]

Research over the past 40 years has also demonstrated that schizophrenia is not merely the summation of psychotic episodes. The model of a developmental disorder as the basis for schizophrenia best fits the data showing sufferers to have emotional, social, cognitive, and neuromotor problems beginning in childhood. Substantial genetic and intrauterine factors contribute to the condition.[101] The psychosis of schizophrenia can be defined in cross-section by the presence of emotional blunting and hallucinations or delusions and longitudinally by the presence of childhood pre-psychotic features. To fit the data, criterion A should be modified to resemble Table 16.2. Each feature should also be operationally defined.[102]

Table 16.2. Proposed revision of criterion A for schizophrenia (all must be present)

1. Emotional blunting (loss of emotional expression and avolition)
2. Any one of the following:
   Hallucinations of voices
   Delusions of passivity
   Formal thought disorder
3. Pre-psychosis features (any two):
   Long-standing emotional aloofness
   Poor peer socialization
   Neuromotor developmental delays or other abnormalities
   Poor sustained attention without hyperactivity
   Cognitive inflexibility
   Odd word usage

Schizophrenia, however, while a traditional term, has no scientific meaning. Bleuler coined it to indicate a splitting of mental functions, a non-specific notion without validity. Heterogeneity is likely among patients with the diagnosis even when defined by the criteria above. Its usage only implies a nonaffective disorder with psychosis. This alternative terminology should be considered.[103]

Schizophreniform psychosis

Karl Langfeldt introduced the concept of schizophreniform psychosis in 1939, referring to patients who initially appeared to have a schizophrenic psychosis but who did not devolve to a chronic defect state. Langfeldt hypothesized a psychogenic origin for the condition. The original concept limited an episode to a few months, but the "less than 6 months, but more than a month" DSM criterion is arbitrary and can only be applied retrospectively.[104] Brief psychotic disorder is a variation of the schizophreniform notion.

In reviewing Langfeldt's original series, Fish concluded the sample was heterogeneous, with patients suffering from manic-depression, cycloid psychosis, and personality disorder.[105] In a five-year follow-up of 123 persons with a first-episode psychosis, for example, those with a schizophreniform diagnosis had more positive symptoms, fewer negative symptoms, and more manic symptoms.[106]

Efforts to distinguish schizophreniform psychosis from schizophrenia focus on first ever episodes. Patients with first episodes lasting only a few weeks (brief psychotic disorder) have a better long-term prognosis than those with first episodes lasting 6 months or longer.[107] The presence of mood disorder features also indicates a better prognosis.[108] Many such patients, however, cannot be meaningfully distinguished from acutely ill manic patients on any clinical or laboratory variable.

Acute manics are typically psychotic, come to medical attention within days or a few weeks of episode onset, and with appropriate treatment remit quickly.[109]

Long-term follow-up studies consistently find that patients identified as having schizophreniform disorder are clinically heterogeneous, that the diagnosis is not stable over time, and that many such patients have recurrences identified as mood disorder or schizoaffective illness, but not schizophrenia.[110] Most such patients benefit from treatments for mood disorder. The category should be discarded.

Schizoaffective disorder

The introduction of the schizoaffective construct was an effort to understand the unexpected variable outcomes of patients diagnosed as schizophrenic.[111] Such patients were defined by a long-term course in between the poor outcomes of schizophrenia and the better outcomes of patients with manic-depression. Its addition to present classification was to provide a class for uncertain diagnosis, not because it was an established condition. Not surprisingly, reliability for the diagnosis is poor.[112] Efforts to refine it have been unsuccessful.

For example, the psychotic episodes of patients with the schizoaffective label and those with schizophrenia and manic-depression reveal overlapping features that do not discriminate the conditions.[113] Long-term follow-up studies find schizoaffective patients to be more like those with manic-depressive illness than like those with schizophrenia. This is particularly so for patients with prominent cross-sectional features of depression or mania. The presence of psychotic features does not predict the course.[114] Patients with the diagnosis also respond best to treatments typically prescribed for those with mood disorder.[115]

Family studies find the first-degree relatives of schizoaffective patients to have increased risks for schizophrenic, manic-depressive, and schizoaffective episodes, suggesting heterogeneity within patient samples.[116] Genetic linkage studies, relying on poorly defined samples, find some overlap between schizophrenia and manic-depressive illness on several chromosomes, roiling meaningful understanding of distinctions among psychotic patients.[117]

Overall, the data support the position that the schizoaffective category should be eliminated or added to the mood disorders as a severity modifier.[118] A recent literature review similarly concluded that schizoaffective disorder "is not a separate, 'bona-fide' disease. Patients diagnosed with [it] likely suffer from a psychotic mood disorder. The diagnosis of schizoaffective disorder, which can result in substandard treatment, should be eliminated".[119]

Cycloid psychosis was introduced by Karl Leonhard as an alternative to the schizophreniform idea. He distinguished it from schizophrenia and manic-depressive illness.[120] Its usage has waxed and waned since its introduction, and interest in it is limited to Europe.

Perris and others[121] characterize the syndrome as of acute onset with perplexity or puzzlement, overwhelming fearfulness alternating with ecstasy, akinetic or hyperactive phases, and delusions and hallucinations of any kind. It is reported to be uncommon, but familial. The construct comes closest to the idea of schizoaffective disorder with patients experiencing intense and multiple psychotic features as well as symptoms of mood disorder. A similar notion is *bouffée délirante* of the French literature, another acute, brief psychotic syndrome. Patients with the cycloid psychosis diagnosis respond best to treatments for mood disorder. The construct has neither clinical nor research value and should not be included in classifications.[122]

Shared psychotic disorder (Folie à deux)

No other medical field creates a distinct illness category based on the fact that two or more persons with close contact have a similar illness. If all members of a family suffer from "a cold" there is no "shared Rhinovirus disorder" in which to lump them. The notion is absurd. Among the scattered case reports, most of the dyads are either siblings or parent–child pairs with a highly heritable disorder, or spouses with a disorder recognized as associated with assortative mating (e.g. patients with similar illnesses are more likely to meet).[123]

Catatonia[124]

Catatonia is a well-defined syndrome of motor dysregulation that is associated with many conditions. Its present primary linkage in classification to schizophrenia is anachronistic and poorly serves the majority of patients with catatonia. Most have associated mood disorder or definable and treatable neurologic disease. It should be in a separate diagnostic class, as are delirium and dementia. The evidence for this has been reviewed extensively.[125]

The primary linkage of catatonia to schizophrenia influences clinicians to think that most, if not all, patients with catatonia are suffering from schizophrenia. Treatments based on this erroneous impression rely on increasing doses of antipsychotic agents for "catatonic schizophrenia". This approach not only fails to relieve catatonia, but may worsen the condition by inducing the *Neuroleptic Malignant Syndrome*, a form of *malignant catatonia*. Further, the more likely causes of catatonia will not be sought or specifically treated.

Systematic studies of catatonic patients in Europe, North America, and Asia from the early 1920s to the present find about 50% to have manic-depression as their primary illness.[126] Among manic patients, 25% or more will have sufficient catatonic features to meet present DSM criteria. In more severely ill manic patients, almost all exhibit catatonic features.[127] Many general medical conditions are associated with catatonia and include metabolic disorders, and infection.[128]

Exposure to antipsychotic drugs and SSRI, benzodiazepine withdrawal, dopaminergic drug withdrawal, opiate intoxication, and the use of many illicit drugs are causes for catatonia.[129] Post-encephalitic states, and basal ganglia and frontal lobe disease are some of the neurologic conditions associated with catatonia.[130] Developmental disorders and epilepsy are frequent causes in children.[131] About 10% of patients with catatonia meet criteria for schizophrenia when that diagnosis requires no evidence of mood disorder.[132] Catalepsy, mannerisms, posturing, and mutism are the features traditionally associated with schizophrenia.

Catatonia is common. Since 1990, systematic surveys of acutely hospitalized psychiatric patients find 10–15% of such patients to be catatonic, even by the restrictive DSM criteria. The recent surveys are consistent with reports from 1920 to 1976 that find the prevalence of catatonia among hospitalized psychiatric patients as 7–37%.[133]

Cognitive disorders

Several established neuro-behavioral syndromes are not delineated in psychiatric classification although such patients are commonly hospitalized in psychiatric facilities. A typical clinical recourse is to force a diagnosis of mood or psychotic disorder or apply the label NOS. Treatments for mood disorder or psychosis are then applied, although more specific pharmacotherapy and rehabilitation care could be offered.

The syndromes with the most supporting evidence involve frontal lobe circuitry, and several of these are detailed in Chapters 3, 13, and 15.[134] The *volitional/apathetic* and the *disinhibited frontal lobe syndromes* should be included as separate categories in the cognitive disorders section of psychiatric classifications.

Obsessive–compulsive disorder (OCD)

Present classification places OCD in the anxiety disorders category. This decision was based primarily on observations that obsessions elicit anxiety while compulsions may reduce anxiety and encourage associated phobic avoidance.[135] Anxiety, however, is a non-specific phenomenon and most patients with Axis I conditions are anxious.

In contrast, the phenomenology, demographics, neurobiology, and treatment evidence that define OCD best characterize it as a separate class that includes tic disorder, body dysmorphic disorders, and most of the present impulse control disorders such as trichotillomania.[136] Anorexia nervosa is also best classified in the OCD category. Pathological gambling appears to be a heterogeneous category, the non-ill mixed in with persons exhibiting many OCD features.[137] Kleptomania and pathological gambling are co-occurring. Non-melancholic depression is also co-occurring but does not appear to be part of the OCD pathophysiology.[138] OCD warrants its own category of *OCD spectrum disorders.*

The OCD spectrum is seen as several clusters – *somatic:* body image, hypochondriasis, body dysmorphic disorder, anorexia nervosa, and binge eating; *impulse control:* some persons with pathological gambling, some paraphilias, trichotillomania, kleptomania, and self-injury; and *repetitive movement:* Gilles de la Tourette's syndrome, and Sydenham's chorea.[139]

Non-melancholic depression (about 20% of patients) is the most common co-occurring condition with OCD. This prevalence is modestly higher than base rates for non-melancholic depression and may reflect demoralization from the OCD and the low bar for the diagnosis of depression in present criteria.[140] Social phobia is also common, but the prevalence rates for other anxiety disorders are within the estimated population base rates (0–10%).[141] In contrast, the prevalence rates for co-occurring spectrum conditions are greater than estimated population base rates (e.g. 5–10% for anorexia nervosa, body dysmorphic disorder, hypochondriasis, and trichotillomania, 5% for sexual compulsions, and 2–4% for Gilles de la Tourette's syndrome). In patients with these spectrum conditions the prevalence rates of OCD is also high.[142] In contrast, patients with anxiety disorder have low rates of the spectrum conditions.[143]

Family and twin studies find substantial heritability for OCD (about 50%).[144] Family, twin and molecular genetic studies, however, are inconclusive, offering little help in resolving the classification of OCD. While increased rates of OCD, anxiety disorders, and mood disorders are reported in the first-degree relatives of patients with OCD,[145] other studies, while finding higher rates of OCD in relatives of OCD patients, find rates of anxiety disorders and mood disorders similar to those of the general population.[146] The separation of depression into melancholia and non-melancholia disorders may clarify this contradiction. Hollander and colleagues conclude from their review that "most anxiety disorders and affective disorders do not have a familial relationship with OCD".[147]

The lifetime risk for tic disorders and Gilles de la Tourette's disorder (GTS) is also greater in relatives of patients with OCD.[148] The prevalence rates of OCD spectrum disorders are also higher in the first-degree relatives of patients with OCD than in controls,[149] as are the rates of spectrum conditions in the relatives of patients with OCD spectrum. Higher rates of classic OCD are reported in the relatives of patients with trichotillomania[150]

However, no increased risk in relatives of OCD patients is found for eating disorders, but anorexia and bulimia are not separated,[151] and others have found an increased risk for OCD spectrum in the relatives of patients with eating disorder.[152]

The neurology of OCD and the proposed OCD variants reveal similar abnormalities in several domains.[153] Functional brain imaging reveals basal ganglia and white matter abnormalities in patients with classic OCD.[154] Reduced basal ganglia and cerebellar volumes are also reported in patients with trichotillomania.[155]

Patients with OCD have similar patterns of impairment on neuropsychological testing as patients with OCD spectrum conditions. These include problems with working memory, cognitive flexibility, and visual–spatial function (e.g. pattern recognition memory).[156]

Serotonin reuptake agents are the recommended pharmacotherapy, and response prevention or exposure the recommended behavioral therapy for OCD.[157] These treatments are also recommended for the OCD variants of body dysmorphic disorder,[158] pathological gambling,[159] kleptomania,[160] trichotillomania,[161] hypochondriasis,[162] anorexia nervosa,[163] GTS,[164] and some patients with paraphilia[165] or posttraumatic stress disorder.[166] This literature, however, is weak, and there are negative as well as positive studies for most of the variants.[167]

The DSM "obsessive–compulsive personality" likely represents a chronic low-grade illness rather than a deviation in personality development and should also be included in the OCD spectrum. The same behaviors that define OCD define obsessive–compulsive personality.[168] The two conditions are co-occurring. Differences among studies assessing this co-morbidity are, however, inconsistent, relying on categorical rather than dimensional diagnostic criteria, and thus undercounting mild forms of obsessive–compulsive personality. In the studies assessing the co-morbidities of obsessive–compulsive personality reviewed by Fineberg and colleagues (2007), anorexia nervosa and OCD were commonly associated conditions. Family studies also find greater than expected rates of obsessive–compulsive personality in the relatives of patients with OCD.[169]

Somatoform disorders

The somatoform disorder category is conceptually flawed in the defining assumption that it represents conditions whose features are poorly explained by medical evaluation. The limits of present medical knowledge should not be a criterion for defining a behavioral condition.[170] Most of the options in this grouping are best classified elsewhere, and are discussed in several previous chapters. About half of patients with the diagnosis, particularly the most common "undifferentiated" type, do not meet somatoform criteria on follow-up, and those that do are most likely to have depressive illness.[171]

Among the conditions included in the category, body dysmorphic disorder is an OCD variant. Hypochondriasis is a symptom, not a syndrome, and does not warrant separate classification. It is a feature of OCD and depressive illness.[172]

Conversion disorder is also a phenomenon associated with several conditions and does not warrant separate classification.[173] The category should be discarded.

Dissociative conditions[174]

Dissociation is a symptom, not a syndrome. Depersonalization and derealization are seen in anxiety disorders and epileptic conditions. Fugue states and multiple personality can only be medically verified as expressions of seizure disorder. Dissociative amnesia is best explained as a syndrome representing several conditions. The category should be discarded.

Impulse control conditions

The category should be eliminated. Impulsiveness is a behavior, not a disease. Kleptomania, pyromania, pathological gambling, and trichotillomania are OCD variants. Intermittent explosive behavior is a symptom, not a syndrome, and is associated with seizure disorder, traumatic brain injury, delirium and dementia, substance abuse, and antisocial personality disorder. It is like fever in infectious disease and is an ill-defined criterion for classification.

Personality disorders

Axis considerations

Data summarized in Chapters 14 and 15 show present personality disorder classifications to be inconsistent with the evidence. Personality disorder reflects deviant trait behavior evolving from maturational factors, but much of the present formulation reflects disease (e.g. all of the DSM cluster A). The trait syndromes that meet the definition (e.g. narcissistic personality) are poorly defined categorically. The severity continuum of the three DSM clusters does not exist. The cluster system is unsupported and should be eliminated. Many of the present Axis II conditions are best placed within other syndromes or classified independently (see below).

The conditions reflecting maturational deviation should be delineated by dimensional criteria so that the number of features and their degree of strength would both be required to reach a rated score. Several dimensional models could replace the present approach, the "5-Factor" and Cloninger temperament–character systems providing opportunities to re-define the personality disorders.[175] Cloninger's terminology offers understandable descriptive terms: *harm avoidance, novelty seeking, reward dependence, persistence, cooperativeness, self-directedness,* and *self-transcendence.* The 5-factor terms are: *extraversion, agreeableness, conscientiousness, neuroticism, openness to experience, social contact, curiosity, honor, power, order, idealism, independence, status, vengeance, romance, family, activity, saving, acceptance, eating,* and *tranquility.* The details of the terms can form the diagnostic criteria for each personality deviation.

Cluster considerations

Cluster A should be eliminated. These entities reflect low-grade chronic illness. *Schizoid personality* is a variant of schizophrenia and should be included in that category as a pre-psychosis trait. *Paranoid personality* is a variant of delusional disorder and should be included in that category as a mild form. *Schizotypal personality* is a heterogeneous class that includes patients with mood disorder, seizure disorder, and psychoses from traumatic brain injury and illicit drug use.[176] It should be labeled as an independent schizotypal disorder in Axis I akin to delirium.

Cluster B mixes disease and trait abnormalities. *Antisocial, histrionic,* and *narcissistic* personality disorders overlap in presentation and in other variables, but are not well-defined categorically.[177] Their pattern of psychopathology also suggests that they are composed of sub-clusters that may indicate heterogeneity.[178] They are better defined dimensionally as deviations on reliably identified and validated temperament traits, sharing high novelty seeking (high behavioral activation), and low harm avoidance (low behavioral inhibition). They should be grouped in an independent class.

Borderline personality is another heterogeneous category[179] and 50–80% of such patients have an Axis I diagnosis that accounts for all their symptoms.[180] About 50% of patients with the borderline diagnosis exhibit features of the "soft bipolar spectrum" construct or manic-depressive illness with a childhood onset. The latter is less episodic, more chronic, and less severe than the classic form and is associated with drug abuse. Symptoms may be misconstrued as trait behaviors.[181] Such patients should be regarded as having a mood disorder and placed in that category.

The remaining persons given the borderline diagnosis should be given independent status, recognizing their heterogeneity.[182] The term borderline should be replaced. It borders nothing and has no scientific meaning. Persons with the label who do not have mood disorder are diagnosed by the consequences of behaviors associated with antisocial, histrionic, and narcissistic personality disorders. A stormy life with self-mutilating behavior is not a pathognomonic pattern and the reliability of such criteria is poor. In addition to mood disorder, diagnoses associated with these features are mild mental retardation and related syndromes (e.g. Asperger's), obsessive–compulsive disorder, chronic drug abuse affecting basal ganglia (stimulants), and epilepsy.[183]

Cluster C is poorly defined categorically. These patients are better delineated dimensionally as sharing low behavioral activation (low novelty seeking) and high behavioral inhibition (high harm-avoidance).[184]

Table 16.3. Proposed Axis II changes

Eliminate the cluster system

Place schizoid in the schizophrenia spectrum

Classify paranoid personality as a mild delusional disorder

Classify the schizotypal syndrome as an independent Axis I class

Reformulate the borderline condition into two groupings, one as a form of mood disorder and one as an independent Axis I class

Group antisocial, histrionic, and narcissistic personality conditions as an independent class defined by dimensional criteria

Group dependent and avoidant personality conditions as an independent class defined by dimensional criteria

Classify obsessive–compulsive personality in the OCD spectrum

Dependent and avoidant personality classes, however, differ from obsessive–compulsive personality in that patients with obsessive–compulsive personality are low in reward dependence (i.e. they are less likely to be influenced by praise, affection, money and power), while patients with dependent and avoidant personalities exhibit high reward dependence and are greatly influenced by the responses of others. Persons with dependent and avoidant personalities experience anxiety associated with sensitivity to the actions of others. Persons with obsessive–compulsive personality exhibit anxiety when they are unable to act independently and control their situation.[185]

There are, however, reports of avoidant and dependent personality disorders co-occurrence with some cluster A conditions. Such persons are said to exhibit low reward dependence, and decreased sentimentality and the need for social contact.[186] In contrast, most persons with avoidant and dependent personality disorders have high reward dependence with increased sentimentality and the need for social contact,[187] suggesting that the reported co-occurrence is superficial and an artifact of assessing personality categorically.

Obsessive–compulsive personality should be classified as part of the OCD spectrum. Avoidant and dependent personality should be independently classified. Table 16.3 summarizes the proposed Axis II changes.

Conclusion

Traditions in psychopathology have served medicine well, delineating disorders that permit the prescription of increasingly more specific treatments. Lithium in the treatment of manic-depression is a classic model. Most recent efforts have reawakened the recognition of catatonia and melancholia and their treatments.[188]

Official classifications, however, have never been fully consistent with the syndromes recognized by clinicians and researchers, but the advent of DSM-III was a sea-change that abandoned the traditional principles of psychopathologic clinical investigation. The change seriously limited the diagnostic acumen of this generation of young psychiatrists worldwide.

Much of what is detailed in this book is not incorporated in present classifications and is not taught in the disciplines responsible for the care of the psychiatrically ill. These formulations, however, have face validity and are supported by many studies. The mastery of it, however, is an on-going, difficult process. Considering the recommended changes in classification offered here and using the detailed psychopathology presented throughout the text in the diagnosis of patients are the beginnings of the effort. It is "the road less taken", but the journey is worthwhile.

NOTES

1 Lewis Carroll (1872). *Through the Looking Glass and What Alice Found There.* London, Macmillan.
2 Fink and Taylor (2003, 2006).
3 Craddock *et al.* (2006); Owen *et al.* (2007).
4 Robert and Plantikow (2005).
5 Adapted from Taylor and Fink (2006, 2007).
6 The DSM-III and -IV formulation was supported by several literature reviews (Rush and Weisenburger, 1994). The conclusions, however, have been challenged (Taylor and Fink, 2007).
7 Rush (2007).
8 Ghaemi *et al.* (2006).
9 Stroup *et al.* (2003).
10 Taylor and Fink (2006, chapter 3).
11 Taylor and Fink (2006).
12 Kendler *et al.* (1996); Kendler and Gardner (1998).
13 Joyce *et al.* (2002).
14 Blazer *et al.* (1988, 1994); Olsson and von Knorring (1999); Ayuso-Mateos *et al.* (2001); Kessler *et al.* (2003).
15 Rorsman *et al.* (1990).
16 Parker and Hadzi-Pavlovic (1996); Taylor and Fink (2006, chapter 3).
17 Taylor and Fink (2006, chapter 14).
18 Carroll *et al.* (1981); Carroll (1982).
19 Nelson and Davis (1997).
20 First and Zimmerman (2006); Taylor and Fink (2006, chapters 3 and 4).

21 Taylor and Fink (2006, chapter 14).

22 Petrides *et al.* (2001); also see Maixner and Taylor (2008).

23 Max Fink, personal communication.

24 Fink (2000).

25 Danish University Antidepressant Group (1986, 1990, 1993); Roose *et al.* (1994); Perry (1996); Nobler and Roose (1998); Thase (2003).

26 Taylor and Fink (2006, chapter 10); Kellner *et al.* (2006).

27 Khan *et al.* (2003, 2005b); STAR*D study (Rush, 2007).

28 Freemantle *et al.* (2000).

29 Barbui and Hotoph (2001). Nortriptyline offers similar efficacy with better tolerability.

30 Anderson (2000).

31 Anderson and Tomenson (1994).

32 Perry (1996); Schatzberg (1998); Navarro *et al.* (2001); Akhondzadeh *et al.* (2003).

33 Hildebrandt *et al.* (2003).

34 Mulsant *et al.* (1997); Petrides *et al.* (2001).

35 Rush and Weisenburger (1994).

36 Parker and Hadzi-Pavlovic (1996); Taylor and Fink (2006, chapter 12).

37 Parker *et al.* (1991); Schatzberg and Rothschild (1992).

38 Kessing (2003).

39 Kantor and Glassman (1977); Petrides *et al.* (2001); Kho *et al.* (2003).

40 Abrams and Taylor (1983); Kendler (1991); Pini *et al.* (2004).

41 Bellini *et al.* (1992).

42 Fink and Taylor (2003).

43 Morrison (1973); Rohland *et al.* (1993).

44 Greden and Carroll (1979).

45 Kruger and Braunig (2000).

46 Benegal *et al.* (1992).

47 Fink and Taylor (2003).

48 Gavin *et al.* (2005).

49 Miller (2002); Freeman *et al.* (2002); Janssen *et al.* (1996); Jones and Craddock (2001).

50 Beck (1996); Robertson *et al.* (2004).

51 Wisner *et al.* (1993, 1995); Hendrick *et al.* (2000).

52 Taylor and Fink (2006, chapters 8 and 9).

53 Protheroe (1969); Brockington *et al.* (1982b); Pfuhlmann *et al.* (1998); Chaudron *et al.* (2001).

54 Murphy-Eberenz *et al.* (2006).

55 Treloar *et al.* (1999).

56 Dean *et al.* (1989).

57 Dean *et al.* (1989).

58 Freeman *et al.* (2002); Jones and Craddock (2002); Jones *et al.* (2002); Chaudron and Pies (2003).

59 Pfuhlmann *et al.* (2002); Robling *et al.* (2000).

60 Platz and Kendell (1988).

61 Rohde and Marneros (1993); Videbech and Gouliaev (1995).

62 Miller (1994).

63 Rosenzweig *et al.* (1997); Bonanno and Kaltman (2001).

64 Zisook and Shuchter (1991, 1993).

65 Latham and Prigerson (2004).

66 Shuchter *et al.* (1986).

67 Ibid.

68 Weller *et al.* (1990).

69 Benazzi (2004a,b).

70 Winokur *et al.* (1969); Angst and Perris (1972).

71 Taylor and Abrams (1980); Taylor *et al.* (1980).

72 Gershon *et al.* (1982); Fieve *et al.* (1984); Tsuang *et al.* (1985); Andreasen *et al.* (1987); Jones *et al.* (2002b).

73 Taylor *et al.* (1980); Bertelsen *et al.* (1977); McGuffin and Katz (1989); Duffy *et al.* (2000); Jones *et al.* (2002b).

74 McGuffin *et al.* (2003); Bertelsen *et al.* (1977); Torgersen (1986).

75 McGuffin *et al.* (2003). Genetic linkage studies have not adequately looked at the bipolar/unipolar issue, but several report linkage to bipolar disorder on a number of chromosomes (Potash *et al.*, 2003; Mathews and Reus, 2003). One study reports a genetic overlap between bipolar and depressive disorder (Hashimoto *et al.*, 2005). Studies also report an overlap between bipolar disorder and schizophrenia (Bramon and Sham, 2001). The findings are inconsistent, however, in large part due to poorly defined phenotypes including failing to consider the relationship between bipolar disorder and melancholia.

76 Goodwin and Jamison (1990, p. 65).

77 Abrams and Taylor (1974).

78 Dorz *et al.* (2003).

79 These studies are numerous. As examples, see: Goldberg *et al.* (2004); Maj *et al.* (2003); Marneros and Goodwin (2005).

80 Angst and Preisig (1985); Mitchell and Malhi (2004).

81 Numerous studies report this. As examples see: DelBello *et al.* (2003); Akiskal *et al.* (1995); Coryell *et al.* (1995).

82 These studies are numerous. As examples see: Angst and Preisig (1985); Benazzi and Akiskal (2001); Benazzi *et al.* (2004).

83 Cassidy *et al.* (1998); Cervantes *et al.* (2001).

84 Rybakowski *et al.* (1999); Matsunaga and Sarai (2000).

85 Matsunaga and Sarai (2000).

86 Sher *et al.* (2003).

87 Cervantes *et al.* (2001).

88 Bearden *et al.* (2001).

89 Bertolino *et al.* (2003).

90 Strakowski *et al.* (2000).

91 Blumberg *et al.* (2000).

92 Blumberg *et al.* (2003a,b).

93 Cipriani *et al.* (2005).

94 Bauer and Dopfmer (1999); also see Taylor and Fink (2006) for discussions of lithium's efficacy as an augmenting agent in depressive illness and in preventing episodes of mood disorder.

95 Alvarez *et al.* (1997).

96 Baethge *et al.* (2003).

97 Kendler *et al.* (1998); Murray *et al.* (2005).

98 Abrams and Taylor (1978); Berenbaum *et al.* (1987); Bassett *et al.* (1993); Amador *et al.* (1999); Moller *et al.* (2000); Fanous *et al.* (2001).

99 Jager *et al.* (2003).

100 Andreasen *et al.* (1990).

101 McClellan and McCurry (1998).

102 See chapters in this text that detail each of the features in this revision of criterion A.

103 Kingdon *et al.* (2007).

104 Jablensky (2001).

105 Fish (1962, pp. 96–7); another old term no longer in use is *pseudoneurotic schizophrenia*, which was said to be a condition that initially presented as multiple neurotic problems of psychogenic origin that then progressed to psychosis (Hoch and Polatin, 1949).

106 Zhang-Wong *et al.* (1995).

107 Zarate *et al.* (2000); Naz *et al.* (2003).

108 Norman *et al.* (2005).

109 Taylor and Abrams (1984).

110 Iancu *et al.* (2002); Naz *et al.* (2003); Benazzi (2003a); Schimmelmann *et al.* (2005); Addington *et al.* (2006).

111 Chapter 2 provides a discussion of the history of this effort.

112 Maj *et al.* (2000).

113 Abrams and Taylor (1976a); Taylor and Amir (1994); Lake and Hurwitz (2007).

114 Jager *et al.* (2004) review these studies and offer a 15-year follow-up of 241 patients initially diagnosed as schizoaffective, schizophrenic, or manic-depressive. Also see Coryell *et al.* (2001).

115 Taylor (1986).

116 Taylor and Abrams (1983); Taylor (1986); Gershon *et al.* (1988); Kendler *et al.* (1995).

117 Kempf *et al.* (2005).

118 Taylor (1984); Kempf *et al.* (2005).

119 Lake and Hurwitz (2007).

120 Leonhard (1979).

121 Brockington *et al.* (1982a); Perris (1986); Zaudig (1990).

122 Peralta and Cuesta (2003b).

123 Reif and Pfuhlmann (2004).

124 For full discussions of the data supporting a separate category for catatonia, see Fink and Taylor (2003) and Taylor and Fink (2003).

125 Fink and Taylor (2003); Taylor and Fink (2003).

126 Fink and Taylor (2003); as examples, also see Abrams and Taylor (1976b); Krüger and Bräunig (2000).

127 Ibid.

128 Gelenberg (1976); Abrams and Taylor (1976b); Taylor (1990); Carroll *et al.* (1994).

129 Fink and Taylor (2003).

130 Gelenberg (1976); Abrams and Taylor (1976b); Primavera *et al.* (1994).

131 Wing and Shah (2000).

132 Hinsie (1932); Chandrasena (1986).

133 Taylor and Fink (2003).

134 Also see Salloway *et al.* (2001).

135 Tynes *et al.* (1990).

136 Bartz and Hollander (2006).

137 Dannon *et al.* (2006).

138 Dannon *et al.* (2004a,b).

139 Hollander *et al.* (2005); Lochner *et al.* (2005a,b). Compulsive shopping and internet usage and autism have also been proposed as OCD-related.

140 Taylor and Fink (2006, chapters 2 and 6).

141 LaSalle *et al.* (2004).

142 Frare *et al.* (2004); Hollander *et al.* (2005); Ruffolo *et al.* (2006).

143 Richter *et al.* (2003).

144 Hanna *et al.* (2005); vanGrootheest *et al.* (2005).

145 Black *et al.* (1995); Nestadt *et al.* (2001).

146 Carter *et al.* (2004).

147 Hollander *et al.* (2005).

148 Grados *et al.* (2001).

149 Bienvenu *et al.* (2000).

150 Lenane *et al.* (1992).

151 Black *et al.* (1994); Lilenfeld *et al.* (1998).

152 Bellodi *et al.* (2001).

153 Stein and Lochner (2006).

154 Calabrese *et al.* (1993); Jenike *et al.* (1996).

155 O'Sullivan *et al.* (1997); Keuthen *et al.* (2007).

156 Chamberlain *et al.* (2007).

157 Hollander and Wong (1995).

158 Hollander *et al.* (1994); Saxena *et al.* (2001).

159 Hollander *et al.* (1998); Lowengrub *et al.* (2006); Grant and Potenza (2006b).

160 Koran *et al.* (2007).

161 Keuthen *et al.* (1998).

162 Perkins (1999).

163 Kaye *et al.* (2001).

164 Eapen *et al.* (1996). However, tics and other abnormal movements may be made worse in some patients.

165 Kraus *et al.* (2006).

166 Gershuny *et al.* (2006).

167 van Minnen *et al.* (2003); Holtkamp *et al.* (2005); Walsh *et al.* (2006).

168 Fineberg *et al.* (2007).

169 Lilenfeld *et al.* (1998); Samuels *et al.* (2000); Nestadt *et al.* (2000, 2001).

170 Kroenke (2006).

171 Lieb *et al.* (2002).

172 See Chapter 12 and Taylor and Fink (2006).

173 Chapter 7 provides a discussion of these features.

174 Chapter 6 provides a discussion of these constructs.

175 De Fruyt *et al.* (2006).

176 Lyons *et al.* (1994).

177 Johansen *et al.* (2004).

178 Fossati *et al.* (2005).

179 Torgerson (1994); Skodol *et al.* (2002).

180 Skodol *et al.* (2002); Paris (2004, 2005).

181 Akiskal *et al.* (1985); Akiskal (1994); Magill (2004).

182 Atre Vaidya and Hussain (1999).

183 Claes and Vandereycken (2007); Klonsky (2007).

184 Fossati *et al.* (2006).

185 Bejerot *et al.* (1998).

186 Rossi *et al.* (2000).

187 Cloninger *et al.* (1994).

188 Fink and Taylor (2003); Taylor and Fink (2006, 2008).

References

Abbate-Daga, G., Fassino, S., Lo Giudice, R., *et al.* (2007). Anger, depression and personality dimensions in patients with migraine without aura. *Psychotherapy and Psychosomatics,* **76**, 122–8.

Abraham, K. (1927). *Selected Papers of Karl Abraham.* Translated by D. Bryan and A. Strachey. London: Hogarth Press, pp. 503–10.

Abramowitz, J.S. (2005). Hypochondriasis, conceptualization, treatment, and relationship to obsessive compulsive disorder. *Annals of Clinical Psychiatry,* **17**, 211–17.

and Braddock, A.E. (2006). Hypochondriasis, conceptualization, treatment, and relationship to obsessive-compulsive disorder. *Psychiatric Clinics of North America,* **29**, 503–19.

Abrams, R. (2002). *Electroconvulsive Therapy,* 4th edn. New York: Oxford University Press.

and Taylor, M.A. (1973). First-rank symptoms, severity of illness and treatment response in schizophrenia. *Comprehensive Psychiatry,* **14**, 353–5.

and Taylor, M.A. (1974). Unipolar and bipolar depressive illness, phenomenology and response to electroconvulsive therapy. *Archives of General Psychiatry,* **30**, 320–1.

and Taylor, M.A. (1976a). Mania and schizo-affective disorder, manic type, a comparison. *American Journal of Psychiatry,* **133**, 1445–7.

and Taylor, M.A. (1976b). Catatonia, a prospective clinical study. *Archives of General Psychiatry,* **33**, 579–81.

and Taylor, M.A. (1978). A rating scale for emotional blunting. *American Journal of Psychiatry,* **135**, 226–9.

and Taylor, M.A. (1981). The importance of schizophrenic symptoms in the diagnosis of mania. *American Journal of Psychiatry,* **138**, 658–61.

and Taylor, M.A. (1983). The importance of mood incongruent psychotic symptoms in melancholia. *Journal of Affective Disorders,* **5**, 179–81.

Taylor, M.A. and Gaztanaga, P. (1974). Paranoid schizophrenia and manic-depressive illness, a phenomenologic family history and treatment response study. *Archives of General Psychiatry,* **31**, 640–2.

Abrams, R., Taylor, M.A., Hayman, M.A. and Krishna, N.R. (1979). Unipolar mania revisited. *Journal of Affective Disorders,* **1**, 59–68.

à Campo, J., Nijman, H., Merckelbach, H. and Evers, C. (2003). Psychiatric comorbidity of gender identity disorders, a survey among Dutch psychiatrists. *American Journal of Psychiatry,* **160**, 1332–6.

Acierno, R., Lawyer, S.R., Rheingold, A., *et al.* (2007). Current psychopathology in previously assaulted older adults. *Journal of Interpersonal Violence*, **22**, 250–8.

Ackroyd, P. (2005). *Shakespeare, The Biography.* New York: Nan A. Talese, Doubleday.

Adams, R.D. and Salam-Adams, M. (1992). Athetosis and the common athetoid syndromes. In A.B. Joseph and R.R. Young, eds., *Movement Disorders in Neurology and Neuropsychiatry.* Boston: Blackwell Scientific Publications, pp. 532–9.

Addington, J., Chaves, A. and Addington, D. (2006). Diagnostic stability over one year in first-episode psychosis. *Schizophrenia Research*, **86**, 335–6.

Addington-Hall, J. and McCarthy, M. (1995). Dying from cancer, results of a national population-based investigation. *Palliative Medicine*, **9**, 295–305.

Adler, L., Lehmann, K., Rader, K. and Schunemann, K.F. (1993). "Running amok" – content analytic study of 196 news presentations from industrialized countries. *Fortschritte der Neurologie-Psychiatrie*, **61**, 424–33.

Adolphs, R., Jansari, A. and Tranel, D. (2001). Hemispheric perception of emotional valence from facial expressions. *Neuropsychology*, **15**, 516–24.

Ahern, G.L., Herring, A.M., Tackenberg, J., *et al.* (1993). The association of multiple personality and temporal lobe epilepsy. Intracarotid amobarbital test observations. *Archives of Neurology*, **50**, 1020–5.

Akhondzadeh, S., Faraji, H. and Sadeghi, M. (2003). Double-blind comparison of fluoxetine and nortriptyline in the treatment of moderate to severe major depression. *Journal of Clinical Pharmacy and Therapeutics*, **28**, 379–84.

Akiskal, H., Chen, S., Glenn, D., *et al.* (1985). Borderline, an adjective in search of a noun. *Journal of Clinical Psychiatry*, **46**, 41–8.

Akiskal, H.S. (1994). The temperamental borders of affective disorders. *Acta Psychiatrica Scandinavica*, **89**, 32–7.

and Pinto, O. (1999). The evolving bipolar spectrum, prototype I, II, III, and IV. In H.S. Akiskal, ed., *Bipolarity, Beyond Classical Mania. Psychiatric Clinics of North America*, **22**, 517–34.

Djenderdjian, A.H., Rosenthal, R.H. and Khani, M.K. (1977). Cyclothymic disorder, validating criteria for inclusion in the bipolar affective group. *American Journal of Psychiatry*, **134**, 1227–33.

Maser, J.D., Zeller, P.J., *et al.* (1995). Switching from "unipolar" to bipolar II. An 11-year prospective study of clinical and temperamental predictors in 559 patients. *Archives of General Psychiatry*, **52**, 114–23.

Albert, U., Venturello, S., Maina, G., *et al.* (2001). Bulimia nervosa with and without obsessive-compulsive syndromes. *Comprehensive Psychiatry*, **42**, 456–60.

al-Din, S.N., Anderson, M., Eeg-Olofsson, O. and Trontelj, J.V. (1994). Neuro-ophthalmic manifestations of the syndrome of ophthalmoplegia, ataxia and areflexia, a review. *Acta Neurologica Scandinavica*, **89**, 157–63.

Alexander, G.E., Crutcher, M.D. and De Long, M.R. (1990). Basal ganglia–thalamocortical circuits. Parallel substrates for motor, oculomotor, "prefrontal," and "limbic" functions. In H.M.B. Ulyings, C.G. Van Eden, J.P.C. De Bruin, *et al.*, eds., *The Prefrontal Cortex, Its Structure, Function, and Pathology in Brain Research*, Vol. **85**. Amsterdam: Elsevier, pp. 119–46.

Alexander, M.P., Fischer, R.S. and Friedman, R. (1992). Lesion localization in apractic agraphia. *Archives of Neurology*, **49**, 246–51.

Ali, S.O., Denicoff, K.D., Ketter, T.A., *et al.* (1997). Psychosensory symptoms in bipolar disorder. *Neuropsychiatry, Neuropsychology, and Behavioral Neurology*, **10**, 223–31.

Allen, G., McColl, R., Barnard, H., *et al.* (2005). Magnetic resonance imaging of cerebellar–prefrontal and cerebellar–parietal functional connectivity. *Neuroimage*, **28**, 39–48.

Allen, J.S., Damasio, H. and Grabowski, T.J. (2002). Normal neuroanatomical variation in the human brain, an MRI-volumetric study. *American Journal of Physical Anthropology*, **118**, 341–58.

Damasio, H., Grabowski, T.J., *et al.* (2003). Sexual dimorphism and asymmetries in the gray-white composition of the human cerebrum. *Neuroimage*, **18**, 880–94.

Allen, L.S. and Gorski, R.A. (1992). Sexual orientation and the size of the anterior commissure in the human brain. *Proceedings of the National Academy of Science*, **89**, 7199–202.

Allen, V.L. and Levine, J.M. (1968). Creativity and conformity. *Journal of Personality*, **36**, 405–19.

Almeida, O.P., Burton, E.J., Ferrier, N., *et al.* (2003). Depression with late onset is associated with right frontal lobe atrophy. *Psychological Medicine*, **33**, 675–81.

Alsobrook, J.P. and Pauls, D.L. (2002). A factor analysis of tic symptoms in Gilles de la Tourette's syndrome. *American Journal of Psychiatry*, **159**, 291–6.

Altshuler, L.L., Bartzokis, G., Grieder, T., *et al.* (1998). Amygdala enlargement in bipolar disorder and hippocampal reduction in schizophrenia, an MRI study demonstrating neuroanatomic specificity. *Archives of General Psychiatry*, **55**, 663–4.

Bartzokis, G., Grieder, T., *et al.* (2000). An MRI study of temporal lobe structures in men with bipolar disorder or schizophrenia. *Biological Psychiatry*, **48**, 147–62.

Alvarez, E., Perez-Sola, V., Perez-Blanco, J., *et al.* (1997). Predicting outcome of lithium added to antidepressants in resistant depression. *Journal of Affective Disorders*, **42**, 179–86.

Amador, X.F., Kirkpatrick, B., Buchanan, R.W., *et al.* (1999). Stability of the diagnosis of deficit syndrome in schizophrenia. *American Journal of Psychiatry*, **156**, 637–9.

Amato, P.R. (1994). Life-span adjustment of children to their parents' divorce. *Future Child*, **4**, 143–64.

American Psychiatric Association. (1952). *Diagnostic and Statistical Manual of Mental Disorders*. Washington, DC: American Psychiatric Association Mental Health Service.

American Psychiatric Association. (1968). *Diagnostic and Statistical Manual of Mental Disorders*, 2nd edn. (DSM-II). Washington, DC: American Psychiatric Association.

American Psychiatric Association. (1980). *Diagnostic and Statistical Manual of Mental Disorders*, 3rd edn. Washington, DC: American Psychiatric Association.

American Psychiatric Association. (1987). *Diagnostic and Statistical Manual of Mental Disorders*, 3rd edn. revised. Washington, DC: American Psychiatric Association.

American Psychiatric Association. (1994). *Diagnostic and Statistical Manual of Mental Disorders*, 4th edn. Washington, DC: American Psychiatric Association.

American Psychiatric Association. (1996). *Practice Guidelines*. Washington, DC: American Psychiatric Association.

American Psychiatric Association. (1997). Practice guidelines for the treatment of patients with schizophrenia. *American Journal of Psychiatry*, **154** (Suppl).

American Psychiatric Association Task Force on Late Neurological Effects of Antipsychotic Drugs. (1979). *American Psychiatric Association Task Force Report No. 18, Tardive Dyskinesia.* Washington, DC: American Psychiatric Association.

Amieva, H., Letenneur, L., Dartigues, J.F., *et al.* (2004). Annual rate and predictors of conversion to dementia in subjects presenting mild cognitive impairment criteria defined according to a population-based study. *Dementia and Geriatric Cognitive Disorders,* **18**, 87–93.

Amos, J.F. (1999). Differential diagnosis of common etiologies of photopsia. *Journal of the American Optometric Association,* **70**, 485–504.

Anderluh, M.B., Tchanturia, K., Rabe-Hesketh, S. and Treasure, J. (2003). Childhood obsessive-compulsive personality traits in adult women with eating disorders, defining a broader eating disorder phenotype. *American Journal of Psychiatry,* **160**, 242–7.

Anderson, C.A., Camp, J. and Filley, C.M. (1998). Erotomania after aneurismal subarachnoid hemorrhage: case report and literature review. *The Journal of Neuropsychiatry and Clinical Neurosciences,* **10**, 330–7.

Anderson, I.M. (2000). Selective serotonin reuptake inhibitors versus tricyclic antidepressants, a meta-analysis of efficacy and tolerability. *Journal of Affective Disorders,* **58**, 19–36.

and Tomenson, B.M. (1994). The efficacy of selective serotonin re-uptake inhibitors in depression, a meta-analysis of studies against tricyclic antidepressants. *Journal of Psychopharmacology,* **8**, 238–49.

Andreasen, N.C. (1977). Reliability and validity of proverb interpretation to assess mental status. *Comprehensive Psychiatry,* **18**, 465–72.

(1982). Negative symptoms in schizophrenia, definition and reliability. *Archives of General Psychiatry,* **39**, 784–8.

(2007). DSM and the death of phenomenology in America, an example of unintended consequences. *Schizophrenia Bulletin,* **33**, 108–12.

Rice, J., Endicott, J., *et al.* (1987). Familial rates of affective disorder. *Archives of General Psychiatry,* **44**, 461.

Flaum, M., Swayze, V.W. II, *et al.* (1990). Positive and negative symptoms in schizophrenia, a critical reappraisal. *Archives of General Psychiatry,* **47**, 615–21.

Angst, J. (1997). Minor and recurrent brief depression. In H.S. Akiskal and G.B. Cassano, eds., *Dysthymia and the Spectrum of Chronic Depressions.* New York: The Guilford Press, pp. 183–90.

(1998). The emerging epidemiology of hypomania and bipolar II disorder. *Journal of Affective Disorders,* **50**, 143–51.

and Perris, C. (1972). The nosology of endogenous depression. Comparison of the results of two studies. *International Journal of Mental Health,* **1**, 145–58.

and Preisig, M. (1985). Course of a clinical cohort of unipolar, bipolar and schizoaffective patients. Results of a prospective study from 1959 to 1985. *Schweizer Archiv für Neurologie und Psychiatrie,* **146**, 5–16.

Anthony, D.T. and Hollander, E. (1992). Sexual compulsions. In E. Hollander, ed., *Obsessive-Compulsive-Related Disorders.* Washington, DC: American Psychiatric Press, pp. 139–50.

Arango-Lasprilla, J.C., Rogers, H., Lengenfelder, J., *et al.* (2006). Cortical and subcortical diseases, do true neuropsychological differences exist? *Archives of Clinical Neuropsychology,* **21**, 29–40.

Arbelle, S., Magharious, W., Auerbach, J.G., *et al.* (1997). Formal thought disorder in offspring of schizophrenic parents. *Israel Journal of Psychiatry and Related Sciences,* **34,** 210–21.

Arroyo, S., Santamaria, J., Lomena, F., *et al.* (2001). Nocturnal paroxysmal dystonia related to a prerolandic dysplasia. *Epilepsy Research,* **43,** 1–9.

Asarnow, R.F., Nuechterlein, K.H., Fogelson, D., *et al.* (2001). Schizophrenia and schizophrenia-spectrum personality disorders in the first-degree relatives of children with schizophrenia. *Archives of General Psychiatry,* **58,** 581–8.

Asbahr, F.R., Negrao, A.B., Gentil, V., *et al.* (1998). Obsessive–compulsive and related symptoms in children and adolescents with rheumatic fever with and without chorea. A prospective 6-month study. *American Journal of Psychiatry,* **155,** 1122–4.

Askin-Edgar, S., White, K.E. and Cummings, J.L. (2004). Neuropsychiatric aspects of Alzheimer's disease and other dementing illnesses. In S.C. Yudofsky and R.E. Hales, eds., *Essentials of Neuropsychiatry and Clinical Neurosciences.* Washington, DC: American Psychiatric Publishing, pp. 432–5.

Athwal, B.S., Halligan, P.W., Fink, G.R. and Frackowiak, R.S. (2001). Imaging hysterical paralysis. In P.W. Halligan, C. Bass, and J.C. Marshall, eds., *Contemporary Approaches to the Study of Hysteria.* Oxford: Oxford University Press, pp. 216–34.

Atre Vaidya, N. and Hussain, S. (1999). Borderline personality disorder and bipolar mood disorder: two distinct disorders or a continuum? Brief Report. *The Journal of Nervous and Mental Disease,* **187,** 313–15.

  and Taylor, M.A. (1997). The sensitization hypothesis and importance of psychosensory features in mood disorder. A review. *Journal of Neuropsychiatry,* **9,** 525–33.

  and Taylor, M.A. (2004). *Psychiatry Rounds, Practical Solutions to Clinical Challenges.* Miami, FL: MedMaster.

  and Taylor, M.A. (2006). The DSM, should it have a future? *Psychiatric Times,* **24,** 73–9.

  Taylor, M.A., Seidenberg, M.S., *et al.* (1998). Cognitive deficits, psychopathology, and psychosocial functioning mood disorders. *Neuropsychiatry, Neuropsychology and Behavioral Neurology,* **11,** 120–6.

Augustine, J.R. (1996). Circuitry and functional aspects of the insula lobe in primates including humans. *Brain Research Reviews,* **22,** 229–44.

Austin, M.P., Mitchell, P., Wilhelm, K., *et al.* (1999). Cognitive function in depression, a distinct patten of frontal impairment in melancholia? *Psychological Medicine,* **29,** 73–85.

Ayuso-Mateos, J.L., Vazquez-Barquero, J.L., Dowrick, C., *et al.* and the ODIN Group. (2001). Depressive disorders in Europe, prevalence figures from the ODIN study. *British Journal of Psychiatry,* **179,** 308–16.

Baethge, C., Grushka, P., Smolka, M.N., *et al.* (2003). Effectiveness and outcome predictors of long-term lithium prophylaxis in unipolar major depressive disorder. *Journal of Psychiatry and Neuroscience,* **28,** 355–61.

Bailey, P. and Cushing, H. (1925). Medulloblastoma cerebelli. A common type of midcerebellar glioma of childhood. *Archives of Neurology of Psychiatry,* **14,** 192–224.

Baillarger, J. (1853). De la melancholia avec stupeur. *Annales Medico-Psychologiques,* **5,** 151–76.

Baldessano, C.F., Datto, S.M., Littman, L. and Lipari, M.A. (2003). What drugs are best for bipolar depression? *Annals of Clinical Psychiatry,* **15,** 225–32.

Baldessarini, R.J. (1970). Frequency of diagnosis of schizophrenia versus affective disorder from 1948 to 1968. *American Journal of Psychiatry*, **127**, 759–63.

Ballerini, M., Bellini, S., Niccolai, C., *et al.* (2002). Neuroleptic-induced dystonia, incidence and risk factors. *European Psychiatry*, **17**, 366–8.

Ban, T.A., Healy, D. and Shorter, E. (2002). *The Rise of Psychopharmacology and the Story of CINP*. Budapest: Animula Publishing.

Bancaud, J. and Talairach, J. (1992). Clinical semiology of frontal lobe seizures. *Advances in Neurology*, **57**, 3–58.

Barash, D. (1979). *The Whisperings Within, Evolution and the Origin of Human Nature*. New York: Harper and Row.

Barbui, C. and Hotopf, M. (2001). Amitriptyline v. the rest, still the leading antidepressant after 40 years of randomized controlled trials. *British Journal of Psychiatry*, **178**, 129–44.

Barret, E.S., Kent, T. and Stanford, M.S. (1995). The role of biological variables in defining and measuring personality. In J.J. Ratey, ed., *Neuropsychiatry of Personality Disorders*. Cambridge, MA: Blackwell Science, pp. 35–49.

Barrough, P. (1583). *The Methode of Phisicke, Conteyning the Causes, Signes, and Cures of Inward Diseases in Mans Body from the Head to the Foot*. London: Vautrollier.

Barta, P.E., Pearlson, G.D., Brill, L.B. II, *et al.* (1997). Planum temporale asymmetry reversal in schizophrenia, replication and relationship to gray matter abnormalities. *American Journal of Psychiatry*, **154**, 661–7.

Bartz, J.A. and Hollander, E. (2006). Is obsessive-compulsive disorder an anxiety disorder? *Progress in Neuropsychopharmacology and Biological Psychiatry*, **30**, 338–52.

Bartzokis, G., Beckson, M., Wirshing, D.A., *et al.* (1999). Choreoathetoid movements in cocaine dependence. *Biological Psychiatry*, **45**, 1630–5.

Basiaux, P., le Bon, O., Dramaix, M., *et al.* (2001). Temperament and Character Inventory (TCI) personality profile and sub-typing in alcoholic patients, a controlled study. *Alcohol and Alcoholism*, **36**, 584–7.

Bassett, A.S., Collins, E.J., Nuttall, S.E. and Honer, W.G. (1993). Positive and negative symptoms in families with schizophrenia. *Schizophrenia Bulletin*, **11**, 9–19.

Bauer, M. and Dopfmer, S. (1999). Lithium augmentation in treatment-resistant depression, meta-analysis of placebo-controlled studies. *Journal of Clinical Psychopharmacology*, **19**, 427–34.

Baumgarten, H.G. and Grozdanovic, Z. (1998). Role of serotonin in obsessive-compulsive disorder. *British Journal of Psychiatry*, **173** (Suppl. 35), 13–20.

Baxter, D.M. and Warrington, E.K. (1986). Ideational agraphia, a single case study. *Journal of Neurology, Neurosurgery of Psychiatry*, **49**, 369–74.

Bear, D.M. and Fedio, P. (1977). Quantitative analysis of interictal behavior in temporal lobe epilepsy. *Archives of Neurology*, **34**, 454–67.

Bearden, C.E., Hoffman, K.M. and Cannon, T.D. (2001). The neuropsychology and neuroanatomy of bipolar affective disorder, a critical review. *Bipolar Disorders*, **3**, 106–50.

Bebbington, P. and Kuipers, L. (1994). The clinical utility of expressed emotion in schizophrenia. *Acta Psychiatrica Scandmavica*, **46** (Suppl. 382), 46–53.

Beck, A.T., Ward, C.H., Mendelson, M., *et al.* (1961). An inventory for measuring depression. *Archives of General Psychiatry*, **4**, 53–63.

Beck, C.T. (1996). A meta-analysis of predictors of postpartum depression. *Nursing Research*, **45**, 297–303.

Becker, E.S., Rinck, M., Turke, V., *et al.* (2007). Epidemiology of specific phobia subtypes, findings from the Dresden mental health study. *European Psychiatry*, **22**, 69–74.

Becker, J., Kocalevent, R.D., Rose, M., *et al.* (2006). Standardized diagnosing, computer-assisted (CIDI) diagnoses compared to clinically-judged diagnoses in a psychosomatic setting. *Psychotherapie, Psychosomatik, Medizinische Psychologie*, **56**, 5–14.

Beckson, M. and Cummings, J.L. (1991). Neuropsychiatric aspects of stroke. *International Journal of Psychiatry in Medicine*, **21**, 1–15.

Beer, M.D. (1996). The dichotomies, psychosis/neurosis and functional/organic, a historical perspective. *History of Psychiatry*, **7**, 231–55.

Bejerot, S., Schlette, P., Ekselius, L., *et al.* (1998). Personality disorders and relationship to personality dimensions measured by the Temperament and Character Inventory in patients with obsessive-compulsive disorder. *Acta Psychiatrica Scandinavica*, **98**, 243–9.

Bell, L. (1849). On a form of disease resembling some advanced stages of mania and fever, but so contradistinguished from any ordinary observed or described combination of symptoms as to render it probable that it may be an overlooked and hitherto unrecorded malady. *American Journal of Insanity*, **6**, 97–127.

Bell, M., Milstein, R., Beam-Goulet, J., *et al.* (1992). The Positive and Negative Syndrome Scale and the Brief Psychiatric Rating Scale. Reliability, comparability, and predictive validity. *Journal of Mental Disorders*, **180**, 723–8.

Bellini, L., Gatti, F., Gasperini, M. and Smeraldi, E. (1992). A comparison between delusional and nondelusional depressives. *Journal of Affective Disorders*, **25**, 129–38.

Bellino, S., Rocca, P., Patria, L., *et al.* (2004). Relationships of age at onset with clinical features and cognitive functions in a sample of schizophrenia patients. *Journal of Clinical Psychiatry*, **65**, 908–14.

Bellodi, L., Cavallini, M.C., Bertelli, S., *et al.* (2001). Morbidity risk for obsessive-compulsive spectrum disorders in first-degree relatives of patients with eating disorders. *American Journal of Psychiatry*, **158**, 563–9.

Benazzi, F. (2003a). Outcome of schizophreniform disorder. *Current Psychiatry Report*, **5**, 192–6.

  (2003b). Diagnosis of bipolar II disorder. A comparison of structured versus semistructured interviews. *Progress in Neuropsychopharmacology and Biological Psychiatry*, **6**, 985–91.

  (2003c). Testing DSM-IV definition of atypical depression. *Annals of Clinical Psychiatry*, **15**, 9–16.

  (2004a). Depressive mixed state, a feature of the natural course of bipolar II (and major depressive) disorder? *Psychopathology*, **7**, 207–12.

  (2004b). Is depressive mixed state a transition between depression and hypomania? *European Archives of Psychiatry and Clinics in Neuroscience*, **254**, 69–75.

  and Akiskal, H.S. (2001). Delineating bipolar II mixed states in the Ravenna–San Diego collaborative study. The relative prevalence and diagnostic significance of hypomanic features during major depressive episodes. *Journal of Affective Disorders*, **67**, 115–22.

  and Rihmer, Z. (2000). Sensitivity and specificity of DSM-IV atypical features for bipolar II disorder diagnosis. *Psychiatry Research*, **93**, 257–62.

Koukopolous, A. and Akiskal, H.S. (2004). Toward a validation of a new definition of agitated depression as a bipolar mixed state (mixed depression). *European Psychiatry*, **19**, 85–90.

Benca, R.M., Obermeyer, W.H., Thisted, R.A. and Gillin, J.C. (1992). Sleep and psychiatric disorders. A meta-analysis. *Archives of General Psychiatry*, **49**, 651–68.

Benedict, R.F. (1934). *Patterns of Culture*. Boston and New York: Houghton Mifflin.

Benegal, V., Hingorani, S., Khanna, S. and Channabasavanna, S.M. (1992). Is stupor by itself a catatonic symptom? *Psychopathology*, **25**, 229–31.

Benson, D.F. and Ardila, A. (1996). Neural basis of language functions. In D.F. Benson and A. Ardila, eds., *Aphasia, A Clinical Perspective*. New York: Oxford University Press, pp. 262–80.

Bentall, R.P., Corcoran, R., Howard, R., *et al.* (2001). Persecutory delusions, a review and theoretical integration. *Clinical Psychology Reviews*, **21**, 1143–92.

Berenbaum, S., Abrams, R., Rosenberg, S. and Taylor, M.A. (1987). The nature of emotional blunting. A factor-analytic study. *Psychiatric Research*, **20**, 57–67.

Berk, M., Malhi, G.S., Cahill, C., *et al.* (2007). The Bipolar Depression Rating Scale (BDRS): its development, validation and utility. *Bipolar Disorders*, **9**, 571–9.

Berrios, G.E. (1991). Musical hallucinations, a statistical analysis of 46 cases. *Psychopathology*, **24**, 356–60.

(1993). Phenomenology and psychopathology, was there ever a relationship? *Comprehensive Psychiatry*, **34**, 213–20.

(1999). Classifications in psychiatry, a conceptual history. *Australia and New Zealand Journal of Psychiatry*, **33**, 145–60.

and Hauser, R. (1988). The early development of Kraepelin's ideas on classification, a conceptual history. *Psychological Medicine*, **18**, 813–21.

and Luque, R. (1995). Cotard's syndrome, analysis of 100 cases. *Acta Psychiatrica Scandinavica*, **91**, 185–8.

Bertelsen, A. (1999). Reflections on the clinical utility of the ICD-10 and DSM-IV classifications and their diagnostic criteria. *Australia and New Zealand Journal of Psychiatry*, **33**, 166–73.

(2002). Schizophrenia and related disorders, experience with current diagnostic systems. *Psychopathology*, **35**, 89–93.

Harvald, B. and Hauge, M. (1977). A Danish twin study of manic-depressive disorders. *British Journal of Psychiatry*, **130**, 330–51.

Berthier, M., Starkstein, S. and Leiguarda, R. (1988). Asymbolia for pain, a sensory-limbic disconnection syndrome. *Annals of Neurology*, **24**, 41–9.

Berthier, M.L., Ruiz, A., Massone, M.I., *et al.* (1991). Foreign accent syndrome. Behavioral and anatomic findings in recovered and non-recovered patients. *Aphasiology*, **5**, 129–47.

Bertolino, A., Frye, M., Callicott, J.H., *et al.* (2003). Neuronal pathology in the hippocampal area of patients with bipolar disorder, a study with proton magnetic resonance spectroscopic imaging. *Biological Psychiatry*, **53**, 906–13.

Bhugra, D. (2005). Sati, a type of nonpsychiatric suicide. *Crisis*, **26**, 73–7.

Bien, C.G., Benninger, F.O., Urbach, H., *et al.* (2000). Localizing value of epileptic visual auras. *Brain*, **123**, 244–53.

Bienvenu, O.J. and Stein, M.B. (2003). Personality and anxiety disorders, a review. *Journal of Personality Disorders*, **17**, 139–51.

Samuels, J.F., Riddle, M.A., *et al.* (2000). The relationship of obsessive-compulsive disorder to possible spectrum disorders, results from a family study. *Biological Psychiatry,* **48**, 287–93.

Binzer, M., Almay, B. and Eisemann, M. (2003). Chronic pain disorder associated with psychogenic versus somatic factors, a comparative study. *Nordic Journal of Psychiatry,* **57**, 61–6.

Black, D.N., Seritan, A.L., Taber, K.H. and Hurley, R.A. (2004). Conversion hysteria. Lessons from functional imaging. *The Journal of Neuropsychiatry and Clinical Neurosciences,* **16**, 245–51.

Black, D.W., Goldstein, R.B., Noyes, R. and Blum, N. (1994). Compulsive behaviors and obsessive-compulsive disorder (OCD), lack of a relationship between OCD, eating disorders, and gambling. *Comprehensive Psychiatry,* **35**, 145–8.

Goldstein, R.B., Noyes, R. and Blum, N. (1995). Psychiatric disorders in relatives of probands with obsessive-compulsive disorder and co-morbid major depression or generalized anxiety disorder. *Psychiatric Genetics,* **5**, 37–41.

Kehrberg, L.L.D., Flumerfelt, D.L. and Schlosser, M.A.T. (1997). Characteristics of 36 subjects reporting compulsive sexual behavior. *American Journal of Psychiatry,* **154**, 243–9.

Blackwood, N.J., Howard, R.J., Ffytche, D.H., *et al.* (2000). Imaging attentional and attributional bias, an fMRI approach to the paranoid delusion. *Psychological Medicine,* **30**, 873–83.

Howard, R.J., Bentall, R.P. and Murray, R.M. (2001). Cognitive neuropsychiatric models of persecutory delusions. *American Journal of Psychiatry,* **158**, 527–39.

Bentall, R.P., Ffytche, D.H., *et al.* (2004). Persecutory delusions and the determination of self-relevance, an fMRI investigation. *Psychological Medicine,* **34**, 591–6.

Blakeley, J. and Jankovic, J. (2002). Secondary causes of paroxysmal dyskinesia. *Advances in Neurology,* **89**, 402–20.

Blair, R.J. (2003). Neurobiological basis of psychopathy. *British Journal of Psychiatry,* **182**, 5–7.

Blais, M.A., Hilsenroth, M.J. and Castlebury, F.D. (1997). Content validity of the DSM-IV borderline and narcissistic personality disorder criteria sets. *Comprehensive Psychiatry,* **38**, 31–7.

Blanke, O., Landis, T. and Seeck, M. (2000). Electrical cortical stimulation of the human prefrontal cortex evokes complex visual hallucinations. *Epilepsy & Behavior,* **1**, 356–61.

Blashfield, R.K. (1984). *The Classification of Psychopathology.* New York: Plenum Press.

Blazer, D., Swartz, M., Woodbury, M., *et al.* (1988). Depressive symptoms and depressive diagnoses in a community population. Use of a new procedure for analysis of psychiatric classification. *Archives of General Psychiatry,* **45**, 1078–84.

Blazer, D.G., Kessler, R.L., McGonagle, K.A. and Swartz, M.S. (1994). The prevalence and distribution of major depression in a national community sample, the National Comorbidity Survey. *American Journal of Psychiatry,* **151**, 979–86.

Bleuler, E. (1950). *Dementia Praecox or the Group of Schizophrenias,* translated by J. Zinkin. New York: International Universities Press.

(1976). *Textbook of Psychiatry,* 1924 (translated by A.A. Brill). New York: Arno Press (reissued).

Bloom, H. (1998). *Shakespeare, The Invention of the Human.* New York: Riverhead Books.

Blum, P. and Jankovic, L. (1991). Stiff-person syndrome, an autoimmune disease. *Movement Disorders,* **6**, 12–20.

Blumberg, H.P., Stern, E., Martinez, D., *et al.* (2000). Increased anterior cingulate and caudate activity in bipolar mania. *Biological Psychiatry*, **48**, 1045–52.

Kaufman, J., Martin, A., *et al.* (2003a). Amygdala and hippocampal volumes in adolescents and adults with bipolar disorder. *Archives of General Psychiatry*, **60**, 1201–08.

Leung, H-C., Skudlarski, P., *et al.* (2003b). A functional magnetic resonance imaging study of bipolar disorder. *Archives of General Psychiatry*, **60**, 601–09.

Blumer, D., Montouris, G. and Davies, K. (2004). The interictal dysphoric disorder, recognition, pathogenesis, and treatment of the major psychiatric disorder of epilepsy. *Epilepsy & Behavior*, **5**, 826–40.

Bodini, B., Iacboni, M. and Lenzi, G.L. (2004). Acute stroke effects on emotions, an interpretation through the mirror system. *Current Opinions in Neurology*, **17**, 55–60.

Bolla, K.I., Cadet, J.L. and London, E.D. (1998). The neuropsychiatry of chronic cocaine abuse. *The Journal of Neuropsychiatry and Clinical Neurosciences*, **10**, 280–9.

Bonanno, G.A. and Kaltman, S. (2001). The varieties of grief experience. *Clinical Psychology Review*, **21**, 705–34.

Bonilha, L. and Li, L.M. (2004). Heavy coffee drinking and epilepsy. *Seizure*, **13**, 284–5.

Bonnet, U., Banger, M., Wolstein, J. and Gastpar, M. (1998). Choreoathetoid movements associated with rapid adjustment to methadone. *Pharmacopsychiatry*, **31**, 143–5.

Bornstein, R.F. (1998). Reconceptualizing personality disorder diagnosis in the DSM-V, the discriminant validity challenge. *Clinical Psychology: Science and Practice*, **5**, 333–43.

Borod, J.C. (1992). Interhemispheric and intrahemispheric control of emotion, a focus on unilateral brain damage. *Journal of Consulting and Clinical Psychology*, **60**, 339–48.

Cicero, B.A., Obler, L.K., *et al.* (1998). Right hemisphere emotional perception, evidence across multiple channels. *Neuropsychology*, **12**, 446–58.

Bottin, P., Sadzot, B. and Hotermans, C. (2005). Primary orthostatic tremor. *Revue Medicale de Liege*, **60**, 96–100.

Bourget, D. and Whitehurst, L. (2004). Capgras syndrome. A review of the neurophysiological correlates and presenting clinical features in cases involving physical violence. *Canadian Journal of Psychiatry*, **49**, 719–25.

Bower, H. (2001). The gender identity disorder in the DSM-IV classification, a critical review. *Australia and New Zealand Journal of Psychiatry*, **35**, 1–8.

Bowie, C.R. and Harvey, P.D. (2005). Cognition in schizophrenia, impairments, determinants, and functional importance. *Psychiatric Clinics of North America*, **28**, 613–33.

Harvey, P.D., Moriarty, P.J., *et al.* (2004). A comprehensive analysis of verbal fluency deficit in geriatric schizophrenia. *Archives of Clinical Neuropsychology*, **19**, 289–303.

Boz, C., Velioglu, S., Ozmenoglu, M., *et al.* (2004). Temperament and character profiles of patients with tension-type headache and migraine. *Psychiatry and Clinical Neurosciences*, **58**, 536–43.

Braam, A.W., Visser, S., Cath, D.C. and Hoogendijk, W.J. (2006). Investigation of the syndrome of apotemnophobia and course of a cognitive-behavior therapy. *Psychopathology*, **39**, 32–7.

Bracha, H.S., Yoshioka, D.T., Masukawa, N.K. and Stockman, D.J. (2005). Evolution of the human fear-circuitry and acute sociogenic pseudoneurological symptoms, the Neolithic balanced-polymorphism hypothesis. *Journal of Affective Disorders*, **88**, 119–29.

Bradley, L. and Tawfiq, N. (2006). The physical and psychological effects of torture in Kurds seeking asylum in the United Kingdom. *Torture*, **16**, 41–7.

Bramon, E. and Sham, P.C. (2001). The common genetic liability between schizophrenia and bipolar disorder, a review. *Current Psychiatry Reports*, **3**, 332–7.

Brandes, M. and Bienvenu, O.J. (2006). Personality and anxiety disorders. *Current Psychiatry Reports*, **8**, 263–269.

Brandt, J. and Van Gorp, W.G. (2006). Functional ("psychogenic") amnesia. *Seminars in Neurology*, **26**, 331–40.

Braslow, J. (1997). *Mental Ills and Bodily Cures*. Berkeley, CA: University of California Press.

Braude, W.M. and Barnes, T.R.E. (1983). Late-onset akathisia – an incident of covert dyskinesia. Two case reports. *American Journal of Psychiatry*, **140**, 611–12.

Braun, C.M.J., Larocque, B.A., Daigneault, S. and Montour-Proulx, I. (1999). Mania, pseudomania, depression, and pseudodepression resulting from focal unilateral cortical lesions. *Neuropsychiatry, Neuropsychology and Behavioral Neurology*, **12**, 35–51.

    Dumont, M., Duval, J., *et al.* (2003). Brain modules of hallucination, an analysis of multiple patients with brain lesions. *Journal of Psychiatry & Neuroscience*, **28**, 432–49.

Bräunig, P., Kruger, S., Shugar, G., *et al.* (2000). The catatonia rating scale I – development, reliability, and use. *Comprehensive Psychiatry*, **41**, 147–58.

Bremner, J.D., Scott, T.M., Delaney, R.C., *et al.* (1993). Deficits in short-term memory in post traumatc stress disorder. *American Journal of Psychiatry*, **150**, 1015–19.

    Randall, P., Scott, T.M., *et al.* (1995). MRI-based measurements of hippocampal volume in patients with combat-related post traumatic stress disorder. *American Journal of Psychiatry*, **152**, 973–81.

Breslau, N., Roth, T., Rosenthal, L. and Andreski, P. (1996). Sleep disturbance and psychiatric disorders: a longitudinal epidemiological study of young adults. *Biological Psychiatry*, **39**, 411–18.

Briken, P., Habermann, N., Berner, W. and Hill, A. (2005). The influence of brain abnormalities on psychosocial development, criminal history and paraphilias in sexual murderers. *Journal of Forensic Science*, **50**, 1204–08.

Briquet, P. (1859). *Traite Clinique et Therapeutique de l'Hysterie*. Paris: J-B Bailliere.

Brockington, I.F., Perris, C., Kendell, R.E., *et al.* (1982a). The course and outcome of cycloid psychosis: *Psychological Medicine*, **12**, 97–105.

    Winokur, G. and Dean, C. (1982b). Puerperal psychosis. In I.F. Brockington and R. Kumar, eds., *Motherhood and Mental Illness*. London: Academic Press, vol. 3, pp. 37–69.

Bromberg, W. (1930). Mental status in chronic encephalitis. *Psychiatr. Quarterly*, **4**, 537–66.

Brown, R.H. (1992). The periodic paralyses, a review. In A.B. Joseph and R.R. Young, eds., *Movement Disorders in Neurology and Neuropsychiatry*. Boston: Blackwell Scientific Publications, pp. 713–27.

Brown, T.A., Di Nardo, P.A., Lehman, C.L. and Campbell, L.A. (2001). Reliability of DSM-IV anxiety and mood disorders. Implications for the classification of emotional disorders. *Journal of Abnormal Psychology*, **110**, 49–58.

Brune, M., Brune-Cohrs, U., McGrew, W.C. and Preuschoft, S. (2006). Psychopathology in great apes, concepts, treatment options and possible homologies to human psychiatric disorders. *Neuroscience and Biobehavioral Reviews*, **30**, 1246–59.

Bryant, R.A. and Panasetis, P. (2005). The role of panic in acute dissociative reactions following trauma. *British Journal of Clinical Psychology*, **44**, 489–94.

Bryson, S.E., McLaren, J., Wadden, N.P. and MacLean, M. (1991). Differential asymmetries for positive and negative emotion, hemisphere or stimulus effects? *Cortex*, **27**, 359–65.

Bulik, C.M., Beidel, D.C., Duchmann, E., *et al.* (1992). Comparative psychopathology of women with bulimia nervosa and obsessive–compulsive disorder. *Comprehensive Psychiatry*, **33**, 262–8.

Burn, D.J. (2006). Cortical Lewy body disease and Parkinson's disease dementia. *Current Opinions in Neurology*, **19**, 572–9.

Burrows, G.M. (1976). *Commentaries on the Causes, Forms, Symptoms, and Treatment, Moral and Medical, of Insanity*. Facsimile of the 1828 edition. New York: Arno Press.

Burton, R. (1621). *The Anatomy of Melancholy, What It Is*. London: Oxford Cripps.

Buss, D.M. and Haselton, M. (2005). The evolution of jealousy. *Trends in Cognitive Neurosciences*, **9**, 506–07.

Bush, G., Fink, M., Petrides, G., *et al.* (1996). Catatonia. I. Rating scale and standardized examination. *Acta Psychiatrica Scandinavica*, **93**, 129–36.

Butler, P.V. (2000). Diurnal variation in Cotard's syndrome (co-present with Capgras delusion) following traumatic brain injury. *Australia and New Zealand Journal of Psychiatry*, **34**, 684–7.

Buydens-Branchey, L., Branchey, M.H. and Noumair, D. (1989). Age of alcoholism onset. I. Relationship to psychopathology. *Archives of General Psychiatry*, **46**, 225–30.

Caffo, E. and Belaise, C. (2003). Psychological aspects of traumatic injury in children and adolescents. *Child and Adolescent Psychiatric Clinics of North America*, **12**, 493–535.

Calabrese, G., Colombo, C., Onfanti, A., *et al.* (1993). Caudate nucleus abnormalities in obsessive-compulsive disorder, measurements of MRI signal intensity. *Psychiatry Research*, **50**, 89–92.

Calaresi, P.A. (2004). Diagnosis and management of multiple sclerosis. *American Family Physician*, **70**, 1935–44.

Calder, A.J., Keane, J., Manes, F., *et al.* (2000). Impaired recognition and experience of disgust following brain injury. *Nature Neuroscience*, **3**, 1077–8.

Lawrence, A.D. and Young, A.W. (2001). Neuropsychology of fear and loathing. *Nature Reviews in Neuroscience*, **2**, 352–63.

Camacho, A. and Akiskal, H.S. (2005). Proposal for a bipolar-stimulant spectrum, temperament, diagnostic validation and therapeutic outcomes with mood stabilizers. *Journal of Affective Disorders*, **85**, 217–20.

Cameron, N. (1947). *The Psychology of the Behavioral Disorders*. Boston: Houghton Mifflin.

Camperio-Ciani, A., Corna, F. and Capiluppi, C. (2004). Evidence for maternally inherited factors favoring male homosexuality and promoting female fecundity. *Proceedings Biological Sciences*, **271**, 2217–21.

Capgras, J. and Reboul-Lachaux, J. (1923). Illusions des soisie dans un délire systématise chronique. *Annales Medico-Psychologiques*, **81**, 186–93.

Caplan, R., Guthrie, D., Tang, B., *et al.* (2000). Thought disorder in childhood schizophrenia, replication and update of concept. *Journal of the American Academy of Childhood and Adolescent Psychiatry*, **39**, 771–8.

Carbeza, R. and Nyberg, L. (2000). Neural bases of learning and memory, functional neuroimaging evidence. *Current Opinions in Neurology* **13**, 415–21.

Carlomagno, S., Pandolfi, M., Marini, A., *et al.* (2005). Coverbal gestures in Alzheimer's type dementia. *Cortex*, **41**, 535–46.

Carlson, G.A. and Goodwin, F.K. (1973). The stages of mania. *Archives of General Psychiatry*, **28**, 221–8.

Bromet, E.J. and Sievers, S. (2000). Phenomenology and outcome of subjects with early- and adult-onset psychotic mania. *American Journal of Psychiatry*, **157**, 213–19.

Carmin, C.N., Wieqart, P.S., Yunus, U. and Gillock, K.L. (2002). Treatment of late-onset OCD following basal ganglia infarct. *Depression & Anxiety*, **15**, 87–90.

Caroff, S.N., Mann, S.C., Francis, A. and Fricchione, G.L., eds. (2004). *Catatonia, From Psychopathology to Neurobiology.* Washington, DC: American Psychiatric Publishing.

Carr, J.E. and Tan, E.K. (1976). In search of the true Amok, Amok as viewed with the Malay culture. *American Journal of Psychiatry*, **133**, 1295–9.

Carrera, E. and Bogousslavsky, J. (2006). The thalamus and behavior, effects of anatomically distinct strokes. *Neurology*, **66**, 1817–23.

Carrington, C.H. (2006). Clinical depression in African-American women, diagnosis, treatment, and research. *Journal of Clinical Psychology*, **62**, 779–91.

Carroll, B.J. (1982). The dexamethasone suppression test for melancholia. *British Journal of Psychiatry*, **140**, 292–304.

Feinberg, M., Greden, J.F., *et al.* (1981). A specific laboratory test for the diagnosis of melancholia. *Archives of General Psychiatry*, **38**, 15–22.

Carroll, B.T., Anfinson, T.J., Kennedy, J.C., *et al.* (1994). Catatonic disorder due to general medical conditions. *Journal of Neuropsychiatry and Clinical Neurosciences*, **6**, 122–33.

Graham, K.T. and Thalassinos, A.J. (2001). A common pathogenesis of the serotonin syndrome, catatonia, and neuroleptic malignant syndrome. *Journal of Neuropsychiatry and Clinical Neurosciences*, **13**, 150 (abstract).

Carter, A.S., Pollack, R.A., Suvak, M.K. and Pauls, D.L. (2004). Anxiety and major depression comorbidity in a family study of obsessive–compulsive disorder. *Depression & Anxiety*, **20**, 165–74.

Carter, N. and Zee, D.S. (1997). The anatomical localization of saccades using functional imaging studies and transcranial magnetic stimulation. *Current Opinions in Neurology*, **10**, 10–17.

Caspi, A., Roberts, B.W. and Shiner, R.L. (2005). Personality development, stability and change. *Annual Review of Psychology*, **56**, 453–84.

Cassano, G.B., Rucci, P., Frank, E., *et al.* (2004). The mood spectrum in unipolar and bipolar disorder. Arguments for a unitary approach. *American Journal of Psychiatry*, **161**, 1264–9.

Cassidy, F., Ritchie, J.C., Carroll, B.J. (1998). Plasma dexamethasone concentration and cortisol response during manic episodes. *Biological Psychiatry*, **43**, 747–54.

Catlin, G. (2001). The role of culture in brief. *Journal of Social Psychology*, **133**, 173–84.

Cavallaro, R., Covedini, P., Mistretta, P., *et al.* (2003). Basal-corticofrontal circuits in schizophrenia and obsessive-compulsive disorder. A controlled, double dissociation study. *Biological Psychiatry*, **54**, 437–43.

Cavedini, P., Cisima, M., Riboldi, G., *et al.* (2001). A neuropsychological study of dissociation in cortical and subcortical functioning in obsessive-compulsive disorder by Tower of Hanoi Task. *Brain & Cognition*, **46**, 357–63.

Cembrowicz, S.P. and Shepherd, J.P. (1992). Violence in the accident and emergency department. *Medicine, Science and the Law*, **32**, 118–22.

Cervantes, P., Gelber, S., Kin, F., *et al.* (2001). Circadian secretion of cortisol in bipolar disorder. *Journal of Psychiatry and Neuroscience*, **26**, 411–16.

Chamberlain, S.R., Fineberg, N.A., Blackwell, A.D., *et al.* (2007). A neuropsychological comparison of obsessive-compulsive disorder and trichotillomania. *Neuropsychologia*, **45**, 654–62.

Chan, J.-L. and Ross, E.D. (1997). Alien hand syndrome, influence of neglect on the clinical presentation of frontal and callosal variants. *Cortex*, **33**, 287–99.

Chandrasena, R. (1986). Catatonic schizophrenia, an international comparative study. *Canadian Journal of Psychiatry*, **31**, 249–52.

Chang, C., Crottaz-Herbette, S. and Menon, V. (2007). Temporal dynamics of basal ganglia response and connectivity during verbal working memory. *Neuroimage*, **34**, 1253–69.

Chapman, J. (1966). The early symptoms of schizophrenia. *British Journal of Psychiatry*, **112**, 225–51.

Chaturvedi, S.K. (1994). Exploration of concerns and role of psychosocial intervention in palliative care – a study from India. *Annals, Academy of Medicine, Singapore*, **23**, 256–60.

Chaudron, L.H. and Pies, R.W. (2003). The relationship between postpartum psychosis and bipolar disorder, a review. *Journal of Clinical Psychiatry*, **64**, 1284–92.

Klein, M.H. and Remington, P. (2001). Predictors, prodromes and incidence of postpartum depression. *Journal of Psychosomatic Obstetrics and Gynaecology*, **22**, 103–12.

Chen, D.K., So, Y.T., Fisher, R.S. (2005). Therapeutics and Technology Assessment Subcommittee of the American Academy of Neurology. Use of serum prolactin in diagnosing epileptic seizures, report of the Therapeutics and Technology Assessment Subcommittee of the American Academy of Neurology. *Neurology*, **65**, 668–75.

Chen, Y.W. and Dilsaver, S.C. (1995). Comorbidity for obsessive-compulsive disorder in bipolar and unipolar disorders. *Psychiatry Research*, **59**, 57–64.

Cheyette, S.R. and Cummings, J.L. (1995). Encephalitis lethargica, lesions for contemporary neuropsychiatry. *Journal of Neuropsychiatry & Clinics in Neuroscience*, **7**, 387–8.

Cheyne, G. (1733). *The English Malady, or A Treatise of Nervous Diseases of all Kinds, as Spleen, Vapours, Lowness of Spirits, Hypochondriacal and Hysterical Distempers, etc.* London: Strahan and Leake.

Chodoff, P. and Lyons, H. (1958). Hysteria, the hysterical personality and hysterical conversion. *American Journal of Psychiatry*, **114**, 734–40.

Chow, T.W. and Cummings, J.L. (1999). Frontal-subcortical circuits. In B.L. Miller and J.L. Cummings, eds., *The Human Frontal Lobes*. New York: The Guilford Press, pp. 3–26.

Christodoulou, G.N. (1976). Delusional hyper-identification of the Fregoli type, organic pathogenic contributors. *Acta Psychiatrica Scandinavica*, **54**, 305–14.

(1991). The delusional misidentification syndromes. *British Journal of Psychiatry*, **159**, 65–9.

Margariti, M.M., Malliaras, D.E. and Alevizou, S. (1995). Shared delusions of doubles. *Journal of Neurology Neurosurgery and Psychiatry*, **58**, 499–501.

Chung, T. and Martin, C.S. (2005). What were they thinking? Adolescents' interpretations of DSM-IV alcohol dependence symptom queries and implications for diagnostic validity. *Drug and Alcohol Dependence*, **80**, 191–200.

Cipriani, A., Barbui, C. and Geddes, J.R. (2005). Suicide, depression, and antidepressants (editorial). *British Medical Journal*, **330**, 373–4.

Claes, L. and Vandereycken, W. (2007). Self-injurious behavior, differential diagnosis and functional differentiation. *Comprehensive Psychiatry*, **48**, 137–44.

Clark, J.M. and Albers, G.W. (1995). Vertical gaze palsies from medial thalamic infarctions without midbrain involvement. *Stroke*, **26**, 1467–70.

Clark, L.A. (2005). Stability and change in personality pathology, revelations of three longitudinal studies. *Journal of Personality Disorders*, **19**, 524–32.

Clarke, B. (1975). *Mental Disorder in Earlier Britain, Exploratory Studies*. Cardiff: University of Wales Press.

Clayton, G.D. and Clayton, F.E., eds. (1981). *Patty's Industrial Hygiene and Toxicology, Vols. 2A, 2B, and 2C*. New York: John Wiley & Sons.

Clayton, P. (1982). Bereavement. In E.S. Paykel, ed., *Handbook of Affective Disorders*. New York: The Guilford Press, pp. 403–15.

Clements, P.T., Vigil, G.J., Manno, M.S., *et al.* (2003). Cultural perspectives of death, grief, and bereavement. *Journal of Psychosocial Nursing and Mental Health Services*, **41**, 18–26.

Cloninger, C.R. (1991). Brain networks underlying personality development. In B.J. Carroll and J.E. Barett, eds., *Psychopathology and the Brain*. American Psychopathological Association Series. New York: Raven Press, pp. 183–208.

Bohman, M. and Sigvardsson, S. (1981). Inheritance of alcohol abuse. Cross-fostering analysis of adopted men. *Archives of General Psychiatry*, **38**, 861–8.

Sigvardsson, S. and Bohman, M. (1988a). Childhood personality predicts alcohol abuse in young adults. *Alcoholism: Clinical and Experimental Results*, **12**, 494–505.

Sigvardsson, S., Gilligan, S.B., *et al.* (1988b). Genetic heterogeneity and the classification of alcoholism. *Advances in Alcohol and Substance Abuse*, **7**, 3–16.

Svrakic, D.M. and Przybeck, T.R. (1993). A psychobiological model of temperament and character. *Archives of General Psychiatry*, **50**, 975–90.

Przybeck, T.R., Svrakic, D.M. and Wetzel, R.D. (1994). *TCI, The Temperament and Character Inventory (TCI), A Guide to its Development and Use*. St. Louis, MO: Washington University Center for the Study of the Psychobiology of Personality.

Sigvardsson, S., Przybeck, T.R. and Svrakic, D.M. (1995). Personality antecedents of alcoholism in a national area probability sample. *European Archives of Psychiatry and Clinical Neuroscience*, **245**, 239–44.

Svrakic, D.M. and Przybeck, T.R. (2006). Can personality assessment predict future depression? A twelve-month follow-up of 631 subjects. *Journal of Affective Disorders*, **92**, 35–44.

Cochran, B.N. and Cauce, A.M. (2006). Characteristics of lesbian, gay, bisexual, and transgender individuals entering substance abuse treatment. *Journal of Substance Abuse Treatment*, **30**, 135–46.

Cohen-Bendhahan, C.C., van de Beek, C. and Berenbaum, S.A. (2005). Prenatal sex hormone effects on child and adult sex-typed behavior, methods and findings. *Neuroscience & Biobehavioral Reviews*, **29**, 353–84.

Cohen-Kettenis, P.T. and Gooren, L.J. (1999). Transsexualism, a review of etiology, diagnosis and treatment. *Journal of Psychosomatic Research*, **46**, 315–53.

Coleman, E. (1992). Is your patient suffering from compulsive sexual behavior? *Psychiatric Annals*, **22**, 320–5.

Coles, M.E., Phillips, K.A., Menard, W., *et al.* (2006). Body dysmorphic disorder and social phobia. Cross-sectional and prospective data. *Depression & Anxiety*, **23**, 26–33.

Contreras, D., Destexhe, A., Sejnowski, T.J. and Stervade, M. (1996). Control of spatiotemporal coherence of a thalamic oscillation by corticothalamic feedback. *Science*, **274**, 771–4.

Cook, S.E., Miyahara, S., Bacanu, S.A., *et al.* (2003). Psychotic symptoms in Alzheimer disease, evidence for subtypes. *American Journal of Geriatric Psychiatry*, **11**, 406–13.

Coolidge, F.L., Thede, L.L. and Young, S.E. (2002). The heritability of gender identify disorder in a child and adolescent twin sample. *Behavior Genetics*, **32**, 251–7.

Coons, P.M., Bowman, E.S. and Milstein, V. (1988). Multiple personality disorder – A clinical investigation of 50 cases. *Journal of Nervous and Mental Disorders*, **176**, 519–27.

Coryell, W., Endicott, J., Maser, J.D., *et al.* (1995). Long-term stability of polarity distinctions in the affective disorders. *American Journal of Psychiatry*, **152**, 385–90.

Leon, A.C., Turvey, C., *et al.* (2001). The significance of psychotic features in manic episodes, a report from the NIMH collaborative study. *Journal of Affective Disorders*, **67**, 79–88.

Costa, P.T., Jr. (1991). Clinical use of the five-factor model. An introduction. *Journal of Personality Assessment*, **57**, 393–8.

and McCrae, R.R. (1985). *The NEO Personality Inventory Manual*. Odessa, FL: Psychological Assessment Resources.

and McCrae, R.R. (1992). The five-factor model of personality and its relevance to personality disorders. *Journal of Personality Disorders*, **6**, 343–59.

and Widiger, T.A., eds. (1994). *Personality Disorders and the Five-Factor Model of Personality*. Washington, DC: American Psychological Association.

Courbon, P. and Fail, G. (1927). Syndrome d' "illusion de Fregoli" et schizophrénie. *Bulletin de la Société Clinique Médécine Mentale*, **15**, 121–5.

Covey, L., Glassman, A.H. and Stetner, F. (1998). Cigarette smoking and major depression. *Journal of Addictive Disorders*, **17**, 35–46.

Covington, E.C. (2000). Psychogenic pain – what it means, why it does not exist, and how to diagnose it. *Pain and Medicine*, **1**, 287–94.

Craddock, N., O'Donovan, M.C. and Owen, M.J. (2006). Genes for schizophrenia and bipolar disorder? Implications for psychiatric nosology. *Schizophrenia Bulletin*, **32**, 9–16.

O'Donovan, M.C. and Owen, M.J. (2006). Genes for schizophrenia and bipolar disorder? Implications for psychiatric nosology. *Schizophrenia Bulletin*, **32**, 9–16.

Craig, A.D., Bushnell, M.C., Zhang, E.T. and Blomqvist, A. (1994). A thalamic nucleus specific for pain and temperature sensation. *Nature*, **372**, 770–3.

Cranefield, P.F. (1961). A 17th century view of mental deficiency and schizophrenia, Thomas Willis on "stupidity or foolishness". *Bulletin of the History of Medicine*, **35**, 291–316.

Creed, F. and Barsky, A. (2004). A systematic review of the epidemiology of somatization disorder and hypochondriasis. *Journal of Psychosomatic Research*, **56**, 391–408.

Critchley, M. (1950). The body image in neurology. *Lancet* **I**, 335–41.

(1953). *The Parietal Lobes*. New York: Hafner.

(1962). Periodic hypersomnia and megaphasia in adolescent males. *Brain*, **85**, 627–56.

Crosson, B. (1985). Subcortical functions in language, a working model. *Brain and Language*, **25**, 257–92.

and Hughes, C.W. (1987). Role of the thalamus in language, is it related to schizophrenic thought disorder? *Schizophrenia Bulletin*, **13**, 605–21.

Cuesta, M.J. and Peralta, V. (1993). Does formal thought disorder differ among patients with schizophrenia, schizophreniform and manic schizoaffective disorders? *Schizophrenia Research*, **10**, 151–8.

Cummings, J.L. (1985a). *Clinical Neuropsychiatry*. Orlando: Grune and Stratton Inc.

(1985b). Organic delusions, phenomenology, anatomical correlations, and review. *British Journal of Psychiatry*, **146**, 184–97.

and Mega, M.S. (2003). *Neuropsychiatry and Behavioral Neuroscience*. New York: Oxford University Press.

Cummings, W.J.K. (1988). The neurobiology of the body schema. *British Journal of Psychiatry*, **153** (Suppl. 2), 7–11.

Cunha, P.J., Nicastri, S., Gomes, L.P., *et al.* (2004). Neuropsychological impairment in crack cocaine-dependent inpatients, preliminary findings. *Revista Brasileira de Psiquiatria*, **26**, 103–06.

Cutting, J. (1989). Hearing voices. *British Medical Journal*, **298**, 769–70.

(1991). Delusional misidentification and the role of the right hemisphere in the appreciation of identity. *British Journal of Psychiatry*, **159** (Suppl. 14), 70–5.

Cyrulnik, B. (2005). Ethology and the biological correlates of mood. *Dialogues in Clinical Neuroscience*, **7**, 217–21.

Dale, R.C., Heyman, I., Surtees, R.A., *et al.* (2004). Dyskinesias and associated psychiatric disorders following streptococcal infections. *Archives of Disease in Childhood*, **89**, 604–10.

Damasio, A. (1999). *The Feeling of What Happens, Body and Emotion in the Making of Consciousness*. New York: Harcourt Brace.

(2003). *Looking for Spinoza, Joy, Sorrow and the Feeling Brain*. New York: Harcourt.

Damasio, A.R. and Damasio, H. (2000). Aphasia and the neural basis of language. In M.-M. Mesulam, ed., *Principles of Behavioral Neurology*, 2nd edn. New York: Oxford University Press, pp. 294–315.

Danish University Antidepressant Group. (1986). Citalopram, clinical effect profile in comparison with clomipramine. A controlled multicenter study. *Psychopharmacology*, **90**, 131–8.

(1990). Paroxetine, a selective serotonin reuptake inhibitor showing better tolerance, but weaker antidepressant effect than clomipramine in a controlled multicenter study. *Journal of Affective Disorders*, **18**, 289–99.

(1993). Moclobemide, a reversible MAO-A inhibitor showing weaker antidepressant effect than clomipramine in a controlled multicenter study. *Journal of Affective Disorders*, **28**, 105–16.

Dannon, P.N., Lowengrub, K.M., Iancu, I. and Kotler, M. (2004a). Kleptomania, comorbid psychiatric diagnoses in patients and their families. *Psychopathology*, **37**, 76–80.

Lowengrub, K., Sasson, M., *et al.* (2004b). Comorbid psychiatric diagnoses in kleptomania and pathological gambling, a preliminary comparison study. *European Psychiatry*, **19**, 299–302.

Lowengrub, K., Aizer, A. and Kotler, M. (2006). Pathological gambling, comorbid psychiatric diagnoses in patients and their families. *Israel Journal of Psychiatry & Related Sciences*, **43**, 88–92.

Daras, M., Koppel, B.S. and Atos-Radzion, E. (1994). Cocaine-induced choreoathetoid movements ("crack dancing"). *Neurology*, **44**, 751–2.

Darwin, C. (1872). *The Expression of the Emotions in Man and Animals*. London: John Murray. [Reprint 1972. New York: AMS Press.]

Das, P., Kemp, A.H., Liddell, B.J., *et al.* (2005). Pathways for fear perception, modulation of amygdala activity by thalamo-cortical systems. *Neuroimage*, **26**, 141–8.

Dauvilliers, Y., Billiard, M. and Montplaisir, J. (2003). Clinical aspects and pathophysiology of narcolepsy. *Clinical Neurophysiology*, **114**, 2000–17.

David, A.S. (1999). Auditory hallucinations, phenomenology, neuropsychology and neuroimaging update. *Acta Psychiatrica Scandinavica*, **395** (Suppl.), 95–104.

Davidson, K. and Bagley, C.R. (1969). Schizophrenia-like psychoses associated with organic disorders of the central nervous system: a review of the literature. In *Current Problems in Neuropsychiatry*. British Journal of Psychiatry, Special publication, no. **4**, 113–84.

Davis, M. and Whalen, P.J. (2001). The amygdala, vigilance and emotion. *Molecular Psychiatry*, **6**, 3–34.

Dean, C., Williams, R.J. and Brockington, I.F. (1989). Is puerperal psychosis the same as bipolar manic-depressive disorder? A family study. *Psychological Medicine*, **19**, 637–47.

De Boucaud, M.D. (1971). Body language and psychopathology. *Bordeaux médicale*, **4**, 2663–72.

Decety, J. and Lamm, C. (2006). Human empathy through the lens of social neuroscience. *Scientific World Journal*, **20**, 1146–63.

Deeb, A., Mason, C., Lee, Y.S. and Hughes, I.A. (2005). Correlation between genotype, phenotype and sex of rearing in 111 patients with partial androgen insensitivity syndrome. *Clinical Endocrinology*, **63**, 56–62.

Defoe, D. (1697). *An Essay Upon Projects*. London: Cockerill.

De Fruyt, F., De Clercq, B.J., van de Wiele, L. and Van Heeringgen, K. (2006). The validity of Cloninger's psychobiological model versus the five-factor model to predict DSM-IV personality disorders in a heterogeneous psychiatric sample, domain facet and residualized facet descriptions. *Journal of Personality*, **74**, 479–510.

de Haan, L., Beuk, N., Hoogenboom, B., *et al.* (2002). Obsessive–compulsive symptoms during treatment with olanzapine and risperidone, a prospective study of 113 patients with recent-onset schizophrenia or related disorders. *Journal of Clinical Psychiatry*, **63**, 104–07.

Hoogenboom, B., Beuk, N., *et al.* (2005). Obsessive–compulsive symptoms and positive, negative, and depressive symptoms in patients with recent-onset schizophrenic disorders. *Canadian Journal of Psychiatry*, **50**, 519–24.

de La Tourette, G. (1885). Etude sur une affection nerveuse, charactérisée par l'incoordination motrice accompagnée d'écholalie et de coprolalie. *Archives of Neurology*, **9**, 158–200.

Delay, J., Deniker, P. and Harl, J-M. (1952). Utilization en therapeutique psychiatrique d'une phenothiazine d'action central elective. *Annales Medico-Psychologiques*, **110**, 112–20.

DelBello, M.P., Carlson, G.A., Tohen, M., *et al.* (2003). Rates and predictors of developing a manic or hypomanic episode 1 to 2 years following a first hospitalization for major depression with psychotic features. *The Journal of Child and Adolescent Psychopharmacology*, **13**, 173–85.

Delgado, P.L. and Moreno, F.A. (1998). Different roles for serotonin in anti-obsessional drug action and the pathophysiology of obsessive-compulsive disorder. *British Journal of Psychiatry*, **35** (Suppl), 21–5.

Dell'Osso, B., Altamura, A.C., Allen, A., *et al.* (2006). Epidemiological and clinical updates on impulse control disorders, a critical review. *European Archives of Psychiatry and Clinical Neuroscience*, **256**, 464–75.

Demirkiran, M. and Jankovic, J. (1995). Paroxysmal dyskinesias. Clinical features and classification. *Annals of Neurology*, **38**, 571–679.

Demyttenaere, K. and De Fruyt, J. (2003). Getting what you ask for; on the selectivity of depression rating scales. *Psychotherapy and Psychosomatics*, **72**, 61–70.

de Pauw, K.W., Szulecka, T.K. and Poltock, T.L. (1987). Fregoli syndrome after cerebral infarction. *Journal of Nervous and Mental Disorders*, **175**, 433–8.

Devinsky, O. and Vazquez, B. (1993). Behavioral changes associated with epilepsy. In R.A. Brumback, ed., *Behavioral Neurology, Neurologic Clinics*, Vol **11**. Philadelphia: WB Saunders, pp. 127–49.

Putman, F., Grafman, J., *et al.* (1989). Dissociative states and epilepsy. *Neurology*, **39**, 835–40.

Mesad, S. and Alper, K. (2001). Nondominant hemisphere lesions and conversion nonepileptic seizures. *The Journal of Neuropsychiatry and Clinical Neurosciences*, **13**, 367–373.

Dewaraja, R. and Sasaki, Y. (1990). A left to right hemisphere callosal transfer deficit of nonlinguistic information in alexithymia. *Psychotherapy and Psychosomatics*, **54**, 201–07.

De Witte, L., Wilssens, I., Engelborghs, S., *et al.* (2006). Impairment of syntax and lexical semantics in a patient with bilateral paramedian thalamic infarction. *Brain and Language*, **96**, 69–77.

Diamond, M. and Watson, L.A. (2004). Androgen insensitivity syndrome and Klinefelter's syndrome, sex and gender considerations. *Child and Adolescent Psychiatric Clinics of North America*, **13**, 623–40.

Dickey, C.C., McCarley, R.W., Xu, M.L., *et al.* (2007). MRI abnormalities of the hippocampus and cavum septi pellucidi in females with schizotypal personality disorder. *Schizophrenia Research*, **89**, 49–58.

Dierks, T., Linden, D.E., Jandl, M., *et al.* (1999). Activation of Heschl's gyrus during auditory hallucinations. *Neuron*, **22**, 615–21.

Diesing, T.S. and Wijdicks, E.F.M. (2006). Arc de cercle and dysautonomia from anoxic injury. *Movement Disorders*, **21**, 868–9.

Dolan, R.J. (2002). Emotion, cognition, and behavior. *Science*, **298**, 1191–4.

Donohoe, G. and Robertson, I.H. (2003). Can specific deficits in executive functioning explain the negative symptoms of schizophrenia? A review. *Neurocase*, **9**, 97–108.

Dorz, S., Borgherini, G., Conforti, D., *et al.* (2003). Depression in inpatients, bipolar vs unipolar. *Psychology Reports*, **92**, 1031–9.

Drake, A.I., McDonald, E.C., Magnus, N.E., *et al.* (2006). Utility of Glasgow Coma Scale – Extended in symptom prediction following mild traumatic brain injury. *Brain Injury*, **20**, 469–75.

Draper, B. (1991). Potentially reversible dementia, a review. *Australia and New Zealand Psychiatry*, **25**, 506–18.

Duara, R., Barker, W. and Luis, C.A. (1999). Frontotemporal dementia and Alzheimer's disease, differential diagnosis. *Dementia and Geriatric Cognitive Disorders*, **10** (Suppl. 1), 37–42.

Dubois, P. (1905). *The Psychic Treatment of Nervous Disorders, The Psychoneuroses and Their Moral Treatment*, translated by S.E. Jelliffe and W.A. White. New York: Funk and Wagnalls Co.

Duda, J.E. (2007). History and prevalence of involuntary emotional expression disorder. *CNS Spectrums*, **12** (Suppl. 5), 6–10.

Dudley, R.E.J., John, C.H., Young, A.W. and Over, D.E. (1997). Normal and abnormal reasoning in people with delusions. *British Journal of Clinical Psychology*, **36**, 243–58.

Duffy, A., Grof, P., Robertson, C. and Alda, M. (2000). The implications of genetic studies of major mood disorders in clinical practice. *Journal of Clinical Psychiatry*, **61**, 630–7.

Duncan, M.E. (1996). Pregnancy and leprosy neuropathy. *Indian Journal of Leprosy*, **68**, 23–34.

Durbin, C.E. and Klein, D.N. (2006). Ten-year stability of personality disorders among outpatients with mood disorders. *Journal of Abnormal Psychology*, **115**, 75–84.

Dyck, I.R., Phillips, K.A., Warshaw, M.G., *et al.* (2001). Patterns of personality pathology in patients with generalized anxiety disorder, panic disorder with and without agoraphobia, and social phobia. *Journal of Personality Disorders*, **15**, 60–71.

Eapen, V., Trimble, M.R. and Robertson, M.M. (1996). The use of fluoxetine in Gilles de la Tourette syndrome and obsessive compulsive behaviors, preliminary clinical experience. *Progress in Neuropsychopharmacology and Biological Psychiatry*, **20**, 737–43.

Earleywine, M., Finn, P.R., Peterson, J.B. and Pihl, R.O. (1992). Factor structure and correlates of the tridimensional personality questionnaire. *Journal of Studies on Alcohol*, **53**, 233–8.

Edelstyn, N.M.J. and Oyebode, F. (1999). A review of the phenomenology and cognitive neuropsychological origins of the Capgras syndrome. *International Journal of Geriatric Psychiatry*, **14**, 48–59.

Egeland, J., Lund, A., Landro, N.I., *et al.* (2005). Cortisol level predicts executive and memory function in depression, symptom level predicts psychomotor speed. *Acta Psychiatrica Scandinavica*, **112**, 434–41.

Eisenman, R., Platt, J.J. and Darbes, A. (1968). Creativity, intelligence, and achievement. *Psychology Reports*, **22**, 749–54.

el Gaddal, Y.Y. (1989). De Clerambault's syndrome (Erotomania) in organic delusional syndrome. *British Journal of Psychiatry*, **154**, 714–16.

Elliott, F.A. (1984). The episodic dyscontrol syndrome and aggression. *Neurology Clinics*, **2**, 113–25.

Ellis, H.D., Young, A.W., Quayle, A.H. and De Pauw, K.W. (1997). Reduced automatic responses to faces in Capgras delusion. *Proceedings of the Royal Society of London B: Biological Sciences*, **264**, 1085–92.

Emery, V.O. and Oxman, T.E. (1992). Update on the dementia spectrum of depression. *American Journal of Psychiatry*, **149**, 305–17.

Endicott, J. and Spitzer, R.L. (1978). A diagnostic interview. The schedule for affective disorders and schizophrenia. *Archives of General Psychiatry*, **35**, 837–44.

Enevoldson, T.P. (2004). Recreational drugs and their neurological consequences. *Journal of Neurology, Neurosurgery and Psychiatry*, **75** (Suppl. III), 9–15.

Enns, M.W., Larsen, D.K. and Cox, B.J. (2000). Discrepancies between self and observer ratings of depression. The relationship to demographic, clinical and personality variables. *Journal of Affective Disorders*, **60**, 33–41.

Erichsen, J.E. (1882). *On Concussion of the Spine, Nervous Shock, and Other Obscure Injuries of the Nervous System*. London: Longmans Green.

Eriksen, M.K., Thomsen, L.L., Andersen, I., *et al.* (2004). Clinical characteristics of 362 patients with familial migraine with aura. *Cephalagia*, **24**, 564–75.

Erlenmeyer-Kimling, L. and Cornblatt, B. (1984). Biobehavioral risk factors in children of schizophrenic parents. *Journal of Autism and Developmental Disorders*, **14**, 357–74.

Eslinger, P.J., Flaherty-Craig, C.V. and Benton, A.L. (2004). Developmental outcomes after early prefrontal cortex damage. *Brain and Cognition*, **55**, 84–103.

Esquirol, J.E.D. (1838). *Des Maladies Mentales Considerées sous les Rapports Medical, Hygienique et Medico-legal*, Vols. 1, 2. Paris: Baillière.

Evers, S. and Ellger, T. (2004). The clinical spectrum of musical hallucinations. *Journal of Neurological Science*, **227**, 55–65.

Evren, C., Evren, B., Yancar, C. and Erkiran, M. (2007). Temperament and character model of personality profile or alcohol- and drug-dependent inpatients. *Comprehensive Psychiatry*, **48**, 283–8.

Eysenck, H.J. (1964). The effects of psychotherapy. *International Journal of Psychiatry*, **1**, 99–144.
(1985). *Personality and Individual Differences, A Natural Science Approach*. New York, NY: Plenum Publishing Corp.
and Rachman, S. (1965). *The Causes and Cures of Neuroses*. London: Routledge and Kegan Paul.

Faber, R. and Reichstein, M.B. (1981). Language dysfunction in schizophrenia. *British Journal of Psychiatry*, **139**, 519–22.
Abrams, R., Taylor, M.A., *et al.* (1983). Comparison of schizophrenic patients with formal thought disorder and neurologically impaired patients with aphasia. *American Journal of Psychiatry*, **140**, 1348–51.

Factor, S.A., Podskalny, G.D. and Molho, E.S. (1995). Psychogenic movement disorders. Frequency, clinical profile, and characteristics. *Journal of Neurology, Neurosurgery and Psychiatry*, **59**, 406–12.

Fahn, S. (1993). Motor and vocal tics. In R. Kurla, ed., *Handbook of Tourette's Syndrome and Related Tic and Behavioral Disorders*. New York: Marcel Dekker, pp. 3–16.

Falkai, P., Bogerts, B., Schneider, T., *et al.* (1995). Disturbed planum temporale asymmetry in schizophrenia, a quantitative post-mortem study. *Schizophrenia Research*, **14**, 161–76.

Fallon, B.A., Qureshi, A.I., Laje, G. and Klein, B. (2000). Hypochondriasis and its relationship to obsessive-compulsive disorder. *Psychiatric Clinics of North America*, **23**, 605–16.

Falret, J. (1854). Mémoire sur la folie circulaire, forme de la maladie mentale caractérisée par la reproduction successive et régulière de l'état maniaque, de l'état mélancolique, et d'un intervalle lucide plus ou moins prolongé. *Bulletin de l'Académie impériale de médecine, Paris*, **19**, 382–400.

Fan, X., Henderson, D.C., Chiang, E., *et al.* (2007). Sexual functioning, psychopathology and quality of life in patients with schizophrenia. *Schizophrenia Bulletin*, **94**, 119–27.

Fanous, A., Gardner, C., Walsh, D. and Kendler, K.S. (2001). Relationship between positive and negative symptoms of schizophrenia and schizotypal symptoms in nonpsychotic relatives. *Archives of General Psychiatry*, **58**, 669–73.

Farah, M. (1995). Current issues in the neuropsychology of image generation. *Neuropsychologia*, **33**, 1455–71.

Faravelli, C., Giugni, A., Salvatoru, S. and Ricca, V. (2004). Psychopathology after rape. *American Journal of Psychiatry*, **161**, 1483–5.

Farges, F., Corcos, M., Speranza, M., *et al.* (2004). Alexithymia, depression and drug addiction. *Encephale*, **30**, 201–11.

Fassino, S., Abbate-Daga, G., Leombruni, P., *et al.* (2001). Temperment and character in Italian men with anorexia nervosa: a controlled study with the Temperament and Character Inventory. *Journal of Nervous and Mental Disorders*, **189**, 788–94.

Feighner, J.P., Robins, E., Guze, S.B., *et al.* (1972). Diagnostic criteria for use in psychiatric research. *Archives of General Psychiatry*, **26**, 47–63.

Fein, D., Joy S., Green, L.A. and Waterhouse, L. (1996). Autism and pervasive developmental disorders. In B.S. Fogel, R.B. Schiffer and S.M. Rao, eds., *Neuropsychiatry*. Baltimore: William and Wilkins, pp. 571–614.

Feinberg, T.E. and Roane, D.M. (2005). Delusional misidentification. *Psychiatric Clinics of North America*, **28**, 665–83.

Schindler, R.J., Flanagan, N.G. and Haber, L.D. (1992). Two alien hand syndromes. *Neurology*, **42**, 19–24.

Feinstein, A., Stergiopoulos, V., Fine, J. and Lang, A.E. (2001). Psychiatric outcome in patients with a psychogenic movement disorder, A prospective study. *Neuropsychiatry, Neuropsychology and Behavioral Neurology*, **14**, 169–76.

Hershkop, S., Ouchterlony, D., *et al.* (2002). Posttraumatic amnesia and recall of a traumatic event following traumatic brain injury. *Journal of Neuropsychiatry and Clinical Neuroscience*, **14**, 25–30.

Fenn, D.S., Moussaoui, D., Hoffman, W.F., *et al.* (1996). Movements in never-medicated schizophrenics. A preliminary study. *Psychopharmacology (Berlin)*, **123**, 206–10.

Ferguson, E. (2004). Personality as a predictor of hypochondriacal concerns, results from two longitudinal studies. *Journal of Psychosomatic Research*, **56**, 307–12.

Fernandez-Alvarez, E. (2005). Movement disorders of functional origin (psychogenic) in children. *Revue Neurologique*, **40** (Suppl. 1), S75–7.

Fielding, J., Georgiou-Karistianis, N. and White, O. (2006). The role of the basal ganglia in the control of automatic visuospatial attention. *Journal of the International Neuropsychological Society*, **12**, 657–67.

Fields, H.L., Malick, A. and Burstein, R. (1995). Dorsal horn projection targets of on and off cells in the rostral ventromedial medulla. *Journal of Neurophysiology*, **74**, 1742–59.

Fieve, R.R., Go, R., Dunner, D.L. and Elston, R. (1984). Search for biological/genetic markers in a long-term epidemiological and morbid risk study of affective disorders. *Journal of Psychiatric Research*, **18**, 425–45.

Fineberg, N.A., Sharma, P., Sivakumaran, T., *et al.* (2007). Does obsessive-compulsive personality disorder belong with the obsessive-compulsive spectrum? *CNS Spectrums*, **12**, 467–82.

Fink, A., Tsai, M.C., Hays, R.D., *et al.* (2002). Comparing the alcohol-related problems survey (ARPS) to traditional alcohol screening measures in elderly outpatients. *Archives of Gerontology*, **34**, 55–78.

Fink, G.R., Halligan, P.W. and Marshall, J.C. (2006). Neuroimaging of hysteria in psychogenic movement disorders. In M. Hallet, C.R. Cloninger, S. Fahn, *et al.*, eds., *Psychogenic Movement Disorders, Neurology and Neuropsychiatry*. Philadelphia: Lippincott Williams and Wilkins, pp. 230–7.

Fink, M. (1996a). Neuroleptic malignant syndrome and catatonia. One entity or two? *Biological Psychiatry*, **39**, 1–4.

(1996b). Toxic serotonin syndrome or neuroleptic malignant syndrome? Case report. *Pharmacopsychiatry*, **29**, 159–61.

(1999). Delirious mania. *Bipolar Disorders*, **1**, 54–60.

(2000). Electroshock revisited. *American Scientist*, **88**, 162–7.

(2007). Complaints of loss of personal memories after electroconvulsive therapy, evidence of a somatoform disorder? *Psychosomatics*, **48**, 290–3.

and Taylor, M.A. (2003). *Catatonia, A Clinician's Guide to Diagnosis and Treatment*. Cambridge: Cambridge University Press.

and Taylor, M.A. (2007). Resurrecting melancholia. *Acta Psychiatrica Scandinavica*, **115** (Suppl. 433), 14–20.

Bush, G. and Francis, A. (1993). Catatonia. A treatable disorder, occasionally recognized. *Directions in Psychiatry*, **13**, 1–8.

Fink, P., Toft, T., Sparle, K.C., *et al.* (2004). A new, empirically established hypochondriasis diagnosis. *American Journal of Psychiatry*, **161**, 1680–91.

Firestone, P., Dixon, K.L., Nunes, K.L. and Bradford, J.M. (2005). A comparison of incest offenders based on victim age. *Journal of the American Academy of Psychiatry and Law*, **33**, 223–32.

First, M.B. and Zimmerman, M. (2006). Including laboratory tests in DSM-V diagnostic criteria. *American Journal of Psychiatry*, **163**, 2041–2.

Pincus, H.A., Levine, J.B., *et al.* (2004). Clinical utility as a criterion for revising psychiatric diagnoses. *American Journal of Psychiatry*, **161**, 946–54.

Fischer, R.S., Alexander, M.P., D'Esposito, M. and Otto, R. (1995). Neuropsychological and neuroanatomical correlates of confabulation. *Journal of Clinical, and Experimental Neuropsychology*, **17**, 20–8.

Fish, B., Marcus, J., Hans, S.L., *et al.* (1992). Infants at risk for schizophrenia, sequelae of a genetic neurointegrative defect. A review and replication analysis of pandysmaturation in the Jerusalem infant development study. *Archives of General Psychiatry*, **409**, 221–35.

Fish, F. (1967). *Clinical Psychopathology, Signs and Symptoms in Psychiatry*. Bristol: John Wright & Sons.

(1968). *An Outline of Psychiatry, For Students and Practitioners*, 2nd edn. Bristol: John Wright & Sons Ltd.

Fish, F.J. (1962). *Schizophrenia*. Bristol: John Wright and Sons, Ltd.

Fishbain, D.A., Goldberg, M., Meagher, B.R., *et al.* (1986). Male and female chronic pain patients categorized by DSM-III psychiatric diagnostic criteria. *Pain*, **26**, 181–97.

Fitzpatrick, K.K., Euton, S.J., Jones, J.N. and Schmidt, N.B. (2005). Gender role, sexual orientation and suicide risk. *Journal of Affective Disorders*, **87**, 35–42.

Flashman, L.A. and Green, M.F. (2004). Review of cognition and brain structure in schizophrenia, profiles, longitudinal course, and effects of treatment. *Psychiatric Clinics of North America*, **27**, 1–18.

Flaum, M., Arndt, S. and Andreasen, N.C. (1991). The reliability of "bizarre" delusions. *Comprehensive Psychiatry*, **32**, 59–65.

Fletcher, J.M., Page, J.B., Francis, D.J., *et al.* (1996). Cognitive correlates of long-term cannabis use in Costa Rican men. *Archives of General Psychiatry*, **6**, 53, 1051–7.

Flexner, J.T. (1969). *George Washington, Anguish and Farewell (1793–1799)*. Boston: Little, Brown and Company.

Floel, A. and Cohen, L.G. (2006). Translational studies in neurorehabilitation, from bench to bedside. *Cognitive and Behavioral Neurology*, **19**, 1–10.

Flor-Henry, P., Fromm-Auch, D., Tapper, M. and Schopflocher, D. (1981). A neuropsychological study of the stable syndrome of hysteria. *Biological Psychiatry*, **16**, 601–26.

Toer, R., Kumpula, I., *et al.* (1990). Neurophysiological and neuropsychological study of two cases of multiple personality syndrome and comparison with chronic hysteria. *International Journal of Psychophysiology*, **10**, 151–61.

Foa, E.B., Stein, D.J. and McFarlane, A.C. (2006). Symptomatology and psychopathology of mental health problems after disaster. *Journal of Clinical Psychiatry*, **67** (Suppl. 2), 15–25.

Fogelson, D.L., Nuechterlein, K.H., Asarnow, R.A., *et al.* (2007). Avoidant personality disorder in a separable schizophrenia-spectrum personality disorder even when controlling for the presence of paranoid and schizotypal personality disorders. *Schizophrenia Research*, **91**, 192–9.

Folstein, M.F., Folstein, S.E. and McHugh, P.R. (1975). Mini-Mental State, a practical method for grading the cognitive state of patients for the clinician. *Journal of Psychiatric Research*, **12**, 189–98. (The Mini Mental State Examination, Psychological Assessment Resources, 2001.)

Fong, C.S. (2005). Claude's syndrome associated with supranuclear horizontal gaze palsy caused by dorsomedial midbrain infraction. *Acta Neurologica Taiwanica*, **14**, 147–50.

Ford, R.A. (1989). The psychopathology of echophenomena. *Psychological Medicine*, **19**, 627–35.

Foroozan, R. and Buono, L.M. (2003). Foggy visual field defect. *Survey of Ophthalmology*, **48**, 447–51.

Forstl, H., Almeida, O.P., Owen, A.M., *et al.* (1991). Psychiatric, neurological and medical aspects of misidentification syndromes, a review of 260 cases. *Psychological Medicine*, **21**, 905–10.

Fossati, A., Beauchaine, T.P., Grazioli, F., *et al.* (2005). A latent structure analysis of Diagnostic Statistical Manual of Mental Disorders, Fourth Edition, Narcissistic Personality Disorder criteria. *Comprehensive Psychiatry*, **46**, 361–7.

Beauchaine, T.P., Grazioli, F., *et al.* (2006). Confirmatory factor analysis of DSM-IV cluster C personality disorder criteria. *Journal of Personality Disorders*, **20**, 186–203.

Foundas, A.L., Leonard, C.M., Gilmore, R., *et al.* (1994). Planum temporale asymmetry and language dominance. *Neuropsychologia*, **32**, 1225–31.

Macauley, B.L., Raymer, A.M., *et al.* (1995). Gesture laterality in aphasic and apraxic stroke patients. *Brain and Cognition*, **29**, 204–13.

Frank, G.K., Bailer, U.F., Henry, S., *et al.* (2004). Neuroimaging studies in eating disorders. *CNS Spectrums*, **9**, 539–48.

Frare, F., Perugi, G., Ruffolo, G. and Toni, C. (2004). Obsessive–compulsive disorder and body dysmorphic disorder, a comparison of clinical features. *European Psychiatry*, **19**, 292–8.

Freeman, D. and Garety, P.A. (2003). Connecting neurosis and psychosis, the direct influence of emotion on delusions and hallucinations. *Behavior Research and Therapy*, **41**, 923–47.

Freeman, M.P., Smith, K.W., Freeman, S.A., *et al.* (2002). The impact of reproductive events on the course of bipolar disorder in women. *Journal of Clinical Psychiatry*, **63**, 284–7.

Freeman, R. (1992). Communication, body language and dental anxiety. *Dental Update*, **19**, 307–09.

Freemantle, N., Anderson, I.M. and Young, P. (2000). Predictive value of pharmacological activity for the relative efficacy of antidepressant drugs. Meta-regression analysis. *British Journal of Psychiatry*, **177**, 292–302.

Frei, A., Vollm, B., Graf, M. and Dittmann, V. (2006). Female serial killing, review and case report. *Criminal Behavior and Mental Health*, **16**, 167–76.

Freud, S. (1984). Mourning and melancholia. In *The Pelican Freud Library, 11*, On Metapsychology, The Theory of Psychoanalysis. London: Penguin, pp. 245–68.

Friedman, R.C. (1999). Homosexuality, psychopathology, and suicidality. *Archives in General Psychiatry*, **56**, 887–8.

Frijda, N. (1986). *Emotions*. Cambridge: Press Syndicate of University of Cambridge.

Fuller, G.N. and Guiloff, R.J. (1987). Migrainous olfactory hallucinations. *Journal of Neurology, Neurosurgery and Psychiatry*, **50**, 1688–90.

Gabe, P. and Sjoquest, K. (2002). Experience and assessment of pain in individuals with cognitive impairments. *Special Care in Dentistry*, **22**, 174–80.

Gacono, C.B., Meloy, J.R., Sheppard, K., *et al.* (1995). A clinical investigation of malingering and psychopathy in hospitalized insanity acquittees. *Bulletin of the American Academy of Psychiatry and the Law*, **23**, 387–97.

Gaillard, M.C. and Borruat, F.X. (2003). Persisting visual hallucinations and illusions in previously drug-addicted patients. *Klinische Monatsblätter für Augenheilkunde*, **220**, 176–80.

Gallassi, R. (2006). Epileptic amnesia syndrome, an update and further considerations. *Epilepsia*, **47** (Suppl. 2), 13–105.

Gambini, O., Abbruzzese, M. and Scarone, S. (1993). Smooth pursuit and saccadic eye movements and Wisconsin Card Sorting Test performance in obsessive-compulsive disorder. *Psychiatry Research*, **48**, 191–200.

Ganser, S. and Shorter, C.E. (translator). (1965). A peculiar hysterical state. *British Journal of Criminology*, **5**, 120–6.

Gardini, S., De Beni, R., Cornoldi, C., *et al.* (2005). Different neuronal pathways support the generation of general and specific mental images. *Neuroimage*, **27**, 544–52.

Gardner-Thorpe, C. and Pearn, J. (2004). The Cotard syndrome. Report of two patients, with a review of the extended spectrum of "delire des negations". *European Journal of Neurology*, **11**, 563–6.

Garety, P.A. and Freeman, D. (1999). Cognitive approaches to delusions, a critical review of theories and evidence. *British Journal of Clinical Psychiatry*, **38**, 113–54.

and Hemsley, D.R. (1994). *Delusions, Investigations into the Psychology of Delusional Reasoning*. Oxford: Oxford University Press.

Garrabe, J. (2005). Obituary Georges Lanteri-Laura (1930–1994). *History of Psychiatry*, **16**, 365–372.

Gavin, N.I., Gaynes, N., Lohr, K.N., *et al.* (2005). Perinatal depression, a systematic review of prevalence and incidence. *Obstetrics and Gynecology*, **106**, 1071–83.

Gavrilets, S. and Rice, W.R. (2006). Genetic models of homosexuality, generating testable predictions. *Proceedings, Biological Sciences*, **273**, 3031–8.

Gazzaniga, M.S. (2000). Cerebral specialization and interhemispheric communication, does the corpus callosum enable the human condition? *Brain*, **133**, 1293–326.

Gazzaniga, M. and LeDoux, J.E. (1978). *The Integrated Mind*. New York: Plenum Press.

Gelenberg, A.J. (1976). The catatonic syndrome. *Lancet*, **1**, 1339–41.

Geller, D.A. (2006). Obsessive–compulsive and spectrum disorders in children and adolescents. *Psychiatric Clinics of North America*, **29**, 353–70.

George, S.M., Trimble, M.R., Ring, A.H. and Robertson, M.M. (1993). Obsessions in obsessive-compulsive disorder with and without Gilles de La Tourette's syndrome. *American Journal of Psychiatry*, **150**, 98–102.

Gershon, E.S., Hamovit, J., Guroff, J.J., *et al.* (1982). A family study of schizoaffective, bipolar I, bipolar II, unipolar and normal control probands. *Archives of General Psychiatry*, **39**, 1157–67.

DeLisi, L.E., Hamovit, J., *et al.* (1988). A controlled family study of chronic psychoses. *Archives of General Psychiatry*, **45**, 328–36.

Gershuny, B.S., Keuthen, N.J., Gentes, E.L., *et al.* (2006). Current posttraumatic stress disorder and history of trauma in trichotillomania. *Journal of Clinical Psychology*, **62**, 1521–9.

Gervais, M. and Wilson, D.S. (2005). The evolution and functions of laughter and humor, a synthetic approach. *Quarterly Review of Biology*, **80**, 395–430.

Ghaemi, S.N., Hsu, D.J., Thase, M.E., *et al.* (2006). Pharmacologic treatment patterns at study entry for the first 500 STEP-BD participants. *Psychiatric Services*, **57**, 660–5.

Ghika-Schmid, F. and Bogousslavsky, J. (2000). Emotional behavior in acute brain lesions. In J. Bogousslavsky and J.L. Cummings, eds., *Behavior and Mood Disorders in Focal Brain Lesions*. Cambridge: Cambridge University Press, pp. 65–94.

Giesbrecht, T., Jongen, E.M.M., Smulders, F.T.Y. and Merckelbach, H. (2006). Dissociation, resting EEG, and subjective sleep experiences in undergraduates. *Journal of Nervous and Mental Disorders*, **194**, 362–8.

Gilleen, J. and David, A.S. (2005). The cognitive neuropsychiatry of delusions, from psychopathology to neuropsychology and back again. *Psychological Medicine*, **35**, 5–12.

Gillis, A.J. and MacDonald, B. (2006). Unmasking delirium. *Canadian Nurse*, **102**, 18–24.

Gjessing, L.R. (1974). A review of periodic catatonia. *Biological Psychiatry*, **8**, 23–45.

Gjessing, R. (1938). Disturbances of somatic functions in catatonia with periodic course and their compensation. *Journal of Mental Sciences*, **84**, 608–21.

Gloor, P. (1990). Experiental phenomena of temporal lobe epilepsy. Facts and hypotheses. *Brain*, **113**, 1673–94.

Olivier, A., Quesney, L.F., *et al.* (1982). The role of the limbic system in experiential phenomena of temporal lobe epilepsy. *Annals of Neurology*, **12**, 129–44.

Glosser, G., Clark, C., Freundlich, B., *et al.* (1995). A controlled investigation of current and premorbid personality, characteristics of Parkinson's disease patients. *Movement Disorders*, **10**, 201–06.

Goadsby, P.J. (2005). Migraine, allodynia, sensitization and all of that. *European Neurology*, **53** (Suppl. 1), 10–16.

Goldberg, J.F., Wankmuller, M.M. and Sutherland, K.H. (2004). Depression with versus without manic features in rapid-cycling bipolar disorder. *Journal of Nervous and Mental Disorders*, **192**, 602–06.

Goldin-Meadow, S. (1999). The role of gesture in communication and thinking. *Trends in Cognitive Sciences*, **3**, 419–29.

and Wagner, S.M. (2005). How our hands help us learn. *Trends in Cognitive Sciences*, **9**, 234–41.

Goldstein, G., Allen, D.N. and Weiner, C.L. (1999). Lateralized brain dysfunction in schizophrenia, a comparison with patients with lateralized structural lesions. *Schizophrenia Research*, **40**, 179–87.

Goldstein, K. (1944/1964). Methodological approach to the study of schizophrenic thought disorder. In J.S. Kasanin, ed., *Language and Thought in Schizophrenia*. New York: Norton, pp. 17–40.

Goldstein, R.Z., Giovannetti, T., Schullery, M., *et al.* (2003). Neurocognitive correlates of response to treatment in formal thought disorder in patients with first-episode schizophrenia. *Neuropsychiatry, Neuropsychology and Behavioral Neurology*, **15**, 88–98.

Gomez, R.G., Fleming, S.H., Keller, J., *et al.* (2006). The neuropsychological profile of psychotic major depression and its relation to cortisol. *Biological Psychiatry*, **60**, 472–8.

Gonzales, G.R. (1995). Central pain, diagnosis and treatment strategies. *Neurology*, **45** (12 Suppl. 9), S11–16.

Goodall, J. and Van Lawick, H. (photographer) (1971). *In the Shadow of Man*. Boston: Houghton Mifflin Company.

Goodarzi, M.A., Wykes, T. and Hemsley, D.R. (2000). Cerebral lateralization of global–local processing in people with schizotypy. *Schizophrenia Research*, **45**, 115–21.

Goodwin, F.K. and Jamison, K.R., eds. (1990). *Manic-Depressive Illness*. New York: Oxford University Press.

Gorelick, D.A., Kussin, S.Z. and Kahn, I. (1978). Paranoid delusions and auditory hallucinations associated with digoxin intoxication. *Journal of Nervous Diseases*, **166**, 817–19.

Gorman, W.F. (1982). Defining malingering. *Journal of Forensic Science*, **27**, 401–07.

Gottwald, B., Wilde, B., Mihajlovic, Z. and Mehdorn, H.M. (2004). Evidence for distinct cognitive deficits after focal cerebellar lesions. *Journal of Neurology, Neurosurgery & Psychiatry*, **75**, 1524–31.

Gould, R., Miller, B.L., Goldberg, M.A. and Benson, D.F. (1986). The validity of hysterical signs and symptoms. *Journal of Nervous and Mental Disorders*, **174**, 593–7.

Gouzoulis-Mayfrank, E., Daumann, J., Tuchtenhagen, F., *et al.* (2000). Impaired cognitive performance in drug free users of recreational ecstasy (MDMA). *Journal of Neurology, Neurosurgery & Psychiatry*, **68**, 719–25.

Grados, M.A., Riddle, M.A., Samuels, J.F., *et al.* (2001). The familial phenotype of obsessive-compulsive disorder in relation to tic disorders, the Hopkins OCD family study. *Biological Psychiatry*, **50**, 559–65.

Graff-Radford, N.R., Russell, J.W. and Rezai, K. (1995). Frontal degenerative dementia and neuroimaging. *Advances in Neurology*, **66**, 37–47.

Graham, N.L., Emery, T. and Hodgers, J.R. (2004). Distinctive cognitive profiles in Alzheimer's disease and subcortical vascular dementia. *Journal of Neurology, Neurosurgery & Psychiatry*, **75**, 61–71.

Grant, J.E. and Phillips, K.A. (2005). Recognizing and treating body dysmorphic disorder. *Annals of Clinical Psychiatry*, **17**, 205–10.

and Potenza, M.N. (2006a). Compulsive aspects of impulse-control disorders. *Psychiatric Clinics of North America*, **29**, 539–51.

and Potenza, M.N. (2006b). Escitalopram treatment of pathological gambling with co-occurring anxiety, an open-label pilot study with double-blind discontinuation. *International Clinical Psychopharmacology*, **21**, 203–09.

Kim, S.W. and Eckert, E.D. (2002). Body dysmorphic disorder in patients with anorexia nervosa, prevalence, clinical features, and delusionality of body image. *International Journal of Eating Disorders*, **32**, 291–300.

Brewer, J.A. and Potenza, M.N. (2006). The neurobiology of substance and behavioral addictions. *CNS Spectrums*, **11**, 924–30.

Gray, J.A. and McNaughton, N. (2000). *The Neuropsychology, of Anxiety, An Enquiry into the Functions of the Septohippocampal System*, 2nd edn., Oxford: Oxford University Press.

Greden, J.F. and Carroll, B.J. (1979). The dexamethasone suppression test as a diagnostic aid in catatonia. *American Journal of Psychiatry*, **136**, 1199–200.

Green, R.C. and Devinsky, O. (1992). Complex motor manifestations and directed aggression in epilepsy. In A.B. Joseph and R.R. Young, eds., *Movement Disorders in Neurology and Neuropsychiatry*. Boston: Blackwell Scientific Publications, pp. 738–48.

Gresty, M. (1977). Eccentric head positions reveal disorders of conjugate eye movement. *Journal of Neurology, Neurosurgery & Psychiatry*, **40**, 992–1002.

Greveson, G.C., Gray, C.S., French, J.M. and James, O.F.W. (1991). Long-term outcome for patients and carers following hospital admission for stroke. *Age and Ageing*, **20**, 337–44.

Griesinger, W. (1862). *Mental Pathology and Therapeutics*, translated by C.L. Robertson and J. Rutherford. London: New Sydenham Society.

Griffiths, T.D. (2000). Musical hallucinosis in acquired deafness. Phenomenology and brain subsrate. *Brain*, **123**, 2065–76.

Grilo, C.M., Skodol, A.E., Gunderson, J.G., *et al.* (2004). Longitudinal diagnostic efficiency of DSM-IV criteria for obsessive-compulsive personality disorder, a 2-year prospective study. *Acta Psychiatrica Scandinavica*, **110**, 64–8.

Grob, G.N. (1991). *From Asylum to Community, Mental Health Policy in Modern America.* Princeton: Princeton UP, pp. 16–23.

Groppel, G., Kapitany, T. and Baumgartner, C. (2000). Cluster analysis of clinical seizure semiology of psychogenic nonepileptic seizures. *Epilepsia*, **41**, 610–14.

Grosberg, B.M., Solomon, S. and Lipton, R.B. (2005). Retinal migraine. *Current Pain and Headache Reports*, **9**, 268–71.

Guillery-Girard, B., Quinette, P., Desgranges, B., *et al.* (2006). Long-term memory following transient global amnesia, an investigation of episodic and semantic memory. *Acta Neurologica Scandinavica*, **114**, 329–33.

Gundogar, D. and Demirci, S. (2006). Multiple sclerosis presenting with fantastic confabulation. *General Hospital Psychiatry*, **28**, 448–51.

Gurland, B.J., Fleiss, J.L., Cooper, J.E., *et al.* (1969). Cross-national study of diagnosis of the mental disorders. Some comparisons of diagnostic criteria from the first investigation. *American Journal of Psychiatry*, **125** (Suppl.), 30–9.

Gutierrez-Lobos, K., Schmid-Siegel, B., Bankier, B. and Walter, H. (2001). Delusions in first-admitted patients, gender, themes and diagnoses. *Psychopathology*, **34**, 1–7.

Hafkenscheid, A. (1993). Reliability of a standardized and expanded Brief Psychiatric Rating Scale: a replication study. *Acta Psychiatrica Scandinavica*, **88**, 305–10.

Halgren, E., Walter, R.D., Cherlow, D.G., *et al.* (1978). Mental phenomena evoked by electrical stimulation of the human hippocampal formation and amygdala. *Brain*, **101**, 83–177.

Halligan, P.W. and Davis, A.S. (2001). Cognitive neuropsychiatry, towards a scientific psychopathology. *Nature Reviews in Neurosciences*, **2**, 209–15.

Hamann, S.B., Ely, T.D., Grafton, S.T. and Kilts, C.D. (1999). Amygdala activity relayed to enhanced memory for pleasant and aversive stimuli. *Nature Neuroscience*, **2**, 289–93.

Hamer, D.H., Hu, S., Magnuson, V.L., Hu, N. and Pattatucci, A.M. (1993). A linkage between DNA markers on the X chromosome and male sexual orientation. *Science*, **261**, 321–7.

Hamilton, M. (1960). A rating scale for depression. *Journal of Neurology, Neurosurgery & Psychiatry*, **23**, 56–62.

Hammond, W.A. (1973). *Treatise on Insanity in its Medical Relations (1883).* In series, *Mental Illness and Social Policy, The American Experience*, New York: D Appleton and Company (1883), New York: Arno Press (1973).

Hampson, S.E. and Goldberg, L.R. (2006). A first large cohort study of personality trait stability over the 40 years between elementary school and midlife. *Journal of Personality and Social Psychology*, **9**, 763–79.

Hanna, G.L., Fischer, D.J., Chadha, K.R., *et al.* (2005). Familial and sporadic subtypes of early-onset obsessive-compulsive disorder. *Biological Psychiatry*, **57**, 895–900.

Hans, S.L., Marcus, J., Nuechterlein, K.H., *et al.* (1999). Neurobehavioral deficits at adolescence in children at risk for schizophrenia. The Jerusalem infant development study. *Archives of General Psychiatry*, **56**, 741–8.

Hantouche, E.G., Angst, J., Demonfaucon, C., *et al.* (2003). Cyclothymic OCD. A distinct form? *Journal of Affective Disorders*, **75**, 1–10.

Harms, E. (1967). *Origins of Modern Psychiatry.* Springfield: Charles C. Thomas, pp. 136–53.

Harrow, M., O'Connell, E.M., Herbener, E.S., *et al.* (2003). Disordered verbalizations in schizophrenia, a speech disturbance or thought disorder? *Comprehensive Psychiatry*, **44**, 353–9.

Hashimoto, R., Okada, T., Kato, T., *et al.* (2005). The breakpoint cluster region gene on chromosome 22q11 is associated with bipolar disorder. *Biological Psychiatry*, **57**, 1097–102.

Haslam, J. (1798). *Observations on Insanity with Particular Remarks on the Disease and an Account of the Morbid Appearance on Dissections.* London: Rivington.

(1809/1976). *Observations on Madness and Melancholy.* London: J. Callow; New York: Arno Press, reprint 1976.

Hawton, K., Salkovskis, P.M., Kirk, J. and Clark, D.M. (1989). *Cognitive Behavior Therapy for Psychiatric Problems, A Practical Guide.* Oxford: Oxford University Press.

Hayashi, R. (2004). Olfactory illusions and hallucinations after right temporal hemorrhage. *European Neurology*, **51**, 240–1.

Hazra, M., Culo, S. and Mamo, D. (2006). High-dose quetiapine and photopsia. *Journal of Clinical Psychopharmacology*, **26**, 546–7.

Healy, D. (2002). *The Creation of Psychopharmacology.* Cambridge, MA: Harvard University Press.

Hecker, E. (1871). Die hebephrenie. *Archives of Pathology, Anatomy Physiology and Clinical Medicine*, **52**, 394–429.

Heilman, K.M., Watson, R.T. and Valenstein, E. (1985). Neglect and related disorders. In K.M. Heilman and E. Valenstein, eds., *Clinical Neuropsychology*, 2nd edn. New York: Oxford University Press, pp. 243–93.

Helmer, C., Peres, K., Letenneur, L., *et al.* (2006). Dementia in subjects aged 75 years or over within the PAQUID cohort, prevalence and burden by severity. *Dementia and Geriatric Cognitive Disorders*, **22**, 87–94.

Helzer, J.E. and Hudziak, J.J., eds. (2002). *Defining Psychopathology in the 21st Century, DSM-V and Beyond.* Washington, DC: American Psychiatric Press Inc.

Kraemer, H.C. and Krueger, R.F. (2006). The feasibility and need for dimensional psychiatric diagnoses. *Psychological Medicine*, **36**, 1671–80.

Hempel, M.S. (1993). Neurological development during toddling age in normal children and children at risk of developmental disorders. *Early Human Development*, **34**, 47–57.

Henderson, S., Byrne, D.G. and Duncon-Jones, P. (1981). *Neurosis and the Social Environment.* Sydney: Academic Press.

Hendrick, V., Altshuler, L., Strouse, T. and Grosser, S. (2000). Postpartum and nonpostpartum depression, differences in presentation and response to pharmacologic treatment. *Depression and Anxiety*, **11**, 66–72.

Hendrickson, J. and Adityanjee, A. (1996). Lilliputian hallucinations in schizophrenia, case report and review of literature. *Psychopathology*, **29**, 35–8.

Hendryx, M.S., Haviland, M.G. and Shaw, D.G. (1991). Dimensions of alexithymia and their relationship to anxiety and depression. *Journal of Personality Assessment*, **56**, 227–37.

Henkin, R.I., Levy, L.M. and Lin, C.S. (2000). Taste and smell phantoms revealed by MRI (fMRI). *Journal of Computer Assisted Tomography*, **24**, 106–23.

Henriksson, K.G. (2003). Hypersensitivity in muscle pain syndromes. *Current Pain and Headache Reports*, **7**, 426–32.

Herdieckerhoff, G. (1985). Body language in the psychoanalytic treatment situation. *Zeitschrift für Psychosomatische Medicin und Psychoanalyse*, **31**, 129–50.

Hermann, B., Seidenberg, M., Sears, L., *et al.* (2004). Cerebellar atrophy in temporal lobe epilepsy affects procedural memory. *Neurology*, **63**, 2129–31.

Hermesh, H., Konas, S., Shiloh, R., *et al.* (2004). Musical hallucinations, prevalence in psychotic and nonpsychotic outpatients. *Journal of Clinical Psychiatry*, **65**, 191–7.

Heruti, R. J., Reznik, J., Adunski, A., *et al.* (2002). Conversion motor paralysis disorder. Analysis of 34 consecutive referrals. *Spinal Cord*, **40**, 335–40.

Hickie, I., Naismith, S., Ward, P. B., *et al.* (2005). Reduced hippocampal volumes and memory loss in patients with early- and late-onset depression. *British Journal of Psychiatry*, **186**, 197–202.

Hildebrandt, M. G., Steyerberg, E. W., Stage, K. B., *et al.* and The Danish University Antidepressant Group. (2003). Are gender differences important for the clinical effects of antidepressants? *American Journal of Psychiatry*, **160**, 1643–50.

Hill, C. G. (1907). How can we best advance the study of psychiatry? *American Journal of Psychiatry*, **64**, 1–8.

Hiller, W., Dichtl, G., Hecht, H., *et al.* (1994a). Evaluating the new ICD-10 categories of depressive episode and recurrent depressive disorder. *Journal of Affective Disorders*, **31**, 49–60. Dichtl, G., Hecht, H., *et al.* (1994b). Testing the comparability of psychiatric diagnoses in ICD-10 and DSM-III-R. *Psychopathology*, **27**, 19–28.

Hines, M. E., Kubu, C. S., Roberts, R. J. and Varney, N. R. (1995). Characteristics and mechanisms of epilepsy spectrum disorder, an explanatory model. *Applied Neuropsychology*, **2**, 1–6.

Hinsie, L. E. (1932). The catatonic syndrome in dementia praecox. *Psychiatric Quarterly*, **6**, 457–68.

Hirschfeld, R. M. (2001). Bipolar spectrum disorder, improving recognition and diagnosis. *Journal of Clinical Psychiatry*, **62** (Suppl. 14), 5–9.

Hirstein, W. and Ramachandran, V. S. (1997). Capgras syndrome, a novel probe for understanding the neural representation of the identity and familiarity of persons. *Proceedings, Biological Sciences*, **264**, 437–44.

Hoch, A. (1921). *Benign Stupors, A Study of a New Manic-Depressive Reaction Type*. New York: Macmillan Co.

Hoch, P. H. and Polatin, P. (1949). Pseudoneurotic forms of schizophrenia. *Psychiatric Quarterly*, **23**, 248–76.

Hodges, J. R. and Warlow, C. P. (1990). The aetiology of transient global amnesia. A case control study of 114 cases with perspective follow-up. *Brain*, **113**, 639–57.

Hodgins, S., Hiscoke, U. L. and Freese, R. (2003). The antecedents of aggressive behavior among men with schizophrenia, a prospective investigation of patients in community treatment. *Behavioral Science & the Law*, **21**, 523–46.

Holden, C. (2001). "Behavioral" addictions, do they exist? *Science*, **294**, 980–2.

Holden, N. L. (1987). Late paraphrenia or the paraphrenias? A descriptive study with a 10-year follow-up. *British Journal of Psychiatry*, **150**, 635–9.

Hollander, E. and Wong, C. M. (1995). Body dysmorphic disorder, pathological gambling, and sexual compulsions. *Journal of Clinical Psychiatry*, **56** (Suppl. 4), 7–12.

Cohen, L.J., Simeon, D., *et al.* (1994). Fluvoxamine treatment of body dysmorphic disorder. *Journal of Clinical Psychopharmacology*, **14**, 75–7.

Begaz, T. and DeCaria, C. (1998). Pharmacological approaches in the treatment of pathological gambling. *CNS Spectrums. International Journal of Neuropsychiatric Medicine*, **3**, 72–8.

Friedberg, J.P., Wasserman, S., *et al.* (2005). The case for the OCD spectrum. In J.S. Abramowitz and A.C. Houts, eds., *Handbook of Controversial Issues in Obsessive–Compulsive Disorder.* Dordrecht: Kluwer Academic Press, pp. 95–118.

Holtkamp, K., Konrad, K., Kaiser, N., *et al.* (2005). A retrospective study of SSRI treatment in adolescent anorexia nervosa, insufficient evidence for efficacy. *Journal of Psychiatric Research*, **39**, 303–10.

Hooley, J.M. and Delgado, M.L. (2001). Pain insensitivity in the relatives of schizophrenic patients. *Schizophrenia Research*, **47**, 265–73.

Howard, M.O., Kivlahan, D. and Walker, R.D. (1997). Cloninger's tridimensional theory of personality and psychopathology, applications to substance use disorders. *Journal of Studies on Alcoholism*, **58**, 48–66.

Howard, R.J., Almeida, O., Levy, R., *et al.* (1994). Quantitative magnetic resonance imaging volumetry distinguishes delusional disorder from late-onset schizophrenia. *British Journal of Psychiatry*, **165**, 474–80.

Humphrey, D.H. and Dahlstrom, W.G. (1995). The impact of changing from the MMPI to the MMPI-2 on profile configurations. *Journal of Personality Assessments*, **64**, 428–39.

Hunter, M.D., Eickhoff, S.B., Miller, T.W., *et al.* (2006). Neural activity in speech-sensitive auditory cortex during silence. *Proceedings of the National Academy of Science*, **103**, 189–94.

T.D. Griffiths, T.F. Farrow, *et al.* (2003). A neural basis for perception of voices in external auditory space. *Brain*, **126**, 161–9.

Hunter, R. and Macalpine, I. (1963). *Three Hundred Years of Psychiatry, 1535–1860.* London: Oxford University Press.

Husain, M., Mannan, S., Hodgson, T., *et al.* (2001). Impaired spatial working memory across saccades contributes to abnormal search in parietal neglect. *Brain*, **124**, 941–52.

Huse, E., Larbig, W., Birdaumer, N. and Flor, H. (2001). Cortical reorganization and pain. Empirical findings and therapeutic implication using the example of phantom limb. *Der Schmerz*, **15**, 131–7.

Hutton, S.B., Huddy, V., Barnes, T.R., *et al.* (2004). The relationship between antisaccades, smooth pursuit, and executive dysfunction in first-episode schizophrenia. *Biological Psychiatry*, **56**, 553–9.

Iancu, I., Dannon, P.N., Ziv, R. and Lepkifker, E. (2002). A follow-up of patients with DSM-IV schizophreniform disorder. *Canadian Journal of Psychiatry*, **47**, 56–60.

Levin, J., Dannon, P.N., *et al.* (2007). Prevalence of self-reported specific phobia symptoms in an Israeli sample of young conscripts. *Journal of Anxiety Disorders*, **21**, 762–9.

Ichimiya, T., Okubo, Y., Suhara, T. and Sudo, Y. (2001). Reduced volume of the cerebellar vermis in neuroleptic-naive schizophrenia. *Biological Psychiatry*, **49**, 20–7.

Ilkjaer, K., Kortegaard, L., Hoerder, K., *et al.* (2004). Personality disorders in a total population twin cohort with eating disorders. *Comprehensive Psychiatry*, **45**, 261–67.

Insel, T.R. and Akiskal, H.S. (1986). Obsessive–compulsive disorder with psychotic features. A phenomenologic analysis. *American Journal of Psychiatry*, **143**, 1527–33.

Ishii, R., Canuet, L., Iwase, M., *et al.* (2006). Right parietal activation during delusional state in episodic interictal psychosis of epilepsy, a report of two cases. *Epilepsy and Behavior*, **9**, 367–72.

Jablensky, A. (2001). Classification of nonschizophrenic psychotic disorders, a historical perspective. *Current Psychiatry Reports*, **3**, 326–31.

(2002). The classification of personality disorders, critical review and need for rethinking. *Psychopathology*, **35**, 112–16.

Jager, M., Bottlender, R., Strauss, A. and Moller, H.J. (2003). On the descriptive validity of ICD-10 schizophrenia. Empirical analyses in the spectrum of non-affective functional psychoses. *Psychopathology*, **36**, 152–9.

Bottlender, R., Strauss, A. and Moller, H.J. (2004). Fifteen-year follow-up of ICD-10 schizoaffective disorders compared with schizophrenia and affective disorders. *Acta Psychiatrica Scandinavica*, **109**, 30–7.

James, E. (1991). *Catching Serial Killers*. Lansing, MI: Forensic Services.

Jampala, V.C., Abrams, R.A. and Taylor, M.A. (1985). Mania with emotional blunting. Affective disorder or schizophrenia? *American Journal of Psychiatry*, **142**, 608–12.

Taylor, M.A. and Abrams, R. (1989). The diagnostic implications of formal thought disorder in mania and schizophrenia. A reassessment. *American Journal of Psychiatry*, **146**, 459–63.

Janet, P. (1901). *The Mental State of Hystericals*, translated by C.R. Corson. New York: GP Putmam.

(1907). *The Major Symptoms of Hysteria*. London: Macmillan.

Janssen, H.J.E.M., Cuisinier, M.C.J., Hoogduin, K.A.L. and deGraaw, K.P. (1996). Controlled prospective study on the mental health of women following pregnancy loss. *American Journal of Psychiatry*, **153**, 226–30.

Jaspers, K. (1963). *General Psychopathology* [seven editions between 1913 and 1959], translated by J. Hoenig and M.W. Hamilton. Chicago: University of Chicago Press.

Jedrzejczak, J., Owczarek, K. and Majkowski, J. (1999). Psychogenic pseudoseizures, clinical and electroencephalogram (EEG) video-tape recordings. *Neurology*, **6**, 473–9.

Jehel, L., Duchet, C., Paterniti, S., *et al.* (2001). [Prospective study of post-traumatic stress in victims of terrorist attacks]. *Encephale*, **27**, 393–400.

Jenike, M.A., Breiter, H.C., Baer, L., *et al.* (1996). Cerebral structural abnormalities in obsessive-compulsive disorder. A quantitative morphometric magnetic resonance imaging study. *Archives of General Psychiatry*, **53**, 625–32.

Johansen, M., Karterud, S., Pedersen, G., *et al.* (2004). An investigation of the prototype validity of the borderline DSM-IV construct. *Acta Psychiatrica Scandinavica*, **109**, 289–98.

Johansson, P., Kerr, M. and Andershed, H. (2005). Linking adult psychopathy with childhood hyperactivity–impulsivity–attention problems and conduct problems through retrospective self-reports. *Personality Disorders*, **19**, 94–101.

Johnson, M.D. and Ojemann, G.A. (2000). The role of the human thalamus in language and memory, evidence from electrophysiological studies. *Brain and Cognition*, **42**, 218–30.

Johnston, P.J., Stojanov, W., Devir, H. and Schall, U. (2005). Functional MRI of facial emotion recognition deficits in schizophrenia and their electrophysiological correlates. *European Journal of Neuroscience*, **22**, 1221–32.

Jones, I. and Craddock, N. (2001). Familiality of the puerperal trigger in bipolar disorder, results of a family study. *American Journal of Psychiatry*, **158**, 913–17.

and Craddock, N. (2002). Do puerperal psychotic episodes identify a more familial subtype of bipolar disorder? Result from a family history study. *Psychiatry and Genetics*, **12**, 177–80.

Kent, L. and Craddock, N. (2002). The genetics of affective disorders. In P. McGuffin, M.J. Owen and I.I. Gottesman, eds., *Psychiatric Genetics and Genomics*. Oxford: Oxford University Press, pp. 211–45.

Jorden, E. (1603). *A Briefe Discourse of a Disease Called the Suffocation of the Mother*. London: Windet.

Joseph A.B. and Sainte-Hilaire, M-H. (1992). Startle syndromes. In A.B. Joseph and R.R. Young, eds., *Movement Disorders in Neurology and Neuropsychiatry*. Boston: Blackwell Scientific Publications, pp. 487–92.

Joseph, R. (1999). Frontal lobe psychopathology, mania, depression, confabulation, catatonia, perseveration, obsessive compulsions and schizophrenia. *Psychiatry*, **62**, 138–72.

Joyce, P.R., Mulder, R.T., Luty, S.E., *et al.* (2002). Melancholia. Definitions, risk factors, personality, neuroendocrine markers and differential antidepressant response. *Australia and New Zealand Journal of Psychiatry*, **36**, 376–83.

McKenzie, J.M., Luty, S.E., *et al.* (2003). Temperament, childhood environment and psychopathology as risk factors for avoidant and borderline personality disorders. *Australia and New Zealand Journal of Psychiatry*, **37**, 756–64.

Kahlbaum, K.L. (1863). *Die Gruppierung der Psychischen Krankheiten und die Einteilung der Seelenstorungen* (The Classification of Mental Illnesses and the Division of Emotional Disturbances). Danzig: AW Kafemann.

(1973). *Catatonia 1874*, reprinted, translated by Y. Levij and T. Pridan. Baltimore: The Johns Hopkins University Press.

Kales, H.C., Neighbors, H.W., Blow, F.C., *et al.* (2005). Race, gender, and psychiatrists' diagnosis and treatment of major depression among elderly patients. *Psychiatric Services*, **56**, 721–8.

Kalia, M. (2005). Neurobiological basis of depression. An update. *Metabolism*, **54** (Suppl. 1), 24–7.

Kantor, S.J. and Glassman, A.H. (1977). Delusional depressions, natural history and response to treatment. *British Journal of Psychiatry*, **131**, 351–60.

Kaptsan, A., Meodownick, C. and Lerner, V. (2000). Oneiroid syndrome. A concept of use for which Western psychiatry. *Israel Journal of Psychiatry and Related Sciences*, **37**, 278–85.

Kardiner, A. and Spiegel, H. (1941). *War Stress and Neurotic Illness*. London: Paul B Hoeber.

Karila, L., Ferreri, M., Coscas, S., *et al.* (2007). Self-mutilation induced by cocaine abuse, the pleasure of bleeding. *Presse Medicale*, **36**, 235–7.

Kasai, K., Shenton, M.E., Salisbury, D.F., *et al.* (2003a). Progressive decrease of left superior temporal gyrus gray matter volume in patients with first-episode schizophrenia. *American Journal of Psychiatry*, **160**, 156–64.

Shenton, M.E., Salisbury, D.F., *et al.* (2003b). Differences and similarities in insular and temporal pole MRI gray matter volume abnormalities in first-episode schizophrenia and affective psychosis. *Archives of General Psychiatry*, **60**, 1069–77.

Kasanin, J. (1933). The acute schizoaffective psychoses. *American Journal of Psychiatry*, **13**, 97–126.

Kashiwase, H. and Kato, M. (1997). Folie a deux in Japan – analysis of 97 cases in the Japanese literature. *Acta Psychiatrica Scandinavica*, **96**, 231–4.

Katz, W.A. and Rothenberg, R. (2005). Section 3, The nature of pain, pathophysiology. *Journal of Clinical Rheumatology*, **11** (Suppl. 2), S11–15.

Katzman, D.K., Christensen, B., Young, A.R. and Zipursky, R.B. (2001). Starving the brain, structural abnormalities and cognitive impairment in adolescents with anorexia nervosa. *Seminars in Clinical Neuropsychiatry*, **6**, 146–52.

Kaufman, D.M. (1995). *Clinical Neurology for Psychiatrists*, 4th edn. Philadelphia: WB Saunders.

Kaufman, K.R. and Sachdeo, R.C. (2003). Caffeinated beverages and decreased seizure control. *Seizure*, **12**, 519–21.

Kayahan, B., Ozturk, O., Veznedaroglu, B. and Eraslan, D. (2005). Obsessive–compulsive symptoms in schizophrenia, prevalence and clinical correlates. *Psychiatry Clinics and Neuroscience*, **59**, 291–5.

Kaye, W.H., Nagata, T., Weltzin, T.E., *et al.* (2001). Double-blind placebo-controlled administration of fluoxetine in restricting- and restricting-purging-type anorexia nervosa. *Biological Psychiatry*, **49**, 644–52.

Bulik, C.M., Thornton, L., *et al.* (2004). Comorbidity of anxiety disorders with anorexia and bulimia nervosa. *American Journal of Psychiatry*, **161**, 2215–21.

Keane, J.R. (1989). Hysterical gait disorders, 60 cases. *Neurology*, **39**, 586–9.

Keedy, S.K., Ebens, C.L., Keshavan, M.S. and Sweenet, J.A. (2006). Functional magnetic resonance imaging studies of eye movements in first episode schizophrenia, smooth pursuit, visually guided saccades and the oculomotor delayed response task. *Psychiatry Research*, **146**, 199–211.

Keller, M.B., Klein, D.N., Hirschfeld, R.M., *et al.* (1995). Results of the DSM-IV mood disorder field trial. *American Journal of Psychiatry*, **152**, 843–9.

Hanks, D.L., Klein, D.N. (1996). Summary of the DSM-IV mood disorders field trial and issue overview. *Psychiatric Clinics of North America*, **19**, 1–28.

Coventry, W.L., Heath, A.C. and Martin, N.G. (2005). Widespread evidence for non-additive genetic variation in Cloninger's and Eysenck's personality dimensions using a twin plus sibling design. *Behavioral Genetics*, **35**, 707–21.

Kellinghaus, C., Loddenkemper, T., Dinner, D.S., *et al.* (2004). Non-epileptic seizures of the elderly. *Journal of Neurology*, **251**, 704–09.

Kellner, C.H., Knapp, R.G., Petrides, G., *et al.* (2006). Continuation ECT versus pharmacotherapy for relapse prevention in major depression, a multi-site study from Consortium for Research in Electroconvulsive Therapy (CORE). *Archives of General Psychiatry*, **63**, 1337–44.

Kelly, B.D. (2005). Erotomania, epidemiology and management. *CNS Drugs*, **19**, 657–9.

Kempf, L., Hussain, N. and Potash, J.B. (2005). Mood disorder with psychotic features, schizoaffective disorder, and schizophrenia with mood features. Trouble at the borders. *International Review of Psychiatry*, **17**, 9–19.

Kendell, R. and Jablensky, A. (2003). Distinguishing the validity and utility of psychiatric diagnoses. *American Journal of Psychiatry*, **160**, 4–12.

Kendler, K.S. (1991). Mood-incongruent psychotic affective illness. *Archives of General Psychiatry*, **48**, 362–9.

and Gardner, C.O. (1998). Boundaries of major depression, an evaluation of DSM-IV criteria. *American Journal of Psychiatry*, **155**, 172–7.

McGuire, M., Gruenberg, A.M. and Walsh, D. (1995). Examining the validity of DSM-III-R schizoaffective disorder and its putative subtypes in the Roscommon family study. *American Journal of Psychiatry*, **152**, 755–64.

Eaves, L.J., Walters, E.E., *et al.* (1996). The identification and validation of distinct depressive syndromes in a population-based sample of female twins. *Archives of General Psychiatry*, **53**, 391–9.

Karkowski, L.M. and Walsh, D. (1998). The structure of psychosis, latent class analysis of probands from the Roscommon Family Study. *Archives of General Psychiatry*, **55**, 492–9.

Thornton, L.M., Gilman, S.E. and Kessler, R.C. (2000). Sexual orientation in a U.S. national sample of twin and non-twin sibling pairs. *American Journal of Psychiatry*, **157**, 1843–6.

Czajkowski, N., Tambs, K., *et al.* (2006). Dimensional representations of DSM-IV Cluster A personality disorders in a population-based sample of Norwegian twins, a multivariate study. *Psychological Medicine*, **36**, 1583–91.

Kennard, C., Crawford, T.J. and Henderson, I. (1994). A pathophysiological approach to saccadic eye movements in neurological and psychiatric disease. *Journal of Neurology, Neurosurgery & Psychiatry*, **57**, 881–5.

Kennedy, S.P., Baraff, L.J., Suddath, R.L. and Asarnow, J.R. (2004). Emergency department management of suicidal adolescents. *Annals of Emergency Medicine*, **43**, 452–60.

Kerns, J.G. and Berenbaum, H. (2002). Cognitive impairments associated with formal thought disorder in people with schizophrenia. *Journal of Abnormal Psychology*, **111**, 211–24.

Kessing, L.V. (2003). Subtypes of depressive episodes according to ICD-10. Prediction of risk and relapse and suicide. *Psychopathology*, **36**, 285–91.

(2005a). Diagnostic stability in depressive disorder as according to ICD-10 in clinical practice. *Psychopathology*, **38**, 32–7.

(2005b). Diagnostic stability in bipolar disorder in clinical practice as according to ICD-10. *Journal of Affective Disorders*, **85**, 293–9.

Kessler, R.C. (2003). Epidemiology of women and depression. *Journal of Affective Disorders*, **74**, 5–13.

Keuthen, N.J., O'Sullivan, R.L., Goodchild, P., *et al.* (1998). Retrospective review of treatment outcome for 63 patients with trichotillomania. *American Journal of Psychiatry*, **155**, 560–1.

Makris, N., Schlerf, J.E., *et al.* (2007). Evidence for reduced cerebellar volumes in trichotillomania. *Biological Psychiatry*, **61**, 374–81.

Khan, A., Detke, M., Khan, S.R.F. and Mallinckrodt, C. (2003). Placebo response and antidepressant clinical trial outcome. *Journal of Nervous and Mental Disorders*, **191**, 211–18.

Kolts, R.L., Rapaport, M.H., *et al.* (2005b). Magnitude of placebo response and drug-placebo differences across psychiatric disorders. *Psychological Medicine*, **35**, 743–9.

Khan, A.A., Jacobson, K.C., Gardner, C.O., *et al.* (2005a). Personality and comorbidity of common psychiatric disorders. *British Journal of Psychiatry*, **186**, 190–6.

Kho, K.H., van Vreeswijk, M.F., Simpson, S. and Zwinderman, A.H. (2003). A meta-analysis of electroconvulsive therapy efficacy in depression. *The Journal of ECT*, **19**, 139–47.

Kim, J.S. (2002). Post-stroke emotional incontinence after small lenticulocapsular stroke, correlation with lesion location. *Journal of Neurology*, **249**, 805–10.

Kim, T.S., Pae, C.U., Jeong, J.T., *et al.* (2006). Temperament and character dimensions in patients with atopic dermatitis. *Journal of Dermatology*, **33**, 10–15.

Kimhy, D., Goetz, R., Yale, S., *et al.* (2005). Delusions in individuals with schizophrenia, factor structure, clinical correlates, and putative neurobiology. *Psychopathology*, **38**, 338–44.

Kingdon, D.G., Kinoshita, Y., Naeem, F., *et al.* (2007). Schizophrenia can and should be renamed. *British Medical Journal*, **334**, 221–2.

Kirby, G.H. (1913). The catatonic syndrome and its relation to manic-depressive insanity. *Journal of Nervous and Mental Disorders*, **40**, 694–704.

Kirk, S.A. and Kutchins, H. (1992). *The Selling of DSM: The Rhetoric of Science in Psychiatry.* New York: De Gruyter.

Kirkcaldy, B.D. and Siefen, G. (1991). Personality correlates of intelligence in a clinical group. *Psychology Reports*, **69**, 947–52.

Kirshner, H.S. and Lavin, P.J. (2006). Posterior cortical atrophy, a brief review. *Current Neurology & Neuroscience Reports*, **6**, 477–80.

Kiyosawa, M., Ishii, K., Inoue, C., *et al.* (1996). Positron emission tomography in diagnosing brainstem vascular lesions that cause abnormal gaze movements. *American Journal of Ophthalmology*, **122**, 557–67.

Kleifield, E.I., Sunday, S., Hurt, S. and Halmi, K.A. (1993). Psychometric validation of the Temperamental Personality Questionnaire, application to subgroups of eating disorders. *Comprehensive Psychiatry*, **34**, 249–53.

Klein, D.A. and Greenfield, D.P. (1999). Chronic benign pain. *CNS Spectrums*, **4**, 24–31.

Klein, D.F. (1989). The pharmacological validation of psychiatric diagnosis. In L.N. Robins and J.E., Barrett, eds., *The Validity of Psychiatric Diagnosis.* New York: Raven Press, pp. 177–201. and Davis, J.M. (1969). *Diagnosis and Drug Treatment of Psychiatric Disorders.* Baltimore, MD: Williams & Wilkins.

Kleist, K. (1914). Aphasie und Geisteskrankheit (Aphasia and Mental Illness). *Munchever Medizinische Wochenschrift*, **61**, 8–12.

Klonsky, E.D. (2007). The functions of deliberate self-injury, a review of the evidence. *Clinical Psychology Reviews*, **27**, 226–39.

Knight, R.A. and Valner, J.B. (1993). Affective deficits. In C.G. Costello, ed., *Symptoms of Schizophrenia.* New York: John Wiley and Sons, pp. 145–200.

Kobayashi, Y., Miyamoto, M., Miyamoto, T., *et al.* (2002). Narcolepsy manifesting initially as cataplexy and sleep paralysis, Usefulness of CSF hypocretin-1 examination for early diagnosis. *Rinsho Shinkeigaku*, **42**, 233–6.

Koehler, P.J. (2003). Freud's comparative study of hysterical and organic paralyses, how Charcot's assignment turned out. *Archives of Neurology*, **60**, 1646–50.

Kojima, S., Nagai, N., Nakabeppu, Y., *et al.* (2005). Comparison of regional cerebral blood flow in patients with anorexia nervosa before and after weight gain. *Psychiatry Research*, **140**, 251–8.

Kolb, B. and Whishaw, I.Q. (1996). *Fundamentals of Human Neuropsychiatry*, 4th edn. New York: WH Freeman and Co.

Kolmel, H.W. (1993). Visual illusions and hallucinations. *Baillières Clinical Neurology*, **2**, 243–64.

Kon, Y. (1994). Amok. *British Journal of Psychiatry*, **165**, 685–9.

Koo, M.S., Dickey, C.C., Park, H.J., *et al.* (2006a). Smaller neocortical gray matter and larger sulcal cerebrospinal fluid volumes in neuroleptic-naive women with schizotypal personality disorder. *Archives of General Psychiatry*, **63**, 1090–100.

Levitt, J.J., McCarley, R.W., *et al.* (2006b). Reduction of caudate nucleus volumes in neuroleptic-naive female subjects with schizotypal personality disorder. *Biological Psychiatry*, **60**, 40–8.

Kopala, L.C., Good, K.P. and Honer, W.G. (1994). Olfactory hallucinations and olfactory identification ability in patients with schizophrenia and other psychiatric disorders. *Schizophrenia Research*, **12**, 205–11.

Kopelman, M.D. (1996). Transient disorders of memory and consciousness. In B.S. Fogel, R.B. Schiffer and S.M. Rao, eds., *Neuropsychiatry*. Baltimore: William & Wilkins, pp. 615–24.

Korach, K.S. (1994). Insights from the study of animals lacking functional estrogen receptor. *Science*, **266**, 1524–7.

Koran, L.M., Aboujaoude, E.N. and Gamel, N.N. (2007). Escitalopram treatment of kleptomania, an open-label trial followed by double-blind discontinuation. *Journal of Clinical Psychiatry*, **68**, 422–7.

Koroshetz, W.J., Myers, R.H. and Martin, J.B. (1992). The neurology of Huntington's disease. In A.B. Joseph and R.R. Young, eds., *Movement Disorders in Neurology and Neuropsychiatry*. Boston: Blackwell Scientific Publications, pp. 167–77.

Kotagal, P., Costa, M., Wyllie, E. and Wolgamuth, B. (2002). Paroxysmal nonepileptic events in children and adolescents. *Pediatrics*, **110**, e46.

Kozubski, W. (2005). Basilar-type migraine, Pathophysiology, symptoms and signs, and treatment. *Neurologià i Neurochirurgià Polska*, **39** (4 Suppl. 1), S65–7.

Kraepelin, E. (1896). *Psychiatrie*, 5th edn. Leipzig: Johann Ambrosius Barth.

(1913). *Psychiatrie*, vol. **3**, 8th edn. Leipzig: Johann Ambrosius Barth.

(1921/1976). *Manic-depressive Insanity and Paranoia*, translated by R.M. Barclay edited by G.M. Robertson. Edinburgh: E. and S. Livingstone, reprinted by Arno Press, New York.

(1968). *Lectures in Clinical Psychiatry*, 1904 edition facsimile, edited by T. Johnstone. New York: Hafner Publishing Company.

(1971). *Dementia Praecox and Paraphrenia*, translated by R.M. Barclay, edited by G.M. Robertson, facsimile 1919 edition. Huntington, NY: Robert E. Krieger Publishing Co. Inc.

(1987). *Emil Kraepelin Memoirs*, edited by H. Hippius, G. Peters, D. Ploog, P. Hoff, Kreuter, translated by C. Wooding-Deane. Berlin and Heidelberg: Springer-Verlag.

Kraus, C., Strohm, K., Hill, A., *et al.* (2006). Selective serotonin reuptake inhibitors (SSRI) in the treatment of paraphilia. *Fortschritte des Neurologie Psychiatrie*, **75**, 351–6.

Krem, M.M. (2004). Motor conversion disorders reviewed from a neuropsychiatric perspective. *Journal of Clinical Psychiatry*, **65**, 783–90.

Kretschmer, E. (1925). *Physique and Character*. New York: Harcourt Brace.

Kroenke, K. (2006). Physical symptom disorder, a simpler diagnostic category for somatization-spectrum conditions. *Journal of Psychosomatic Research*, **60**, 335–9.

Kropp, S., Schulz-Schaeffer, W.J., Finkenstaedt, M. *et al.* (1999). The Heidenhain variant of Creutzfeldt–Jakob disease. *Archives of Neurology*, **56**, 55–61.

Krueger, R.B. and Kaplan, M.S. (2001). The paraphilic and hypersexual disorders, an overview. *Journal of Psychiatric Practice*, **7**, 391–403.

Krüger, S. and Bräunig, P. (2000). Catatonia in affective disorder. New findings and a review of the literature. *CNS Spectrums*, **5**, 48–53.

Kuljic-Obradovic, D.C. (2003). Subcortical aphasia, three different language disorder syndromes? *European Journal of Neurology*, **10**, 445–8.

Kumral, E., Kocaer, T., Sagduyu, A., *et al.* (1995). Callosal infarction after bilateral occlusion of the internal carotid arteries with hemineglect syndrome and astasia–abasia. *Reviews in Neurology*, **151**, 202–05.

Kunkel, R.S. (2005). Migraine aura without headache: Benign, but a diagnosis of exclusion. *Cleveland Clinic Journal of Medicine*, **72**, 529–34.

Kupfer, D.J., First, M.B. and Regier, D.A., eds. (2002). *A Research Agenda for DSM-V.* Washington DC: American Psychiatric Press Inc.

Kurlan, R., Como, P.G., Miller, B., *et al.* (2002). The behavioral spectrum of tic disorders. A community-based study. *Neurology*, **59**, 414–20.

Lafforgue, P., Toussirot, E., Bille, F. and Acquaviva, P.C. (1993). Astasia–abasia revealing a primary Sjogren's syndrome. *Clinical Rheumatology*, **12**, 261–4.

Lake, C.R. and Hurwitz, N. (2007). Schizoaffective disorder merges schizophrenia and bipolar disorders as one disease – there is no schizoaffective disorder. *Current Opinions in Psyhiatry*, **20**, 365–79.

Lalonde, J.K., Hudson, J.I., Gigante, R.A. and Pope, H.G. Jr. (2001). Canadian and American psychiatrists' attitudes toward dissociative disorders diagnosis. *Canadian Journal of Psychiatry*, **46**, 407–12.

Lambert, M.V., Sierra, M., Phillips, M.L. and David, A.S. (2002). The spectrum of organic depersonalization. A review plus four new cases. *Journal of Neuropsychiatry and Clinical Neuroscience*, **14**, 141–54.

Lamberti, P., De Mari, M., Zenzola, A., *et al.* (2002). Frequency of apraxia of eyelid opening in the general population and in patients with extrapyramidal disorders. *Neurological Science*, **23** (Suppl. 2), S81–2.

Lanczik, M. and Keil, G. (1991). Carl Wernicke's localization theory and its significance for the development of scientific psychiatry. *History of Psychiatry*, **2**, 171–80.

Landre, J.K. and Taylor, M.A. (1995). Formal thought disorder in schizophrenia: Linguistic, attentional, and intellectual correlates. *Journal of Nervous and Mental Disorders*, **183**, 673–80.

Landre, N., Taylor, M.A. and Kerns, K. (1992). Language functioning in schizophrenic and aphasic patients. *Neuropsychiatry, Neuropsychology and Behavioral Neurology*, **5**, 7–14.

Lang, A. (2006). General overview of psychogenic movement disorders. Epidemiology, diagnosis and prognosis in psychogenic movement disorders. In M. Hallet, C.M. Cloninger, S. Fahn, *et al.*, eds., *Psychogenic Movement Disorders, Neurology and Neuropsychiatry.* Philadelphia: Lippincott Williams and Wilkins, pp. 35–41.

Lang, D.J., Khorram, B., Goghari, V.M., *et al.* (2006). Reduced anterior internal capsule and thalamic volumes in first-episode psychosis. *Schizophrenia Research*, **87**, 89–99.

Langdon, R. and Coltheart, M. (2000). The cognitive neuropsychology of delusions. *Mind and Language*, **15**, 184–218.

Langevin, R. (2006). Sexual offenses and traumatic brain injury. *Brain and Cognition*, **60**, 206–07.

Langfeldt, G. (1939). *The Schizophreniform State*. Copenhagen: Munksgaard.

Laroche, C., Buge, A., Escourolle, R., *et al.* (1976). "Astasia–abasia," unilateral left-sided apraxia, and touch disorders in an astrocytoma of the corpus callosum. A clinico-pathological report. *Annales de Medicine Interne*, **127**, 1–10.

Larson, J.K., Brand, N., Bermond, B. and Hijman, R. (2003). Cognitive and emotional characteristics of alexithymia, a review of neurobiological studies. *Journal of Psychosomatic Research*, **54**, 533–41.

LaSalle, V.H., Cromer, K.R., Nelson, K.N., *et al.* (2004). Diagnostic interview assessed neuropsychiatric disorder comorbidity in 334 individuals with obsessive-compulsive disorder. *Depression and Anxiety*, **19**, 163–73.

Lasegue, C. and Falret, J. (1877). La folie a deux (ou folie communiqué). *Annales Medico-Psychologique*, **18**, 321–55. (English translation and bibliography by R. Michaud (1964). *American Journal of Psychiatry*, **121** (Suppl. 4).)

Lasser, R.A., Nasrallah, H., Helldin, L., *et al.* (2007). Remission in schizophrenia, applying recent consensus criteria to refine the concept. *Schizophrenia Bulletin*, **30**, 223–31.

Latham, A.E. and Prigerson, H.G. (2004). Suicidality and bereavement, complicated grief as psychiatric disorder presenting greatest risk for suicidality. *Suicide and Life Threatening Behavior*, **34**, 350–62.

La Vega-Talbot, M., Duchowny, M. and Jayakar, P. (2006). Orbitofrontal seizures presenting with ictal visual hallucinations and interictal psychosis. *Pediatric Neurology*, **35**, 78–81.

Lazarus, R.S. (1991). Progress on a cognitive–motivational–relational theory of emotion. *American Psychologist*, **46**, 819–34.

Leopold, D. (2002). Distortion of olfactory perception, diagnosis and treatment. *Chemical Senses*, **27**, 611–15.

Lester, D. (2006). Sexual orientation and suicidal behavior. *Psychology Reports*, **99**, 923–4.

Le Vay, S. (1991). A difference in hypothalamic structure between heterosexual and homosexual men. *Science*, **253**, 1034–7.

Leckman, J.F., Rauch, S.L. and Mataix-Cols, D. (2007). Symptom dimensions in obsessive-compulsive disorder, implications for the DSM-V. *CNS Spectrums*, **12**, 376–87.

Lee, G.P., Meador, K.J., Loring, D.W., *et al.* (2004). Neural substrates of emotion as revealed by functional magnetic resonance imaging. *Cognitive and Behavioral Neurology*, **17**, 9–17.

Lejoyeux, M. and Ada, S.J. (1997). Anidepressant discontinuation, a review of the literature. *Journal of Clinical Psychiatry*, **58** (Suppl. 7), 11–15.

Lempert, T. and von Brevern, M. (2005). Episodic vertigo. *Current Opinions in Neurology*, **18**, 5–9.

Brandt, T., Dieterich, M. and Huppert, D. (1991). How to identify disorders of stance and gait. A video study of 37 patients. *Journal of Neurology*, **238**, 140–6.

Lemus, C.Z. and Lieberman, J.A. (1992). Antidepressant-induced myoclonus. In A.B. Joseph and R.R. Young, eds., *Movement Disorders in Neurology and Neuropsychiatry*. Boston: Blackwell Scientific Publications, pp. 146–54.

Lenane, M.C., Swedo, S.E., Rapoport, J.L., *et al.* (1992). Rates of obsessive compulsive disorder in first degree relatives of patients with trichotillomania, a research note. *Journal of Child Psychology and Psychiatry*, **33**, 925–33.

Leonhard, K. (1979). *The Classification of Endogenous Psychoses*, 5th edn, edited by E. Robins, translated by R. Berman. New York: Irvington Publishers, Inc.

Lepore, M., Conson, M., Ferringno, A., *et al.* (2004). Spatial transportations across tasks and response modalities, exploring representational allochiria. *Neurocase*, **10**, 386–92.

Leslie, K.R., Johnson-Frey, S.H. and Grafton, S.T. (2004). Functional imaging of face and hand imitation, towards a motor theory of empathy. *Neuroimage*, **21**, 601–07.

Lesson, V.C., Simpson, A., McKenna, P.J. and Laws, K.R. (2005). Executive inhibition and semantic association in schizophrenia. *Schizophrenia Research*, **74**, 61–7.

Levin, B. and Duchowny, M. (1991). Childhood obsessive-compulsive disorder and cingulate epilepsy. *Biological Psychiatry*, **30**, 1049–55.

Levin, H.S., High, W.M., Meyers, C.A., *et al.* (1985). Impairment of remote memory after closed head injury. *Journal of Neurology, Neurosurgery & Psychiatry*, **48**, 556–63.

Levine, J.B., Gruber, S.A., Baird, A.A. and Yurgelun-Todd, D. (1998). Obsessive-compulsive disorder among schizophrenic patients, an exploratory study using functional magnetic resonance imaging data. *Comprehensive Psychiatry*, **39**, 308–11.

Levy, R. and Czernecki, V. (2006). Apathy and the basal ganglia. *Journal of Neurology*, **253** (Suppl. 7), vii, 54–61.

and Dubois, B. (2006). Apathy and the functional anatomy of the prefrontal cortex–basal ganglia circuits. *Cerebral Cortex*, **16**, 916–28.

Lewis, A.J. (1934). Melancholia, a historical review. *Journal of Mental Sciences*, **80**, 1–42.

Lewis, G., Croft-Jeffreys, C. and David, A. (1990). Are British psychiatrists racist? *British Journal of Psychiatry*, **157**, 410–15.

Lewis, R. (2004). Should cognitive deficit be a diagnostic criterion for schizophrenia? *Journal of Psychiatry and Neuroscience*, **29**, 102–13.

Lezak, M.D., Howieson, D.B., Loring, D.W., *et al.* (2004). *Neuropsychological Assessment*, 4th edn. New York: Oxford University Press.

Libon, D.J., Bogdanoff, B., Leopold, N., *et al.* (2001). Neuropsychological profiles associated with subcortical white matter alterations and Parkinson's disease – implications for the diagnosis of dementia. *Archives of Clinical Neuropsychology*, **16**, 19–32.

Lieb, R., Zimmermann, P., Friis, R.H., *et al.* (2002). The natural course of DSM-IV somatoform disorders and syndromes among adolescents and young adults, a prospective-longitudinal community study. *European Psychiatry*, **17**, 321–31.

Likitcharoen, Y. and Phanthumchinda, K. (2004). Environmental reduplication in a patient with right middle cerebral artery occlusion. *Journal of the Medical Association of Thailand*, **87**, 1526–9.

Lilenfeld, L.R., Kaye, W.H., Greeno, C.G., *et al.* (1998). A controlled family study of anorexia nervosa and bulimia nervosa, psychiatric disorders in first-degree relatives and effects of proband comorbidity. *Archives of General Psychiatry*, **55**, 603–10.

Lilienfeld, S.O., Van Valkenburg, C., Larntz, K. and Akiskal, H.S. (1986). The relationship of histrionic personality disorder to antisocial personality and somatization disorders. *American Journal of Psychiatry*, **143**, 718–22.

Lilly, R., Cummings, J.L., Benson, D.F. and Frankel, M. (1983). The human Klüver–Bucy syndrome. *Neurology*, **33**, 1141–5.

Linde, J.A. and Clark, L.A. (1998). Diagnostic assignment of criteria. Clinicians and DSM-IV. *Journal of Personality Disorders*, **12**, 126–37.

Lindstrom, T.C. (2002). "It ain't necessarily so" ... Challenging mainstream thinking about bereavement. *Family and Community Health*, **25**, 11–21.

Lipowski, Z.J. (1987). Somatization, the experience and communication of psychological distress as somatic symptoms. *Psychotherapeutics and Psychosomatics*, **47**, 160–7.

Livesley, W.J., Jang, K.L. and Vernon, P.A. (1998). Phenotypic and genetic structure of traits delineating personality disorder. *Archives of General Psychiatry*, **55**, 941–8.

Lloyd-Richardson, E.E., Perrine, N., Dierker, L. and Kelley, M.L. (2007). Characteristics and functions of non-suicidal self-injury in a community sample of adolescents. *Psychology and Medicine*, **37**, 1183–92.

Lochner, C., Hemmings, S.M., Kinnear, C.J., *et al.* (2005a). Cluster analysis of obsessive-compulsive spectrum disorders in patients with obsessive-compulsive, clinical and genetic correlates. *Comprehensive Psychiatry*, **46**, 14–19.

Kinnear, C.J., Hemmings, S.M., *et al.* (2005b). Hoarding in obsessive-compulsive disorder, clinical and generic correlates. *Journal of Clinical Psychiatry*, **66**, 1155–60.

Loeb, C. and Meyer, J.S. (1996). Vascular dementia, still a debatable entity? *Journal of Neurological Sciences*, **143**, 31–40.

Lopez, F., Akil, H. and Watson, S.J. (1999). Neural circuits mediating stress. *Biological Psychiatry*, **46**, 1461–71.

Lopez, M.N., Charter, R.A., Mostafavi, B., *et al.* (2005). Psychometric properties of the Folstein Mini-Mental State Examination. *Assessment*, **12**, 137–44.

Lopez-Pousa, S., Garre-Olmo, J., Turon-Estrada, A., *et al.* (2002). The clinical incidence of frontal dementia. *Reviews in Neurology*, **34**, 216–22.

Lowengrub, K., Iancu, I., Aizer, A., *et al.* (2006). Pharmacotherapy of pathological gambling, review of new treatment modalities. *Expert Research in Neurotherapeutics*, **6**, 1845–51.

Ludlow, C.L. and Loucks, T. (2003). Stuttering, a dynamic motor control disorder. *Journal of Fluency Disorders*, **28**, 273–95.

Lundeberg, T. and Ekholm, J. (2002). Pain – from periphery to brain. *Disability and Rehabilitation*, **24**, 402–06.

Luria, A.R. (1963). *The Working Brain, An Introduction to Neuropsychology*. New York: Basic Books.

Lyons, M.J., Toomey, R., Faraone, S.V. and Tsuang, M.T. (1994). Comparison of schizotypal relatives of schizophrenic versus affective probands. *American Journal of Medical Genetics (Neuropsychiatric Genetics)*, **54**, 279–85.

Ma, N., Tan, L.W., Wang, Q., *et al.* (2007). Lower levels of whole blood serotonin in obsessive-compulsive disorder and in schizophrenia with obsessive-compulsive symptoms. *Psychiatry Research*, **150**, 61–9.

Ma, Q.P. and Woolf, C.J. (1996). Progressive tactile hypersensitivity, an inflammation-induced incremental increase in the excitability of the spinal cord. *Pain*, **67**, 97–106.

Macaskill, N., Geddes, J. and Macaskill, A. (1991). DSM-III in the training of British psychiatrists. A national survey. *International Journal of Social Psychiatry*, **37**, 182–6.

Mace, C.J. and Trimble, M.R. (1996). Ten-year prognosis of conversion disorder. *British Journal of Psychiatry*, **169**, 282–8.

MacLullich, A.M., Edmond, C.L., Ferguson, K.J., *et al.* (2004). Size of the neocerebellar vermis is associated with cognition in healthy elderly men. *Brain and Cognition*, **56**, 344–8.

Magill, C.A. (2004). The boundary between borderline personality disorder and bipolar disorder, current concepts and challenges. *Canadian Journal of Psychiatry*, **49**, 551–6.

Mailis-Gagnon, A., Giannoylis, I., Downar, J., *et al.* (2003). Altered central somatosensory processing in chronic pain patients with "hysterical" anesthesia. *Neurology*, **60**, 1501–07.

Maixner, D. and Taylor, M.A. (2008). The efficacy and safety of electroconvulsive therapy. In P. Tyrer and K.R. Silk, eds., *Cambridge Textbook of Effective Treatment in Psychiatry*. Cambridge: Cambridge University Press, pp. 57–82.

Maj, M., Pirozzi, R., Formicola, A.M., *et al.* (2000). Reliability and validity of the DSM-IV diagnostic category of schizoaffective disorder. Preliminary data. *Journal of Affective Disorders*, **57**, 95–8.

Pirozzi, R., Magliano, L. and Bartoli, L. (2003). Agitated depression in bipolar I disorder, prevalence, phenomenology, and outcome. *American Journal of Psychiatry*, **160**, 2134–40.

Malloy, P., Bihrle, A., Duffy, J. and Cimino, C. (1993). The orbitomedial frontal syndrome. *Archives of Clinical Neuropsychology*, **8**, 185–201.

Malloy, P.F. and Richardson, E.D. (1994). The frontal lobes and content-specific delusions. *Neuropsychiatry and Clinical Neurosciences*, **6**, 455–66.

Malone, G.L. and Leiman, H.I. (1983). Differential diagnosis of palinacousis in a psychiatric patient. *American Journal of Psychiatry*, **140**, 1067–8.

Manford, M. and Andermann, F. (1998). Complex visual hallucinations, clinical and neurobiological insights. *Brain*, **121**, 1819–40.

Fish, D.R. and Shorvon, S.D. (1996). An analysis of clinical seizure patterns and their localizing value in frontal and temporal lobe epilepsies. *Brain*, **119**, 17–40.

Mankoff, R., ed. (2004). *The Complete Cartoons of The New Yorker*. New York: Black Dog and Leventhal Publishers.

Marien, P., Saerens, J., Nanhoe, R., *et al.* (1996). Cerebellar induced aphasia, case report of cerebellar induced prefrontal aphasic language phenomena supported by SPECT findings. *Journal of Neurological Sciences*, **144**, 34–43.

Markowitsch, H.J. (1999). Functional neuroimaging correlates of functional amnesia. *Memory*, **7**, 561–83.

Marks, I.M. (1969). *Fears and Phobias*. London: Academic Press.

Marneros, A. and Goodwin, F. (2005). *Bipolar Disorders, Mixed States, Rapid Cycling and Atypical Forms*. Cambridge: Cambridge University Press.

Marshall, J.C., Halligan, P.W., Fink, G.R., *et al.* (1997). The functional anatomy of a hysterical paralysis. *Cognition*, **64**, B1–8.

Martin, M.L.S. (1999). Running amok, a modern perspective on a culture-bound syndrome. *Primary Care Journal: Clinical Psychiatry*, **1**, 66–70.

Maruff, P., Wood, S.J., Velakoulis, D., *et al.* (2005). Reduced volume of parietal and frontal association areas inpatients with schizophrenia characterized by passivity delusions. *Psychological Medicine*, **35**, 783–9.

Marvel, C.L. and Paradiso, S. (2004). Cognitive and neurological impairment in mood disorders. *Psychiatric Clinics of North America*, **27**, 19–26.

Schwartz, B.L. and Isaacs, K.L. (2004). Word production deficits in schizophrenia. *Brain and Language*, **89**, 182–91.

Masi, G., Perugi, G., Toni, C., *et al.* (2004). Obsessive-compulsive bipolar comorbidity, focus on children and adolescents. *Journal of Affective Disorders*, **78**, 175–83.

Mason, L. (2000). Body language – non-verbal cues. *British Journal of Perioperative Nursing*, **10**, 512–18.

Masson, C., Koskas, P., Cambier, J. and Masson, M. (1991). Left pseudothalamic cortical syndrome and pain asymbolia. *Reviews in Neurology*, **147**, 668–70.

Mathews, C.A. and Reus, V.I. (2003). Genetic linkage in bipolar disorder. *CNS Spectrums*, **8**, 891–904.

Matsunaga, H. and Sarai, M. (2000). Low-dose (0.5 mg) DST in manic and major depressive episodes, in relation to the severity of symptoms. *Seishin Shinkeigaku Zasshi*, **102**, 367–98.

Kiriike, N., Miyata, A. *et al.* (1999). Prevalence and symptomatology of comorbid obsessive-compulsive disorder among bulimic patients. *Psychiatry and Clinical Neuroscience*, **53**, 661–6.

Maudsley, H. (1867). *The Physiology and Pathology of the Mind*. New York: D. Appleton & Co.

Max, J.E., Robertson, B.A.M. and Lansing, A.E. (2001). The phenomenology of personality change due to traumatic brain injury in children and adolescents. *Journal of Neuropsychiatry and Clinical Neurosciences*, **13**, 161–70.

Mayberg, H.S., Liotti, M., Brannan, S.K., *et al.* (1999). Reciprocal limbic-cortical function and negative mood, converging PET findings in depression and normal sadness. *American Journal of Psychiatry*, **156**, 675–82.

Mayberry, R.I. and Jacques, J. (2000). Gesture production during stuttered speech. Insights into the nature of gesture-speech integration. In D. McNeill, ed., *Language and Gesture*. Cambridge: Cambridge University Press, pp. 199–214.

Mayer-Gross, W., Slater, E. and Roth, M. (1969). *Clinical Psychiatry*, 3rd edn. Baltimore: Williams and Wilkins.

McAbee, G., Sagan, A. and Winter, L. (2000). Olfactory hallucinations during migraine in an adolescent with MRI temporal lobe lesion. *Headache*, **40**, 592–4.

McAllister, T.W. (1992). Neuropsychiatric sequelae of head injuries. *Psychiatric Clinics of North America*, **114**, 395–413.

McCabe, M.S. (1975). Reactive psychosis. A clinical and genetic investigation. *Acta Psychiatrica Scandinavica*, **259** (Suppl.), 1–133.

McCann, J. and Peppe, S. (2003). Prosody in autism spectrum disorders, a critical review. *International Journal of Language and Communication Disorders*, **4**, 325–50.

McClellan, J. and McCurry, C. (1998). Neurodevelopmental pathways in schizophrenia. *Seminars in Clinical Neuropsychiatry*, **3**, 320–32.

McCrae, R.R., Yang, J., Costa, P.T., Jr., *et al.* (2001). Personality profiles and the prediction of categorical personality disorders. *Journal of Personality*, **69**, 155–74.

McCreadie, R.G., Srinivasan, T.N., Padmavati, R. and Thara, R. (2005). Extrapyramidal symptoms in unmedicated schizophrenia. *Journal of Psychiatric Research*, **39**, 261–6.

McDonald, W.M., Richard, I.H. and DeLong, M.R. (2003). Prevalence, etiology, and treatment of depression in Parkinson's disease. *Biological Psychiatry*, **54**, 363–75.

McElroy, S.L., Kotwal, R. and Keck, P.E. (2006). Comorbidity of eating disorders with bipolar disorder and treatment implications. *Bipolar Disorders*, **8**, 686–95.

McEwen, B.S. (2006). Protective and damaging effects of stress mediators, central role of the brain. *Dialogues in Clinical Neuroscience*, **8**, 367–81.

McGlashan, T.H., Grilo, C.M., Sanislow, C.A., *et al.* (2005). Two-year prevalence and stability of individual DSM-IV criteria for schizotypal, borderline, avoidant, and obsessive-compulsive personality disorders, toward a hybrid model of axis II disorders. *American Journal of Psychiatry*, **162**, 883–9.

McGuffin, P. and Katz, R. (1989). The genetics of depression and manic-depressive disorder. *British Journal of Psychiatry*, **155**, 294–304.

Rijsdijk, F., Andrew, M., *et al.* (2003). The heritability of bipolar affective disorder and the genetic relationship to unipolar depression. *Archives of General Psychiatry*, **60**, 497–502.

McGuire, P.K., Quested, D.J., Spence, S.A., *et al.* (1998). Pathophysiology of "positive" thought disorder in schizophrenia. *British Journal of Psychiatry*, **173**, 231–5.

McKee, A.C., Levine, D.N., Kowall, N.W. and Richardson, E.P., Jr. (1990). Peduncular hallucinosis associated with isolated infarction of the substantia nigra reticulate. *Annals of Neurology*, **27**, 500–04.

McKendrick, A.M., Vingrys, A.J., Badcock D.R. and Heywood, J.T. (2000). Visual field losses in subjects with migraine headaches. *Investigative Ophthalmology and Visual Science*, **41**, 1239–47.

Vingrys, A.J., Badcock, D.R. and Heywood, J.T. (2001). Visual dysfunction between migraine events. *Investigative Ophthalmology and Visual Science*, **42**, 626–633.

McKhann, G.M., Albert, M.S., Grossman, M., *et al.* (2001). Clinical and pathological diagnosis of frontotemporal dementia, report of the Work Group on Frontotemporal Dementia and Picks Disease. *Archives of Neurology*, **58**, 1803–09.

Meeren, H.K., van Heijnsbergen, C.C. and de Gelder, B. (2005). Rapid perceptual integration of facial expression and emotional body language. *Proceedings of the National Academy of Science USA*, **102**, 16,518–23.

Meloy, J.R. (1984). Thought organization and primary process in the parents of schizophrenics. *British Journal of Medical Psychology*, **57**, 279–81.

Mendez, M.F., Doss, R.C. and Taylor, J.L. (1993a). Interictal violence in epilepsy. Relationship to behavior and seizure variables. *Journal of Nervous and Mental Disoders*, **181**, 566–9.

Doss, R.C., Taylor, J.L. and Arguello, R. (1993b). Relationship of seizure variables to personality disorders in epilepsy. *Journal of Neuropsychiatry and Clinical Neurosciences*, **5**, 283–6.

Chen, A.K., Shapira, J.S. and Miller, B.L. (2005). Acquired sociopathy and frontotemporal dementia. *Dementia and Geriatric Cognitive Disorders*, **20**, 99–104.

Mergl, R., Seidscheck, I., Allgaier, A.K., *et al.* (2007). Depressive, anxiety, and somatoform disorders in primary care, prevalence and recognition. *Depression and Anxiety,* **24**, 185–95.

Merskey, H. and Buhrich, N. (1975). Hysteria and organic brain disorders. *British Journal of Medical Psychology,* **48**, 359–66.

Mertz, L.B. and Ostergaard, J.R. (2006). Neurological aspects of stuttering. *Ugeskrift for Laeger,* **168**, 3109–13.

Meston, C.M. and Frohlich, P.F. (2000). The neurobiology of sexual function. *Archives of General Psychiatry,* **57**, 1012–30.

Mesulam, M-M. (1981). Dissociative states with abnormal temporal lobe EEG. Multiple personality and the illusion of possession. *Archives of Neurology,* **38**, 176–81.

(2000). *Principles of Behavioral and Cognitive Neurology,* 2nd edn. New York: Oxford University Press.

Meyer, J.S., Shirai, T. and Akiyama, H. (1996). Neuroimaging for differentiating vascular from Alzheimer's dementias. *Cerebrovascular and Brain Metabolism Reviews,* **8**, 1–10.

Meynert, T. (1968). *Psychiatry, A Clinical Treatise on Diseases of the Fore-Brain Based Upon A Study of its Structure, Functions, and Nutrition, Part I. The Anatomy, Physiology, and Chemistry of the Brain,* translated by B. Sachs. New York: GP Putnam's and Sons, The Knickerbocker Press, 1885. Republished by Hafner Publishing Company, New York.

Mezzich, J.E. (2002). International surveys on the use of ICD-10 and related diagnostic systems. *Psychopathology,* **35**, 72–5.

Miceli, G., Capasso, R., Ivella, A. and Caramazza, A. (1997). Acquired dysgraphia in alphabetic and stenographic handwriting. *Cortex,* **33**, 355–67.

Middleton, W.Q., Raphael, B., Burnett, P. and Martinek, N. (1998). A longitudinal study comparing bereavement phenomena in recently bereaved spouses, adult children and parents. *Australia and New Zealand Journal of Psychiatry,* **32**, 235–41.

Mihalik, J.P., Stump, J.E., Collins, M.W., *et al.* (2005). Posttraumatic migraine characteristics in athletes following sports-related concussion. *Journal of Neurosurgery,* **102**, 850–5.

Miller, K. and Franz, E.A. (2005). Bimanual gestures. Expressions of spatial representations that accompany speech processes. *Laterality,* **10**, 243–65.

Miller, L.J. (1994). Use of electroconvulsive therapy during pregnancy. *Hospital and Community Psychiatry,* **45**, 444–50.

(2002). Postpartum depression. *Journal of the American Medical Association,* **287**, 762–5.

Miller, N.S. (1991). *Comprehensive Handbook of Drug and Alcohol Addiction.* New York: Marcell Dekker.

Mitchell, P.B. and Malhi, G.S. (2004). Bipolar depression, phenomenological overview and clinical characteristics. *Bipolar Disorders,* **6**, 530–9.

Mitchell, R.L.C. and Crow, T.J. (2005). Right hemisphere language functions and schizophrenia, the forgotten hemisphere? *Brain,* **128**, 963–78.

Miyashita, Y. (2004). Cognitive memory, cellular and network machineries and their top-down control. *Science,* **306**, 435–40.

Modan-Moses, D., Yaroslavsky, A., Novikov, I., *et al.* (2003). Stunting of growth as a major feature of anorexia nervosa in male adolescents. *Pediatrics,* **111**, 270–6.

Moene, F.C., Landberg, E.H., Hoogduin, K.A., *et al.* (2000). Organic syndromes diagnosed as conversion disorder. Identification and frequency in a study of 85 patients. *Journal of Psychosomatic Research*, **49**, 7–12.

Moller, H.J., Bottlender, R., Wegner, U., *et al.* (2000). Long-term course of schizophrenic, affective and schizoaffective psychosis, focus on negative symptoms and their impact on global indicators of outcome. *Acta Psychiatrica Scandinavica*, **407** (Suppl.), 54–7.

Molnar, B.E., Buka, S.L. and Kessler, R.C. (2001). Child sexual abuse and subsequent psychopathology, results from the National Comorbidity Survey. *American Journal of Public Health*, **91**, 753–60.

Monday, K. and Jankovic, J. (1993). Psychogenic myoclonus. *Neurology*, **43**, 349–52.

Montagna, P. (2004). Sleep-related non-epileptic motor disorders. *Journal of Neurology*, **251**, 781–94.

Montanes, F. and de Lucas Taracena, M.T. (2006). Evolutionary aspects of affective disorders, critical review and proposal of a new model. *Actas españoles de Psiquiatria*, **34**, 264–76.

Montgomery, S.A. and Asberg, M. (1979). A new depression scale designed to be sensitive to change. *British Journal of Psychiatry*, **134**, 382–9.

Moore, D.J., Atkinson, J.H., Akiskal, H., *et al.* (2005). Temperament and risky behaviors, a pathway to HIV? *Journal of Affective Disorders*, **85**, 191–200.

Mora, G. (1992). The history of psychiatry in the United States, historiographic and theoretical considerations. *History of Psychiatry*, **3**, 187–201.

Morana, H.C., Stone, M.H. and Abdalla-Filho, E. (2006). [Personality disorders, psychopathology and serial killers]. *Revista Brasilenia de Psiquiatria*, **28** (Suppl. 2), S74–9.

Morrison, D.P. (1990). Abnormal perceptual experiences in migraine. *Cephalagia*, **10**, 273–7.

Morrison, J.R. (1973). Catatonia. Retarded and excited types. *Archives of General Psychiatry*, **28**, 39–41.

Morsella, E. and Krauss, R.M. (2004). The role of gestures in spatial working memory and speech. *American Journal of Psychology*, **117**, 411–24.

Mortimer, A.M. (2007). Symptom rating scales and outcome in schizophrenia. *British Journal of Psychiatry*, **50** (Suppl.), s7–14.

Moss, G.C. (1967). Mental disorder in antiquity. In D. Brothwell and A.T. Sandison, eds., *Diseases in Antiquity*. Springfield: Charles C. Thomas, pp. 709–22.

Mullen, P.E. (2007). A modest proposal for another phenomenological approach to psychopathology. *Schizophrenia Bulletin*, **33**, 113–21.

Mulsant, B.H., Haskett, R.F., Prudic, J., *et al.* (1997). Low use of neuroleptic drugs in the treatment of psychotic major depression. *American Journal of Psychiatry*, **154**, 559–61.

Mungas, D. (1982). Interictal behavior abnormality in temporal lobe epilepsy. A specific syndrome or nonspecific psychopathology? *Archives of General Psychiatry*, **39**, 108–11.

Murphy, T.K., Husted, D.S. and Edge, P.J. (2006). Preclinical/clinical evidence of central nervous system infectious etiology in PANDAS. *Advances in Neurology*, **99**, 148–58.

Murphy-Eberenz, K., Zandi, P.P., March, D., *et al.* (2006). Is perinatal depression familial? *Journal of Affective Disorders*, **90**, 49–55.

Murray, V., McKee, I., Miller, P.M., *et al.* (2005). Dimensions and classes of psychosis in a population cohort, a four-class dimension model of schizophrenia and affective psychoses. *Psychological Medicine*, **35**, 499–510.

Nachev, P. and Husain, M. (2006). Disorders of visual attention and the posterior parietal cortex. *Cortex*, **42**, 766–73.

Narita, M., Yoshida, T., Nakajima, M., *et al.* (2006). Direct evidence for spinal cord microglia in the development of a neuropathic pain-like state in mice. *Journal of Neurochemistry*, **97**, 1337–48.

Nathaniel-James, D.A. and Frith, C.D. (1996). Confabulation in schizophrenia, evidence of a new form? *Psychological Medicine*, **26**, 391–9.

Navarro, V., Gasto, C., Torres, X., Marcos, T. and Pintor, L. (2001). Citalopram versus nortriptyline in late-life depression, a 12-week randomized single-blind study. *Acta Psychiatrica Scandinavica*, **103**, 435–40.

Naz, B., Bromet, E.J. and Mojtabai, R. (2003). Distinguishing between first admission schizophreniform disorder and schizophrenia. *Schizophrenia Research*, **62**, 51–8.

Nelson, J.C. and Charney, D.S. (1981). The symptoms of major depressive illness. *American Journal of Psychiatry*, **138**, 1–13.

and Davis, J.M. (1997). DST studies in psychotic depression, a meta-analysis. *American Journal of Psychiatry*, **154**, 1497–503.

Nestadt, G., Samuels, J., Riddle, M.A., *et al.* (2000). A family study of obsessive-compulsive disorder. *Archives of General Psychiatry*, **57**, 358–63.

Samuels, J., Riddle, M.A., *et al.* (2001). The relationship between obsessive-compulsive disorder and anxiety and affective disorders, results from the John Hopkins OCD Family Study. *Psychological Medicine*, **31**, 481–7.

Neuhauser, H., Leopold, M., von Brevern, M., *et al.* (2001). The interrelations of migraine, vertigo, and migrainous vertigo. *Neurology*, **56**, 436–41.

Neugebauer, R. (1979). Medieval and early modern theories of mental illness. *Archives of General Psychiatry*, **36**, 477–83.

Neumann, H. (1859). *Lehrbuch der Psychiatrie*. Erlangen, Germany: Ferdinand Enke.

Nierenberg, A.A., Ostacher, M.J., Calabrese, J.R., *et al.* (2006). Treatment-resistant bipolar depression, a STEP-BD equipoise randomized effectiveness trial of antidepressant augmentation with lamotrigine, inositol, or rispiridone. *American Journal of Psychiatry*, **163**, 210–16.

Nishitani, N., Schurmann, M., Amunts, K. and Hari, R. (2005). Broca's region, from action to language. *Physiology*, **20**, 60–9.

Nixon, R.D., Nishith, P. and Resick, P.A. (2004). The accumulative effect of trauma exposure on short-term and delayed verbal memory in a treatment-seeking sample of female rape victims. *Journal of Trauma and Stress*, **17**, 31–5.

Nobler, M.S. and Roose, S.P. (1998). Differential response to antidepressants in melancholic and severe depression. *Psychiatric Annals*, **28**, 84–8.

Nopoulos, P.C., Ceeilley, J.W., Gailis, E.A. and Andreasen, N.C. (1999). An MRI study of cerebellar vermis morphology in patients with schizophrenia. Evidence in support of the cognitive dysmetria concept. *Biological Psychiatry*, **46**, 703–11.

Nordeen, E.J. and Yahr, P. (1982). Hemispheric asymmetries in the behavioral and hormonal effects of sexually differentiating mammalian brain. *Science*, **218**, 391–3.

Norman, R.M., Scholten, D.J., Malla, A.K. and Ballageer, T. (2005). Early signs in schizophrenia spectrum disorders. *Journal of Nervous and Mental Disorders*, **193**, 17–23.

North, C.S., Nixon, S.J., Shariat, S., *et al.* (1999). Psychiatric disorders among survivors of the Oklahoma City bombing. *Journal of the American Medical Association*, **282**, 755–62.

Norton, J.W. and Corbett, J.J. (2000). Visual perceptual abnormalities, hallucinations and illusions. *Seminars in Neurology*, **20**, 111–21.

Nurnberg, H.G., Raskin, M., Levine, P.E., *et al.* (1991). The comorbidity of borderline personality disorder and other DSM-III-R axis II personality disorders. *American Journal of Psychiatry*, **148**, 1371–7.

Nys, G.M., van Zandvoort, M.J., van der Worp, H.B., *et al.* (2005). Early depressive symptoms after stroke, neuropsychological correlates and lesion characteristics. *Journal of Neurological Science*, **228**, 27–33.

O'Brien, K.M. and Vincent, N.K. (2003). Psychiatric comorbidity in anorexia and bulimia nervosa, nature, prevalence, and casual relationships. *Clinical Psychology Reviews*, **23**, 57–74.

Ochsner, K.N., Kosslyn, S., Cosgrove, G.R., *et al.* (2001). Deficits in visual cognition and attention following bilateral anterior cingulotomy. *Neuropsychologia*, **39**, 219–39.

O'Driscoll, G.A., Lenzenwenger, M.F. and Holzman, P.S. (1998). Antisaccades and smooth eye tracking and schizotype. *Archives of General Psychiatry*, **55**, 837–43.

O'Gorman, R.L., Kumari, V., Williams, S.C., *et al.* (2006). Personality factors correlate with regional cerebral perfusion. *Neuroimage*, **31**, 489–95.

Oh, T.M., McCarthy, R.A. and McKenna, P.J. (2002). Is there a schizophasia? A study applying the single case approach to formal thought disorder in schizophrenia. *Neurocase*, **8**, 233–44.

Ohayon, M.M. (2000). Prevalence of hallucinations and their pathological associations in the general population. *Psychiatry Research*, **97**, 153–64.

Olsson, G.I., von Knorring, A.L. (1999). Adolescent depression, prevalence in Swedish high-school students. *Acta Psychiatrica Scandinavica*, **99**, 324–31.

Ono, T., Nishijo, H. and Nishijo, H. (2000). Functional role of the limbic system and basal ganglia in motivated behaviors. *Journal of Neurology*, **247** (Suppl. 5), V23–32.

Onuma, T. (2000). Classification of psychiatric symptoms in patients with epilepsy. *Epilepsia*, **41** (Suppl. 9), 43–8.

Osman, O.T. and Loschen, E.L. (1992). Self-injurious behavior in the developmentally disabled, pharmacologic treatment. *Psychopharmacology Bulletin*, **28**, 439–49.

O'Sullivan, R.L., Rauch, S.L., Breiter, H.C., *et al.* (1997). Reduced basal ganglia volumes in trichotillomania measured via morphometric magnetic resonance imaging. *Biological Psychiatry*, **42**, 39–45.

Osuji, I.J. and Cullum, C.M. (2005). Cognition in bipolar disorder. *Psychiatric Clinics of North America*, **28**, 427–41.

Ovanesov, K.B. (1998). The effect of caffeine on the color-discriminating function of the retina in volunteers. *Eksperimentalnaia Klinicheskaia Farmakologiia*, **61**, 17–19.

Overall, J.E. and Hollister, L.E. (1979). Comparative evaluation of research diagnostic criteria for schizophrenia. *Archives of General Psychiatry*, **36**, 1198–205.

Ovsiew, F. (1997). Bedside neuropsychiatry. Eliciting the clinical phenomena of neuropsychiatric illness. In S.C. Yudofsky and R.E Hales, eds., *The American Psychiatric Press Textbook of Neuropsychiatry, 3rd edn*. Washington, DC: American Psychiatric Press, Inc., p. 127.

Owen, M.J., Craddock, N. and Jablensky, A. (2007). The genetic deconstruction of psychosis. *Schizophrenia Bulletin*, **33**, 905–11.

Pal, S. (1997). Mental disorders in abnormal offenders in Papua New Guinea. *Medicine and the Law*, **16**, 87–95.

Pally, R. (2002). The neurobiology of borderline personality disorder. The synergy of "nature and nurture." *Journal of Psychiatric Practice*, **8**, 133–42.

Panzarino, P.J., Jr. (2000). Psychiatric training and practice under managed care. *Administration and Policy in Mental Health*, **28**, 51–9.

Papageorgiou, C.C., Alevizos, B., Ventouras, E., *et al.* (2004). Psychophysiological correlates of patients with delusional misidentification syndromes and psychotic major depression. *Journal of Affective Disorders*, **81**, 147–52.

Paris, J. (2004). Gender differences in personality traits and disorders. *Current Psychiatry Reports*, **6**, 71–4.

(2005). Borderline personality disorder. *Canadian Medical Association Journal*, **72**, 1579–83.

Parker, G. and Hadzi-Pavlovic, D. (1996). *Melancholia, A Disorder of Movement and Mood*. Cambridge: Cambridge University Press.

Hadzi-Pavlovic, D., Hickie, I., *et al.* (1991). Distinguishing psychotic and non-psychotic melancholia. *Journal of Affective Disorders*, **22**, 135–48.

Hadzi-Pavlovic, D., Brodaty, H., *et al.* (1993). Psychomotor disturbance in depression. Defining the constructs. *Journal of Affective Disorders*, **27**, 255–65.

Parks, S.M. and Feldman, S.M. (2006). Self-injurious behavior in the elderly. *The Consultant Pharmacist*, **21**, 905–10.

Parnell, R.W. (1958). *Behavior and Physique*. London: Arnold.

Parr, L.A., Waller, B.M. and Fugate, J. (2005). Emotional communication in primates, implications for neurobiology. *Current Opinions in Neurobiology*, **15**, 716–20.

Parvizi, J. and Damascio, A.R. (2001). Consciousness and the brain stem. *Cognition*, **79**, 135–59.

Arciniegas, D.B., Bernardini, G.L., *et al.* (2006). Diagnosis and management of pathological laughter and crying. *Mayo Clinic Proceedings*, **81**, 1482–96.

Patel, A.S., Arnone, D. and Ryan, W. (2004). Folie a deux in bipolar affective disorder. A case report. *Bipolar Disorders*, **6**, 162–5.

Pavlov, I.P. (1941). *Conditioned Reflexes and Psychiatry*, translated by W.H. Gantt. New York: International Universities Press.

Pearn, J. and Gardner-Thorpe, C. (2002). Jules Cotard (1840–1889). His life and the unique syndrome which bears his name. *Neurology*, **58**, 1400–03.

Pehlivanturk, B. and Unal, F. (2002). Conversion disorder in children and adolescents. A 4-year follow-up study. *Journal of Psychosomatic Research*, **52**, 187–91.

Peleg, T. and Shalev, A.Y. (2006). Longitudinal studies of PTSD, overview of findings and methods. *CNS Spectrums*, **11**, 573–4.

Pelegrin Valero, C., Gomez Hernandez, R., Munoz Cespedes, J.M., *et al.* (2001). Nosologic aspects of personality change due to head trauma. *Reviews in Neurology*, **32**, 681–7.

Penfield, W. and Faulk, M.E. (1955). The insula, further observations of its function. *Brain*, **78**, 445–70.

and Perot, P. (1963). The brain's record of auditory and visual experience. *Brain*, **86**, 595–696.

Peralta, V. and Cuesta, M.J. (1999). Diagnostic significance of Schneider's first-rank symptoms in schizophrenia. Comparative study between schizophrenic and non-schizophrenic psychotic disorders. *British Journal of Psychiatry*, **174**, 243–8.

and Cuesta, J. (2003a). The nosology of psychotic disorders, a comparison among competing classification systems. *Schizophrenia Bulletin*, **29**, 413–25.

and Cuesta, M.J. (2003b). Cycloid psychosis, a clinical and nosological study. *Psychological Medicine*, **33**, 443–53.

Cuesta, M.J. and de Leon, J. (1992). Formal thought disorder in schizophrenia, a factor analytic study. *Comprehensive Psychiatry*, **33**, 105–10.

Perico, C.A., Skaf, C.R., Yamada, A., *et al.* (2005). Relationship between regional cerebral blood flow and separate symptom clusters of major depression, a single photon emission computed tomography study using statistical parametric mapping. *Neuroscience Letters*, **384**, 265–70.

Perkins, A., Fitzgerald, J.A. and Moss, G.E. (1995). A comparison of LH secretion and brain estradiol receptors in heterosexual and homosexual rams and female sheep. *Hormones and Behavior*, **29**, 31–41.

Perkins, R.J. (1999). SSRI antidepressants are effective for treating delusional hypochondriasis. *Medical Journal of Australia*, **170**, 140–1.

Perris, C. (1986). The case for the independence of cycloid psychotic disorder from schizoaffective disorder. In A. Marneros and M. Tsuang, eds., *Schizoaffective Psychoses*. Berlin: Springer, pp. 272–308.

Perry, P.J. (1996). Pharmacotherapy for major depression with melancholic features, relative efficacy of tricyclic versus selective serotonin reuptake inhibitor antidepressants. *Journal of Affective Disorders*, **20**, 391–6.

Persaud, R. and Cutting, J. (1991). Lateralized anomalous perceptual experiences in schizophrenia. *Psychopathology*, **24**, 365–8.

Perugi, G. and Akiskal, H.S. (2005). Emerging concepts of mixed states, a longitudinal perspective. In A. Marneros and F.K. Goodwin, eds., *Bipolar Disorders, Mixed States, Rapid-Cycling, and Atypical Forms*. Cambridge: Cambridge University Press, pp. 45–60.

Akiskal, H.S., Pfanner, C., *et al.* (1997). The clinical impact of bipolar and unipolar affective disorder comorbidity on obsessive-compulsive disorder. *Journal of Affective Disorders*, **46**, 15–23.

Akiskal, H.S., Toni, C., *et al.* (2001). The temporal relationship between anxiety disorders and (hypo)mania, a retrospective examination of 63 panic, social phobic and obsessive-compulsive patients with comorbid bipolar disorder. *Journal Affective Disorders*, **67**, 199–206.

Toni, C., Frare, F., *et al.* (2002). Obsessive-compulsive–bipolar comorbidity, a systematic exploration of clinical features and treatment outcome. *Journal of Clinical Psychiatry*, **63**, 1129–34.

Petrides, G., Fink, M., Husain, M.M., *et al.* (2001). ECT remission rates in psychotic versus nonpsychotic depressed patients, a report from CORE. *Journal of ECT*, **17**, 244–53.

Pfuhlmann, B., Stober, G., Franzek, E., *et al.* (1998). Cycloid psychoses predominate in severe postpartum psychiatric disorders. *Journal of Affective Disorders*, **50**, 125–34.

Stober, G. and Beckmann, H. (2002). Postpartum psychoses, prognosis, risk factors, and treatment. *Current Psychiatry Reports*, **4**, 185–90.

Phelps, E.A., O'Connor, K.J., Gatenby, C., *et al.* (2001). Activation of the left amygdala to a cognitive representation of fear. *Nature Neuroscience*, **4**, 437–41.

Phillips, B. (2004). Movement disorders. A sleep specialist's perspective. *Neurology*, **62**, S9–16.

Phillips, K.A. and Kaye, W.H. (2007). The relationship of body dysmorphic disorder and eating disorders to obsessive-compulsive disorder. *CNS Spectrums*, **12**, 347–58.

Menard, W., Fay, C. and Weisberg, R. (2005). Demographic characteristics, phenomenology, comorbidity, and family history in 200 hundred individuals with body dysmorphic disorder. *Psychosomatics*, **46**, 317–25.

Menard, W., Pagano, M.E., *et al.* (2006). Delusional versus nondelusional body dysmorphic disorder. Clinical features and course of illness. *Journal of Psychiatric Research*, **40**, 95–104.

Phillips, M.L., Drevets, W.C., Rauch, S.L. and Lane, R. (2003). Neurobiology of emotion perception II. Implications for major psychiatric disorders. *Biological Psychiatry*, **54**, 515–28.

Pichot, P. (1983). *A Century of Psychiatry*. Basle: F. Hoffmann-La Roche and Co.

Pillard, R.C. and Weinrich, J.D. (1986). Evidence of familial nature of male homosexuality. *Archives of General Psychiatry*, **43**, 808–12.

Pinel, P. (1791). Observations sur une espece particuliere de melancholie qui conduit au suicide. *La Medecine Eclairee par Les Sciences Physiques*. Paris, vol. **1**, p. 154.

(1962). *A Treatise on Insanity*, translated by D.D. Davis. London: Cadell and Davies, 1806, reprinted under the auspices of The Library of the New York Academy of Medicine, New York, Hafner Publishing Company.

Pini, S., de Queiroz, V., Dell'Osso, L., *et al.* (2004). Cross-sectional similarities and differences between schizophrenia, schizoaffective disorder and mania or mixed mania with mood-incongruent psychotic features. *European Psychiatry*, **19**, 8–14.

Pinto, A., Mancebo, M.C., Eisen, J.L., *et al.* (2006). The Brown Longitudinal Obsessive Compulsive Study, clinical features and symptoms at intake. *Journal of Clinical Psychiatry*, **67**, 703–11.

Piper, A. Jr. (1994). Multiple personality disorder. *British Journal of Psychiatry*, **164**, 600–12.

and Merskey, H. (2004). The persistence of folly: Critical examination of dissociative identity disorder. Part II. The defense and decline of multiple personality or dissociative identity disorder. *Canadian Journal of Psychiatry*, **49**, 678–83.

Pitts, F.N., Jr. and McClure, J.N., Jr. (1967). Lactate metabolism in anxiety neurosis. *New England Journal of Medicine*, **277**, 1329–36.

Platz, C. and Kendell, R.E. (1988). A matched-control follow-up and family study of puerperal psychoses. *British Journal of Psychiatry*, **153**, 90–4.

Ploman, R. and Bergeman, C.S. (1991). The nature of nurture: Genetic influence on "environmental" measures. *Behavioral and Brain Sciences*, **14**, 373–427.

Podell, K. and Robinson, D. (2000). Illusory splitting as visual aura symptom in migraine. *Cephalagia*, **20**, 228–32.

and Robinson, D. (2001). Recurrent Lilliputian hallucinations as visual aura symptom in migraine. *Cephalagia*, **21**, 990–2.

Lovell, M. and Goldberg, E. (2001). Lateralization of frontal lobe functions. In S. P. Salloway, P. F. Malloy and J. D. Duffy, *The Frontal Lobes and Neuropsychiatric Illness*. Washington, DC: American Psychiatric Publishing, pp. 83–99.

Ebel, H., Robinson, D. and Nicola, U. (2002). Obligatory and facultative symptoms of the Alice in Wonderland syndrome. *Minerva Medica*, **4**, 287–93.

Polatin, P. B., Kinney, R. K., Gatchel, R. J., *et al.* (1993). Psychiatric illness and chronic low-back pain. The mind and the spine – which goes first? *Spine*, **18**, 66–71.

Pollmann, W., Feneberg, W. and Erasmus, L. P. (2004). Pain in multiple sclerosis – a still underestimated problem. The 1 year prevalence of pain syndromes, significance and quality of care of multiple sclerosis inpatients. *Des Nervenarzt*, **75**, 135–40.

Pope, H. G., Poliakoff, M. B., Parker, M. P., *et al.* (2007). Is dissociative amnesia a culture-bound syndrome? Findings from a survey of historical literature. *Psychological Medicine*, **37**, 225–33.

Popescu, I. and Vaidya, N. (2007). An isolated inability to write cursively following transient ischemic attack (TIA). *Cognitive and Behavioral Neurology*, **20**, 131–5.

Potash, J. B., Zandi, P. P., Willour, V. L., *et al.* (2003). Suggestive linkage to chromosomal regions 13q31 and 22q12 in families with psychotic bipolar disorder. *American Journal of Psychiatry*, **160**, 680–6.

Pranzatelli, M. R. (2003). Myoclonus in childhood. *Seminars in Pediatric Neurology*, **10**, 41–51.

Prasad, K. M., Patel, A. R., Muddasani, S., *et al.* (2004a). The entorhinal cortex in first-episode psychotic disorders, a structural magnetic resonance imaging study. *American Journal of Psychiatry*, **161**, 1612–19.

Rohm, B. R. and Keshavan, M. S. (2004b). Parahippocampal gyrus in first episode psychotic disorders, a structural magnetic resonance imaging study. *Progress in Neuropsychopharmacology and Biological Psychiatry*, **28**, 651–8.

Prevey, M. L., Delaney, R. C. and Mattson, R. H. (1988). Metamemory in temporal lobe epilepsy, self-monitoring of memory functions. *Brain and Cognition*, **7**, 298–311.

Prichard, J. C. (1833). *A Treatise on Insanity*. London: Marchant.

Primeau, F. and Fontaine, R. (1987). Obsessive disorders with self-mutilation, A subgroup responsive to pharmacotherapy. *Canadian Journal of Psychiatry*, **32**, 699–701.

Primavera, A., Fonti, A., Novello, P., *et al.* (1994). Epileptic seizures in patients with acute catatonic syndrome. *Journal of Neurology, Neurosurgery & Psychiatry*, **57**, 1419–22.

Protheroe, C. (1969). Puerperal psychoses. A long term study 1927–1961. *British Journal of Psychiatry*, **115**, 9–30.

Proverbio, A. M., Zani, A. and Avella, C. (1997). Hemispheric asymmetries for spatial frequency discrimination in a selective attention task. *Brain and Cognition*, **34**, 311–20.

Provine, R. R. (2000). *Laughter, A Scientific Investigation*. New York: Viking.

Purcell, R., Maruff, P., Kyrios, M. and Pantelis, C. (1998). Cognitive deficits in obsessive-compulsive disorder on tests of frontal–striatal function. *Biological Psychiatry*, **43**, 348–57.

Quinette, P., Guillery-Girard, B., Dayan, J., *et al.* (2006). What does transient global amnesia mean? Review of the literature and thorough study of 142 cases. *Brain*, **129**, 1640–58.

Quraishi, S. and Frangou, S. (2002). Neuropsychology of bipolar disorder, a review. *Journal of Affective Disorders*, **72**, 209–26.

Rabe-Jablonska Jolanta, J. and Sobow Tomasz, M. (2000). The links between body dysmorphic disorder and eating disorders. *European Psychiatry*, **15**, 302–05.

Rabkin, J.G., Ferrando, S.J., Jacobsberg, L.B. and Fishman, B. (1997). Prevalence of axis I disorders in an AIDS cohort, a cross-sectional, controlled study. *Comprehensive Psychiatry*, **38**, 146–54.

Radanovic, M. and Scaff, M. (2003). Speech and language disturbances due to subcortical lesions. *Brain and Language*, **84**, 337–52.

Azambuja, M., Mansur, L.L., *et al.* (2003). Thalamus and language, interface with attention, memory and executive functions. *Arquivos de Neuro-Psiquiatria*, **61**, 34–42.

Ramsey, B.J. (1999). Frontal lobe epilepsy presenting as a psychotic disorder with delusions and hallucination, a case study. *CNS Spectrums*, **4**, 64–82.

Rao, V. and Lyketsos, C.G. (1998). Delusions in Alzheimer's disease, a review. *Journal of Neuropsychiatry and Clinical Neuroscience*, **10**, 373–82.

Rapoport, J.L., Ryland, D.H. and Kriete, M. (1996). Drug treatment of canine acral lick, an animal model of obsessive-compulsive disorder. *Archives of General Psychiatry*, **49**, 517–21.

Rapoport, M.J., Leonov, Y. and Leibovitz, A. (1995). Body language in the emergency room. *Lancet*, **345**, 1060.

Raymond, N.C., Coleman, E. and Miner, M.H. (2003). Psychiatric comorbidity and compulsive/impulsive traits in compulsive sexual behavior. *Comprehensive Psychiatry*, **44**, 370–80.

Read, T.R., Hocking, J., Sinnott, V. and Hellard, M. (2007). Risk factors for incident HIV infection in men having sex with men, a case-control study. *Sexual Health*, **4**, 35–9.

Reay, J.L., Hamilton, C., Kennedy, D.O. and Scholey, A.B. (2006). MDMA polydrug users show process-specific central executive impairments coupled with impaired social and emotional judgment processes. *Journal of Psychopharmacology*, **20**, 385–8.

Regier, D.A., Meyer, J.K., Kramer, M., *et al.* (1984). The NIMH Epidemiologic Catchment Area program, historic context, major objections and study population. *Archives of General Psychiatry*, **41**, 934–41.

Kaelber, C.T., Roper, M.T., *et al.* (1994). The ICD-10 clinical field trial for mental and behavioral disorders, results in Canada and the United States. *American Journal of Psychiatry*, **151**, 1340–50.

Reichel, G., Kirchofer, U. and Stenner, A. (2001). Camptocormia–segmental dystonia. Proposal of a new definition for an old disease. *Der Nervenarzt*, **72**, 281–5.

Reif, A. and Pfuhlmann, B. (2004). Folie a deux versus genetically driven delusional disorder. Case reports and nosological considerations. *Comprehensive Psychiatry*, **45**, 155–60.

Reinders, A.A.T.S., Nijenhuis, E.R.S., Paans, A.M.J., *et al.* (2003). One brain, two selves. *Neuroimage*, **20**, 2119–25.

Richard, I. and Kurlan, R. (2002). Anxiety and panic. In S.A. Factor and W.J. Weiner, eds., *Parkinson's Disease, Diagnosis and Treatment*. New York: Demos Medical Publishing, pp. 161–72.

Richardson, E.D., Malloy, P.F. and Grace, J. (1991). Othello syndrome secondary to right cerebrovascular infarction. *Journal of Geriatric Psychiatry and Neurology*, **4**, 160–5.

Richter, J.C., Waydhas, C. and Pajonk, F.G. (2006). Incidence of post traumatic stress disorder after prolonged surgical intensive care unit treatment. *Psychosomatics*, **47**, 223–30.

Richter, M.A., Summerfeldt, L.J., Antony, M.M. and Swinson, R.P. (2003). Obsessive-compulsive spectrum conditions in obsessive-compulsive disorder and other anxiety disorders. *Depression and Anxiety*, **18**, 118–27.

Riddle, M. (1998). Obsessive-compulsive disorder in children and adolescents. *British Journal of Psychiatry*, **173** (Suppl. 35), 91–6.

Ries, R.K., Demirsoy, A., Russo, J.E., *et al.* (2001). Reliability and clinical utility of DSM-IV substance-induced psychiatric disorders in acute psychiatric inpatients. *American Journal of Addiction*, **10**, 308–18.

Rissmiller, D.J., Wayslow, A., Madison, H., *et al.* (1998). Prevalence of malingering in inpatient suicide ideators and attempters. *Crisis*, **19**, 62–6.

Rizzo, S., Venneri, A. and Papagno, C. (2002). Famous face recognition and naming test, a normative study. *Neurological Sciences*, **23**, 153–9.

Robert, J.S. and Plantikow, T. (2005). Genetics, neuroscience and psychiatric classification. *Psychopathology*, **38**, 215–18.

Roberts, B.W., Walton, K.E. and Viechtbauer, W. (2006). Patterns of mean-level change in personality traits across the life course. A meta-analysis of longitudinal studies. *Psychological Bulletin*, **132**, 1–25.

Roberts, R.J., Gorman, L.L., Lee, G.P., *et al.* (1992). The phenomenology of multiple partial seizure-like symptoms without stereotyped spells, an epilepsy spectrum disorder? *Epilepsy Research*, **13**, 167–77.

Robertson, E., Grace, S., Wallington, T. and Stewart, D.E. (2004). Antenatal risk factors for postpartum depression, a synthesis of recent literature. *General Hospital Psychiatry*, **26**, 289–95.

Robertson, E.M. (2004). Skill learning. Putting procedural consolidation in context. *Current Biology*, **14**, R1061–3.

Robins, E. and Guze, S.B. (1970). Establishment of diagnostic validity in psychiatric illness, its application to schizophrenia. *American Journal of Psychiatry*, **126**, 983–7.

Robinson, D.S., Nies, A., Ravaris, C.L. and Lamborn, K.R. (1973). The monoamine oxidase inhibitor, phenelzine, in the treatment of depressive-anxiety states. A controlled clinical trial. *Archives of General Psychiatry*, **29**, 407–13.

Robinson, R.G. and Starkstein, S.E. (1989). Mood disorders following stroke, new findings and future directions. *Journal of Geriatric Psychiatry*, **22**, 1–15.

Robling, S.A., Paykel, E.S., Dunn, V.J., Abbott, R. and Katona, C. (2000). Long-term outcome of severe puerperal psychiatric illness. *Psychological Medicine*, **30**, 1263–71.

Rodriguez-Ferrera, S., McCarthy, R.A. and McKenna, P.J. (2001). Language in schizophrenia and its relationship to formal thought disorder. *Psychological Medicine*, **31**, 197–205.

Rodway, P., Wright, L. and Hardie, S. (2003). The valence-specific laterality effect in free viewing conditions, the influence of sex, handedness, and response bias. *Brain and Cognition*, **53**, 452–63.

Roeltgen, D.P., Sevush, S. and Heilman, K.M. (1983). Pure Gerstmann's syndrome from a focal lesion. *Archives of Neurology*, **40**, 46–7.

Rogers, D. (1985). The motor disorders of severe psychiatric illness, a conflict of paradigms. *British Journal of Psychiatry*, **146**, 221–32.

Rohde, A. and Marneros, A. (1993). Prognosis of puerperal psychoses, follow-up and outcome after an average of 26 years. *Der Nervenarzt*, **64**, 175–80.

Rohland, B.M., Carroll, B.T. and Jacoby, R.G. (1993). ECT in the treatment of the catatonic syndrome. *Journal of Affective Disorders*, **29**, 255–61.

Romanos, M. (2004). Migrainous complex hallucinations in 10-year old patient – a case report and review. *Zeitschrift für Kinder und Jungendpsychiatrie und Psychotherapie*, **32**, 201–07.

Ron, M. (2001). Examining the unexplained. Understanding hysteria. *Brain*, **124**, 1065–6.

Ronthal, M. (1992). Myoclonus and asterixis. In A.B. Joseph and R.R. Young, eds., *Movement Disorders in Neurology and Neuropsychiatry*. Boston: Blackwell Scientific Publications, pp. 479–86.

Rooks, J.K., Roberts, D.J. and Scheltema, K. (2000). Tattoos, their relationship to trauma, psychopathology, and other myths. *Minnesota Medicine*, **83**, 24–7.

Roose, S.P., Glassman, A.H., Attia, E. and Woodring, S. (1994). Comparative efficacy of selective serotonin reuptake inhibitors and tricyclics in the treatment of melancholia. *American Journal of Psychiatry*, **151**, 1735–39.

Rorsman, B., Grasbeck, A., Hagnell, O., *et al.* (1990). A prospective study of first-incidence depression. The Lundby Study, 1957–72. *British Journal of Psychiatry*, **156**, 336–42.

Rosenham, D.L. (1973). On being sane in insane places. *Science*, **179**, 250–8.

Rosenzweig, A., Prigerson, H., Miller, M.D. and Reynolds, C.F. III (1997). Bereavement and late-life depression, grief and its complications in the elderly. *Annual Review of Medicine*, **48**, 421–8.

Ross, E.D. (2000). Affective prosody and the aprosodias. In M.-M. Mesulam, ed., *Principles of Behavioral and Cognitive Neurology, 2nd edn.*. New York: Oxford University Press, pp. 316–31.

Edmondson, J.A., Seibert, G.B. and Homan, R.W. (1988). Acoustic analysis of affective prosody during right-sided Wada test, a within subjects verification of the right hemisphere's role in language. *Brain and Language*, **33**, 128–45.

Homan, R.W. and Buck, R. (1994). Differential hemispheric lateralization of primary and social emotions. *Neuropsychiatry, Neuropsychology & Behavioral Neurology*, **7**, 1–19.

Ross, T.A. (1941). *Lectures on War Neuroses*. London: Edward Arnold.

Rosse, R.B., Collins, J.P., Fay-McCarthy, M., *et al.* (1994). Phenomenologic comparison of the idiopathic psychosis of schizophrenia and drug-induced cocaine and phencyclidine psychoses, a retrospective study. *Clinical Neuropharmacology*, **17**, 359–69.

Rossell, S.L., Shapleske, J. and David, A.S. (1998). Sentence verification and delusions, a content-specific deficit. *Psychological Medicine*, **28**, 1189–98.

Rossi, A., Marinanjeli, M.G., Butti, G., *et al.* (2000). Pattern of comorbidity among anxious and odd personality disorders, the case of obsessive-compulsive personality disorder. *CNS Spectrums*, **5**, 23–6.

Roth, M. (1959). The phobic anxiety–depersonalization syndrome. *Proceedings of the Royal Society of Medicine*, **52**, 587–95.

Roth, R.M., Baribeau, J., Milovan, D., *et al.* (2004). Procedural and declarative memory in obsessive-compulsive disorder. *Journal of the International Neuropsychological Society*, **10**, 647–54.

Rubino, F.A. (2002). Gait disorders. *Neurologist*, **8**, 254–62.

Ruffolo, J.S., Phillips, K.A., Menard, W., *et al.* (2006). Comorbidity of body dysmorphic disorder and eating disorders. Severity of psychopathology and body image disturbance. *International Journal of Eating Disorders*, **39**, 11–19.

Rush, A.J. (2007). STAR*D, What have we learned? *American Journal of Psychiatry*, **164**, 201–04.
and Weisenburger, J.E. (1994). Melancholic symptom features and DSM-IV. *American Journal of Psychiatry*, **151**, 489–98.
Trivedi, M.H., Wisniewski, S.R., *et al.* (2006). Bupropion-SR, Sertraline, or venlafaxine-XR after failure of SSRIs for depression. *New England Journal of Medicine*, **354**, 1231–42.

Rybakowski, J.K. and Twardowska, K. (1999). The dexamethasone/corticotropin-releasing hormone test in depression in bipolar and unipolar affective illness. *Journal of Psychiatry Research*, **33**, 363–70.

Sabri, O., Erkwoh, R., Schreckenberger, M., *et al.* (1997). Correlation of positive symptoms exclusively to hyperperfusion or hypoperfusion of cerebral cortex in never-treated schizophrenics. *Lancet*, **349**, 1735–39.

Saint-Cyr, J.A., Taylor, A.E. and Nicholson, K. (1995). Behavior and the basal ganglia. *Advances in Neurology*, **65**, 1–28.

Saint-Hilaire, M-H. and Feldman, R.G. (1992). The "on–off" phenomenon in Parkinson's disease. In A.B. Joseph and R.R. Young, eds., *Movement Disorders in Neurology and Neuropsychiatry*. Boston: Blackwell Scientific Publications, pp. 204–08.

Salloway, S.P., Malloy, P.F. and Duffy, J.D. (2001). *The Frontal Lobes and Neuropsychiatric Illness*. Washington, DC: American Psychiatric Publishing Inc.

Salpolsky, R.M., Uno, H., Rebert, C.S. and Finch, C.E. (1990). Hippocampal damage associated with prolonged glucocorticoid exposure in primates. *Journal of Neuroscience*, **10**, 2897–902.

Samuels, J., Nestadt, G., Bienvenu, O.J., *et al.* (2000). Personality disorders and normal personality dimensions in obsessive-compulsive disorder. *British Journal of Psychiatry*, **177**, 457–62.

Sanchez, L., Hagino, O., Weller, E. and Weller, R. (1999). Bipolarity in children. *Psychiatric Clinics of North America*, **22**, 629–48.

Sanchez-Roman, S., Tellez-Zenteno, J.F., Zermrno-Phols, F., *et al.* (2007). Personality in patients with migraine evaluated with the "Temperament and Character Inventory." *Journal of Headache and Pain*, **8**, 94–104.

Sandifer, M.G., Hordern, A., Timbury, G.C. and Green, L.M. (1969). Similarities and differences in patient evaluation by U.S. and U.K. psychiatrists. *American Journal of Psychiatry*, **126**, 206–12.

Sandler, J.Z. and Fulford, B. (2004). Should patients and their families contribute to the DSM-V process? *Psychiatric Services*, **55**, 133–8.

Sandor, P. (1993). Gilles de la Tourette syndrome. A neuropsychiatric disorder. *Journal of Psychosomatic Research*, **37**, 211–26.

Sanfilipo, M., Lafargue, T., Rusinek, H., *et al.* (2000). Volumetric measure of the frontal and temporal lobe regions in schizophrenia, relationship to negative symptoms. *Archives of General Psychiatry*, **57**, 471–80.

Santhouse, A.M., Howard, R.J. and Ffytche, D.H. (2000). Visual hallucinatory syndromes and the anatomy of the visual brain. *Brain*, **123**, 2055–64.

Santor, D.A., Ascher-Svanum, H., Lindenmayer, J.P. and Obenchain, R.L. (2007). Item response analysis of the Positive and Negative Syndrome Scale. *BMC Psychiatry*, **7**, e66.

Santos, C.O., Caeiro, L., Ferro, J.M., *et al.* (2006). Anger, hostility and aggression in the first days of acute stroke. *European Journal of Neurology*, **13**, 351–8.

Santos, S., Lopez del Val, J., Tejero, C., *et al.* (2000). Transient global amnesia, a review of 58 cases. *Review of Neurology*, **30**, 1113–17.

Sapara, A., Cooke, M., Fannon, D., *et al.* (2007). Prefrontal cortex and insight in schizophrenia, a volumetric MRI study. *Schizophrenia Research*, **89**, 22–34.

Sartorius, N., Kaelber, C.T., Cooper, J.E., *et al.* (1993). Progress toward achieving a common language in psychiatry. Results from the field trial of the clinical guidelines accompanying the WHO classification of mental and behavioral disorders in ICD-10. *Archives of General Psychiatry*, **50**, 115–24.

Ustun, T.B., Korten, A., *et al.* (1995). Progress toward achieving a common language in psychiatry, II. Results from the international field trials of the ICD-10 diagnostic criteria for research for mental and behavioral disorders. *American Journal of Psychiatry*, **152**, 1427–37.

Sato, W., and Aoki, S. (2006). Right hemispheric dominance in processing of unconscious negative emotion. *Brain and Cognition*, **62**, 261–6.

Sato, Y. and Berrios, G.E. (2003). Extracampine hallucinations. *Lancet*, **361**, 1479–80.

Saucier, D.M. and Elias, L.J. (2001). Lateral and sex differences in manual gesture during conversation. *Laterality*, **6**, 239–45.

Savitz, J., Solms, M., Piertersen, E., *et al.* (2004). Dissociative identity disorder associated with mania and change in handedness. *Cognitive and Behavioral Neurology*, **17**, 233–7.

Saxe, G.N., Vasile, R.G., Hill, T.C., *et al.* (1992). SPECT imaging and multiple personality disorder. *Journal of Nervous and Mental Disorders*, **180**, 662–3.

Saxena, S., Brody, A.L., Schwartz, J.M. and Baxter, L.R. (1998). Neuroimaging and frontal–subcortical circuitry in obsessive-compulsive disorder. *British Journal of Psychiatry*, **173** (Suppl. 35), 26–37.

Winograd, A., Dunkin, J.J., *et al.* (2001). A retrospective review of clinical characteristics and treatment response in body dysmorphic disorder versus obsessive-compulsive disorder. *Journal of Clinical Psychiatry*, **62**, 67–72.

Sbrana, A., Dell'osso, L., Benvenuti, A., *et al.* (2005). The psychotic spectrum, validity and reliability of the Structured Clinical Interview for the Psychotic Spectrum. *Schizophrenia Research*, **75**, 375–87.

Scarr, S. and McCartney, K. (1983). How people make their own environments, a theory of genotype greater than environment effects. *Child Development*, **54**, 424–35.

Schatzberg, A.F. (1998). Noradrenergic versus serotonergic antidepressants, predictors of treatment response. *Journal of Clinical Psychiatry*, **59** (Suppl. 14), 15–18.

and Rothschild, A.J. (1992). Psychotic (delusional) major depression, Should it be included as a distinct syndrome in DSM-IV?. *American Journal of Psychiatry*, **149**, 733–45.

Scheibel, A. (1997). The thalamus and neuropsychiatric disease. *Journal of Neuropsychiatry and Clinical Neuroscience*, **9**, 342–53.

Scheibel, A.B. and Wechler, A.F., eds. (1990). *Neurobiology of Higher Cortical Function.* New York: Guilford Press.

Schimmelmann, B.G., Conus, P., Edwards, J., *et al.* (2005). Diagnostic stability 18 months after treatment initiation for first-episode psychosis. *Journal of Clinical Psychiatry,* **66**, 1239–46.

Schmahmann, J.D. (2004). Disorders of the cerebellum. Ataxia, dysmetria of thought, and the cerebellar cognitive affective syndrome. *Journal of Neuropsychiatry and Clinical Neuroscience,* **16**, 367–78.

Schneider, B., Maurer, K., Sargk, D., *et al.* (2004). Concordance of DSM-IV Axis I and II diagnoses by personal and informant's interview. *Psychiatry Research,* **127**, 121–36.

Schneider, C. (1942). *Die Schizophrenen Symptomverbande* (The Schizophrenic Symptom Groups). Berlin: Springer.

Schneider, K. (1950). *Psychopathic Personalities,* 9th edn., translated by M.W. Hamilton. London: Cassell.

(1959). *Clinical Psychopathology,* translated by M.W. Hamilton . New York: Grune and Stratton.

Schneider, L.S., Tariot, P.N., Lyketsos, C.G., *et al.* (2001). National Institute of Mental Health Clinical Antipsychotic Trials of Intervention Effectiveness (CATIE), Alzheimer disease trial methodology. *American Journal of Geriatric Psychiatry,* **9**, 346–60.

Schrag, A., Trimble, M., Quinn, N. and Bhatia, K. (2004). The syndrome of fixed dystonia. An evaluation of 103 patients. *Brain,* **127**, 2360–72.

Schulz-Stubner, S. (2004). Panic attacks and hyperventilation may mimic local anesthesia toxicity. *Regional Anesthesia and Pain Medicine,* **29**, 617–19.

Schutter, D.J. and van Honk, J. (2005). The cerebellum on the rise in human emotion. *Cerebellum,* **4**, 290–4.

Schweitzer, I., Tuckwell, V., Ames, D. and O'Brien, J. (2001). Structrual neuroimaging studies in late-life depression, a review. *World Journal of Biological Psychiatry,* **2**, 83–8.

Scull, A. (1981). The social history of psychiatry in the Victorian Era. In A. Scull, ed., *Madhouses, Mad-Doctors, and Madmen, The Social History of Psychiatry in the Victorian Era.* Philadelphia: University of Pennsylvania.

Sedler, M.J. and Dessain, E.C. (1983). Falret's discovery, The origin of the concept of bipolar affective illness. *American Journal of Psychiatry,* **140**, 1127–33.

and Schoelly, M-L. (1985). The legacy of Ewald Hecker, a new translation of "*Die Hebephrenie*". *American Journal of Psychiatry,* **142**, 1265–71.

Serdaru, M., Gray, F., Lyon-Caen, O., *et al.* (1982). Parinaud's syndrome and tonic vertical gaze deviation. 3 anatomo-clinical observations. *Revue Neurologique (Paris),* **138**, 601–17.

Sergent, J. (1982). Influence of luminance on hemisphere processing. *Bulletin of the Psychonomic Society,* **20**, 221–3.

Serra Catafau, J., Rubio, F. and Serra, J. (1992). Peduncular hallucinosis associated with posterior thalamic infarction. *Journal of Neurology,* **239**, 89–90.

Sharp, H.M., Fear, C.F. and Healy, D. (1997). Attributional style and delusions, an investigation based on delusional content. *European Psychiatry,* **12**, 1–7.

Shapero, A.K., Shapero, E.S., Young, J.G. and Feinberg, T.E. (1988). *Gilles de la Tourette Syndrome,* 2nd edn. New York: Raven Press.

Shapero, D. (1965). *Neurotic Styles.* New York: Basic Books.

Shefner, J.M. (1992). Ballism. In A.B. Joseph and R.R. Young, eds., *Movement Disorders in Neurology and Neuropsychiatry*. Boston: Blackwell Scientific Publications, pp. 503–10.

Sheldon, W.H. and Stevens, S.S. (1942). *The Varieties of Temperament, A Psychology of Constitutional Differences*. New York: Harper.

Shenton, M.E., Dickey, C.C., Frumin, M. and McCarley, R.W. (2001). A review of MRI findings in schizophrenia. *Schizophrenia Research*, **49**, 1–52.

Sheline, Y.I. (2000). 3D MRI studies of neuroanatomic changes in unipolar major depression, the role of stress and medical comorbidity. *Biological Psychiatry*, **48**, 791–800.

Sher, L., Oquendo, M.A., Li, S., *et al.* (2003). Prolactin response to fenfluramine administration in patients with unipolar and bipolar depression and healthy controls. *Psychoneuroendocrinology*, **28**, 559–73.

Shockley, K., Santana, M.V. and Fowler, C.A. (2003). Mutual interpersonal postural constraints are involved in cooperative conversation. *Journal of Experimental Psychology: Human Perception and Performance*, **29**, 326–32.

Shorter, E. (1992). *From Paralysis to Fatigue, A History of Psychosomatic Illness in the Modern Era*. New York: The Free Press.

(1997). *A History of Psychiatry, From the Era of the Asylum to the Age of Prozac*. New York: John Wiley & Sons.

(2005). *A Historical Dictionary of Psychiatry*. Oxford: Oxford University Press.

and Healy, D. (2007). *Shock Therapy, A History of Electroconvulsive Treatment in Mental Illness*. New Brunswick: Rutgers University Press.

Shuchter, S.R., Zisook, S., Kirkorowicz, C. and Risch, C. (1986). The dexamethasone suppression test in acute grief. *American Journal of Psychiatry*, **143**, 879–81.

Siebel, U., Michels, R., Hoff, P., *et al.* (1997). Multi-axial system of chapter V (F) of ICD-10. Initial results of a multicenter practicability and reliability study. *Der Nervenarzt*, **68**, 231–8.

Sierles, F.S. and Taylor, M.A. (1995). Medical student career choice in psychiatry, the US decline and what to do about it. *American Journal of Psychiatry*, **152**, 1416–26.

Sierra, M. and Berrios, G.E. (1999). Flashbulb memories and other repetitive images, a psychiatric perspective. *Comprehensive Psychiatry*, **40**, 115–25.

Siever, L.J. (1994). Biologic factors in schizotypal personal disorders. *Acta Psychiatrica Scandinavica*, **384** (Suppl.), 45–50.

and Davis, K.L. (2004). The pathophysiology of schizophrenia disorders, perspectives from the spectrum. *American Journal of Psychiatry*, **161**, 398–413.

Silva, J.A., Leong, G.B. and Wine, D.B. (1993). Misidentification delusions, facial recognition, and right brain injury. *Canadian Journal of Psychiatry*, **38**, 239–41.

Silveira, J.M. and Seeman, M.V. (1995). Shared psychotic disorder. A critical review of the literature. *Canadian Journal of Psychiatry*, **40**, 389–95.

Silver, J.M., Yudofsky, S.C. and Hales, R.E. (2004). *Neuropsychiatry of Traumatic Brain Injury*. Washington, DC: American Psychiatric Press.

Silver, L.J. and Davis, K.L. (1991). A psychobiological perspective on the personality disorders. *American Journal of Psychiatry*, **148**, 1647–58.

Simeon, D., Stanley, B., Frances, A., *et al.* (1992). Self-mutilation in personality disorders, psychological and biological correlates. *American Journal of Psychiatry,* **149**, 221–6.

Knutelska, M., Yehuda, R. *et al.* (2007). Hypothalamic-pituitary-adrenal axis function in dissociative disorders, posttraumatic stress disorder and healthy volunteers. *Biological Psychiatry,* **61**, 966–73.

Simon, D.K., Nishino, S. and Scammell, T.E. (2004). Mistaken diagnosis of psychogenic gait disorder in a man with status cataplecticus ("limp man syndrome"). *Movement Disorders,* **19**, 838–40.

Sims, A. (1995). *Symptoms in the Mind, An Introduction to Descriptive Psychopathology,* 2nd edn. London: WB Saunders Company LTD.

Singh, M.K., Giles, L.L. and Nasrallah, H.A. (2006). Pain insensitivity in schizophrenia, trait or state marker? *Journal of Psychiatric Practice,* **12**, 90–102.

Skaf, C.R., Yamada, A., Garrido, G.E., *et al.* (2002). Psychotic symptoms in major depressive disorder are associated with reduced regional cerebral blood flow in the subgenual anterior cingulate cortex, a voxel-based single photon emission computed tomography (SPECT) study. *Journal of Affective Disorders,* **68**, 295–305.

Skinner, B.F. (1948). *Walden Two.* New York: Macmillan.

Skodol, A.E., Gunderson, J.G., Pfohl, B., *et al.* (2002). The borderline diagnosis I: Psychopathology, comorbidity, and personality structure. *Biological Psychiatry,* **51**, 936–50.

Slade, T. and Andrews, G. (2001). DSM-IV and ICD-10 generalized anxiety disorder, discrepant diagnoses and associated disability. *Social Psychiatry and Psychiatric Epidemiology,* **36**, 45–51.

Slater, E. (1965). Diagnosis of "hysteria". *British Medical Journal,* **1**, 1395–9.

and Glithero, E. (1965). A follow-up of patients diagnosed as suffering from "hysteria". *Journal of Psychosomatic Research,* **9**, 9–13.

Smith, C.D., Walton, A., Loveland, A.D., *et al.* (2005a). Memories that last in old age, motor skill learning and memory preservation. *Neurobiology and Aging,* **26**, 883–90.

Smith, D.J., Duffy, L., Stewart, M.E., *et al.* (2005b). High harm avoidance and low self-directedness in euthymic young adults with recurrent, early-onset depression. *Journal of Affective Disorders,* **87**, 83–9.

Smith, G.R. Jr., Golding, J.M., Kashner, T.M. and Rost, K. (1991). Antisocial personality disorder in primary care patients with somatization disorder. *Comprehensive Psychiatry,* **32**, 367–72.

Smith, R.C., Hussain, M.I., Chowdhury, S.A. and Stearns, A. (1999). Stability of neurological soft signs in chronically hospitalized schizophrenic patients. *Journal of Neuropsychiatry and Clinical Neuroscience,* **11**, 91–6.

Smith, S.D. and Bulman-Fleming, M.B. (2005). An examination of the right-hemisphere hypothesis of the lateralization of emotion. *Brain and Cognition,* **57**, 210–13.

Snowden, J.S., Thompson, J.C. and Neary, D. (2004). Knowledge of famous faces and names in semantic dementia. *Brain,* **127**, 860–72.

Soloff, P.H., Lis, J.A., Kelly, T.R., *et al.* (1994). Risk factors for suicidal behavior in borderline personality disorder. *American Journal of Psychiatry,* **151**, 1316–23.

Sorene, E.D., Heras-Palou, C. and Burke, F.D. (2006). Self-mutilation of a healthy hand, a case of body integrity identity disorder. *Journal of Hand Surgery (British European Volume),* **31B**, 6, 593–5.

Sorensen, M.J., Mors, O. and Thomsen, P.H. (2005). DSM-IV or ICD-10 diagnoses in child and adolescent psychiatry, does it matter? *European Child and Adolescent Psychiatry,* **14**, 335–40.

Soyka, M., Naber, G. and Volcker, A. (1991). Prevalence of delusional jealousy in different psychiatric disorders. An analysis of 93 cases. *British Journal of Psychiatry,* **158**, 549–53.

Spatt, J. (2002). Déjà Vu. Possible parahippocampal mechanisms. *Journal of Neuropsychiatry and Clinical Neuroscience,* **14**, 6–10.

Spence, S.A., Crimlisk, H.L., Cope, H., *et al.* (2000). Discrete neurophysiological correlates in prefrontal cortex during hysterical and feigned disorder of movement. *Lancet,* **355**, 1243–4.

Speranza, M., Corcos, M., Godart, N., *et al.* (2001). Obsessive compulsive disorders in eating disorders. *Eating Behaviors,* **2**, 193–207.

Spitzer, R.L. and Endicott, J. (1968). DIAGNO, a computer program for converting diagnoses to the new nomenclature of the American Psychiatric Association. *American Journal of Psychiatry,* **125**, 151–2.

and Fleiss, J.L. (1974). A re-analysis of the reliability of psychiatric diagnosis. *British Journal of Psychiatry,* **125**, 341–7.

Endicott, J. and Robins, E. (1980). *Research Diagnostic Criteria (RDC) for a Selected Group of Functional Disorders.* New York: NY State Psychiatric Institute.

Spitzka, E.C. (1887/1973). *Insanity, Its Classification, Diagnosis and Treatment.* 1887 facsimile. New York: Arno Press.

Sprock, J. (2003). Dimensional versus categorical classification of prototypic and nonprototypic cases of personality disorder. *Journal of Clinical Psychology,* **59**, 991–1014.

Squire, L.R. and Zola, S.M. (1997). Amnesia, memory and brain systems. *Philosophical Transactions of the Royal Society London B. Biological Sciences,* **352** (1362), 1663–73.

Stamouli, S. and Lykouras, L. (2006). Quetiapine-induced obsessive-compulsive symptoms, a series of five cases. *Journal of Clinical Psychopharmacology,* **26**, 396–400.

Stanton, D., Volness, L.J. and Beatty, W.W. (2007). Diagnosis and classification of pediatic bipolar disorder. *Journal of Affective Disorders,* **105**, 205–12.

Starkstein, S.E. and Robinson, R.G. (1997). Mechanism of disinhibition after brain lesions. *Journal of Nervous and Mental Disorders,* **183**, 108–14.

and Manes, F. (2000). Apathy and depression following stroke. *CNS Spectrums,* **5**, 43–50.

Boston, J.D. and Robinson, R.G. (1988a). Mechanisms of mania after brain injury. *Journal of Nervous and Mental Disorders,* **176**, 87–100.

Robinson, R.G., Berthier, M.L., *et al.* (1988b). Differential mood changes following basal ganglia versus thalamic lesions. *Archives of Neurology,* **45**, 725–30.

Robinson, R.G. and Price, T.R. (1988c). Comparison of patients with and without post-stroke major depression matched for size and location of lesion. *Archives of General Psychiatry,* **45**, 247–52.

Fedoroff, J.P., Price, T.R., *et al.* (1992). Anosognosia in patients with cerebrovascular lesions. A study of causative factors. *Stroke,* **23**, 1446–53.

Steiger, H. and Bruce, K.R. (2007). Phenotypes, endophenotypes, and genotypes in bulimia spectrum eating disorders. *Canadian Journal of Psychiatry,* **52**, 220–7.

Stein, D.J. and Lochner, C. (2006). Obsessive-compulsive spectrum disorders, a multidimensional approach. *Psychiatric Clinics of North America,* **29**, 343–51.

Stephane, M., Barton, S. and Boutros, N.N. (2001). Auditory verbal hallucinations and dysfunction of the neural substrates of speech. *Schizophrenia Research*, **50**, 61–78.

Stewart, L., von Kriegstein, K., Warren, J.D. and Griffiths, T.D. (2006). Music and the brain, disorders of musical listening. *Brain*, **129**, 2533–53.

Stickler, G.B. and Cheung-Patton, A. (1989). Astasia–abasia. A conversion reaction. Prognosis. *Clinical Pediatrics*, **28**, 12–16.

Stippich, C., Blatow, M., Durst, A., *et al.* (2006). Global activation of primary motor cortex during voluntary movements in man. *Neuroimage*, **27**, 1227–37.

Stone, J., Sharpe, M., Carson, A., *et al.* (2002). Are functional motor and sensory symptoms more frequent on the left? A systematic review. *Journal of Neurology, Neurosurgery and Psychiatry*, **73**, 578–81.

Sharpe, M., Rothwell, P.M. and Warlow, C.P. (2003). The 12 year prognosis of unilateral functional weakness and sensory disturbance. *Journal of Neurology, Neurosurgery and Psychiatry*, **74**, 591–6.

Sharpe, M. and Bimzer, M. (2004). Motor conversion symptoms and pseudoseizures. A clinical comparison of characteristics. *Psychosomatics*, **45**, 492–9.

Smyth, A.C., Prescott, R., *et al.* (2005). Systematic review of misdiagnosis of conversion symptoms and "hysteria". *British Medical Journal*, **331**, e989–984.

Strakowski, S.M., DelBello, M.P., Adler, C., *et al.* (2000). Neuroimaging in bipolar disorder. *Bipolar Disorders*, **2**, 148–64.

Stromgren, E. (1974). Psychogenic psychoses. In S.R. Hirsch and M. Shepherd, eds., *Themes and Variations in European Psychiatry*. Bristol: John Wright and Sons, pp. 102–25.

Stroup, T.S., McEvoy, J.P., Swartz, M.S., *et al.* (2003). The National Institute of Mental Health Clinical Antipsychotic Trials of Intervention Effectiveness (CATIE) project, schizophrenia trial design and protocol development. *Schizophrenia Bulletin*, **29**, 15–31.

Stubhaug, B., Tveito, T.H., Eriksen, H.R. and Ursin, H. (2005). Neurasthenia, subjective health complaints and sensitization. *Psychoneuroendocrinology*, **30**, 1003–09.

Stubner, S., Rustenbeck, E., Grohmann, R., *et al.* (2004). Severe and uncommon involuntary movement disorders due to psychotropic drugs. *Pharmacopsychiatry*, **37** (Suppl. 1), S54–64.

Stunell, H., Power, R.E., Floyd, M. Jr. and Quinlan, D.M. (2006). Genital self-mutilation. *International Journal of Urology*, **13**, 1358–60.

Styron, W. (1990). *Darkness Visible, A Memoir of Madness*. New York: Random House.

Suhail, K. (2003). Phenomenology of delusions in Pakistani patients, effect of gender and social class. *Psychopathology*, **36**, 195–9.

Surguladze, S., Brammer, M.J., Keedwell, P., *et al.* (2005). A differential pattern of neural response toward sad versus happy facial expressions in major depressive disorder. *Biological Psychiatry*, **57**, 201–09.

Suzuki, K., Takei, N., Kawai, M., *et al.* (2003). Is Taijin Kyofusho a culture-bound syndrome? *American Journal of Psychiatry*, **160**, 1358.

Sveinbjornsdottir, S. and Duncan, J.S. (1993). Parietal and occipital lobe epilepsy, a review. *Epilepsia*, **35**, 467.

Svrakic, D.M., Whitehead, C., Przybeck, T.R. and Cloninger, C.R. (1993). Differential diagnosis of personality disorders by the seven-factor model of temperament and character. *Archives of General Psychiatry*, **50**, 991–9.

Swaab, D.F., Gooren, L.J. and Hofman, M.A. (1992). Gender and sexual orientation in relation to hypothalamic structures. *Hormone Research*, **38** (Suppl. 2), 51–61.

Gooren, L.J. and Hofman, M.A. (1995). Brain research, gender and sexual orientation. *Journal of Homosexuality*, **28**, 283–301.

Swartz, C.M. and Shen W.W. (1999). Is episodic obsessive compulsive disorder bipolar? A report of four cases. *Journal of Affective Disorders*, **56**, 61–6.

Szasz, T.S. (1974). *The Myth of Mental Illness, Foundations of a Theory of Personal Conduct* (rev. edn). New York: Harper and Row.

Tadokoro, Y., Oshima, T. and Kanemoto, K. (2006). Postictal autoscopy in a patient with partial epilepsy. *Epilepsy and Behavior*, **9**, 535–40.

Takaoka, K. and Takata, T. (1999). "Alice in Wonderland" syndrome and Lilliputian hallucinations in a patient with substance-related disorder. *Psychopathology*, **32**, 47–9.

Talbot, N.L., Duberstein, P.R., King, D.A., *et al.* (2000). Personality traits of women with a history of childhood sexual abuse. *Comprehensive Psychiatry*, **41**, 130–6.

Tamietto, M., Latini Corrazzini, L., *et al.* (2006). Functional asymmetry and interhemispheric cooperation in the perception of emotions from facial expressions. *Experimental Brain Research*, **171**, 389–404.

Tantam, D. (1988). Lifelong eccentricity and social isolation. II, Asperger's syndrome or schizoid personality disorder? *British Journal of Psychiatry*, **153**, 783–91.

Tateno, A., Jorge, R.E. and Robinson, R.G. (2004). Pathological laughing and crying following traumatic brain injury. *Journal of Neuropsychiatry and Clinical Neuroscience*, **16**, 426–34.

Tavares, H., Zilberman, M.L., Hodgins, D.C. and el-Guebaly, N. (2005). Comparison of craving between pathological gamblers and alcoholics. *Alcoholism: Clinical and Experimental Research*, **29**, 1427–31.

Taylor, K.I., Brugger, P. and Schwarz, U. (2005). Audiovisual peduncular hallucinations, a release of cross-modal integration sites? *Cognitive and Behavioral Neurology*, **18**, 135–6.

Taylor, M.A. (1972). Schneiderian first-rank symptoms and clinical prognostic features in schizophrenia. *Archives of General Psychiatry*, **26**, 64–7.

(1981). The diagnosis of schizophrenia. A new look at an old label. *American Journal of Psychiatry.*, **2**, 7–14.

(1984). Schizo-affective and allied disorders. In R.M. Post and J.C. Ballenger, *The Neurobiology of Manic-Depressive Illness*. Baltimore: Williams and Wilkins, pp. 136–56.

(1986). The validity of schizo-affective disorders: Treatment and prevention studies. In A. Maneros and M.T. Tsuang, *Schizo-Affective Psychoses*: Berlin-Heidelberg, Springer-Verlag, pp. 94–113.

(1990). Catatonia. A review of a behavioral neurologic syndrome. *Neuropsychiatry, Neuropsychology and Behavioral Neurology*, **3**, 48–72.

(1991). The role of the cerebellum in the pathogenesis of schizophrenia. *Neuropsychiatry, Neuropsychology and Behavioral Neurology*, **4**, 251–80.

(1999). *The Fundamentals of Clinical Neuropsychiatry*. New York: Oxford University Press.

and Heiser, J.F. (1971). Phenomenology: An alternative approach to diagnosis of mental disease. *Comprehensive Psychiatry*, **5**, 480–5.

and Abrams, R. (1973). The phenomenology of mania. A new look at some old patients. *Archives of General Psychiatry*, **29**, 520–2.

and Abrams, R.A. (1975a). Acute mania. *Archives of General Psychiatry*, **32**, 863–5.

and Abrams, R. (1975b). Manic-depressive illness and "good prognosis" schizophrenia. *American Journal of Psychiatry*, **132**, 741–2.

and Abrams, R. (1978). The prevalence of schizophrenia. A reassessment using modern diagnostic criteria. *American Journal of Psychiatry*, **135**, 945–8.

and Abrams, R. (1980). Reassessing the bipolar–unipolar dichotomy. *Journal of Affective Disorders*, **2**, 195–217.

and Abrams, R. (1983). Schizo-affective disorder, manic type. *Psychiatria Clinica*, **16**, 234–44.

and Abrams, R. (1984). Cognitive impairment in schizophrenia. *American Journal of Psychiatry*, **141**, 196–201.

and Amir, N. (1994). Are schizophrenia and affective disorder related? The problem of schizoaffective disorder and the discrimination of the psychoses by signs and symptoms. *Comprehensive Psychiatry*, **35**, 420–9.

and Fink, M. (2003). Catatonia in psychiatric classification. A home of its own. *American Journal of Psychiatry*, **160**, 1233–41.

and Fink, M. (2006). *Melancholia, The Diagnosis, Pathophysiology, and Treatment of Patients with Depressive Illness*. Cambridge: Cambridge University Press.

and Fink, M. (2008). Restoring melancholia in the classification of mood disorders. *Journal of Affective Disorders*, **105**, 1–14.

and Vaidya, N.A. (2005). Psychopathology in neuropsychiatry, DSM and beyond. *Journal of Neuropsychiatry and Clinical Neuroscience*, **17**, 246–9.

Abrams, R. and Gaztanaga, P. (1974). Manic-depressive illness and acute schizophrenia. A clinical, family history and treatment response study. *American Journal of Psychiatry*, **131**, 678–82.

Abrams, R. and Gaztanaga, P. (1975). Manic-depressive illness and schizophrenia. A partial validation of research diagnostic criteria utilizing neuropsychological testing. *Comprehensive Psychiatry*, **16**, 91–6.

Abrams, R. and Hayman, M. (1980). The classification of affective disorder. A reassessment of the bipolar–unipolar dichotomy. Part 1, A clinical, laboratory and family study. *Journal of Affective Disorders*, **2**, 95–109.

Redfield, J. and Abrams, R. (1981). Neuropsychological dysfunction in schizophrenia and affective disease. *Biological Psychiatry*, **16**, 467–78.

Reed, R. and Berenbaum, S. (1994). Patterns of speech disorders in schizophrenia and mania. *Journal of Nervous and Mental Disorders*, **182**, 319–26.

Teeney, N.H., Schotte, C.K., Denys, D.A., *et al.* (2003). Assessment of DSM-IV personality disorders in obsessive-compulsive disorder. Comparison of clinical diagnosis, self-report questionnaire, and semi-structured interview. *Journal of Personality Disorder*, **17**, 550–61.

Teive, H.A.G., Germiniani, F.M.B., Della Coletta, M.V. and Werneck, L.C. (2001). Tics and Tourette's syndrome. Clinical evaluation of 44 cases. *Arquivos de Neuro-psiquiatria*, **59**, 725–8.

Tekin, S. and Cummings, J.L. (2002). Frontal–subcortical neuronal circuits and clinical neuropsychiatry, an update. *Journal of Psychosomatic Research*, **53**, 647–54.

Tenback, D.E., van Harten, P.N., Slooff, C.J., *et al.* (2007). Worsening of psychosis in schizophrenia is longitudinally associated with tardive dyskinesia in the European Scizophrenia Outpatient Health Outcomes Study. *Comprehensive Psychiatry*, **48**, 436–40.

Thaker, G.K., Cassady, S., Adami, H., *et al.* (1996). Eye movements in spectrum personality disorders, comparison of community subjects and relatives of schizophrenic patients. *American Journal of Psychiatry*, **153**, 362–8.

Thase, M.E. (2003). Effectiveness of antidepressants, comparative remission rates. *Journal of Clinical Psychiatry*, **64** (Suppl. 2), 3–7.

Thomas, C.L., ed. (1997). *Taber's Cyclopedic Medical Dictionary*, 18th edn. Philadelphia: F.A. Davis Company.

Thomke, F. and Hopf, H.C. (1999). Pontine lesions mimicking acute peripheral vestibulopathy. *Journal of Neurology, Neurosurgery & Psychiatry*, **66**, 340–9.

Thompson, C., ed. (1987). *The Origins of Modern Psychiatry*. Chichester: John Wiley and Sons.

Thompson, K.M., Crosby, R.D., Wonderlich, S.A., *et al.* (2003). Psychopathology and sexual trauma in childhood and adulthood. *Journal of Traumatic Stress*, **16**, 35–8.

Thompson, P.A., Buckley, P.F. and Meltzer, H.Y. (1994). The brief psychiatric rating scale: effect of scaling system on clinical response assessment. *Journal of Clinical Psychopharmacology*, **14**, 344–6.

Thorup, A., Peterson, L., Jeppesen, P. and Nordentoft, M. (2007). Frequency and predictive values of first rank symptoms at baseline among 362 young adult patients with first-episode schizophrenia. Results from the Danish OPUS study. *Schizophrenia Research*, **13**, 60–7.

Tien, A.Y., Pearlson, G.D., Machlin, S.R., *et al.* (1992). Oculomotor performance in obsessive-compulsive disorder. *American Journal of Psychiatry*, **149**, 641–6.

Ross, D.E., Pearlson, G.D. and Strauss, M.E. (1996). Eye movements and psychopathology in schizophrenia and bipolar disorder. *Journal of Nervous and Mental Disorders*, **184**, 331–8.

Tippett, W.J. and Sergio, L.E. (2006). Visuomotor integration is impaired in early stage Alzheimer's disease. *Brain Research*, **1102**, 92–102.

Todd, R.D., Joyner, C.A., Heath, A.C., *et al.* (2003). Reliability and stability of a semistructured DSM-IV interview designed for family studies. *Journal of the American Academy of Childhood and Adolescent Psychiatry*, **42**, 1460–8.

Todes, C.J. and Lees, A.J. (1985). The premorbid personality of patients with Parkinson's disease. *Journal of Neurology, Neurosurgery & Psychiatry*, **48**, 97–100.

Todorov, A., Mandisodza, A.N., Goren, A. and Hall, C.C. (2005). Inferences of competence from faces predict election outcomes. *Science*, **308**, 1623–6.

Tohen, M., Tsuang, M.T. and Goodwin, D.C. (1992). Prediction of outcome in mania by mood-congruent or mood-incongruent psychotic features. *American Journal of Psychiatry*, **149**, 1580–4.

Torgersen, S. (1986). Genetic factors in moderately severe and mild affective disorders. *Archives of General Psychiatry*, **43**, 222–6.

(1994). Genetics in borderline conditions. *Acta Psychiatrica Scandinavica*, **379** (Suppl.), 19–25.

(2005). Behavioral genetics of personality. *Current Psychiatry Reports*, **7**, 51–6.

Lygren, S., Oien, P.A., *et al.* (2000). A twin study of personality disorders. *Comprehensive Psychiatry*, **41**, 416–25.

Treloar, S.A., Martin, N.G., Bucholz, P.A., *et al.* (1999). Genetic influences on post-natal depressive symptoms, finding from an Australian twin sample. *Psychological Medicine*, **29**, 645–54.

Tremeau, F., Malaspina, D., Duval, F., *et al.* (2005). Facial expressiveness in patients with schizophrenia compared to depressed patients and nonpatient comparison subjects. *American Journal of Psychiatry*, **162**, 92–101.

Trimble, M. (2004). *Somatoform Disorders, A Medicolegal Guide.* Cambridge: Cambridge University Press.

Trimble, M.R. (2002). Clinical presentations in neuropsychiatry. *Seminars in Clinical Neuropsychiatry*, **7**, 11–17.

Truong, H.M., Kellogg, T., Klausner, J.D., *et al.* (2006). Increases in sexually transmitted infections and sexual risk behavior without a concurrent increase in HIV incidence among men who have sex with men in San Francisco, a suggestion of HIV serosorting? *Sexually Transmitted Infections*, **82**, 461–6.

Tsuang, M.T., Faraone, S.V. and Fleming, J.A. (1985). Familial transmission of major affective disorders, is there evidence supporting the distinction between unipolar and bipolar disorders? *British Journal of Psychiatry*, **146**, 268–71.

Tucker, D.M., Luu, P., Pribram and K.H. (1995). Social and emotional self-regulation. *Annals of the New York Academy of Science*, **769**, 213–39.

Tynes, L.L., White, K. and Steketee, G.S. (1990). Toward a new nosology of obsessive-compulsive disorder. *Comprehensive Psychiatry*, **31**, 465–80.

Tyrer, P. and Alexander, J. (1979). Classification of personality disorder. *British Journal of Psychiatry*, **135**, 163–7.

Udell, E.T. (1994). Malingering behavior in private medical practice. *Clinics in Podiatric Medicine and Surgery*, **11**, 65–72.

Uher, R. and Treasure, J. (2005). Brain lesions and eating disorders. *Journal of Neurology, Neurosurgery and Psychiatry*, **76**, 852–7.

Uhlhaas, P.J. and Mishara, A.L. (2007). Perceptual anomalies in schizophrenia, integrating phenomenology and cognitive neuroscience. *Schizophrenia Bulletin*, **33**, 142–56.

Ungvari, G.S. and Rankin, A.F. (1990). Speech-prompt catatonia. A case report and review of the literature. *Comprehensive Psychiatry*, **30**, 56–61.

Vaever, M.S., Licht, D.M., Moller, L., *et al.* (2005). Thinking within the spectrum, schizophrenic thought disorder in six Danish pedigrees. *Schizophrenia Research*, **72**, 137–49.

Vaina, L.M., Cowey, A., LeMay, M., *et al.* (2002). Visual deficits in a patient with "kaleidoscope disintegration of the visual world". *European Journal of Neurology*, **9**, 463–77.

Vakil, E., Blachstein, H. and Soroker, N. (2004). Differential effect of right and left basal ganglionic infarctions on procedural learning. *Cognitive and Behavioral Neurology*, **17**, 62–73.

Valenza, N., Murray, M.M., Ptak, R. and Vuilleumier, P. (2004). The space of senses. Impaired crossmodal interactions in a patient with Balint syndrome after bilateral parietal damage. *Neuropsychologia*, **42**, 1737–48.

Vanderzant, C.W., Giordani, S., Dreifuss, F.E., Sackellares, J.C. (1986). Personality of patients with pseudoseizures. *Neurology*, **36**, 664–8.

van der Zwaard, R. and Polak, M.A. (2001). Pseudohallucinations, a pseudoconcept? A review of the validity of the concept, related to associate symptomatology. *Comprehensive Psychiatry*, **42**, 42–50.

vanGrootheest, D.S., Cath, D.C., Beekman, A.T. and Boomsma, D.L. (2005). Twin studies in obsessive-compulsive disorder, a review. *Twin Research and Human Genetics*, **8**, 450–8.

Van Loey, N.E. and Van Son, M.J. (2003). Psychopathology and psychological problems in patients with burn scars, epidemiology and management. *American Journal of Clinical Dermatology*, **4**, 245–72.

van Minnen, A., Hoogduin, K.A., Keijsers, G.P., *et al.* (2003). Treatment of trichotillomania with behavioral therapy or fluoxetine, a randomized, waiting-list controlled study. *Archives of General Psychiatry*, **60**, 517–22.

van't Wout, M., Aleman, A., Bermond, B. and Kahn, R.S. (2007). No words for feelings, alexithymia in schizophrenic patients and first-degree relatives. *Comprehensive Psychiatry*, **48**, 27–33.

Varambally, S., Venkatasubramanian, G., Thirthalli, J., *et al.* (2006). Cerebellar and other neurological soft signs in antipsychotic-naïve schizophrenia. *Acta Psychiatrica Scandinavica*, **114**, 352–6.

Varon, D., Pritchard, P.B. III., Wagner, M.T. and Topping, K. (2003). Transient Klüver–Bucy syndrome following complex partial status epilepticus. *Epilepsy and Behaviour*, **4**, 348–51.

Vataja, R., Leppavuori, A., Pohjasvaara, T., *et al.* (2004). Poststroke depression and lesion location revisited. *Journal of Neuropsychiatry and Clinical Neuroscience*, **16**, 156–62.

Vazquez, B. and Devinsky, O. (2003). Epilepsy and anxiety. *Epilepsy and Behaviour*, **4** (Suppl. 4), S20–5.

Venna, N. and Sabin, T.D. (1992). Senile gait disorders. In A.B. Joseph and R.R. Young, eds., *Movement Disorders in Neurology and Neuropsychiatry*. Boston: Blackwell Scientific Publications, pp. 301–09.

Verheul, R. and Widiger, T.A. (2004). A meta-analysis of the prevalence and usage of the personality disorder not otherwise specified (PDNOS) diagnosis. *Journal of Personality Disorders*, **18**, 309–19.

Vermetten, E., Schmahl, C., Linder, S., *et al.* (2006). Hippocampal and amygdala volumes in dissociative identity disorder. *American Journal of Psychiatry*, **163**, 630–6.

Vetter, P.H., von Pritzbuer, J., Jungmann K., *et al.* (2001). The validity of the ICD-10 classification of recurrent affective disorders, do endogenous and psychogenic depressions form a homogeneous diagnostic group? *Psychopathology*, **34**, 36–42.

Videbech, P. and Gouliaev, G. (1995). First admission with puerperal psychosis, 7–14 years of follow-up. *Acta Psychiatrica Scandinavica*, **91**, 167–73.

Vinamaki, H., Tanskanen, A., Honkalampi, K., *et al.* (2004). Is the Beck Depression Inventory suitable for screening major depression in different places of disease? *Nordic Journal of Psychiatry*, **58**, 49–53.

Volavka, J. (2002). *The Neurobiology of Violence*, 2nd edn. Washington, DC: American Psychiatric Publishing.

Volchan, E., Pereira, M.G., Oliveira, L.D.L., *et al.* (2003). Emotional stimuli, sensory processing and motor responses. *Revista Brasileira de Psiquiatria*, **25** (Suppl. 2), 29–32.

Vuilleumier, P. (2005). Hysterical conversion and brain function. *Progress in Brain Research*, **150**, 309–29.

Wade, J.B., Taylor, M.A., Kasprisin, A., *et al.* (1987). Tardive dyskinesia and cognitive impairment. *Biological Psychiatry*, **22**, 393–5.

Wagner, A., Greer, P., Bailer, U.F., *et al.* (2006). Normal brain tissue volumes after long-term recovery in anorexia and bulimia nervosa. *Biological Psychiatry*, **59**, 291–3.

Wahler, R.G., Herring, M. and Edwards, M. (2001). Co-regulation of balance between children's prosocial approaches and acts of compliance, A pathway to mother–child cooperation? *Journal of Clinical Child Psychology*, **30**, 473–8.

Wakefield, J.C. (1997). Diagnosing DSM-IV – Part I: DSM-IV and the concept of disorder. *Behaviour Research and Therapy*, **35**, 633–49.

Walsh, B.T., Kaplan, A.S., Attia, E., *et al.* (2006). Fluoxetine after weight restoration in anorexia nervosa, a randomized controlled trial. *Journal of the American Medical Association*, **295**, 2605–12.

Walker, E. and Lewine, R.J. (1990). Prediction of adult-onset schizophrenia from childhood home movies of the patients. *American Journal of Psychiatry*, **147**, 1052–6.

Wang, Q., Gu, Y., Ferguson, J.M., *et al.* (2003). Cytogenetic analysis of obsessive-compulsive disorder (OCD), identification of a FRAXE fragile site. *American Journal of Medical Genetics*, **118**, 25–8.

Watson, D. (2001). Dissociations of the night, individual differences in sleep-related experiences and their relation to dissociation and schizotypy. *Journal of Abnormal Psychology*, **110**, 526–35.

Watson, R.T. and Heilman, K.M. (1979). Thalamic neglect. *Neurology*, **29**, 690–4.

Weber, P., Ruof, H. and Jourdan, S. (2005). Differential diagnosis of visual hallucinations. *Klinische Padiatrie*, **217**, 25–30.

Weinberger, D.R. (1987). Implications for normal brain development for the pathogenesis of schizophrenia. *Archives of General Psychiatry*, **44**, 660–9.

Weinstock, A., Giglio, P., Kerr, S.L., *et al.* (2003). Hyperkinetic seizures in children. *Journal of Child Neurology*, **18**, 517–24.

Weissman-Fogel, I., Sprecher, E., Granovsky, Y. and Yarnitsky, D. (2003). Repeated noxious stimulation of the skin enhances cutaneous pain perception of migraine patients in-between attacks, clinical evidence for continuous sub-threshold increase in membrane excitability of central trigeminovascular neurons. *Pain*, **104**, 693–700.

Weller, E.B., Weller, R.A., Fristad, M.A. and Bowes, J.M. (1990). Dexamethasone suppression test and depressive symptoms in bereaved children, a preliminary report. *Journal of Neuropsychiatry and Clinical Neuroscience*, **2**, 418–21.

Wellman, C.L., Izquierdo, A., Garrett, J.E., *et al.* (2007). Impaired stress-coping and fear extinction and abnormal corticolimbic morphology in serotonin transporter knock-out mice. *Journal of Neuroscience*, **27**, 684–91.

Wernicke, C. (1906). *Fundamentals of Psychiatry*. Leipzig: Thieme.

Widiger, T.A. and Samuel, D.B. (2005). Evidence based assessment of personality disorders. *Psychological Assessments*, **17**, 278–87.

Widiger, T.A., Frances, A.J., Spitzer, R.L. and Williams, J.B.W. (1988). The DSM-III-R personality disorders, an overview. *American Journal of Psychiatry*, **145**, 786–95.

Wijeratne, C., Hickie, I. and Schwartz, R. (1997). Erotomania associated with temporal lobe abnormalities following radiotherapy. *Australia and New Zealand Journal of Psychiatry*, **31**, 765–8.

Wilhelm, D., Palmer, S. and Koopman, P. (2007). Sex differentiation and gonadal development in mammals. *Physiology Reviews*, **87**, 1–28.

Willemse, G.R., Van Yperen, T.A. and Rispens, J. (2003). Reliability of the ICD-10 classification of adverse familial and environmental factors. *Journal of Child Psychology and Psychiatry*, **44**, 202–13.

Williams, J.H., Waiter, G.D., Gilchrist, A., *et al.* (2006a). Neural mechanisms of imitation and "mirror neuron" functioning in autistic spectrum disorder. *Neuropsychologia*, **44**, 610–21.

Williams, L.M., Das, P., Liddell, B.J., *et al.* (2006b). Mode of functional connectivity in amygdala pathways dissociated level of awareness for signals of fear. *Journal of Neuroscience*, **26**, 9264–71.

Wilson, W.H. (1989). Reassessment of state hospital patients diagnosed with schizophrenia. *Journal of Neuropsychiatry and Clinical Neuroscience*, **1**, 394–7.

Wilcox, J.A. (1992). The predictive value of thought disorder in manic psychosis. *Psychopathology*, **25**, 161–5.

Wing, L. and Shah, A. (2000). Possible causes of catatonia in austic spectrum disorders. *British Journal of Psychiatry*, **177**, 180–1 (Reply to Chaplin).

Winger, G., Woods, J.H., Galuska, C.M. and Wade-Galuska, T. (2005). Behavioral perspectives on the neuroscience of drug addiction. *Journal of the Experimental Analysis of Behavior*, **84**, 667–81.

Winokur, G., Clayton, P. and Reich, T. (1969). *Manic Depressive Illness*. St. Louis: CV Mosby. Coryell, W., Keller, M., *et al.* (1995). A family study of manic-depressive illness (bipolar I). Is it a distinct disease separable from primary unipolar depression? *Archives of General Psychiatry*, **52**, 367–73.

Winslow, H., Mickey, B. and Frohman, E.M. (2006). Sympathetic-induced kaleidoscopic visual illusion associated with reversible splenium lesion. *Archives of Neurology*, **63**, 135–7.

Wirthrington, R.H. and Wynn-Parry, C.B. (1985). Rehabilitation of conversion paralysis. *Journal of Bone and Joint Surgery, British*, **67**, 635–7.

Wise, T.N. and Kalyanam, R.C. (2000). Amputee fetishism and genital mutilation, case report and literature review. *Journal of Sex and Marital Therapy*, **26**, 339–44.

Wisner, K.L., Peindl, K.P. and Hanusa, B.H. (1993). Relationship of psychiatric illness to childbearing status, a hospital-based epidemiologic study. *Journal of Affective Disorders*, **28**, 39–50. Peindl, K.P. and Hanusa, B.H. (1995). Psychiatric episodes in women with young children. *Journal of Affective Disorders*, **34**, 1–11.

Wittchen, H-U., Muhlig, S. and Pezawas, L. (2003). Natural course and burden of bipolar disorders. *International Journal of Neuropsychopharmacology*, **6**, 145–54.

Wolpe, J. (1958). *Psychotherapy by Reciprocal Inhibition*. Stanford: Stanford University Press.

Wonderlich, S.A., Crosby, R.D., Mitchell, J.E., *et al.* (2001). Sexual trauma and personality, developmental vulnerability and additive effects. *Journal of Personality Disorders*, **15**, 496–504. Rosenfeldt, S., Crosby, R.D., *et al.* (2007). The effects of childhood trauma on daily mood lability and comorbid psychopathology in bulimia nervosa. *Journal of Trauma and Stress*, **20**, 77–87.

Woo, B.S. and Rey, J.M. (2005). The validity of the DSM-IV subtypes of attention-deficit/hyperactivity disorder. *Australia and New Zealand Journal of Psychiatry*, **39**, 344–53.

Woodruff, P.W.R., Wright, I.C., Bullmore, E.T., *et al.* (1997). Auditory hallucinations and the temporal cortical response to speech in schizophrenia, a functional magnetic resonance imaging study. *American Journal of Psychiatry*, **154**, 1676–82.

Woodruff, R.A., Goodwin, D.W. and Guze, S.B. (1974). *Psychiatric Diagnosis*. New York: Oxford University Press.

Woodward, S.H., Kaloupek, D.G., Streeter, C.C., *et al.* (2006). Hippocampal volume, PTSD, and alcoholism in combat veterams. *American Journal of Psychiatry*, **163**, 674–81.

Yamamoto, M., Okudaira, A., Kohira, I., *et al.* (1993). Pure sensory seizures. *Seizure*, **2**, 49–51.

Yan, S-M., Chen, D.B.M., Chao, Y.Z., *et al.* (1982). Prevalence and characteristics of mania in Chinese inpatients, a prospective study. *American Journal of Psychiatry*, **139**, 1150–53.

Yaryura-Tobias, J.A. and Neziroglu, F.A. (1991). Organicity in obsessive-compulsive disorder. *Biological Psychiatry*, **29** (Suppl.), 337S.

and Neziroglu, F.A. (1997). *Obsessive-Compulsive Disorder Spectrum*. Washington, DC: American Psychiatric Press, Inc.

Neziroglu, F.A. and Kaplan, S. (1995). Self-mutilation, anorexia, and dysmenorrhea in obsessive-compulsive disorder. *International Journal of Eating Disorders*, **17**, 33–38.

Yasuno, F., Nishikawa, T., Nakagawa, T., *et al.* (2000). Functional anatomic study of psychogenic amnesia. *Psychiatry Research*, **99**, 43–57.

Yates, A.J. (1970). *Behavior Therapy*. New York: John Wiley and Sons.

Yazici, K.M. and Kostakoglu, L. (1998). Cerebral blood flow changes in patients with conversion disorder. *Psychiatry Research*, **83**, 163–8.

Demirci, M., Demir, B. and Ertugrul, A. (2004). Abnormal somatosensory evoked potentials in two patients with conversion disorder. *Psychiatry and Clinical Neuroscience*, **58**, 222–5.

Yehuda, R. (2004). Risk and resilience in posttraumatic stress disorder. *Journal of Clinical Psychiatry*, **65** (Suppl. 1), 29–36.

Yin, W., He, S. and Weekes, B.S. (2005). Acquired dyslexia and dysgraphia in Chinese. *Behavioral Neurology*, **16**, 159–67.

Young, A.W., Leafhead, K.M. and Szulecka, T.K. (1994). The Capgras and Cotard delusions. *Psychopathology*, **27**, 226–31.

Young, M.A., Abrams, R., Taylor, M.A. and Meltzer, H.Y. (1983). Establishing diagnostic criteria for mania. *Journal of Nervous and Mental Disorders*, **171**, 676–82.

Zald, D.H. and Kim, S.W. (1996a). Anatomy and function of the orbital frontal cortex I, anatomy, neurocircuitry, and obsessive-compulsive disorder. *Journal of Neuropsychiatry and Clinical Neuroscience*, **8**, 125–38.

and Kim, S.W. (1996b). Anatomy and function of the orbital frontal cortex II, function and relevance to obsessive-compulsive disorder. *Journal of Neuropsychiatry and Clinical Neuroscience*, **8**, 249–61.

Zanarini, M.C. and Frankenburg, F.R. (2001). Attainment and maintenance of reliability of axis I and II disorders over the course of a longitudinal study. *Comprehensive Psychiatry*, **42**, 369–74.

Zarate, C.A. Jr., Tohen, M. and Land, M.L. (2000). First-episode schizophreniform disorder, comparisons with first-episode schizophrenia. *Schizophrenia Research*, **46**, 31–4.

Zaudig, M. (1990). Cycloid psychoses and schizoaffective psychoses – a comparison of different diagnostic classification systems and criteria. *Psychopathology*, **23**, 233–42.

Zhang-Wong, J., Beiser, M., Bean, G. and Iacono, W.G. (1995). Five-year course of schizophreniform disorder. *Psychiatry Research*, **59**, 109–17.

Zhou, J.N., Hofman, M.A., Gooren, L.J. and Swaab, D.F. (1995). A sex difference in the human brain and its relation to transsexuality. *Nature*, **378**, 68–70.

Zielinski, C.M., Taylor, M.A. and Juzwin, K.R. (1991). Neuropsychological deficits in obsessive-compulsive disorder. *Neuropsychiatry, Neuropsychology and Behavioral Neurology*, **4**, 110–26.

Zilboorg, G. (1967). *A History of Medical Psychology*. New York: WW Norton and Company, Inc.

Zimmerman, M., Chelminski, L. and Posternak, M. (2004). A review of studies of the Montgomery–Asberg Depression Rating Scale in controls: implications for the definition of remission in treatment studies of depression. *International Clinics in Psychopharmacology*, **19**, 1–7.

Zisook, S. and Shuchter, S.R. (1991). Depression through the first year after the death of a spouse. *American Journal of Psychiatry*, **148**, 1346–52.

  and Shuchter, S.R. (1993). Uncomplicated bereavement. *Journal of Clinical Psychiatry*, **54**, 365–72.

Zutshi, A., Kamath, P. and Reddy, Y.C. (2007). Bipolar and nonbipolar obsessive-compulsive disorder, a clinical exploration. *Comprehensive Psychiatry*, **48**, 245–51.

Index

Sutton's Law, diagnosis 102
Sydenham, Thomas 27
symptom rating scales 118–119
symptomatology
    pattern and primacy of symptom features
        100–101
    rate of sequence of emergence 98–100
synesthesia 254
Szasz, Thomas 83

tactile hallucinations 79–80, 259–260
talking-past-the-point 236
tangential speech 234
tardive dyskinesia (TD) 175–176
tarentism, "dancing mania" 166
Taylor, M.A. 166, 207, 373–374
temperament
    aid to diagnosis 148
    high heritability of 338
    see also personality
temporal lobe functions 65
terminal illness, effect on normal personality
    344–345
terminology
    importance of precise 94–97
    of emotion 197–198
terrorist attack, effect on personality 347
test selection
    dementia syndrome tests 319–321
    guidelines for 316
thalamus, function of 65–66, 69
"theory of the mind" concept 81–82
thought blocking 232
thought disorder see formal thought
    disorder (FTD)
thought echo (écho de la pensée) 263
tics 176, 299
tobacco use 127, 367
topographic orientation, testing early
    Alzheimer's disease 324
torture, effects on personality 347
Tourette's syndrome see Gilles de La Tourette's
    syndrome (GTS)
training
    descriptive psychopathology 5
    in psychiatry, post World War II in USA 41
transient global amnesia (TGA) 141–142
transsexualism 342
trauma, sexual, effect on personality 346
traumatic brain injury (TBI), personality
    changes associated with 359, 360
treatment
    for melancholia 376–377
    monitoring, reason for cognitive assessment 315
    weak relationship between diagnosis and
        response 40
tremor 173, 178
trichotillomania 296
tricyclic antidepressants (TCAs) versus SSRIs
    for melancholic depression 377

Tuke, Daniel Hack 32
Tyrer, P. 335

unconscious, the 25–26
unipolar disorder see bipolar and unipolar
    disorder
unitary psychosis model 31
utilization behavior 177

validity of current diagnostic systems 8
vegetative functions, adverse effect of
    melancholia 211–212
ventral emotion system 71–72
verbal absurdities, cognitive testing 321
verbal automatic obedience 162
verbal hallucinations 79
verbal negativism 162, 236
verbal stereotypy 232
Verbigeration 162, 232
violence
    during neuropsychiatric evaluation
        behavioral signs of 115
        behavioral strategies to reduce and control 115
        risk factors 112–116
        safety in examination setting 109
    and homicidal thoughts 288–289
    self-injury 297–298
viscous personality 358
vision loss from retinal migraine 267–269
visual hallucinations 78, 258–259
visual imagery, brain correlates of 55
visual–motor coordination, shape
    copying test 320
visual–spatial function, assessment of early
    Alzheimer's disease 324
voice hallucinations 261–262, 263
von Hohenheim, T.B. 25
Vorbeireden 162, 236

war neuroses 28
waxy flexibility, cataleptic patients 163
Wechsler Memory Scale batteries 331
Weissenburger, J.E. 156
Wernicke, Carl 32, 261
Wechsler Adult Intelligence Scale (WAIS) 330
Whytt, Robert 27
Willis, Thomas 27, 30
Winokur, G. 215, 380
Witzelsucht 202
working memory, assessment of 326
World Health Organization (WHO)
    ICD-6 39–40
    see also ICD-10
World War II, leading to changes in psychiatry
    40–42
writing difficulties 229–230

Zebra Principle, diagnosis 102
Zimmerman, M. 374
Zinkin, Joseph 41–42